TEXTBOOK OF NEUROANAESTHESIA AND CRITICAL CARE

DEDICATION

To our patients

TEXTBOOK OF NEUROANAESTHESIA AND CRITICAL CARE

Edited by

Basil F Matta MB BCh BA BOA DA FRCA

Consultant in Anaesthesia and Neuro-Critical Care
Director of Neuroanaesthetic Services
Addenbrookes Hospital
University of Cambridge
UK

David K Menon PhD MD MBBS FRCP FRCA FmedSci

Lecturer in Anaesthesia
University of Cambridge
Director of Neurocritical Care
Addenbrookes Hospital
University of Cambridge
UK

John M Turner MBBS FRCA

Consultant in Anaesthesia and Neuro-intensive Care
Addenbrookes Hospital
Associate Lecturer
University of Cambridge
UK

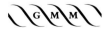

GMM

© 2000

GREENWICH MEDICAL MEDIA LTD
137 Euston Road
London
NW1 2AA

ISBN 1 900151 73 1

First Published 2000

Typeset by Saxon Graphics Ltd, Derby
Printed in Spain by Grafos

Contents

SECTION 5   ANAESTHESIA FOR NEUROIMAGING

Contributors

Mark J Abrahams
MBBS
SPECIALIST REGISTRAR IN ANAESTHESIA
Addenbrookes Hospital
Cambridge, UK

Simon J Boniface
MD MA BSc MRCP
CONSULTANT IN NEUROPHYSIOLOGY
DEPARTMENT OF CLINICAL NEUROPHYSIOLOGY
Addenbrookes Hospital
Cambridge, UK

Rowan M Burnstein
FRCA
RESEARCH FELLOW
MRC Brain Repair Centre
Cambridge, UK

Alasdair J Coles
MRCP PhD
SPECIALIST REGISTRAR IN NEUROLOGY
Addenbrookes Hospital
Cambridge, UK

Marek Czosnyka
PhD
LECTURER IN NEUROPHYSICS
Academic Neurosurgical Unit
Addenbrookes Hospital
Cambridge, UK

Patrick W Doyle
MBBS FRCA
SPECIALIST REGISTRAR IN ANAESTHESIA
Addenbrookes Hospital
Cambridge, UK

Catherine Duffy
MD FRCP(C)
CLINICAL FELLOW IN NEUROANAESTHESIA
Addenbrookes Hospital
Cambridge, UK

Richard E Erskine
MBBS FRCA
CONSULTANT IN ANAESTHESIA
Addenbrookes Hospital
Cambridge, UK

Fay Gilder
FRCA
SPECIALIST REGISTRAR
Department of Anaesthesia
Addenbrookes Hospital
Cambridge, UK

Leisha S Godsiff
MBBS FRCA
SPECIALIST REGSITRAR IN ANAESTHESIA
Addenbrookes Hospital
Cambridge, UK

Kevin E J Gunning
FRCA
CONSULTANT IN INTENSIVE CARE AND ANAESTHESIA
Department of Anaesthesia
Addenbrookes Hospital
Cambridge, UK

Arun Gupta
MBBS FRCA
CONSULTANT IN ANAESTHESIA AND NEURO-INTENSIVE CARE
Addenbrookes Hospital
Cambridge, UK

Sanjeeva Gupta
MBBS FRCA
SPECIALIST REGISTRAR IN ANAESTHESIA
Addenbrookes Hospital
Cambridge, UK

Karen J Heath
MBBS FRCA
SPECIALIST REGISTRAR IN ANAESTHESIA
Addenbrookes Hospital
Cambridge, UK

Peter J A Hutchinson
MBBS FRCS
SPECIALIST REGISTRAR IN ANAESTHESIA
Addenbrookes Hospital
Cambridge, UK

Peter J Kirkpatrick
FRCS
CONSULTANT NEUROSURGEON
Academic Department of Neurosurgery
Addenbrookes Hospital
Cambridge, UK

Robert Macfarlane
MD, FRCS
CONSULTANT NEUROSURGEON
Department of Neurosurgery
Addenbrookes Hospital
Cambridge, UK

Brian McNamara
MD BSc MRCP(Irl)
REGISTRAR IN NEUROPHYSIOLOGY
Department of Clinical Neurophysiology
Addenbrookes Hospital
Cambridge, UK

Basil F Matta
MB BCh BA BOA DA FRCA
CONSULTANT IN ANAESTHESIA AND NEURO-CRITICAL CARE
DIRECTOR OF NEUROANAESTHETIC SERVICES
Addenbrookes Hospital
Cambridge, UK

David Menon
PhD MD MBBS FRCP FRCA FmedSci
LECTURER IN ANAESTHESIA
University of Cambridge
DIRECTOR OF NEUROCRITICAL CARE
Addenbrookes Hospital
Cambridge, UK

Pawanjit S Minhas
FRCA
SPECIALIST REGISTRAR IN NEUROSURGERY
University Department of Neurosurgery
Addenbrookes Hospital
Cambridge, UK

Mark T O'Connell
PhD
SENIOR RESEARCH ASSOCIATE
MRC Brain Repair Centre
Cambridge, UK

Mayesh Prabhu
MBBS
SPECIALIST REGISTRAR IN ANAESTHESIA
Addenbrookes Hospital
Cambridge, UK

Robert L Ross-Russell
MB BCh MRCP
DIRECTOR OF PAEDIATRIC INTENSIVE CARE
Addenbrookes Hospital
Cambridge, UK

Richard Seinge
FRCA
SPECIALIST REGISTRAR IN ANAESTHESIA
Department of Anaesthesia
Addenbrookes Hospital
Cambridge, UK

Helen L Smith
MB BS FRCA
SPECIALIST REGISTRAR IN ANAESTHESIA
Department of Anaesthesia
Addenbrookes Hospital
Cambridge, UK

Andrew C Summors
MBBS FRCA
SPECIALIST REGISTRAR IN ANAESTHESIA
Addenbrookes Hospital
Cambridge, UK

John M Turner
MBBS FRCA
CONSULTANT IN ANAESTHESIA AND NEURO-INTENSIVE CARE
Addenbrookes Hospital
ASSOCIATE LECTURER
University of Cambridge

Sarah Walsh
MBBS FRCA
SPECIALIST REGISTRAR IN ANAESTHESIA
Addenbrookes Hospital
Cambridge, UK

Liz A Warburton
MA DM MRCP
CONSULTANT PHYSICIAN
Addenbrookes Hospital
Cambridge, UK

Preface

Neuroanaesthesia, perhaps more than any other field of anaesthesia has represented an area where the expertise and competence of the anaesthetist can influence patient outcome. Indeed, developments in neurosurgery, neurointensive care and neuroradiology have only been possible due to concomitant advances in neuroanaesthesia. These advances in clinical practice have always been underpinned by experimental research, and there has also been a tradition of high quality clinical research in our specialty. The development continues, and the availability of novel drugs and monitoring modalites represent both an opportunity and a challenge. They represent an opportunity because the use of modern imaging, novel monitoring modalities and multimodality integration of such data provide exciting insights into disease mechanisms and pathophysiology, and allow the specific selection of appropriate therapies. They also represent a challenge because there is a danger that we may confuse the aim of improved clinical management with the technological means of achieving it.

We hope therefore, that this book will provide not only an understanding of the science that underpins modern clinical practice in neuroanaesthesia and neurointensive care, but also the clinical context in which such concepts are best applied. Wherever possible, we have attempted to base our recommendations on high quality clinical research with outcome evaluation. Where paucity of such data or rapid advances in the understanding of disease makes this inappropriate, we have based our management on personal experience and data regarding clinical pathophysiology. While we expect that future studies addressing clinical pathophysiology and outcome will modify practice, this book is a distillation of current knowledge, experience and prejudices, as viewed from Cambridge.

Basil F Matta
David K Menon
John M Turner
October, 1999

Acknowledgements

We would like to thank all our anaesthetic, neuro-surgical and nursing colleagues for their help and encouragement during the preparation of this book.

SECTION 1

NEUROPHYSIOLOGY AND NEUROPHARMACOLOGY

1

ANATOMICAL CONSIDERATIONS IN NEUROANAESTHESIA

Robert Macfarlane

INTRODUCTION

There are a multitude of anatomical details which influence the way in which neurosurgeons approach specific problems and which are likely to impinge upon anaesthesia. This chapter provides an overview of some of the more important ones, but without burdening the reader with excessive detail that can be found in standard anatomical texts.

THE CRANIUM

ANATOMY OF THE CSF PATHWAYS

The lateral ventricles are C-shaped cavities within the cerebral hemispheres. Each drains separately into the third ventricle via the foramen of Monro, which is situated just in front of the anterior pole of the thalamus. The third ventricle is a midline slit, bounded laterally by the thalami and inferiorly by the hypothalamus. It drains via the narrow aqueduct of Sylvius through the dorsal aspect of the midbrain to open out into the diamond-shaped fourth ventricle. This has the cerebellum as its roof and the dorsal aspect of the pons and medulla as its floor. The fourth ventricle opens into the basal cisterns via a midline foramen of Magendie, which sits posteriorly between the cerebellar tonsils, and laterally into the cerebellopontine angle via the foraminae of Luschka.

Approximatley 80% of the cerebrospinal fluid (CSF) is produced by the choroid plexus in the lateral, third and fourth ventricles. The remainder is formed around the cerebral vessels and from the ependymal lining of the ventricular system. The rate of CSF production (500–600ml per day in the adult) is independent of intraventricular pressure, until intracranial pressure (ICP) is elevated to the point at which cerebral blood flow (CBF) is compromised. Absorption, however, is largely by bulk flow and is therefore pressure-related. Most of the CSF is reabsorbed via the arachnoid villi into the superior sagittal sinus, while some is reabsorbed in the lumbar theca. CSF flow across the ventricular wall into the brain extracellular space is not an important mechanism under physiological conditions.

Hydrocephalus

Obstruction to CSF flow results in hydrocephalus. This is divided clinically into communicating and non-communicating types (otherwise known as obstructive/non-obstructive), depending upon whether the ventricular system communicates with the subarachnoid space in the basal cisterns. The distinction between the two is important when considering treatment (see below). Examples of communicating hydrocephalus include subarachnoid haemorrhage (either traumatic or spontaneous, both of which silt up the arachnoid villi), meningitis and sagittal sinus thrombosis. In contrast, aqueduct stenosis, intraventricular haemorrhage and intrinsic tumours are common causes of non-communicating hydrocephalus.

The diagnosis is usually made by the appearance on CT or MRI scan. The features which suggest active hydrocephalus rather than *ex vacuo* dilatation of the ventricular system secondary to brain atrophy are:

- dilatation of the temporal horns of the lateral ventricles (>2mm width);
- rounding of the third ventricle or ballooning of the frontal horns of the lateral ventricles;
- low density surrounding the frontal horns of the ventricles. This is caused by transependymal flow of CSF and is known as periventricular lucency (PVL). However, in the elderly this sign may be misleading as it is also seen after multiple cerebral infarcts.

Management of hydrocephalus

If the hydrocephalus is communicating then CSF can be drained from either the lateral ventricles or the lumbar theca. Generally, this will involve the insertion of a permanent indwelling shunt unless the cause for the hydrocephalus is likely to be transient, infection is present or blood within the CSF is likely to block the shunt. Under such circumstances, either an external ventricular or lumbar drain or serial lumbar punctures may be appropriate.

Obstructive hydrocephalus requires CSF drainage from the ventricular system. Lumbar puncture is potentially dangerous because of the risk of coning if a pressure differential is created between the cranial and spinal compartments. A single drainage catheter is adequate if the lateral ventricles communicate with each other (the majority of cases) but bilateral catheters are needed if the blockage lies at the foramen of Monro.

Many forms of non-communicating hydrocephalus can now be treated by endoscopic third ventriculostomy, obviating the need for a prosthetic shunt. An artificial outlet for CSF is created in the floor of the third ventricle between the mamillary bodies and the infundibulum, via an endoscope introduced through the frontal horn of the lateral ventricle and foramen of Monro. This allows CSF to drain directly from the third ventricle into the basal cisterns, where it emerges between the posterior clinoid processes and the basilar artery.

BRAIN STRUCTURE AND FUNCTION

Disorders of different lobes of the brain produce characteristic clinical syndromes, dependent not only on site but also side. Almost all right-handed patients (93%–99%) are left hemisphere dominant, as are the majority of left-handers and those who are ambidextrous (ranging from 50% to 92% in various studies; for review, see [1]).

Intracranial mass lesions generally present in one of three ways: focal neurological deficit, symptoms or signs of raised intracranial pressure, or with epilepsy. A very simple guide to the neurological deficits which may develop in association with disorders of the cerebral or cerebellar hemispheres is as follows.

The frontal lobe

The frontal lobe is the hemisphere anterior to the Rolandic fissure (central sulcus; Fig. 1.1). Important areas within it are the motor strip, Broca's speech area (in the dominant hemisphere) and the frontal eye fields. Patients with bilateral frontal lobe dysfunction typically present with personality disorders, dementia, apathy and disinhibition. The anterior 7 cm of one frontal lobe can be resected without significant neurological sequelae, providing that the contralateral hemisphere is normal. Resections more posterior than this in the dominant hemisphere are likely to damage the anterior speech area.

Temporal lobe

The temporal lobe lies anteriorly below the Sylvian fissure and becomes the parietal lobe posteriorly at the angular gyrus (Fig. 1.1). The uncus forms its medial border and is of particular clinical importance because it overhangs the tentorial hiatus adjacent to the midbrain. When intracranial pressure rises in the supratentorial compartment, it is the uncus of the temporal lobe which transgresses the tentorial hiatus, compressing the third nerve, midbrain and posterior cerebral artery.

There are many functions to the temporal lobe including memory, the cortical representation of olfactory, auditory and vestibular information, some aspects of emotion and behaviour, Wernicke's speech area (in the dominant hemisphere) and parts of the visual field pathway.

Like the frontal lobe, lesions in the temporal lobe may present with memory impairment or personality change. Seizures are common, with prodromal symptoms linked typically to the function of the temporal lobe (e.g. olfactory, auditory or visual hallucinations, unpleasant visceral sensations, bizarre behaviour or déjà vu).

The anterior 5–6 cm of one temporal lobe (approximately at the junction of the Rolandic and Sylvian fissures) may be resected. Usually the upper part of the superior temporal gyrus is preserved to protect the branches of the middle cerebral artery lying in the Sylvian fissure. More posterior resection may damage the speech area in the dominant hemisphere. Care is needed if resecting the medial aspect of the uncus because of proximity to the optic tract. In some patients undergoing temporal lobectomy (the majority of epilepsy cases, for example), it may be appropriate to undertake a sodium amytal test preoperatively, to both confirm laterality of language and establish whether the patient is likely to suffer significant memory impairment as a result of the procedure. This investigation, otherwise known as the Wada test, involves selective catheterization of each internal carotid artery in turn. Whilst the hemisphere in question is anaesthetized with sodium amytal (effectiveness is confirmed by the onset of contralateral hemiplegia), the patient's ability to speak is evaluated. They are then presented with a series of words and images which they are asked to recall once the hemiparesis has recovered, thereby assessing the strength of verbal and non-verbal memory in the contralateral hemisphere.

Parietal lobes

These extend from the Rolandic fissure to the parieto-occipital sulcus posteriorly and to the temporal lobe inferiorly. The dominant hemisphere shares speech function with the adjacent temporal lobe, while both sides contain the sensory cortex and visual association areas.

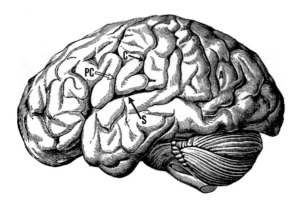

Figure 1.1   Topography of the brain. A = Angular gyrus; C = Central sulcus (Rolandic fissure); PC = Precentral sulcus; S = Sylvian fissure.

Parietal lobe dysfunction may produce cortical sensory loss or sensory inattention. In the dominant hemisphere the result is dysphasia and in the non-dominant, dyspraxia (e.g. difficulty dressing, using a knife and fork or difficulty with spatial orientation). Involvement of the visual association areas may give rise to visual agnosia (inability to recognize objects) or to alexia (inability to read).

Occipital lobes

Lesions within the occipital lobe typically present with a homonymous field defect which does not spare the macula. Visual hallucinations (flashes of light, rather than the formed images which are typical of temporal lobe epilepsy) may develop.

Resection of the occipital lobe will result in a contralateral homonymous hemianopia. The extent of resection is restricted to 3.5cm from the occipital pole in the dominant hemisphere because of the angular gyrus, where lesions can produce dyslexia, dysgraphia and acalculia. In the non-dominant hemisphere, up to 7cm may be resected.

Surgical resections may be undertaken in eloquent parts of the brain either by remaining within the confines of the disease process (intracapsular resection) or by employing some form of cortical mapping. This involves either cortical stimulation in awake patients under neuroleptanalgesia or preoperative functional MR which is then linked to an intraoperative image guidance system.

Cerebellum

The cerebellum consists of a group of midline structures, the lingula, vermis and flocculonodular lobe, and two laterally placed hemispheres.

Lesions affecting midline structures typically produce truncal ataxia, which may make it difficult for the patient to stand or even to sit. Vertigo may result from damage to the vestibular reflex pathways. Obstructive hydrocephalus is common. Nystagmus is typically the result of involvement of the flocculonodular lobe. Invasion of the floor of the fourth ventricle may give rise to effortless vomiting or cranial nerve dysfunction. In contrast, lesions within the hemispheres usually cause ipsilateral limb ataxia. Hypotonia, dysarthria and pendular reflexes are other features associated with disorders of the cerebellum.

Surface markings of the brain

The precise position of intracranial structures varies, but a rough guide to major landmarks is as follows.

Draw an imaginary line in the midline between the nasion and inion (external occipital protuberance). The Sylvian fissure runs in a line from the lateral canthus to three-quarters of the way from nasion to inion. The central sulcus (separating the motor from the sensory cortex) lies 2cm behind the midpoint from nasion to inion and joins the Sylvian fissure at a point vertically above the condyle of the mandible.

THE CEREBRAL CIRCULATION

Arterial

The arterial anastomosis in the suprasellar cistern is named after Thomas Willis (Fig. 1.2), who published his dissections in 1664, with illustrations by the architect Sir Christopher Wren. The cerebral circulation is divided into two parts. The anterior circulation is fed by the internal carotid arteries, while the posterior circulation derives from the vertebral arteries (the vertebrobasilar circulation). A detailed account of the normal and abnormal anatomy of the cerebral vasculature can be found in Yasargil.[2]

The internal carotid artery has no branches in the neck but gives off two or three small vessels within the cavernous sinus before entering the cranium just medial to the anterior clinoid process. It gives off the ophthalmic and posterior communicating arteries before reaching its terminal bifurcation, where it divides to become the anterior and middle cerebral arteries (Fig. 1.3). The anterior choroidal artery, the blood supply to the internal capsule, generally arises

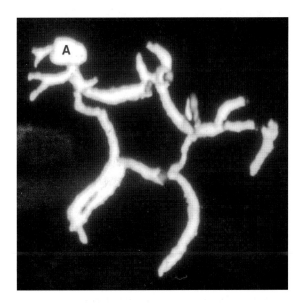

Figure 1.2   CT angiogram of the circle of Willis. There is an aneurysm of the middle cerebral artery bifurcation (A).

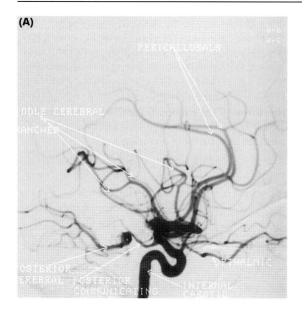

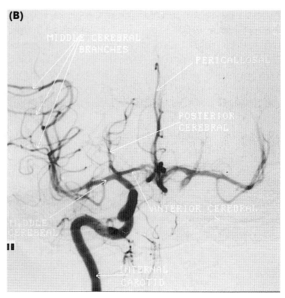

Figure 1.3   Subtraction angiogram of the internal carotid circulation. (A) Lateral projection. (B) AP projection.

from the distal internal carotid artery just beyond the posterior communicating artery. The anterior cerebral artery passes over the optic nerve and is connected with the vessel of the opposite side in the interhemispheric fissure by the anterior communicating artery (ACoA). The segment of the anterior cerebral artery proximal to the ACoA is known as the A1 segment and that beyond it as the A2 (until it branches again to form the pericallosal and callosal marginal arteries). The anterior cerebral artery supplies the orbital surface of the frontal lobe and the medial surface of the hemisphere above the corpus callosum back to the parieto-occipital sulcus. It extends onto the lateral surface of the hemisphere superiorly, where it meets the territory supplied by the middle cerebral artery. The motor and sensory cortex to the lower limb are within its territory of supply.

The middle cerebral artery is the largest branch of the circle of Willis. It passes laterally behind the sphenoid ridge and up through the Sylvian fissure where it divides into frontal and temporal branches. These then turn sharply in a posterosuperior direction to reach the insula. The main trunk of the middle cerebral is known as the M1 segment and its first branches at the trifurcation are the M2 segments. It supplies much of the lateral aspect of the hemisphere, with the exception of the superior frontal and inferior temporal gyrus and the occipital cortex (Fig. 1.4). Within its territory of supply are the internal capsule, speech and auditory areas and the motor and sensory areas for the opposite side, with the exception of the lower limbs.

The posterior circulation comprises the vertebral arteries, which join at the clivus to form the basilar artery. This gives off multiple branches to the brainstem and cerebellum before bifurcating near the level of the posterior clinoids to become the posterior cerebral arteries (Fig. 1.5). The first large branch of the posterior cerebral is the posterior communicating artery (PCoA), thus connecting the anterior and posterior circulations. The segment of the posterior cerebral artery proximal to the PCoA is known as the P1 and that which is distal to it as the P2. The P2 then curves posterolaterally around the cerebral peduncle to enter the ambient cistern and cross the tentorial hiatus. It is here that the artery may be occluded when intracranial pressure is high (Fig. 1.6). Its territory of supply is the inferior and inferolateral surface of the temporal lobe and the inferior and most of the lateral surface of the occipital lobe. The contralateral visual field lies entirely within its territory.

Arterial anomalies

In postmortem series, a fully developed arterial circle of Willis exists in about 96% of cadavers, although the communicating arteries will be small in some.[3] Because haemodynamic anomalies are associated with an increased risk of berry aneurysm formation, an incomplete circle of Willis is likely to be more common in neurosurgical patients than in the general population.

Hypoplasia or absence of one or more of the communicating arteries can be particularly important at times

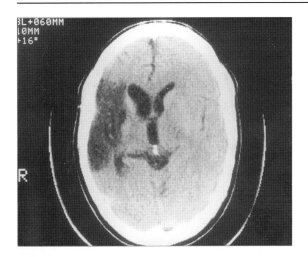

Figure 1.4   CT head scan showing infarction of the right middle cerebral artery territory. Midline structures are slightly displaced towards the side of the lesion, indicating loss of brain volume and that the infarct is therefore long-standing.

when one of the major feeding arteries is temporarily occluded, for example during carotid endarterectomy or when gaining proximal control of a ruptured intracranial aneurysm. Under such conditions the anastomotic circle cannot be relied upon to maintain adequate perfusion to parts of the ipsilateral or contralateral hemisphere. This situation will be compounded by atherosclerotic narrowing of the vessels or by systemic hypotension. The areas particularly vulnerable to ischaemia are the watersheds between vascular territories. Some estimate of flow

across the ACoA can be obtained angiographically by the cross-compression test. During contrast injection, the contralateral carotid is compressed in the neck, thereby reducing distal perfusion and encouraging flow of contrast from the ipsilateral side (Fig. 1.7). Transcranial Doppler provides a more quantitative assessment. Trial balloon occlusion in the conscious patient is a further method of evaluating crossflow and tolerance of permanent occlusion.

The A1 segments are frequently disparate in size (60–80% of patients). In approximately 5% of the population one A1 sement will be severely hypoplastic or aplastic. The ACoA is very variable in nature, having developed embryologically from a vascular network. It exists as a single channel in 75% of subjects but may be duplicated or occasionally absent (2%). The PCoA is less than 1mm diameter in approximately 20% of patients. In almost 25% of people the PCoA is larger than the P1 segment and the posterior cerebral arteries are therefore supplied primarily (or entirely) by the internal carotid rather than the vertebral arteries. Because the posterior cerebral artery derives embryologically from the internal carotid artery, this anatomical variant is known as a persistent foetal-type posterior circulation.

If both the ACoA and PCoA arteries are hypoplastic then the middle cerebral territory is supplied only by the ipsilateral internal carotid artery (the so-called 'isolated middle cerebral artery'; Fig. 1.8). Such a patient will be very vulnerable to ischaemia if the internal carotid is temporarily occluded during surgery. Should it be necessary to occlude the internal

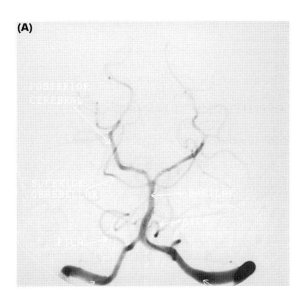

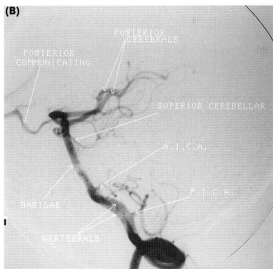

Figure 1.5   Subtraction vertebral angiogram. (A) AP projection. (B) Lateral projection.

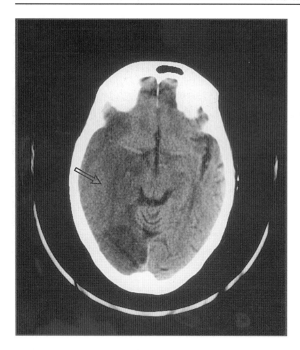

Figure 1.6   CT head scan showing extensive infarction (low density) in the territory of the posterior cerebral artery (open arrow). This was the result of compression of the vessel where it crossed the tentorial hiatus due to raised intracranial pressure.

carotid artery permanently, for example in a patient with an intracavernous aneurysm, some form of bypass graft will be required. Usually this is between the superficial temporal artery and a branch of the middle cerebral artery (an extracranial–intracranial artery [EC-IC] bypass). The small perforating vessels which arise from the circle of Willis to enter the base of the brain are known as the central rami. Those from the anterior and middle cerebral arteries supply the lentiform and caudate nuclei and internal capsule, whilst those from the communicating arteries and posterior cerebrals supply the thalamus, hypothalamus and mesencephalon. Damage to any of these small perforators at surgery may result in significant neurological deficit.

Microscopic anatomy

An understanding of the histology of cerebral arteries is particularly relevant to subarachnoid haemorrhage. Unlike systemic muscular arteries, cerebral vessels possess only a rudimentary tunica adventitia. Whereas clot surrounding a systemic artery will not result in the development of delayed vasospasm, it is likely that the lack of an adventitia allows blood breakdown products access to smooth muscle of the tunica media of cerebral vessels, thereby giving rise to late constriction.

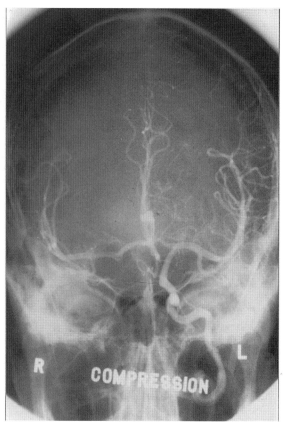

Figure 1.7   The cross-compression test. Contrast has been injected into the left internal carotid artery whilst the right is occluded by external compression in the neck. This shows that the distal vessels on the right will fill from the left if the right ICA is occluded and that the ACoA and A1 segments are therefore patent. However, this test alone is not a reliable way of determining that neurological deficit will not ensue if the contralateral carotid artery is permanently occluded.

The tunica media of both large and small cerebral arteries has its muscle fibres orientated circumferentially. This results in a point of potential weakness at the apex of vessel branches and may lead to aneurysm formation. Approximately 85% of berry aneurysms develop in the anterior circulation.

Venous

Unlike many other vascular beds, cephalic venous drainage does not follow the arterial pattern. There are superficial and deep venous systems which, like the internal jugular veins, are valveless (Fig. 1.9).

The basal ganglia and adjacent structures drain via the internal cerebral veins, which lie in the roof of the third ventricle, and the basal veins which pass around

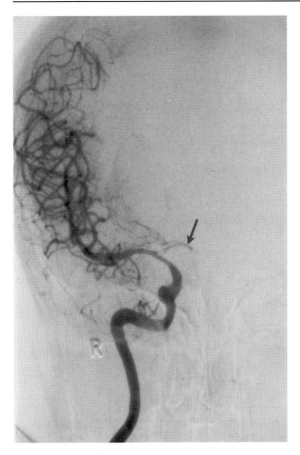

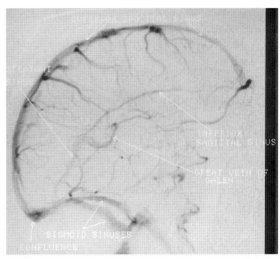

Figure 1.9 Venous phase angiography, showing the major superficial and deep venous drainage of the brain.

Figure 1.8 Only the middle cerebral artery territory fills following right internal carotid angiography in this patient. The A1 segment (arrow) is very narrow (in this instance as a consequence of vasospasm from an anterior communicating artery aneurysm rather than hypoplasia). In this patient the circle of Willis would be unable to maintain right MCA blood flow if perfusion were to be reduced in the ipsilateral ICA.

the cerebral peduncles. The internal cerebral and basal veins join to form the great cerebral vein of Galen beneath the splenium of the corpus callosum. This short vein joins the inferior sagittal sinus (which runs in the free edge of the falx) to form the straight sinus.

In general, the venous drainage of the hemispheres is into the nearest venous sinus. The superior sagittal sinus occupies the convex margin of the falx and is triangular in cross-section. Because of its semirigid walls, the sinus does not collapse when venous pressure is low, resulting in a high risk of air embolism during surgery if the sinus is opened with the head elevated. Venous lakes are sometimes present within the diploë of the skull adjacent to the sinus, and can result in excessive bleeding or air embolus when a craniotomy flap is being turned.

The lateral margin of the superior sagittal sinus contains arachnoid villi responsible for the reabsorption of CSF into the venous circulation. It begins at the floor of the anterior cranial fossa at the crista galli and extends back in the midline, increasing progressively in size, until it reaches the level of the internal occipital protuberence. Here it turns to one side, usually the right, as the transverse sinus. The straight sinus turns to form the opposite transverse sinus at this point. An anastomosis of variable size connects the two and is known as the confluence of the sinuses or torcular Herophili.

The superior cerebral veins (usually 8–12 in number) lie beneath the arachnoid on the surface of the cerebral cortex and drain the superior and medial surface of the hemisphere into the superior sagittal sinus. To do this, they must bridge the subdural space (hence the alternative name of 'bridging veins'). If the hemisphere is atrophic and therefore relatively mobile within the cranium, these veins are likely to be torn by even minor head injury, giving rise to chronic subdural haematoma. A large acute subdural haematoma may also displace the hemisphere sufficiently to avulse the bridging veins, provoking brisk venous bleeding from multiple points in the sinus when the clot is evacuated. Tearing of bridging veins may also occur during or early after neurosurgical procedures in which there has been excessive shrinkage of the brain or loss of CSF. This phenomenon is thought to account for some cases in which haemorrhages develop postoperatively in regions remote from the operative site.[4,5]

Although venous anastomoses exist on the lateral surface of the hemisphere, largely between the superior anastomotic vein (draining upwards in the central sulcus to the superior sagittal sinus – the vein of Trolard), the Sylvian vein (draining downwards in the Sylvian fissure to the sphenoparietal sinus) and the angular or inferior anastomotic vein (draining via the vein of Labbé into the transverse sinus), sudden occlusion of large veins or a patent venous sinus may result in brain swelling or even venous infarction. As a general rule, the anterior one-third of the superior sagittal sinus may be ligated, but only one bridging vein should be divided distal to this if complications are to be avoided. If the sinus has been occluded gradually, for example by a parasagittal meningioma, then there is time for venous collaterals to develop but it then becomes all the more important that these anastomotic veins are not divided during removal of the tumour. Venous phase angiography is particularly useful in planning the operative approach to tumours adjacent to the major venous sinuses or to the vein of Galen and thereby determining whether the sinus is completely occluded and can be resected *en bloc* with the tumour or whether the sinus is patent and requires reconstruction.

Anastomotic venous channels allow communication between intracranial and extracranial tissues via diploic veins in the skull. These may allow infection from the face or paranasal air sinuses to spread to the cranium, resulting in subdural empyema, cerebral abscess or a spreading cortical venous or sinus thrombosis.

INNERVATION OF THE CEREBRAL VASCULATURE. NEUROGENIC INFLUENCES ON CEREBRAL BLOOD FLOW

Sympathetic

The sympathetic innervation to the cerebral vasculature is largely from the superior cervical ganglion. In addition to the catecholamines, sympathetic nerve terminals contain another potent vasoconstrictor, neuropeptide Y. This 36 amino acid neuropeptide is found in abundance in both the central and peripheral nervous systems.

Only minor (5–10%) reductions in CBF accompany electrical stimulation of sympathetic nerves, far less than that seen in other vascular beds.[6] Although feline pial arterioles vasoconstrict in response to topical noradrenaline and the response is blocked by the α-blocker phenoxybenzamine, application of the latter alone at the same concentration has no effect on vessel calibre. This and other observations from denervation studies indicate that the sympathetic nervous system does not exert a significant tonic influence on cerebral vessels under physiological conditions. Neither does the sympathetic innervation contribute to CBF regulation under conditions of hypotension or hypoxia. However, Harper and colleagues[7] observed that sympathetic stimulation does produce a profound fall in CBF if cerebral vessels have been dilated by hypercapnia. From this study came the 'dual control' hypothesis, proposing that the cerebral circulation comprises two resistances in series. Extraparenchymal vessels are thought to be regulated largely by the autonomic nervous system, whilst intraparenchymal vessels are responsible for the main resistance under physiological conditions and are governed primarily by intrinsic metabolic and myogenic factors.

As well as exerting a significant influence on cerebral blood volume, the sympathetic innervation has been shown to protect the brain from the effects of acute severe hypertension. When blood pressure rises above the limits of autoregulation, activation of the sympathetic nervous system attenuates the anticipated rise in CBF and reduces the plasma protein extravasation which follows breakdown of the blood–brain barrier. The autoregulatory curve is 'reset' such that both the upper and lower limits are raised. This is an important physiological mechanism by which the cerebral vasculature is protected from injury during surges in arterial blood pressure.[8] Whilst cerebral vessels escape from the vasoconstrictor response to sympathetic stimulation under conditions of normotension, this does not occur during acute hypertension. It also follows from this that CBF is better preserved by drug-induced than haemorrhagic hypotension for the same perfusion pressure, because circulating catecholamine levels are high in the case of the latter.

Sympathetic nerves are also thought to exert trophic influences upon the vessels which they innervate. Sympathectomy reduces the hypertrophy of the arterial wall which develops in response to chronic hypertension. Denervation has been shown to increase the susceptibility of stroke-prone spontaneously hypertensive rats to bleed into the cerebral hemisphere which has been sympathectomized.[9]

Parasympathetic

The cerebrovascular parasympathetic innervation derives from multiple sources, which include the sphenopalatine and otic ganglia and small clusters of ganglion cells within the cavernous plexus, Vidian and lingual nerves. Vasoactive intestinal polypeptide (VIP), a potent 28 amino acid polypeptide vasodilator which is non-EDRF dependent, has been localized immunohistochemically within parasympathetic nerve endings, as has nitric oxide synthase, the enzyme which forms nitric oxide from L-arginine.

Although stimulation of parasympathetic nerves does elicit a rise in cortical blood flow, there is, like the sympathetic nervous system, little to suggest that cholinergic mechanisms contribute significantly to CBF regulation under physiological conditions. Nor are parasympathetic nerves involved in the vasodilatory response to hypercapnia. However, chronic parasympathetic denervation increases infarct volume by 37% in rats subjected to permanent middle cerebral artery occlusion, primarily because of a reduction in CBF under situations when perfusion pressure is reduced.[10] This suggests that parasympathetic nerves may help to maintain perfusion at times of reduced CBF and may in part explain why patients with autonomic neuropathy, such as diabetics, are at increased risk of stroke.

SENSORY NERVES AND HEAD PAIN

The anatomy of the sensory innervation to the cranium is important for an understanding of the basis of certain types of headache. Furthermore, the sensory innervation to the cerebral vasculature has been shown to influence CBF under a variety of pathological conditions.

Anatomy

The pain-sensitive structures within the cranium are the dura mater, the dural venous sinuses and the larger cerebral arteries ($>50 \mu$m diameter). The structures that lie within the supratentorial compartment and rostral third of the posterior fossa are innervated predominantly by small myelinated and unmyelinated nerve fibres which emanate from the ophthalmic division of the trigeminal nerve (with a small contribution from the maxillary division). The caudal two-thirds of the posterior fossa is innervated by the C1 and C2 dorsal roots. With the exception of midline structures, the innervation is strictly unilateral. Although each individual neurone has divergent axon collaterals which innervate both the cerebral vessels and dura mater, the extracranial and intracranial trigeminal innervation are separate peripherally. Centrally, however, they synapse onto single interneurones in the trigeminal nucleus caudalis.

This arrangement accounts for the strictly unilateral nature of some types of headache. The pain is poorly localized because of large receptive fields, and is referred to somatic areas. In many respects, headache is little different from the pain experienced in association with inflammation of other viscera. Just as appendicitis is accompanied by referred pain to the umbilicus and abdominal muscle rigidity, so headache is generally referred to the frontal (ophthalmic) or cervicooccipital

(C2) regions and is associated with tenderness in the temporalis and cervical musculature. It is because of this arrangement that tumours in the upper posterior fossa may present with frontal headache and why patients with raised pressure within the posterior fossa and impending herniation of the cerebellar tonsils through the foramen magnum may complain of neck pain and exhibit nuchal rigidity. Central projections of the trigeminal nerve to the nucleus of the tractus solitarius account for the autonomic responses (sweating, hypertension, tachycardia and vomiting) which may accompany headache (for review, see [11]).

Sensory nerves form a fine network on the adventitial surface of cerebral arteries. Several neuropeptides, including substance P (SP), neurokinin A (NKA) and calcitonin gene-related peptide (CGRP), are contained within vesicles in the naked nerve endings. All three are vasodilators, whilst SP and NKA promote plasma protein extravasation and an increase in vascular permeability. Neurotransmitter release can follow both orthodromic stimulation and axon reflex-like mechanisms. Trigeminal perivascular sensory nerve fibres have been found to contribute significantly to the hyperaemic responses which follow reperfusion after a period of cerebral ischaemia and which accompany acute severe hypertension, seizures and bacterial meningitis.[12,13] There is now considerable evidence to support the notion that neurogenic inflammation in the dura mater resulting from the release of sensory neuropeptides is the fundamental basis for migraine.

ANATOMICAL CONSIDERATIONS IN SURGICAL ACCESS TO THE CRANIUM

There are a number of factors that require consideration when planning an operative approach. The most direct route to the pathology via the smallest possible exposure is not necessarily the technique which offers the best outcome. As well as cosmetic considerations, other factors which require thought when planning a surgical approach include the following:-

Eloquent areas of the brain

It is self-evident that an approach should be chosen which minimizes the risk of creating additional neurological deficit. Where applicable, approaches to extra-axial midline structures are generally via the non-dominant hemisphere. Stereotactic or image-guided methods may be appropriate to assist the surgeon when planning the trajectory. On occasions, cranial surgery is performed on awake patients so that cortical mapping can be used to avoid eloquent areas. Where appropriate, cortical incisions are made through the sulci rather than gyri.

Degree of retraction

The brain is intolerant of retraction, particularly if it is prolonged or over a narrow area. Brain swelling and intraparenchymal haemorrhage are the consequences of injudicious use of brain retractors. Although a good anaesthetic is fundamental for providing satisfactory operating conditions which minimize the need for retraction, it is also important that the patient has been positioned correctly to reduce venous pressure and that adequate bone has been removed to allow the surgeon to displace the brain as little as possible. A number of skull base and craniofacial exposures have been developed to improve access without excessive brain retraction. Examples include excision of a large acoustic neuroma via the labyrinth to minimize displacement of the cerebellum, or osteotomy of the zygomatic arch in the subtemporal approach to a basilar apex aneurysm. Early cerebrospinal fluid drainage is another manoeuvre which may assist surgical exposure.

Brain swelling

A large bone flap is generally appropriate if the brain is likely to be swollen at the time of surgery. Not only can the bone be omitted and the dura left open widely at the end of the procedure in order to provide a decompression which reduces intracranial pressure, but there is less risk with a large opening that brain herniation through the defect will obstruct the pial vessels at the dural margin and result in ischaemia or infarction of the prolapsing tissue. Preservation of the draining veins is another factor which should be considered when planning the approach in order to minimize postoperative swelling.

Epilepsy

Some areas of the brain are more epileptogenic than others and this may at times be a factor to consider. Access to the lateral ventricle via the frontal lobe is, for example, more likely to induce seizures than is an interhemispheric route through the corpus callosum.

THE SPINE

ASSESSING STABILITY OF THE VERTEBRAL COLUMN

A stable spine is one in which normal movements will not result in displacement of the vertebrae. In an unstable spine, be it from trauma, infection, tumour, degenerative changes or inflammatory disease, alterations in alignment may occur with movement.

However, the degree of bone destruction or spinal instability does not always correlate with the extent of any associated spinal cord injury.

The concept of the 'three column' spine, as proposed by Holdsworth[14] and refined by Denis,[15] is widely accepted as a means of assessing stability. The anterior column of the spine is formed by the anterior longitudinal ligament, the anterior annulus fibrosus of the intervertebral disc and the anterior part of the vertebral body. The middle column is formed by the posterior longitudinal ligament, the posterior annulus fibrosus of the intervertebral disc and the posterior wall of the vertebral body. The posterior column is formed by the posterior arch, supraspinous and interspinous ligaments and the ligamentum flavum. If only one of the columns is disrupted then the spine remains stable but if two or more are involved then the spine is potentially unstable.

Plain radiographs showing normal vertebral alignment in a neutral position do not necessarily indicate stability and views in flexion and extension may be necessary to assess the degree of ligamentous or bony damage (Fig. 1.10). While an unstable spine should generally be maintained in a fixed position, not all movements will necessarily risk compromising neurological function. For example, if a vertebral body has collapsed because of infection or tumour but the posterior elements are preserved then the spine will be stable in extension, but flexion will increase the deformity and may force diseased tissue or the buckled posterior longitudinal ligament into the spinal canal.

The mechanism of the injury has an important bearing on spinal stability after trauma. As a general rule, wedge compression fractures to the spine are stable but flexion–rotation injuries cause extensive ligamentous damage posteriorly and are therefore unstable. In the cervical spine, hyperextension injuries are nearly always stable. Hyperextension is a very uncommon mechanism of injury in the thoracolumbar spine but is invariably unstable because there is disruption of the anterior longitudinal ligament and intervertebral disc and an associated fracture of the vertebral body.

THE SPINAL CORD

The adult spinal cord terminates at about the lower border of L1 as the conus medullaris. Below this the spinal canal contains peripheral nerves known as the cauda equina. Lesions above this level produce upper motor neurone signs and those below it, a lower motor neurone pattern. Lesions of the conus itself may produce a mixed picture.

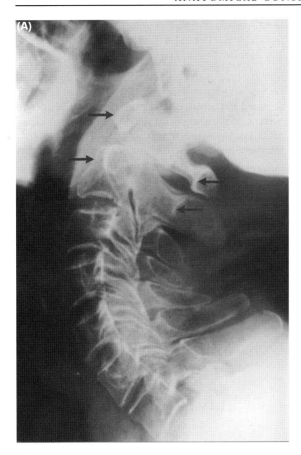 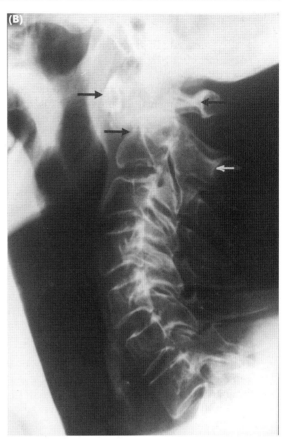

Figure 1.10   Non-union of a fracture of the dens. (A) Vertebral alignment is satisfactory in extension (arrows). (B) Flexion of the neck causes subluxation of C1 on C2, thereby severely compromising the spinal canal

A detailed account of the ascending and descending pathways is beyond the scope of this chapter but can be found in all standard anatomical texts. However, like the cerebrum, there are several common patterns of involvement.

Extrinsic spinal cord compression

Classically, this produces symmetrical corticospinal ('pyramidal') involvement, with upper motor neurone weakness below the level of the compression (increased tone, clonus, little or no muscle wasting, no fasciculation, exaggerated tendon reflexes and extensor plantar responses), together with a sensory loss. If, however, the mass is laterally placed then the pattern may initially be of hemisection of the cord – the Brown–Sequard syndrome. This produces ipsilateral pyramidal weakness, loss of fine touch and impaired proprioception but contralateral impairment of pain and temperature sensation.

Central cord syndromes

Syringomyelia or intramedullary tumours affecting the cervicothoracic region will first involve the pain and temperature fibres which decussate near the midline before ascending in the lateral spinothalamic tracts. The result of central cord involvement is therefore a 'suspended' sensory loss, with a cape-type distribution of loss of sensitivity to pain in the upper limbs and trunk but with sparing of the lower limbs.

Cauda equina compression

This may result, for example, from a lumbar disc prolapse. Usually but not invariably, it is accompanied by sciatica, which may be bilateral or unilateral and there may be weakness or sensory loss in a radicular distribution. In addition, there is perineal sensory loss in a saddle distribution, painless retention of urine with dribbling overflow incontinence and loss of anal tone.

Blood supply

The blood supply to the spinal cord is tenuous. The anterior and posterior spinal arteries form a longitudinal anastomotic channel which is fed by spinal branches of the vertebral, deep cervical, intercostal and lumbar arteries. In the neck, there is usually a feeder which comes from the thyrocervical trunk and accompanies either the C3 or C4 root. The largest radicular artery arises from the lower thoracic or upper lumbar region and supplies the spinal cord below the level of about T4. Its position is variable but is generally on the left side (two-thirds of cases) and arises between T10 and T12 in 75% of patients. In 15% it lies between T5 and T8 and in 10% at L1 or L2. As in the cervical region, it accompanies one of the nerve roots and is known as the artery of Adamkewicz. It has a characteristic hairpin appearance on angiography because it ascends up the nerve root and then splits into a large caudal and a small cranial branch when it reaches the cord.

This vessel is vulnerable to damage during operations on the thoracic spine, particularly during excision of neurofibromas or meningiomas or if an intercostal vessel is divided during excision of a thoracic disc. The artery is also vulnerable to injury during surgery to the descending thoracic aorta, during nephrectomy or even intercostal nerve blocks. Atherosclerotic disease of the radicular artery or prolonged hypotension may induce infarction of the anterior half of the cord up to mid-dorsal level, producing paraplegia, incontinence and spinothalamic sensory loss. However, joint position sense and light touch are preserved. Posterior spinal artery occlusion does not often produce a classic distribution of deficit because the vessel is part of a plexus and the territory of supply is variable. Because the arterial supply to the cord is not readily apparent at operation, surgery to the lower thoracic spine is often preceded by spinal angiography to determine the precise location of the artery of Adamkewicz. However, this procedure itself carries a very small risk of spinal cord infarction.

REFERENCES

1. Hamani C. Language dominance in the cerebral hemispheres. Surg Neurol 1997; 47: 81–83.

2. Yasargil MG. Microneurosurgery, vol I. Springer Verlag, Stuttgart, 1984.

3. Fawcett E, Blachford JV. The circle of Willis. An examination of 700 specimen. J Anat 1906; 40: 63–70.

4. Papanastassiou V, Kerr R, Adams C. Contralateral cerebellar hemorrhagic infarction after pterional craniotomy: report of five cases and review of the literature. Neurosurgery 1996; 39: 841–852.

5. Toczek MT, Morrell MJ, Silverberg GA, Lowe GM. Cerebellar hemorrhage complicating temporal lobectomy. Report of four cases. J Neurosurg 1996; 85: 718–722.

6. Kobayashi S, Waltz AG, Rhoton AL. Effects of stimulation of cervical sympathetic nerves on cortical blood flow and vascular reactivity. Neurology 1971; 21: 297–230.

7. Harper AM, Deshmukh VD, Rowman JO, Jennett WB. Influence of sympathetic nervous activity in cerebral blood flow. Arch Neurol 1972; 27: 1–6.

8. Heistad DD, Marcus M, Busija D, Sadoshima S. Protective effects of sympathetic nerves in the cerebral circulation. In: Heistad DD, Marcus ML (eds), Cerebral blood flow: effect of nerves and neurotransmitters. Elsevier, New York, 1982, pp 267–273.

9. Mueller SM, Heistad DD. Effect of chronic hypertension on the blood–brain barrier. Hypertension 1980; 2: 809–812.

10. Kano M, Moskowitz MA, Yokota M. Parasympathetic denervation of rat pial vessels significantly increases infarction volume following middle cerebral artery occlusion. J Cereb Blood Flow Metab, 1991; 11: 628–637.

11. Moskowitz MA, Macfarlane R. Neurovascular and molecular mechanisms in migraine headaches. Cerebrovasc Brain Metab Rev, 1993; 5: 159–177.

12. Macfarlane R, Moskowitz MA, Sakas DE, Tasdemiroglu E, Wei EP, Kontos HA. The role of neuroeffector mechanisms in cerebral hyperperfusion syndromes. J Neurosurg 1991; 75: 845–855.

13. Macfarlane R, Moskowitz MA. The innervation of pial blood vessels and their role in cerebrovascular regulation, In: Caplan LR (ed) Brain ischemia: basic concepts and clinical relevance. Springer Verlag, London, 1995, pp. 247–259.

14. Holdsworth F. Fractures, dislocations and fracture-dislocations of the spine. J Bone Joint Surg 1970; 52A: 1534–1551.

15. Denis F. The three column spine and its significance in the classification of acute thoracolumbar spinal injuries. Spine 1983; 8: 817–831.

2

THE CEREBRAL CIRCULATION

David K. Menon

INTRODUCTION

The brain receives 15% of the resting cardiac output (700 ml/min in the adult) and accounts for 20% of basal oxygen consumption. Mean resting cerebral blood flow (CBF) in young adults is about 50 ml/100 g brain/min. This mean value represents two very different categories of flow: 70 and 20 ml/100g/min for grey and white matter respectively. Regional CBF (rCBF) and glucose consumption decline with age, along with marked reductions in brain neurotransmitter content and less consistent decreases in neurotransmitter binding.[1]

FUNCTIONAL ANATOMY OF THE CEREBRAL CIRCULATION

ARTERIAL SUPPLY

Blood supply to the brain is provided by the two internal carotid arteries and the basilar artery. The anastomoses between these two sets of vessels give rise to the circle of Willis. While a classic 'normal' polygonal anastomotic ring is found in less than 50% of brains,[2] certain patterns of regional blood supply from individual arteries are generally recognized. Global cerebral ischaemia, such as that associated with systemic hypotension, classically produces maximal lesions in areas where the zones of blood supply from two vessels meet, resulting in 'watershed' infarctions. However, the presence of anatomical variants may substantially modify patterns of infarction following large vessel occlusion. For example, in some individuals, the proximal part of one anterior cerebral artery is hypoplastic and flow to the ipsilateral frontal lobe is largely provided by the contralateral anterior cerebral, via the anterior communicating artery. Occlusion of the single dominant anterior cerebral in such a patient may result in massive infarction of both frontal lobes: the unpaired anterior cerebral artery syndrome.

MICROCIRCULATION

The cerebral circulation is protected from systemic blood pressure surges by a complex branching system and two resistance elements: the first of these lies in the large cerebral arteries and the second in vessels of diameter less than 100 μm. The cerebrovascular microarchitecture is highly organized and follows the columnar arrangement seen with neuronal groups and physiological functional units.[3] Pial surface vessels give rise to arterioles that penetrate the brain at right angles to the surface and give rise to capillaries at all laminar levels. Each of these arterioles supplies a hexagonal column of cortical tissue, with intervening boundary zones, an arrangement that is responsible for columnar patterns of local blood flow, redox state[4] and glucose metabolism seen in the cortex during hypoxia or ischaemia.[5] Capillary density in the cortex is one-third of adult levels at birth, doubles in the first year and reaches adult levels at four years. At maturity capillary density is related to the number of synapses, rather than number of neurones or mass of cell bodies in a given region,[6] and can be closely correlated with the regional level of oxidative metabolism.[7,8]

Conventionally, functional activation of the brain is thought to result in 'capillary recruitment', implying that some parts of the capillary network are non-functional during rest. However, recent evidence suggests that all capillaries may be persistently open[8] and 'recruitment' involves changes in capillary flow rates with homogenization of the perfusion rate in a network.[9]

VENOUS DRAINAGE

The brain is drained by a system of intra- and extra-erebral venous sinuses, which are endothelialized channels in folds of dura mater. These sinuses drain into the internal jugular veins which, at their origin, receive minimal contributions from extracerebral tissues. Measurement of oxygen saturation in the jugular bulb ($SjvO_2$) thus provides a useful measure of cerebral oxygenation. It has been suggested that the supratentorial compartment is preferentially drained by the right internal jugular vein, while the infratentorial compartment is preferentially drained by the left internal jugular vein. However, more recent data suggest considerable interindividual variation in cerebral venous drainage.[10]

CEREBRAL BLOOD VOLUME: PHYSIOLOGY AND POTENTIAL FOR THERAPEUTIC INTERVENTION

Most of the intracranial blood volume of about 200 ml is contained in the venous sinuses and pial veins, which constitute the capacitance vessels of the cerebral circulation. Reduction in this volume can buffer rises in the volume of other intracranial contents (the brain and CSF). Conversely, when compensatory mechanisms to control intracranial pressure (ICP) have been exhausted, even small increases in cerebral blood volume can result in steep rises in ICP (Fig. 2.1).

The position of the system on this curve can be expressed in terms of the pressure–volume index (PVI), which is defined as the change in intracranial volume that produces a 10-fold increase in ICP. This is

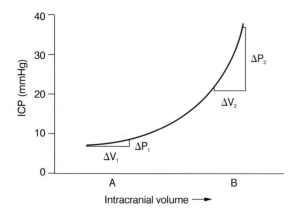

Figure 2.1   Intracranial pressure–volume curve (see text).

normally about 26 ml[11] but may be markedly lower in patients with intracranial hypertension, who are on the steep part of the intacranial pressure–volume curve.

With the exception of oedema reduction by mannitol, the only intracranial constituent whose volume can be readily modified by the anaesthetist by physiological or pharmacological interventions is the CBV. Although the CBV forms only a small part of the intracranial volume and such interventions only produce small absolute changes (typically $\simeq$ 10 ml or less), they may result in marked reductions in ICP in the presence of intracranial hypertension. Conversely, inappropriate anaesthetic management may cause the CBV to increase. Again, although the absolute magnitude of such increase may be small, it may result in steep rises in ICP in the presence of intracranial hypertension.

The appreciation that pharmacological and physiological modulators may have independent effects on CBV and CBF is important for two reasons. First, interventions aimed at reducing CBV in patients with intracranial hypertension may have prominent effects on CBF and result in cerebral ischaemia.[12] Conversely, drugs that produce divergent effects on CBF may have similar effects on CBV and using CBF measurement to infer effects on CBV and hence ICP may result in erroneous conclusions.[13]

THE CEREBRAL PERFUSION PRESSURE

The inflow pressure to the brain is equal to the mean arterial pressure (MAP) measured at the level of the brain. The outflow pressure from the intracranial cavity depends on the ICP, since collapse of intracerebral veins is prevented by the maintainance of an intraluminal pressure 2–5 mmHg above ICP. The difference between the MAP and the ICP thus provides an estimate of the effective cerebral perfusion pressure (CPP):

$$CPP = MAP - ICP$$

MICROCIRCULATORY TRANSPORT AND THE BLOOD–BRAIN BARRIER

Endothelial cells in cerebral capillaries contain few pinocytic vesicles and are sealed with tight junctions, with no anatomical gap. Consequently, unlike other capillary beds, the endothelial barrier of cerebral capillaries presents a high electrical resistance and is remarkably non-leaky, even to small molecules such as mannitol (molecular weight (MW) 180 daltons). This property of the cerebral vasculature is termed the blood–brain barrier (BBB) and resides in three cellular components (the endothelial cell, astrocyte and pericyte) and one non-cellular structure (the endothelial basement membrane). A fundamental difference between brain endothelial cells and the systemic circulation is the presence of interendothelial tight junctions termed the *zona occludens*.

The BBB is a function of the cerebral microenvironment rather than an intrinsic property of the vessels themselves and leaky capillaries from other vascular beds develop a BBB if they are transplanted to the brain or exposed to astrocytes in culture.[14] Passage through the BBB is not simply a function of MW; lipophilic substances traverse the barrier relatively easily and several hydrophilic molecules (including glucose) cross the BBB via active transport systems to enter the brain interstitial space[15] (Fig. 2.2). In addition, the BBB maintains a tight control of relative ionic distribution in the brain extracellular fluid.

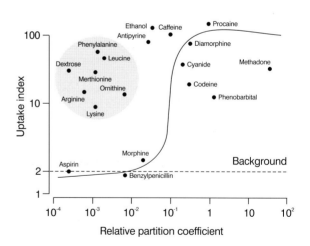

Figure 2.2   Correlation between brain uptake index and oil/water partition coefficients for different substrates. While BBB permeability, in general, increases with lipid solubility, note that several substances including glucose and amino acids show high penetration due to active transport or facilitated diffusion (after Oldendorf[12]).

These activities require energy and thus the mitochondrial density is exceptionally high in these endothelial cells, accounting for 10% of cytoplasmic volume.[16] Several endogenous substances, including catecholamines[17] and vascular endothelial growth factor,[18] can dynamically modulate BBB permeability. Although the BBB is disrupted by ischaemia, this process takes hours or days rather than minutes and much of the cerebral oedema seen in the initial period after ischaemic insults is cytotoxic rather than vasogenic. Consequently, mannitol retains its ability to reduce cerebral oedema in the early phases of acute brain injury.

MEASUREMENT OF rCBF

All clinical and many laboratory methods of measuring CBF or rCBF are indirect and may not produce directly comparable measurements. It is also important to treat results from any one method with caution and attribute any observed phenomena to physiological effects only when demonstrated by two or more independent techniques. Methods of measuring CBF may be regional or global and applicable either to humans or primarily to experimental animals. All of these methods have advantages and disadvantages All methods that provide absolute estimates of rCBF use one of two principles: they either measure the distribution of a tracer or estimate rCBF from the wash-in or wash-out curve of an indicator. Other techniques do not directly estimate rCBF but can be used to either measure a related flow variable (such as arterial flow velocity) or infer changes in flow from changes in metabolic parameters. These issues are addressed in detail in Chapter 00.

PHYSIOLOGICAL DETERMINANTS OF RCBF AND RCBV

FLOW–METABOLISM COUPLING

Increases in local neuronal activity are accompanied by increases in regional cerebral metabolic rate (rCMR). Until recently, the increases in rCBF and oxygen consumption produced during such functional activation were thought to be closely coupled to the cerebral metabolic rate of utilization of O_2 ($CMRO_2$) and glucose (CMR_{glu}). However, it has now been clearly shown that increases in rCBF during functional activation tend to track glucose utilization but may be far in excess of the increase in oxygen consumption.[19] This results in regional *anaerobic* glucose utilization and a consequent local decrease in oxygen extraction

ratio and increase in local haemoglobin saturation. The resulting local decrease in deoxyhaemoglobin levels is used by functional MRI techniques to image the changes in rCBF produced by functional activation. Despite this revision of the proportionality between increased rCBF and $CMRO_2$ during functional activation in the brain, the relationship between rCBF and CMR_{glu} is still accepted to be linear.

The cellular mechanisms underlying these observations are elucidated by recent publications which have highlighted the role played by astrocytes in the regulation of cerebral metabolism.[20] These data suggest that astrocytes utilize glucose glycolytically and produce lactate which is transferred to neurones, where it serves as a fuel in the citric acid cycle.[21] Astrocytic glucose utilization and lactate production appear to be, in large part, coupled by the astrocytic reuptake of glutamate released at excitatory synapses (Fig. 2.3).

The regulatory changes involved in flow–metabolism coupling have a short latency ($\simeq 1$ s) and may be mediated by either metabolic or neurogenic pathways. The former category includes the increases in perivascular K^+ or adenosine concentrations that follow neuronal depolarization. The cerebral vessels are richly supplied by nerve fibres and the mediators thought to play an important part in neurogenic flow–metabolism coupling are acetylcholine[22] and nitric oxide,[23] although roles have also been proposed for 5-hydroxytryptamine, substance P and

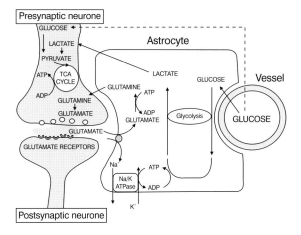

Figure 2.3 Relationship of astrocytes to oxygen and energy metabolism in the brain. Glucose taken up by astrocytes undergoes glycolysis for generation of ATP to meet astrocytic energy requirements (for glutamate reuptake, predominantly). The lactate that this process generates is shuttled to neurones, which utilize it aerobically in the citric acid cycle.

neuropeptide Y. More recent publications implicate dopamineric neurones (see later).

AUTOREGULATION

Autoregulation refers to the ability of the cerebral circulation to maintain CBF at a relatively constant level in the face of changes in CPP by altering cerebrovascular resistance (CVR) (Fig. 2.4). While autoregulation is maintained irrespective of whether changes in CPP arise from alterations in MAP or ICP, autoregulation tends to be preserved at lower levels when falls in CPP are due to increases in ICP rather than decreases in MAP due to hypovolaemia.[24,25] One possible reason for this may be the cerebral vasoconstrictive effects of the massive levels of catecholamines secreted in haemorrhagic hypotension, since lower MAP levels are tolerated in hypotension if the fall in blood pressure is induced by sympatholytic agents[26,27] or occurs in the setting of autonomic failure.[28] Autoregulatory changes in CVR probably arise from myogenic reflexes in the resistance vessels but these may be modulated by activity of the sympathetic system or the presence of chronic systemic hypertension.[29] Thus, sympathetic blockade or cervical sympathectomy shifts the autoregulatory curve to the left while chronic hypertension or sympathetic activation shifts it to the right. These modulatory effects may arise from angiotensin-mediated mechanisms. Primate studies suggest that nitric oxide is unlikely to be important in pressure autoregulation.[30]

In reality, the clearcut autoregulatory thresholds seen with varying CPP in Figure 2.4A are not observed; the autregulatory 'knees' tend to be more gradual and there may be wide variations in rCBF at a given value of CPP in experimental animals and even in neurologically normal individuals.[31] It has been demonstrated that symptoms of cerebral ischaemia appear when the MAP falls below 60% of an individual's lower autoregulatory threshold.[32] However, generalized extrapolation from such individualized research data to the production of 'safe' lower limits of MAP for general clinical practice is hazardous for several reasons. First, there may be wide individual scatter in rCBF autoregulatory efficiency, even in normal subjects. Second, the coexistence of fixed vascular obstruction (e.g. carotid atheroma or vascular spasm) may vary the MAP level at which rCBF reaches critical levels in relevant territories. Third, the autoregulatory curve may be substantially modulated by the mechanisms used to produce hypotension. Earlier discussion made the distinction between reductions in CPP produced by haemorrhagic hypotension, intracranial hypertension and pharmacological hypotension. The effects on autoregulation may also vary with the pharmacological agent used to produce hypotension. Thus, neuronal function is better preserved at similar levels of hypotension produced by halothane, nitroprusside or isoflurane in comparison with trimetaphan.[33] Finally, autoregulatory responses are not immediate: estimates of the latency for compensatory changes in rCVR range from 10 to 60 s.[34]

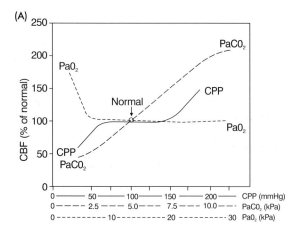

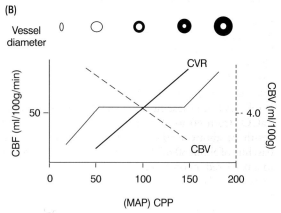

Figure 2.4 Effect of changes in CPP, $PaCO_2$ and PaO_2 on CBF. (A) Note the increase in slope of the $CBF/PaCO_2$ curve as basal CBF increases from 20 ml/100g/min (white matter) to 50–70 ml/100g/min (grey matter). (B) Note that maintenance of CBF with reductions in CPP are achieved by cerebral vasodilatation which results in reductions in cerebrovascular resistance. This leads to an increase in CBV, which has no detrimental effects in healthy subjects. However, these CBV increases may cause critical ICP increases in patients with intracranial hypertension, who operate on the steep part of the intracranial pressure–volume curve.

Some recent studies suggest that, especially in patients with impaired autoregulation, the cardiac output and pulsatility of large vessel flow may be more important determinants of rCBF than CPP itself.[35]

PaCO$_2$

CBF is proportional to PaCO$_2$, subject to a lower limit below which vasoconstriction results in tissue hypoxia and reflex vasodilatation and an upper limit of maximal vasodilatation (Fig. 2.4A). On average, in the middle of the physiological range, each kPa change in PaCO$_2$ produces a change of about 15 ml/100g/min in CBF. However, the slope of the PaCO$_2$/CBF relationship depends on the baseline normocapnic rCBF value, being maximal in areas where it is high (e.g. grey matter: cerebrum) and least in areas where it is low (e.g. white matter: cerebellum and spinal cord). Moderate hypocapnia (PaCO$_2$ $\approx$3.5 kPa) has long been used to reduce CBV in intracranial hypertension but this practice is under review for two reasons. The CO$_2$ response is directly related to the change in perivascular pH; consequently, the effect of a change in PaCO$_2$ tends to be attenuated over time (hours) as brain ECF bicarbonate levels fall to normalize interstitial pH.[36] Second, it has now been shown that 'acceptable' levels of hypocapnia in head-injured patients can result in dangerously low rCBF levels.[12,37] Prostaglandins may mediate the vasodilatation produced by CO$_2$[38] and more recent work suggests that nitric oxide may also be involved,[39] perhaps in a permissive capacity.[40]

PaCO$_2$: effects on CBV and ICP (Fig. 2.5)

Grubb et al[41] studied the CBF/PaCO$_2$ response curve in primates and demonstrated that the CBF changed by approximately 1.8 ml/100g/min for each mmHg change in PaCO$_2$. However, in the same experiment, the CBV/PaCO$_2$ curve was much flatter (about 0.04 ml/100g/mmHg (0.3ml/100g/kPa) change in PaCO$_2$). It follows from these figures that while a reduction in PaCO$_2$ from 40 to 30 mmHg (5.3 to 4 kPa) would result in about a 40% reduction in CBF (from a baseline of about 50 ml/100g/min), it would only result in a 0.4% reduction in intracranial volume. This may seem trivial but in the presence of intracranial hypertension, the resultant 5 ml decrease in intracranial volume in an adult brain could result in a halving of ICP since the system operates on the steep part of the intracranial compliance curve.[42]

PaO$_2$ AND CaO$_2$

Classic teaching is that CBF is unchanged until PaO$_2$ levels fall below approximately 7 kPa but rises sharply

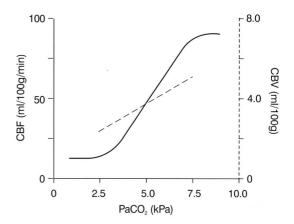

Figure 2.5 Relative effects of PaCO$_2$ on CBF and CBV. Hyperventilation is aimed at reducing CBV in patients with intracranial hypertension but may be detrimental because of its effects on CBF. Note that the slope of CBF reactivity to PaCO$_2$ is steeper than that for CBV ($\approx$25%/kPa PaCO$_2$ vs 20%/kPa PaCO$_2$ respectively).

with further reductions[43] (Fig. 2.4A). However, recent TCD data from humans suggest cerebral thresholds for cerebral vasodilatation as high as 8.5 kPa ($\approx$89–90% SaO$_2$).[44] This non-linear behaviour is because tissue oxygen delivery governs CBF and the sigmoid shape of the haemoglobin–O$_2$ dissociation curve means that the relationship between CaO$_2$ (arterial O$_2$ content) and CBF is inversely linear. These vasodilator responses to hypoxaemia appear to show little adaptation with time[45] but may be substantially modulated by PaCO$_2$ levels.[46,47] Nitric oxide does not appear to play a role in the vasodilatory response to hypoxia.[39]

Some studies suggest that hyperoxia may produce cerebral vasoconstriction, with a 10–14% reduction on CBF with inhalation of 85–100% O$_2$ and a 20% reduction in CBF with 100% O$_2$ at 3.5 atmospheres.[48] Human data suggest that this effect is not *clinically* significant.[49]

HAEMATOCRIT

As in other organs, optimal O$_2$ delivery in the brain depends on a compromise between the oxygen-carrying capacity and flow characteristics of blood; previous experimental work suggests that this may be best achieved at a haematocrit of about 40%. Some recent studies in the setting of vasospasm following subarachnoid haemorrhage have suggested that modest haemodilution to a haematocrit of 30–35% may improve neurological outcome by improving rheological characteristics and increasing rCBF. However, this may result in a reduction in O$_2$ delivery if maximal vasodilatation is already present and since clinical results in the setting of acute ischaemia have not been uniformly successful, this approach must be viewed with caution.

AUTONOMIC NERVOUS SYSTEM

The autonomic nervous system mainly affects the larger cerebral vessels, up to and including the proximal parts of the anterior, middle and posterior cerebral arteries. β_1-adrenergic stimulation results in vasodilatation while α_2-adrenergic stimulation vaso-constricts these vessels. The effect of systemically administered α or β-agonists is less significant. However, significant vasoconstriction can be produced by extremely high concentrations of cate-cholamines (e.g. in haemorrhage) or centrally acting α_2-agonists (e.g. dexmedetomidine).

PHARMACOLOGICAL MODULATION OF CBF

INHALED ANAESTHETICS

All the potent fluorinated agents have significant effects on CBF and CMR. The initial popularity of halothane as a neurosurgical anaesthetic agent was reversed by the discovery that it was a potent cerebral vasodilator, producing decreases of 20–40% in cere-brovascular resistance in normocapnic individuals at 1.2–1.5 MAC.[50,51] In another study, 1% halothane was shown to result in clinically significant elevations in ICP in patients with intracranial space-occupying lesions.[52] Preliminary studies with enflurane and isoflurane suggested that these agents might produce smaller increases in cerebrovascular resistance (CVR) at equivalent doses.[53] Since enflurane may produce epileptogenic activity, its use in the context of neuroanaesthesia decreased.

However, several studies compared the effects of isoflurane and halothane on CBF, with conflicting results. While some studies showed that halothane produced larger decreases in CVR, others found no difference. Examination of the patterns of rCBF produced by these two agents provides some clues to the origin of this discrepancy. Halothane selectively increases cortical rCBF while markedly decreasing subcortical rCBF, while isoflurane produces a more generalized reduction in rCBF.[54,55] A review of published comparisons of the CBF effects of the two agents suggests that studies that estimated CBF using techniques that preferentially looked at the cortex (e.g.[133]Xe wash-out) tended to show that halothane was a more potent vasodilator, while most studies that

used more global measures of hemispheric CBF (e.g. the Kety–Schmidt technique) have found little difference between the two agents at levels of around 1 MAC (Fig. 2.6).

Both agents tend to reduce global CMR but the regional pattern of such an effect may vary, with isoflurane producing greater cortical metabolic suppression[56] (reflected by its ability to produce EEG burst suppression at higher doses). Both the rCBF and rCMR effects of the two anaesthetics are markedly modified by baseline physiology and other pharmaco-logical agents. Thus, CBF increases produced by both agents are attenuated by hypocapnia (more so with isoflurane[57,58]) and thiopentone attenuates the relative preservation of cortical rCBF seen with halothane. It is difficult to predict accurately what the effect of either agent would be on CBF in a given clinical situation but this would be a balance of its suppressant effects on rCMR (with autoregulatory vasoconstriction) and its direct vasodilator effect (which is partially mediated via both endothelial and neuronal nitric oxide[39]).

Although initial reports suggested that halothane could 'uncouple' flow and metabolism,[59] more recent studies clearly show that at concentrations commonly used for neuroanaesthesia neither halothane,[59] isoflurane[60,61] or

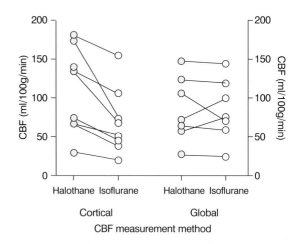

Figure 2.6 Comparison of mean + SD CBF in animals anaesthetized with 0.5–1.5 MAC isoflurane or halothane, either in the same study or in comparable studies from a single research group with identical methodology within a single publication.[149–160] In studies shown on the left, CBF was estimated using techniques likely to be biased towards cortical flow (e.g. [133]Xe wash-out) and show that halothane produces greater increases in CBF. In studies on the right, CBF was estimated using techniques that measured global cerebral blood flow (e.g. Kety–Schmidt method); the difference in effects on CBF between the two agents is much less prominent.

desflurane[62] completely disrupts flow–metabolism coupling, although their vasodilator effects may alter the slope of this relationship, due to changes in the flow:metabolism ratio with increases in anaesthetic concentration. Thus, though increases in metabolism are matched by increases in flow at all levels of anaesthesia, flow is higher at higher volatile anaesthetic concentrations at the same level of metabolism. In practice, the metabolic suppressant effects of the anaesthetics are more prominent at lower concentrations and when no other metabolic suppressants are used. Conversely, these vasodilator effects may become more prominent at higher concentrations or when the volatile agents are introduced on a baseline of low or suppressed cerebral metabolism (such as that produced by intravenous anaesthesia).

In equi-MAC doses, nitrous oxide is probably a more powerful vasodilator than either halothane or isoflurane.[63,64] Since N_2O has been shown to produce cerebral stimulation with increases in $CMRO_2$, glucose utilization and coupled increase in CBF,[65] its pharmacodynamic profile is particularly unfavourable in patients with raised ICP.[66,67] Further, the vasodilatation produced by nitrous oxide is not decreased by hypocapnia[68] although the resulting increases in ICP can be attenuated by the administration of other CMR depressants such as the barbiturates.[69]

While initial studies suggested that desflurane[70] and sevoflurane[71] had effects on the cerebral vasculature that appear very similar to isoflurane, more recent studies have shown distinct differences between these agents.

While high-dose desflurane, like isoflurane, can produce EEG burst suppression, this effect may be attenuated over time.[72] It is not known whether this adaptation represents a pharmacokinetic or pharmacodynamic effect. Initial clinical reports suggest that desflurane may cause a clinically significant rise in ICP in patients with supratentorial lesions,[73] despite its proven ability to reduce $CMRO_2$ as documented by EEG burst supression.[72,74] These increases in ICP, which are presumably related to cerebral vasodilatation, appear to be independent of changes in systemic haemodynamics.[75]

In humans, sevoflurane produces some increase in TCD flow velocities at high doses ($\geq$1.5 MAC) but these appear to be less marked than desflurane and were reported to be unassociated with increases in ICP in patients with supratentorial space-occupying lesions.[76] In other studies 1.5 MAC sevoflurane caused no increase in middle cerebral artery flow velocities[77] and did not affect CO_2 reactivity or pressure autoregulation.[78–80] This may be partially explained by sevoflurane's weak direct vasodilator effect, especially in humans.[81–82]

INTRAVENOUS ANAESTHETICS

Thiopentone,[83] etomidate[84] and propofol[85,86] all reduce global CMR to a minimum of approximately 50% of baseline, with a coupled reduction in CBF, although animal studies suggest small differences in the distribution of rCBF changes with individual agents. Decreases in CBV have been demonstrated with barbiturates[87] and probably occur with propofol and etomidate as well. Maximal reductions in CMR are reflected in an isoelectric EEG, although burst suppression is associated with only slightly less CMR depression.[83] Initial doubts that CBF reductions produced by propofol were secondary to falls in MAP have proved to be unfounded.[85,86] Even high doses of thiopentone[87] or propofol[88] do not appear to affect autoregulation, CO_2 responsiveness or flow–metabolism coupling.

OPIATES

Although high doses (3 mg/kg) of morphine and moderate doses of fentanyl (15 µg/kg) have little effect on CBF and CMR, high doses of fentanyl (50–100 µg/kg)[89] and sufentanil[90] depress CMR and CBF. Results with alfentanil, in doses of 0.32 mg/kg, show no reduction in rCBF.[91] These effects are variable and may only be prominent in the presence of nitrous oxide, where CMR may be reduced by 40% from baseline.[92] Bolus administration of large doses of fentanyl or alfentanil may be associated with increases in ICP in patients with intracranial hypertension,[93] probably due to reflex increases in CBF that follow an initial decrease in CBF (due to reductions in MAP and cardiac output produced by large bolus doses of these agents). These effects are unlikely to be clinically significant if detrimental haemodynamic and blood gas changes can be avoided. Opioids do not appear to affect autoregulation.

OTHER DRUGS

Ketamine can produce increases in global CBF and ICP,[94] with specific increases in rCMR and rCBF in limbic structures, which may be partially attenuated by hypocapnia, benzodiazepines or halothane.[95] The ICP and CBF increases produced by ketamine are also attenuated by general anaesthetic agents.[96] Sedative doses of benzodiazepines tend to produce small decreases in CMR and CBF;[97] however, there is a ceiling effect and increasing doses do not produce greater reductions in these variables.[98] α_2-agonists such as dexmedetomidine reduce CBF in man.[99] There are good data, in animal models at least,[100] that CBF reductions produced by intraventricular dexmedetomidine are probably direct vascular effects of the agent and not exclusively the consequence of either systemic hypotension or coupled falls in rCBF arising from reductions in neuronal metabolism.

Most non-depolarizing neuromuscular blockers have little effect on CBF or CMR, although large doses of d-tubocurarine may increase CBV and ICP secondary to histamine release and vasodilatation. In contrast, succinylcholine can produce increases in ICP, probably secondary to increases in CBF mediated via muscle spindle activation. However, these effects are transient and mild[101,102] and can be blocked by prior precurarization[103] if necessary; they provide no basis for avoiding succinylcholine in patients with raised ICP when its rapid onset of action is desirable for clinical reasons.

CBF IN DISEASE

ISCHAEMIA

Graded reductions in CBF are associated with specific electrophysiological and metabolic consequences (Table 2.1). Some of these thresholds for metabolic events are well recognized but others, such as the development of acidosis, cessation of protein synthesis and the failure of osmotic regulation, have only recently received attention.[104] Ischaemia is thus a continuum between normal cellular function and cell death; cell death, however, is not merely a function of the severity of ischaemia but is also dependent on its duration and several other circumstances that modify its effects. Thus, the effects of ischaemia may be ameliorated by the CMR depression produced by hypothermia or drugs, exacerbated by increased metabolic demand associated with excitatory neurotrans-

mitter release or compounded by other mechanisms of secondary neuronal injury (such as cellular calcium overload or reperfusion injury) (Fig. 2.7).

HEAD INJURY

Severe head injury is accompanied by both direct and indirect effects on cerebral blood flow and metabolism, which show both temporal and spatial variations. CBF may be high, normal or low soon after the ictus but is typically reduced.[105] Thirty percent of patients undergoing CBF studies within 6–8 h of a head injury have significant cerebral ischaemia.[106] Global hypoperfusion in these studies was associated with a 100% mortality at 48 h and regional ischaemia with significant deficits. CBF patterns also vary with relation to the time after injury[107] (Fig. 2.8). Initial reductions are replaced, especially in patients who achieve good outcomes, by a period of relative increase in CBF which, towards the end of the first week post ictus, may be replaced by reductions in CBF which are the consequence of vasospasm associated with subarachnoid haemorrhage.[108] CBF changes are non-uniform in the injured brain (Fig. 2.9). Blood flow tends to be reduced in the immediate vicinity of intracranial contusions[109,110] and cerebral ischaemia associated with hyperventilation may be extremely regional and not reflected in global monitors of cerebrovascular adequacy[111] (Fig. 2.10).

Elevations in intracranial pressure result in reductions in CPP and cerebral ischaemia, which lead to secondary neuronal injury. There is strong evidence that maintenance of a CPP above 60 mmHg improves outcome in patients with head injury and raised ICP.[112] Traditionally, patients with intracranial hypertension have been nursed head up in an effort to reduce ICP. It is important to realize, however, that such manoeuvres will also reduce the effective MAP at the level of the head and run the risk of reducing CPP. Feldman et

Table 2.1 Electrophysiological and metabolic consequences of graded reductions in CBF	
CBF (ml/100g/min)	Electrophysiological/metabolic consequence
> 50	Normal neuronal function
?	Immediate early gene activation
?	Cessation of protein synthesis
?	Cellular acidosis
20–23	Reduction in electrical activity
12–18	Cessation of electrical activity
8–10	ATP rundown, loss of ionic homeostasis
<8	Cell death (also depends on other modifiers: duration, CMR, etc.)

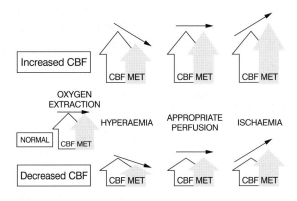

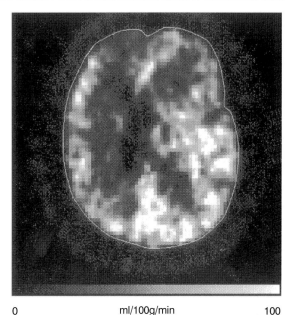

Figure 2.7 Relationship of cerebral blood flow to the presence of ischaemia under conditions of varying metabolism. Changes in CBF levels compared to physiological levels may be misleading, since a diagnosis of ischaemia or hyperaemia demands that CBF levels be assessed in the context of metabolic requirements.

al[113] suggest that a 30° head-up elevation may provide the optimal balance by reducing ICP without decreasing CPP.

HYPERTENSIVE ENCEPHALOPATHY

Current concepts of the causation of hypertensive encephalopathy are based on the forced vasodilatation hypothesis.[114] Severe acute or sustained elevations in mean arterial pressure overcome autoregulatory vasoconstriction in the resistance vessels and result in forced vasodilatation. These vasodilated vessels, exposed to high intraluminal pressures, leak fluid and protein and result in cerebral oedema, which is multifocal and later diffuse.

Figure 2.9 PET images of cerebral blood flow in a patient with a left temporoparietal contusion following head injury. Note the marked heterogeneity in CBF values in the region of the contusion.

SUBARACHNOID HAEMORRHAGE

Cerebral autoregulation and CO_2 responsiveness are grossly distorted after SAH, more so in patients in worse clinical grades[115] (Fig. 2.11). Such patients may be unable to compensate for reductions in MAP produced by anaesthetic agents and develop clinically

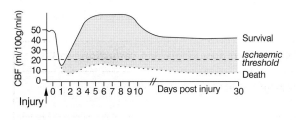

Figure 2.8 Spectrum of CBF patterns following severe head injury. Following an initial period of ischaemia lasting <24 h, CBF begins to rise and may exceed normal values on day 2–4. CBF may fall to subnormal levels at later time points, chiefly due to the presence of vasospasm secondary to traumatic subarachnoid haemorrhage. CBF levels may never rise in some patients, especially those who have a poor outcome. (Redrawn from Bullock R. Injury on cell function. In Reilly P, Bullock R (Eds). Head injury. London Chapman & Hall 1997.)

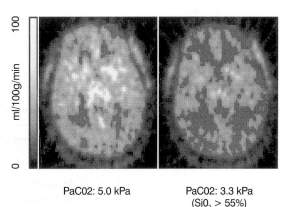

Figure 2.10 PET CBF image showing the effect of hyperventilation within the first 24 h after head injury. Despite the maintenance of SjO_2 values at acceptable levels, hyperventilation results in increases in the volume of brain tissue where CBF falls below recognized thresholds of ischaemia.

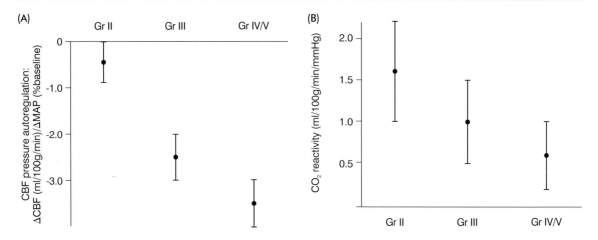

Figure 2.11   Effect of Hunt and Hess grade of aneurysmal subarachnoid haemorrhage on (A) CBF reactivity to changes in $PaCO_2$ and (B) pressure autoregulation. (Drawn from data in Ref. 115)

significant deficits.[116] Clinically significant vasospasm after SAH occurs in up to 30–40%[117] of patients, typically several days after the initial bleed, and may be due to one or more of several mechanisms. Nitric oxide (NO) may be taken up by haemoglobin in the extravasated blood or be inactivated to peroxynitrite (ONOO⁻) by superoxide radicals (O⁻•) produced during ischaemia and reperfusion. Alternatively, spasm may be secondary to lipid peroxidation of the vessel wall by various oxidant species including superoxide and peroxynitrite. Other authors have proposed a role for endothelin.[118,119] Vasospasm tends to be worst in patients with the largest amounts of subarachnoid blood,[120] suggesting that the blood in itself contributes to the phenomenon. Vasospasm is associated with parallel reductions in rCBF and $CMRO_2$ in the regions affected.

The clinical impact of late vasospasm has been substantially modified by the routine use of Ca^{++} channel blockers such as nimodipine[121] and by the routine use of hypertensive hypervolaemic haemodilution[122] (triple H therapy). Triple H (3H) therapy involves the use of colloid administration (with venesection if needed) to increase filling pressures and reduce haematocrit to 30–35%. If moderate hypertension is not achieved with volume loading, vasopressors and inotropes are used to maintain systolic blood pressures as high as 120–140 mmHg. The hypertensive element of this therapy protects non-autoregulating portions of the cerebral vasculature from hypoperfusion, while the haemodilution improves rheological characteristics of blood and facilitates flow through vessels whose calibre is reduced by spasm. Such interventions have been shown to produce clinically useful improvements in rCBF in

regions of ischaemia[123] in the setting of SAH, but not in stroke.

MECHANISMS IN CBF CONTROL

Some of the mechanisms involved in cerebrovascular control are shown in Figure 2.12. Several of these have been referred to earlier. In addition, the level of free Ca^{2+} is important in determining vascular tone and arachidonate metabolism can produce prostanoids that are either vasodialators (e.g. PGI_2) or vasoconstrictive (e.g. TXA_2). Endothelin (ET), produced by endothelin-converting enzyme (ECE) in endothelial cells, balances the vasodilator effects of nitric oxide in a tonic matter by exerting its influences at ET_A receptors in the vascular smooth muscle.

NITRIC OXIDE IN THE REGULATION OF CEREBRAL HAEMODYNAMICS[37]

Recent interest has focused on the role of nitric oxide (NO) in the control of cerebral haemodynamics. NO is synthesized in the brain from the amino acid L-arginine by the constitutive form of enzyme nitric oxide synthase (NOS). This form of the enzyme is calmodulin dependent and requires Ca^{++} and tetrahydrobiopterin for its activity and differs from the inducible form of the enzyme which is present in mononuclear blood cells and is activated by cytokines. Under basal conditions, endothelial cells synthesize NO which diffuses into the muscular layer and, via a cGMP-mediated mechanism, produces relaxation of vessels. There is strong evidence to suggest that NO exerts a tonic dilatory influence on cerebral vessels. It is important to emphasize that data on NO obtained

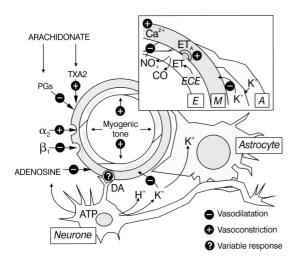

Figure 2.12 Mechanisms involved in the regulation of rCBF in health and disease. The diagram shows a resistance vessel in the brain in the vicinity of a neurone and an astrocyte. E = endothelium; M = muscular layer; PGs = prostaglandins; TXA_2 = thromboxane A_2; ET = endothelin; ECE = endothelin-converting enzyme; ET_A = ET_A receptor; NO = nitric oxide; CO = carbon monoxide; DA = dopmaine. The inset box shows the detail of the vessel wall and adjacent glial cell process. See text for details.

from peripheral vessels cannot always be translated to the cerebral vasculature; for example, some of the endothelium-derived relaxant factor (EDRF) activity in cerebral vessels may be due to compounds other than NO. There is growing evidence that carbon monoxide (CO) produced by heme oxygenase may be responsible for significant cerebral vasodilatation, especially when NO production is reduced.[124]

NO plays an important role in cerebrovascular responses to functional activation, excitatory amino acids, hypercapnia, ischaemia and subarachnoid haemorrhage. Further, it may play an important part in mediating the vasodilatation produced by volatile anaesthetic agents[37] although other mechanisms, including a direct effect on the vessel wall, cannot be excluded.

NEUROGENIC FLOW–METABOLISM COUPLING

While the last 10 years have focused on flow–metabolism coupling being effected by a diffusible extracellular mediator, there is now accumulating evidence to suggest that dopaminergic neurones may play a major part in such events[125] and, additionally, may control blood–brain barrier permeability.[17]

REFERENCES

1. Edvinsson L, Mackenzie ET, McCulloch J. The aged brain. In: Cerebral blood flow and metabolism. Raven Press, New York, 1993, pp 647–660.

2. Alpers BJ, Berry RG, Paddison RM. Anatomical studies in the circle of Willis in normal brains. Arch Neurol Psychiatr 1959; 81: 409–418.

3. Collins RC. Intracortical localization of 2-deoxyglucose metabolism on-off metabolic columns. In: Passonneau JV, Hawkins RA, Lust WD, Welsh FA (eds) Cerebral metabolism and neural function. Williams and Wilkins, Baltimore, 1980, pp 338–351.

4. Welsh FA. Regional evaluation of ischaemic metabolic alterations. J Cereb Blood Flow Metab 1984; 4: 309–316.

5. Pulsinelli WA, Duffy TE. Local cerebral glucose metabolism during controlled hypoxaemia in rats. Science 1979; 204: 626–629.

6. Dunning HS, Wolff HG. The relative vascularity of various parts of the central and peripheral nervous system in the cat and its relation to function. J Comp Neurol 1937; 67: 433–450.

7. Sokoloff L, Reivich M, Kennedy C et al. The [14C]-deoxyglucose method for measurement of local cerebral glucose utilization: theory, procedure, and normal values in the conscious and anesthetized albino rat. J Neurochem 1977; 28: 897–916.

8. Göbel U, Theilen H, Kuschinsky W. Congruence of total and perfused capillary network in rat brains. Circ Res 1990; 66: 271–281.

9. Kuschinsky W, Paulson OB. Capillary circulation in the brain (review). Cerebrovasc Brain Metab Rev 1992, 4: 261–286.

10. Beards SC, Yule S, Kassner A, Jackson A. Anatomical variation of cerebral venous drainage: the theoretical effect on jugular bulb blood samples. Anaesthesia 1998; 53: 627–633.

11. Shapiro K, Marmarou A, Shulman K. Characterization of clinical CSF dynamics and neural axis compliance using the pressure-volume index. I. The normal pressure-volume index. Ann Neurol 1980; 7: 508–513.

12. Chesnut RM. Hyperventilation in traumatic brain injury: Friend or foe? Crit Care Med 1997; 25: 1275–1278.

13. Todd MM, Weeks J. Comparative effect of propofol, pentobarbital and isoflurane on cerebral blood flow and volume. J Neurosurg Anesthesiol 1996; 8: 296–303.

14. Janzer RC, Raff MC. Astrocytes induce blood–brain barrier properties in endothelial cells. Nature 1987; 325: 253–257.

15. Oldendorf WH. Lipid solubility and drug penetration of the blood brain barrier. Proc Soc Exp Biol Med 1974; 147: 813–816.

16. Oldendorf WH, Cornford ME, Brown WJ. The large apparent work capability of the blood brain barrier: a

study of the mitochondrial content of capillary endothelial cells in brain and other tissues of the rat. Ann Neurol 1977; 1: 409–417.

17. Raichle ME, Hartman BK, Eichling JO, Sharpe LG. Central noradrenergic regulation of cerebral blood flow and vascular permeability. Proc Natl Acad Sci USA 1975; 72: 3726–3730.

18. Neufeld G, Cohen T, Grengrinovitch S, Poltorak Z. Vascular endothelial growth factor and its receptors. FASEB J 1999; 13: 9–22.

19. Fox PT, Raichle ME, Mintun MA, Dence C. Nonoxidative glucose consumption during focal physiologic neural activity. Science 1988; 241: 462–464.

20. Tsacopoulos M, Magistretti PJ. Metabolic coupling between glia and neurons. J Neurosci 1996; 16: 877–885.

21. Pellerin L, Magistretti PJ. Glutamate uptake into astrocytes stimulates anaerobic glycolysis: a mechanism coupling neuronal activity to glucose utilization. Proc Natl Acad Sci USA 1994; 91: 10625–10629.

22. Edvinsson L, Mackenzie ET, McCulloch J. Perivascular nerve fibres in brain vessels. In: Cerebral blood flow and metabolism. Raven Press, New York, 1993, pp 57–91.

23. Kontos HA. Nitric oxide and nitrosothiols in cerebrovascular and neuronal regulation (review). Stroke 1993; 24: 1155–1158.

24. Miller JD, Stanek A, Langfitt TW. Concepts of cerebral perfusion pressure and vascular compression during intracranial hypertension. Prog Brain Res 1972; 35: 411–432.

25. Miller JD, Stanek AE, Langfitt TW. Cerebral blood flow regulation during experimental brain compression. J Neurosurg 1973; 39: 186–196.

26. Fitch W, MacKenzie ET, Harper AM. Effects of decreasing arterial blood pressure on cerebral blood flow in the baboon: influence of the sympathetic nervous system. Circ Res 1975; 37: 550–557.

27. Heistad DD, Marcus ML, Sandberg S, Abboud FM. Effect of sympathetic nerve stimulation on cerebral blood flow and on large cerebral arteries of dogs. Circ Res 1977; 41: 342–350.

28. Thomas D, Bannister RG. Preservation of autoregulation of cerebral blood flow in autonomic failure. J Neurol Sci 1980; 44: 205–212.

29. Strandgaard S, Olesen J, Skinhoj E, Jassen NA. Autoregulation of brain circulation in severe arterial hypertension. BMJ 1973; 1: 507–510.

30. Thompson BG, Pluta RM, Girton ME, Oldfield EH. Nitric oxide mediation of chemoregulation but not autoregulation of cerebral blood flow in primates. J Neurosurg 1996; 84: 71–78.

31. Bentsen N, Larsen B, Lassen NA. Chronically impaired autoregulation of cerebral blood flow in long-term diabetics. Stroke 1975; 6: 497–502.

32. Strandgaard S. Autoregulation of CBF in hypertensives. The modifying influence of prolonged antihypertensive treatment on the tolerance to acute, drug induced hypotension. Circulation 1976; 53: 720–727.

33. Michenfelder JD, Theye RA. Canine systemic and cerebral effects of hypotension induced by hemorrhage, trimethaphan, halothane, or nitroprusside. Anesthesiology 1977; 46: 188–195.

34. Aaslid R, Lindegaard K-F, Sorteberg W, Nornes H. Cerebral autoregulation dynamics in humans. Stroke 1989; 20: 45–52.

35. Davis DH, Sundt TM Jr. Relationship of cerebral blood flow to cardiac output, mean arterial pressure, blood volume, and alpha and beta blockade in cats. J Neurosurg 1980; 52: 745–754.

36. Koehler RC, Traystman RJ. Bicarbonate ion modulation of cerebral blood flow during hypoxia and hypercapnia. Am J Physiol 1982, 243: H33–40.

37. Stringer WA, Hasso AN, Thompson JR, Hinshaw DB, Jordan KG. Hyperventilation-induced cerebral ischaemia in patients with acute brain lesions: demonstration by xenon-enhanced CT. Am J Neuroradiol 1993; 14: 465–484.

38. Pickard JD, MacKenzie ET. Inhibition of prostaglandin synthesis and the response of baboon cerebral circulation to carbon dioxide. Nature (New Biol) 1973; 245: 187–188.

39. Maktabi MA. Role of nitric oxide in regulation of cerebral circulation in health and disease. Curr Opin Anaesthesiol 1993, 6: 799–783.

40. Okamoto H, Hudetz AG, Roman RJ, Bosnjak ZJ, Kampine JP. Neuronal NOS-derived NO plays permissive role in cerebral blood flow response to hypercapnia. Am J Physiol 1997; 272: H559–H566.

41. Grubb RL Jr, Raichle ME, Eichling JO, Ter-Pogossian MM. The effects of changes in $PaCO_2$ on cerebral blood volume, blood flow and vascular mean transit time. Stroke 1974; 5: 630–639.

42. Kosteljanetz M. Acute head injury: pressure-volume relations and cerebrospinal fluid dynamics. Neurosurgery 1986; 18: 17–24.

43. McDowall DG. Interrelationships between blood oxygen tension and cerebral blood flow. In: Payne JP, Hill DW (eds) Oxygen measurements in blood and tissues. Churchill, London, 1966, pp 205–214.

44. Gupta AK, Menon DK, Czosnyka M, Smielewski P, Jones JG. Thresholds for hypoxic cerebral vasodilatation in volunteers. Anesth Analg 1997; 85: 817–820.

45. Krasney JA, Jensen JB, Lassen NA. Cerebral blood flow does not adapt to sustained hypoxia. J Cereb Blood Flow Metab 1990; 10: 759–764.

46. Krasney JA, McDonald B, Matalon S. Regional circulatory responses to 96 hours of hypoxia in conscious sheep. Respir Physiol 1984; 57: 73–88.

47. Krasney JA, Hajduczok G, Miki K, Matalon S. Peripheral circulatory responses to 96 hours of eucapnic hypoxia in conscious sheep. Respir Physiol 1985; 59: 197–211.

48. Purves MJ. The physiology of the cerebral circulation. Cambridge University Press, Cambridge, 1972.

49. Matta BF, Lam AM, Mayberg TS. The influence of arterial hyperoxygenation on cerebral venous oxygen content during hyperventilation. Can J Anaesth 1994; 41: 1041–1046.

50. Christensen MS, Hoedt-Rasmussen K, Lassen NA. Cerebral vasodilation by halothane anesthesia in man and its potentiation by hypotension and hypercapnia. Br J Anaesth 1967; 39: 927.

51. Wollman H, Alexander SC, Cohen PJ, Chase PE, Melman E, Behar MG. Cerebral circulation of man during halothane anesthesia. Effects of hypocarbia and of d-tubocurarine. Anesthesiology 1964; 25: 180–184.

52. Jennett WB, Barker J, Fitch W, McDowall DG. Effects of anaesthesia on intracranial pressure in patients with space-occupying lesions. Lancet 1969; i: 61–64.

53. Murphy FL, Kennell EM, Johnstone RE. The effects of enflurane, isoflurane, and halothane on cerebral blood flow and metabolism in man. Abstracts of the Meeting of The American Society of Anesthesiologists, 1974, pp 61–62.

54. Hansen TD, Warner DS, Todd MM, Vust LJ, Trawick DC. Distribution of cerebral blood flow during halothane versus isoflurane anesthesia in rats. Anesthesiology 1988; 69: 332–337.

55. Hansen TD, Warner DS, Todd MM, Vust LJ. Effects of nitrous oxide and volatile anaesthetics on cerebral blood flow. Br J Anaesth 1989; 63: 290–295.

56. Scheller MS, Todd MM, Drummond JC. Isoflurane, halothane and regional cerebral blood flow at various levels of $PaCO_2$ in rabbits. Anesthesiology 1986; 64: 598–604.

57. Drummond JC, Todd MM. The response of the feline cerebral circulation to PaCO2 during anesthesia with isoflurane and halothane and during sedation with nitrous oxide. Anesthesiology 1985; 62: 268–273.

58. Okamoto H, Meng W, Ma J et al. Isoflurane-induced cerebral hyperaemia in neuronal nitric oxide synthase gene deficient mice. Anesthesiology 1997; 86: 875–884.

59. Kuramoto T, Oshita S, Takeshita H, Ishikawa T. Modification of the relationship between cerebral metabolism, blood flow, and the EEG by stimulation during anesthesia in the dog. Anesthesiology 1979; 51: 211–217.

60. Hansen TD, Warner DS, Todd MM, Vust LJ. The role of cerebral metabolism in determining the local cerebral blood flow effects of volatile anaesthetics: evidence for persistent flow-metabolism coupling. J Cereb Blood Flow Metab 1989; 9: 323–328.

61. Maekawa T, Tommasino C, Shapiro HM, Kiefer-Goodman J, Kohlenberger RW. Local cerebral blood flow and glucose utilisation during isoflurane anesthesia in the rat. Anesthesiology 1986; 65: 144–151.

62. Lam AM, Matta BF, Mayberg TS, Strebel S. Changes in cerebral blood flow velocity with onset of EEG silence during inhalational anesthesia in humans: evidence of flow-metabolism coupling? J Cereb Blood Flow Metab 1995; 15: 714–717.

63. Sakabe T, Kuramoto T, Kumagae S, Takeshita H. Cerebral responses to the addition of nitrous oxide to halothane in man. Br J Anaesth 1976; 48: 957–962.

64. Lam AM, Mayberg TS, Eng CC, Cooper JO, Bachenberg KL, Mathisen TL. Nitrous oxide-isoflurane anesthesia causes more cerebral vasodilation than an equipotent dose of isoflurane in humans. Anesth Analg 1994; 78: 462–468.

65. Matta BF, Lam AM. Nitrous oxide increases cerebral blood flow velocity during pharmacologically-induced EEG silence in humans. J Neurosurg Anesthesiol 1995; 7: 89–93.

66. Henriksen HT, Jorgensen PB. The effect of nitrous oxide on intracranial pressure in patients with intracranial disorders. Br J Anaesth 1973; 45: 486–492.

67. Moss E, McDowall DG. ICP increases with 50% nitrous oxide in oxygen in severe head injuries with controlled ventilation. Br J Anaesth 1979; 51: 757–761.

68. Kaieda R, Todd MM, Warner DS. The effects of anesthetics and $PaCO_2$ on the cerebrovascular, metabolic, and electroencephalographic responses to nitrous oxide in the rabbit. Anesth Analg 1989; 68: 135–143.

69. Phirman JR, Shapiro HM. Modification of nitrous oxide induced intracranial hypertension by prior induction of anesthesia. Anesthesiology 1977; 46: 150–151.

70. Young WL. Effects of desflurane on the central nervous system. Anesth Analg 1992; 75 (suppl 4): 32–37.

71. Scheller MS, Tateishi A, Drummond JC, Zornow MH. The effects of sevoflurane on cerebral blood flow, cerebral metabolic rate for oxygen, intracranial pressure and the electroencephalogram are similar to those of isoflurane in the rabbit. Anesthesiology 1988; 68: 548–551.

72. Lutz LJ, Milde JH, Milde LN. The cerebral functional, metabolic, and hemodynamic effects of desflurane in dogs. Anesthesiology 1990; 73: 125–131.

73. Muzzi DA, Losasso TJ, Dietz NM, Faust RJ, Cucchiara RF, Milde LN. The effect of desflurane and isoflurane on cerebrospinal fluid pressure in humans with supra-tentorial mass lesions. Anesthesiology 1992; 76: 720–724.

74. Rampil IJ, Lockhart SH, Eger EI, Weiskopf RB. Human EEG dose response to desflurane. Anesthesiology 1990; 73: A1218.

75. Tonner PH, Scholz J, Krause T, Paris A, Von Knobelsdroff G, Schulte an Esch J. Administration of sufentanil and nitrous oxide blunts cardiovascular responses to desflurane but does not prevent an increase in middle cerebral artery flow velocity. Eur J Anaesthesiol 1997; 14: 389–396.

76. Bundgaard H, Von Oettingen G, Larsen KM et al. Effects of sevoflurane on intracranial pressure, cerebral blood flow and cerebral metabolism. A dose-response

study in patients subjected to craniotomy for cerebral tumours. Acta Anaesthesiol Scand 1998; 42: 621–627.

77. Summors A, Gupta A, Matta BF. Dynamic cerebral autoregulation during sevoflurane anaesthesia: a comparison with isoflurane. Anesth Analg 1999; 88: 341–345.

78. Gupta S, Heath K, Matta BF. The effect of incremental doses of sevoflurane on cerebral pressure autoregulation in humans: a transcranial Doppler study. Br J Anaesth 1997; 79: 469–472.

79. Matta BF, Mayberg TS, Lam AM. Direct cerebrovasodilatory effects of halothane, isoflurane and desflurane during propofol-induced isoelectric encephalogram in humans. Anesthesiology 1995; 83: 980–985.

80. Heath K, Gupta S, Matta BF. Direct cerebral vasodilatory effect of sevoflurane. Anesthesiology 1997; 87: A177.

81. Heath KJ, Gupta S, Matta BF. The effects of sevoflurane on cerebral hemodynamics during propofol anesthesia. Anesth Analg 1997; 85: 1284–1287.

82. Gupta S, Heath K, Matta BF. Effect of incremental doses of sevoflurane on cerebral pressure autoregulation in humans. Br J Anaesth 1997; 79: 469–472.

83. Kassel NF, Hitchon PW, Gerk MK, Sokoll MD, Hill TR. Alterations in cerebral blood flow, oxygen metabolism, and electrical activity produced by high dose sodium thiopental. Neurosurgery 1980; 7: 598–603.

84. Milde LN, Milde JH, Michenfelder JD. Cerebral functional, metabolic, and hemodynamic effects of etomidate in dogs. Anesthesiology 1985; 63: 371–377.

85. Ramani R, Todd MM, Warner DS. The cerebrovascular, metabolic and electroencephalographic effects of propofol in the rabbit – a dose response study. J Neurosurg Anesthesiol 1992; 4: 110–119.

86. Van Hemelrijck J, Van Aken H, Plets C, Goffin J, Vermaut G. The effects of propofol on intracranial pressure and cerebral perfusion pressure in patients with brain umours. Acta Anaesthesiol Belg 1989; 40: 95–100.

87. Weeks J, Todd MM, Warner DS, Katz J. The influence of halothane, isoflurane, and pentobarbital on cerebral plasma volume in hypocapnic and normocapnic rats. Anesthesiology 1990; 73: 461–466.

88. Fox J, Gelb AW, Enns J, Murkin JM, Farrar JK, Manninen PH. The responsiveness of cerebral blood flow to changes in arterial carbon dioxide is maintained during propofol-nitrous oxide anesthesia in humans. Anesthesiology 1992; 77: 453–456.

89. Carlsson C, Smith DS, Keykhah MM, Englebach I, Harp JR. The effects of high dose fentanyl on cerebral circulation and metabolism in rats. Anesthesiology 1982; 57: 375–380.

90. Keykhah MM, Smith DS, Carlsson C, Safo Y, Englebach I, Harp JR. Influence of sufentanil on cerebral metabolism and circulation in the rat. Anesthesiology 1985; 63: 274–280.

91. McPherson RW, Krempasanka E, Eimerl D, Traystman RJ. Effects of alfentanil on cerebral vascular reactivity in dogs. Br J Anaesth 1985; 57: 1232–1238.

92. Murkin JM, Ferrar JK, Tweed WA, McKenzie FN, Guiraudon G. Cerebral autoregulation and flow/metabolism coupling during cardiopulmonary bypass: the influence of $PaCO_2$. Anesth Analg 1987; 66: 825–832.

93. Sperry RJ, Bailey PL, Reichman MV, Peterson PB, Pace NL. Fentanyl and sufentanil increase intracranial pressure in head trauma patients. Anesthesiology 1992; 77: 416–420.

94. Åkeson J, Björkman S, Messeter K, Rosén I, Helfer M. Cerebral pharmacodynamics of anaesthetic and subanaesthetic doses of ketamine in the normoventilated pig. Acta Anaesthesiol Scand 1993; 37: 211–218.

95. Menon DK, Burdett NG, Carpenter TA, Hall LD. Functional MRI of ketamine-induced changes in rCBF: an effect at the NMDA receptor? (abstract). Br J Anaesth 1993, 71: 767P.

96. Mayberg TS, Lam AM, Matta BF, Domino K, Winn HR. Ketamine does not increase cerebral blood flow velocity or intracranial pressure during isoflurane-nitrous oxide anesthesia in patients undergoing craniotomy. Anesth Analg 1995; 81: 84–89.

97. Forster A, Juge O, Morel D. Effects of midazolam on cerebral blood flow in human volunteers. Anesthesiology 1982; 56: 453–455.

98. Fleischer JE, Milde JH, Moyer TP, Michenfelder JD. Cerebral effects of high-dose midazolam and subsequent reversal with RO 15–1788 in dogs. Anesthesiology 1988; 68: 234–242.

99. Zornow MH, Fleischer JE, Scheller MS et al. Dexmedetomidine, an alpha 2-adrenergic agonist, decreases cerebral blood flow in the isoflurane anaesthetised dog. Anesth Analg 1990; 70: 624–630.

100. McPherson RW, Koehler RC, Kirsch JR, Traystman RJ. Intraventricular demedetomidine decreases cerebral blood flow during normoxia and hypoxia in dogs. Anesth Analg 1997; 84: 139–147.

101. Ducey JP, Deppe AS, Foley FT. A comparison of the effects of suxamethonium, atracurium and vecuronium on intracranial haemodynamics in swine. Anaesth Intens Care 1989; 17: 448–455.

102. Kovarik WD, Lam AM, Slee TA, Mathisen TL. The effect of succinylcholine on intracranial pressure, cerebral blood flow velocity and electroencephalogram in patients with neurologic disorders (abstract). Anesthesiology 1991; 75: 207.

103. Stirt JA, Grosslight KR, Bedford RF, Vollmer D. 'Defasciculation' with metocurine prevents succinylcholine-induced increases intracranial pressure. Anesthesiology 1987; 67: 50–53.

104. Siesjo B.K. Pathophysiology and treatment of focal cerebral ischaemia. Part I: pathophysiology. J Neurosurg 1992; 77: 169–184.

105. Robertson CS, Contant CF, Gokaslan ZL, Narayan RK, Grossman RG. Cerebral blood flow, arteriovenous

oxygen difference, and outcome in head injured patients. J Neurol Neurosurg Psychiatry 1992; 55: 594–603.

106. Bouma GJ, Muizelaar JP, Stringer WA, Choi SC, Fatouros P, Young HF. Ultra early evaluation of regional cerebral blood flow in severely head-injured patients using xenon-enhanced computerized tomography. J Neurosurg 1992; 77: 360–369.

107. Martin NA, Patwardhan RV, Alexander MJ et al. Characterization of cerebral hemodynamic phases following severe head trauma: hypoperfusion, hyperaemia and vasospasm. J Neurosurg 1997; 87: 9–19.

108. Martin NA, Doberstein C, Zane C, Caron MJ, Thomas K, Becker DP. Posttraumatic cerebral arterial spasm: transcranial Doppler ultrasound, cerebral blood flow and angiographic findings. J Neurosurg 1992; 77: 575–583.

109. Marion DW, Darby J, Yonas H. Acute regional cerebral blood flow changes caused by severe head injuries. J Neurosurg 1991; 74: 407–414.

110. McLaughlin MR, Marion DW. Cerebral blood flow within and around cerebral contusions. J Neurosurg 1996; 85: 871–876.

111. Menon DK, Minhas P, Herrod NJ et al. Cerebral ischaemia associated with hyperventilation: a PET study. Anesthesiology 1997; 87: A176.

112. Chan KH, Dearden NM, Miller JD, Andrews PJ, Midgley S. Multimodality monitoring as a guide to treatment of intracranial hypertension after severe brain injury. Neurosurgery 1993; 32: 547–552.

113. Feldman Z, Kanter MJ, Robertson CS et al. Effect of head elevation on intracranial pressure, cerebral perfusion pressure and cerebral blood flow in head injured patients. J Neurosurg 1992; 76: 207–211.

114. Lassen NA, Agnoli A. The upper limit of autoregulation of cerebral blood flow on the pathogenesis of hypertensive encephalopathy. Scand J Clin Lab Invest 1973; 30: 113–116.

115. Voldby B, Enevoldsen EM, Jensen FT. Cerebrovascular reactivity in patients with ruptured intracranial aneurysm. J Neurosurg 1985; 62: 59–67.

116. Pickard JD, Matheson M, Patterson J, Wyper D. Prediction of late ischemic complications after cerebral aneurysm surgery by the intraoperative measurement of cerebral blood flow. J Neurosurg 1980; 53: 305–308.

117. Kassell NF, Peerless SJ, Durward QJ, Beck DW, Drake CG, Adams HP. Treatment of ischaemic deficits from vasospasm with intravascular volume expansion and induced arterial hypertension. Neurosurgery 1982; 11: 337–343.

118. Yamaura I, Tani E, Maeda Y, Minami N, Shindo H. Endothelin-1 of canine basilar artery in vasospasm. J Neurosurg 1992; 76: 99–105.

119. Clozel M, Watanabe H. BQ-123, a peptidic endothelin ETA receptor antagonist, prevents the early cerebral vasospasm following subarachnoid hemorrhage after intracisternal but not intravenous injection. Life Sci 1993; 52: 825–834.

120. Jakobsen M, Skj¾dt T, Enevoldsen E. Cerebral blood flow and metabolism following subarachnoid hemorrhage: effect of subarachnoid blood. Acta Neurol Scand 1991; 8: 226–233.

121. Pickard JD, Murray GD, Illingworth R et al. Effect of oral nimodipine on cerebral infarction and outcome after subarachnoid hemorrhage: British Aneurysm Nimodipine Trial. BMJ 1989; 298: 636–642.

122. Origitano TC, Wascher TM, Reichman OH, Anderson DE. Sustained increased cerebral blood flow with prophylactic hypervolemic haemodilution ('Triple – H' Therapy) after subarachnoid haemorrhage. Neurosurgery 1990; 27: 729–738.

123. Darby JM, Yonas H, Marks EC, Durham S, Snyder RW, Nemoto EM. Acute cerebral blood flow response to dopamine-induced hypertension after subarachnoid hemorrhage. J Neurosurg 1994; 80: 857–864.

124. Zakhary R, Gaine SP, Dinennan JL et al. Heme oxygenase 2: endothelial and neuronal localisation and role in endothelial-dependent relaxation. Proc Natl Acad Sci USA 1996; 93: 795–798.

125. Iadecola C. Neurogenic control of the cerebral microcirculation: is dopamine mining the store? Nature Neurosci 1998; 1: 363–364.

3

MECHANISMS OF INJURY AND CEREBRAL PROTECTION

Patrick W. Doyle & Arun K. Gupta

Mechanisms of neural injury, cerebral protection and cerebral resuscitation have been an area of intensive research over the last 20 years and the pathophysiological and biochemical processes responsible for the development and propagation of neural injury are becoming clearer. Despite this explosion of research, current approaches to reducing permanent injury have remained largely unchanged over the past few decades. The pathophysiological processes that lead to neuronal cell death and loss of function are similar whether the CNS insult is the consequence of intraoperative injury, stroke or trauma. In its correct terminology, cerebral protection refers to interventions aimed at reducing neural injury that are instituted before a possible ischaemic event, while cerebral resuscitation refers to interventions that occur after such an event.[1] In practice, many of the mechanisms involved in both phases of the process are identical and the following discussion will deal with both forms of intervention as one.

MECHANISMS OF INJURY

All brain injury can be thought of as being constituted of basic primary, secondary and molecular and biochemical processes. Whatever the primary insult, there will always be secondary and molecular damage, not only in the core of the lesion but also in the penumbral region. Central to all mechanisms of injury are cerebral ischaemia and hypoxia. Global ischaemia refers to events which result in complete hypoperfusion of the entire organ or where no potential for recruitment of collateral flow exists. Focal ischaemia refers to the occlusion of an artery distal to the circle of Willis, which permits some collateral flow, thus resulting in a dense ischaemic core with a partially perfused surrounding penumbral zone.[1] Tissues in the penumbral zone may be more salvageable and hence provide a realistic target for neuroprotection.

BASIC MECHANISMS OF INJURY

All the principal types of brain damage that occur clinically can now be reproduced in experimental models.[2,3] These can be classified as traumatic, ischaemic or hypoxic. Traumatic brain injury may be due to the trauma associated with accidents or personal violence. Alternatively, the trauma may be iatrogenic and accompany a variety of operative procedures, including retraction, shear forces, direct tissue destruction, haemorrhage and vessel disruption with subsequent infarction. These injuries are typically followed by brain swelling, leading to an increase in intracranial volume and intracranial pressure and a consequent reduction in cerebral blood flow. In addition to direct tissue injury, acceleration-deceleration forces may result in shearing of nerve fibres and microvascular structures in the process termed *diffuse axonal injury*.[4,5] While this was originally thought to occur at the time of injury, there is accumulating evidence that the event of axonal shearing is the culmination of processes that mature over hours.

Secondary insults are initiated as a consequence of the primary injury but may not be apparent for an interval following the injury. Intracranial haemorrhage is the most common local structural cause of clinical deterioration and death in patients who have experienced a lucid interval after traumatic injury.[6,7,8] The pathophysiology associated with this process may reflect simple physiological consequences of ischaemia arising from pressure effects to underlying and distant brain regions, shift of vital structures and axonal disruption, reductions in cerebral blood flow and metabolism, hydrocephalus and herniation. However, metabolic processes may cause more subtle changes and ischaemia may not just be due to local microcirculatory compression but also the consequence of vasoactive substances released from the haematoma. In addition, glucose utilization has also been found to be markedly increased in pericontusional and perihaemorrhagic regions, possibly due to activation of excitatory neuronal systems.[2,9] In addition, extravasated subarachnoid blood can cause vasospasm both locally and at distant sites with aggravation of ischaemia.

Systemic physiological insults may occur as a consequence of the primary lesion but can contribute to worsening neural injury. These include hypoxia, hypotension, hypercarbia, hyperthermia, anaemia and electrolyte disturbances. Hypoxia may be the result of airway obstruction, aspiration, thoracic injury, primary hypoventilation or pulmonary shunting.[3] Hypotension has been found to occur in 32–35% of patients in emergency departments, which may be due to systemic causes.[7] This causes a decrease in cerebral perfusion pressure, which may be aggravated by a high ICP, disruption of cerebrovascular autoregulation, vasospasm and change in cerebral blood flow patterns. Hyperthermia may be due to infection, thrombophlebitis, drug reactions or a defect in the thermoregulatory system. This results in excessive excitotoxic neurotransmitter release, altered protein kinase C activity and augmented pathophysiological effects of ischaemia. Hypercarbia causes vasodilatation of cerebral blood vessels, with increased ICP, and exacerbation of any mass or oedema effect. It may also be associated with cerebral metabolic acidosis.

Imbalances between cerebral oxygen delivery and demand that arise as a consequence of the systemic and local secondary insults may result in focal or global ischaemia. Even global ischaemia can result in discrete lesions in specific areas due to either haemodynamic patterns or selective neuronal vulnerability[10] in those regions. These include arterial watershed areas, terminal perfusion beds, the hippocampi (especially the CA1 area), Purkinje cells and the small and medium-sized neurones of striatum and layers three, five and six of the cortex.

MOLECULAR AND BIOCHEMICAL ASPECTS OF CEREBRAL INJURY

Central to cerebral injury are ischaemia and the concept of cellular energy failure. While initial ischaemia may be directly responsible for some of this, the situation is complicated by delayed postischaemic hypoperfusion. After restoration of cerebral blood flow, there is an initial period of reactive hyperaemia because of decreased viscosity of the blood relative to the stagnant blood and because of vasoactive substance release during the ischaemia causing decreased vascular tone.[10] Hypoperfusion develops after the period of reactive hyperaemia. The mechanism of this is unclear but it may be due to increased intracellular calcium levels causing smooth muscle contraction,[11] or increased production of thromboxane A_2, a potent vasoconstrictor.

Hypoxia and ischaemia result in impaired oxidative ATP synthesis with threats to cellular function and survival as a consequence of three processes:

1. anaerobic glycolysis, with resultant intra- and extra-cellular acidosis and free radical production;
2. disruption of ion homoeostasis with abnormal Na+, Cl-, K+, and Ca++ fluxes;
3. structural integrity of the cell is threatened via mitochondrial membrane damage and inhibition of protein synthesis.

Excitatory amino acid receptor activation

Glutamate and aspartate are the major physiological excitatory neurotransmitters in the brain and at pathological concentrations can function as potent neurotoxins. These excitatory amino acids (EAA) are normally present at millimolar levels in the intracellular compartment throughout CNS grey matter. They are normally released in small amounts into the extracellular space for synaptic transmission and are then rapidly cleared by energy-dependent cellular uptake mechanisms. In cellular ischaemia-hypoxia, uptake mechanisms fail and toxic levels of EEA accumulate in the extracellular space.[12]

Indeed, it has been demonstrated that there is a massive increase in the amount of glutamate in the selectively vulnerable areas during ischaemia and the reperfusion phase that precedes a cascade of pathogenetic processes.[13,14] This causes a surge of neuronal activity and membrane depolarization of membranes via activation of agonist gated ion channels.

The predominant mechanism for excitation in the brain normally encompasses ion channels gated by glutamate receptors of which there are four subtypes:

1. NMDA;
2. a-amino-3-hydroxy-5-methyl-4 isoxazole propionic acid (AMPA);
3. high-affinity kainate receptors;
4. metabotropic glutamate receptors.[15]

Of these, the NMDA receptor appears to be the main route of Ca^{++} influx into the cytosol. This process is normally blocked by Mg^{++} ions which reside in the ion channel; this block is alleviated by receptor binding to glutamate and glycine. The glycine is a co-factor in the synaptic cleft rather than a neurotransmitter. Cellular depolarization produced by this process is associated with primary Na^+ and Ca^{++} influx and subsequently results in secondary influx of Ca^{++} via voltage-gated channels.[1] Kainate and AMPA receptors probably work by allowing the displacement of Mg^{++} by Na^+ shifts. Excessive activation of these receptors can trigger an avalanche of Ca^{++} influx via multiple Ca^{++} conductances with concomitant increases in permeability for other ions.[16]

Acidosis and hyperglycaemia

The brain is almost totally dependent on exogenous glucose for its cellular energy requirements. During normal metabolism, glucose is anaerobically metabolized via the glycolytic Embden-Myerhof pathway in the cytoplasm to pyruvate, which is then metabolized in the mitochondrion to yield ATP via the tricarboxylic acid (TCA) cycle.[17] During ischaemia, the cell relies on anaerobic glycolysis and reserves of high-energy phosphate bonds. During glycolysis, pyruvate is converted to lactate. The amount of lactate formed depends on the severity and duration of ischaemia and on preexisting stores of glycogen and glucose. The higher the amount of glucose, the more lactate produced. Since lactate appears to be neurotoxic *per se*, this sequence of events underlies the most commonly proposed mechanism by which hyperglycaemia aggravates cerebral injury. Lactate levels must increase to levels greater than 20 μmol/l to produce irreversible damage.[18] If ischaemia is less than complete then supply of glucose can continue and lactate can rise to excessive levels without contributing to neural injury.[19] While the general consensus is that preischaemic hyperglycaemia is deleterious, in some studies it has been shown to delay the onset of ischaemic Ca^{++} influx from the ECF and potentiate reextrusion of Ca^{++} following recirculation. These findings may reflect the modulatory effects of the type of ischaemia (focal versus global), its duration and extent and the completeness of the ischaemic insult.[10,20] It is thought that acidosis enhances production of reactive free radicals, causes oedema, aggravated tissue damage and delayed seizures and prevents recovery of mitochondrial metabolism.[14,19] However, it still remains to be fully established whether exaggerated intra-ischaemic acidosis enhances postischaemic production of reactive oxygen species (ROS).

Ionic pump failure

A variety of membrane ionic pumps, including Na^+-K^+, Na^+-Ca^{++}, and Ca^{++}-H^+, as well as Cl^- and HCO_3^- leakage fluxes, maintain electrical and concentration gradients for various ions across the cell membrane and hence generate the resting membrane potential.[21] Since these are energy-consuming processes, ischaemia-induced decreases in ATP production result in loss of ionic pump function, with changes in transmembrane concentrations of ions and electrical fluxes. Na^+ and Cl^- influxes result in cellular swelling and osmolytic damage, whilst increased cytosolic Ca^{++} sets off a cascade of events that are discussed later in this chapter. K^+ also rapidly leaves cells. Not only must one consider ATP pump failure but in the 'milieu' of ischaemic tissue, local depolarization leads to activation of ionic conductances. The increased energy demands of depolarization may trigger overt energy failure and consequently prolong transient ionic fluxes.[22]

Siësjo and Siësjo describe three major cascades of reactions:[19]

1. sustained perturbation of cell Ca^{++} metabolism;
2. persistent depression of protein synthesis;
3. programmed cell death.

Calcium

Ca ions play an important role in normal membrane excitation and cellular processes.[21] Normally extracellular concentrations are maintained at a higher concentration than free cytosolic concentrations by an ionic ATP-dependent pump. Failure of ATP energy metabolism will have a deleterious effect on this homoeostasis.[23] It is postulated that the primary defect in cells mortally injured by a transient period of

ischaemia is an inability to regulate Ca^{++}.[24] The slow gradual rise in Ca^{++} is caused by the release of glutamate from the presynaptic nerve endings, primarily via activation of receptors of the NMDA type. This leads to excessively high cytosolic Ca^{++} levels. Activation of the AMPA receptors also results in a Na^+- dependent depolarization which causes further Ca^{++} influx via voltage-gated channels. The secondary loss of cell Ca^{++} homoeostasis may also affect the relationship between Ca^{++} leaks and Ca^{++} extrusion across membranes of the sarcoplasmic reticulum. Exposure of mitochondria to excess Ca^{++} causes them to swell and release intramitochondrial components. This reflects a sudden increase in the permeability of the mitochondrial inner membrane which allows the release of H^+, Ca^{++}, Mg^{++}, and other low molecular weight components. There is strong evidence that mitochondrial dysfunction is an early recirculation event following long periods of ischaemia or ischaemia complicated by hyperglycaemia, qualifying as a direct cause of bioenergetic failure.[19] The effects of Ca^{++} are summarized in Figure 3.1.

Depression of protein synthesis

Normal protein synthesis is an early casualty of the ischaemic cascade. Normally the glutamate-induced Ca influx would result in transcription and translation of the immediate early genes (IEGs) c-fos and c-jun. These IEGs regulate the transcription of genes that code for proteins of repair.[19,23] These include the heat shock protein family, nerve growth factors, brain-derived neurotrophic factor, neurotropin-3 and enhanced expression of genes for glucose transports.[25] A block in translation due to focal or global ischaemia may thus affect the production of these stress proteins, trophic factors or enzymes and enhance ischaemic damage (Fig. 3.2).

Programmed cell death (PCD)

PCD, or apoptosis when it occurs during development, is a process that weeds out approximately half of all neurones produced during neurogenesis, leaving only those that make useful functional connections to other neurones and end-organs.[25] It is a cell death characterized by membrane blebbing, cell shrinkage, nuclear condensation and fragmentation. There are considerable data that indicate that the mechanisms leading to apoptotic and necrotic forms of cell injury are very similar.[19] In apoptosis, cells and nuclei shrink, condense and fragment and are rapidly phagocytosed by macrophages. There is no leakage of cellular contents and thus no reactive response. During cell injury, cells swell, burst and necrose. The rupture of

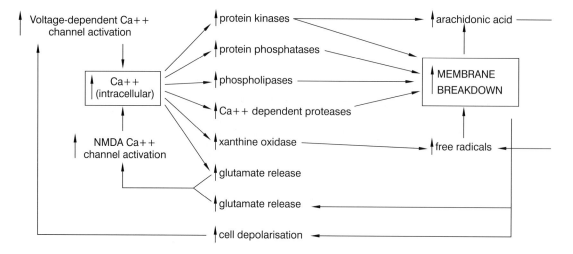

Figure 3.1   Role of Ca++ in neuronal injury (redrawn from Andrews RJ. Mechanisms of injury to the central nervous system. Williams and Wilkins, Baltimore, 1996, pp 7–19).

intracellular contents into the ECF space provides a stimulus for a reactive response.[26] PCD is an active process which requires protein synthesis and is executed by the activation of 'death genes',[27] probably triggered by stimuli such as free radicals, Ca++ accumulation, excitatory amino acids (glutamate), cytokines, antigens, hormones and apoptotic receptor signalling.[16,19] The apoptotic process also involves changes in cell surface chemistry to enable recognition by macrophages. Much of the delayed neuronal necrosis that accounts for cell death hours or days subsequent to reperfusion after ischaemic injury appears to be caused by PCD,[25] and signs of apoptosis are often encountered in the penumbral zone of a focal ischaemic area.[19]

Lipid peroxidation and free radical formation

Free radicals are reactive chemical species that damage DNA, denature structural and functional proteins and result in peroxidation of membrane lipids. Free radicals are formed as a consequence of several processes including phospholipase activation by cytosolic Ca++, transitional metal reactions which involve free iron, arachidonate metabolism and oxidant production by inflammatory cells. These processes result in the formation of superoxide radicals, which are protonated in the ischaemic environment of the ischaemic brain to produce highly reactive hydroxyl radicals. Normally aerobic cells produce free radicals, which are then consumed by free radical scavengers, e.g. a-tocopherol and ascorbic acid, or appropriate enzymes, e.g. superoxide dismutase. In states where enzymatic processes are

disrupted (ischaemia) or hyperoxia occurs (reperfusion), there may be excessive production of oxidants, in particular superoxide, hydrogen peroxide and the hydroxyl radical. These highly reactive oxidant species cause peroxidation of membrane phospholipids, oxidation of cellular proteins and nucleic acids and can attack both neuronal membranes as well as cerebral vasculature.[10] It appears that free radicals target cerebral microvasculature and that with other inflammatory mediators, e.g. platelet-activating factor, cause microvascular dysfunction and blood–brain–barrier disruption.[19] The brain is particularly vulnerable to oxidant attack due to intrinsically low levels of tissue antioxidant activity.

Endothelial nitric oxide (NO) is normally associated with relaxation of vascular endothelium and in this setting may aid recovery from acute ischaemic insults. However, generation of neuronal NO, often triggered by EAAs, may result in cellular injury. One of the mechanisms of such injury involves the combination of NO with hydroxyl radicals to generate the highly reactive peroxynitrite species, which can result in molecular oxidant injury.

Adhesion molecule expression

Acute brain injury is known to be associated with an inflammatory response[29] and there is evidence that leucocytes are involved in the production of brain swelling up to 10 days postinjury. Gupta et al have demonstrated that normal brain endothelial cells express low levels of leucocyte cell adhesion molecules (CAMs), and that these molecules are upregu-

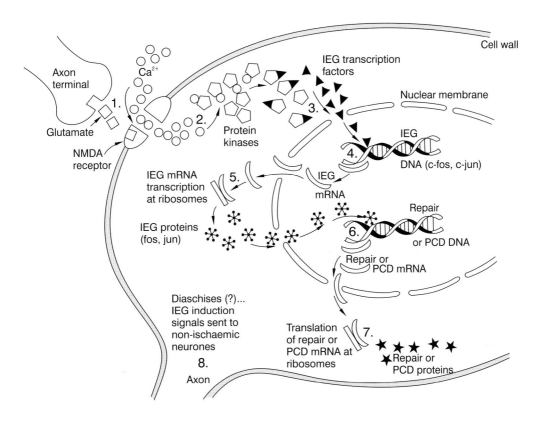

Figure 3.2 (1) Ischaemia causes axon terminals to release excitoxic glutamate, which opens N-methyl-D-aspartate (NMDA) channels, which allow calcium (Ca²⁺) into the neurone. (2) Excess calcium, sodium and other indicators of ischaemia activate protein kinases which (3) phosphorylate immediate early gene (IEG) transcription factors. (4) These travel from the cytoplasm into the nucleus where they induce the transcription of IEG DNA (e.g. *c-fos* and *c-jun*), making IEG mRNA. (5) IEG mRNA leaves the nucleus and is translated at ribosomes into IEG protein (e.g. Fos and Jun families). (6) These gene-specific IEG products travel from the cytoplasm into the nucleus where they initiate transcription of DNA that codes for proteins of repair or the endonucleases that cause programmed cell death (PCD). (7) Repair or PCD mRNA then goes out to ribosomes in the cytoplasm where it is translated into proteins of repair (e.g. heat shock proteins) or PCD endonucleases. (8) Neurones that are distant from the ischaemic area are signalled to induce IEG transcription and translation (redrawn from reference[25]).

lated in a time-dependent manner following head injury in humans.[30] Activation of these CAMs recruits neutrophils to the damaged area, thereby occluding capillaries and enhancing free radical production. This has important implications for the potential strategies using antibodies that have been found experimentally.[31,32]

Brain oedema

Two types of oedema occur: cytotoxic and vasogenic. Cytotoxic oedema is due to failure of ionic pumps with resultant ionic and fluid shifts. Vasogenic oedema is due to the release of mediators that damage endothelial cells, basement membrane matrix and/or glial cells, resulting in blood–brain barrier breakdown. Specific mediators that have been involved in this process include arachidonic acid metabolites, free radicals, bradykinin and platelet-activating factor. The resulting oedema can cause increases in intracranial pressure, with reduction in cerebral perfusion pressure (and cerebral ischaemia) and herniation of brain structures.

CEREBRAL PROTECTION

Cerebral protection implies interventions designed to prevent pathophysiolgical processes from occurring, whilst cerebral resuscitation refers to intervention instituted after onset of the ischaemic insult, in order to interrupt the process.[1] It goes without saying that any form of cerebral or neuroprotection begins with the fundamentals of any resuscitative treatment, i.e. basic airway, respiratory and cardiovascular support. Unless normoxia and normotension are maintained, the application of drugs that antagonize the processes listed above is bound to be ineffective. These basics of clinical management are dealt with in appropriate sections elsewhere.

While this discussion will focus on agents that achieve neuroprotection by reversing one or more of the secondary injury processes listed above, other therapeutic interventions can reduce neuronal injury by optimizing cerebrovascular physiology. Drugs such as mannitol and dexamethasone can reduce posttraumatic and peritumoral oedema respectively and thus augment cerebral perfusion pressure and oxygen delivery. Similarly, the use of haemodynamic augmentation with hypervolaemia and hypertension can enhance cerebral blood flow in the setting of intracranial hypertension or cerebral vasospasm.

ANAESTHETIC AGENTS

Barbiturates

As early as 1966 it was recognized that barbiturates had a neuroprotective effect and they have served as the prototype for anaesthetic protection against cerebral ischaemia. The primary CNS protective mechanism of the barbiturates is attributed to their ability to decrease the cerebral metabolic rate, thus improving the ratio of oxygen supply to oxygen demand.[33] More specifically, these agents appear to selectively reduce the energy expenditure required for synaptic transmission, whilst maintaining the energy required for basic cellular functions.[34] Mechanisms by which these effects may be exerted are listed in Box 3.1.

Maximal metabolic suppression by anaesthetic agents can reduce oxygen demands to approximately 50% of baseline values, since the remaining oxygen utilization is required to support cellular integrity rather than suppressible electrical activity.[36] Barbiturates appear to be particularly protective in conditions of focal ischaemia as even though blood flow may be reduced, some synaptic transmission continues and its suppression can improve oxygen demand/supply relationships.[25] Such electrical activity is absent during global ischaemia and studies to date have failed to demonstrate any improved clinical outcome with anaesthetic neuroprotection following cardiac arrest.[37,38] There is currently considerable caution in assigning neuroprotective properties to agents based on studies conducted before the confounding effects of mild hypothermia were well documented.

1. Reduction in synaptic transmission.
2. Reduction in calcium influx.
3. Ability to block sodium channels and membrane stabilization.
4. Improvement in distribution of regional cerebral blood flow.
5. Suppression of cortical EEG activity.
6. Reduction in cerebral oedema.
7. Free radical scavenging.
8. Potentiate GABA-ergic activity.
9. Alteration of fatty acid metabolism.
10. Suppression of catecholamine-induced hyperactivity.
11. Reduction in CSF secretion.
12. Anaesthesia, deafferentation, and immobilization.
13. Uptake of glutamate in synapses.

Box 3.1   Mechanisms by which anaesthetic agents may exert their neuroprotective effects

However, recent studies do confirm that these agents do have neuroprotective properties.[39,40]

Propofol

Propofol has been widely used for anaesthesia for a number of years now and it is known to decrease neuronal activity on the electroencephalogram (EEG), with an accompanying decrease in cerebral oxygen utilization and cerebral blood flow.[41] As yet, there are few published human clinical trials to show its clinical effectiveness as a neuroprotective agent. There are, however, a number of animal studies that show that this may be the case.[42,43,44] These studies showed that in conditions of incomplete global ischaemia, with hypotension or hypoxia, outcome was improved when animals were treated with doses of propofol that induced burst suppression. These animals maintained better cerebral perfusion, ECF biochemical and electrolyte levels and aerobic metabolism when compared with controls. While it is likely that propofol produces at least some of these neuroprotective effects via metabolic suppression, it has been documented that the agent is a potent free radical scavenger.[44]

Etomidate

Etomidate has been reported to possess similar cerebral metabolic protective effects to the barbiturates, but is disadvantaged by its adrenal suppressant effects and ability to cause myoclonic movements.[45–48] As is the case with barbiturates, no further reduction of

CMR occurs when additional drug is administered beyond a dose sufficient to produce isoelectricity.[49] Again there appears to be no benefit in complete global ischaemic states.[50]

Opioids, ketamine and benzodiazepines

Opioids are not thought generally to have neuroprotective properties but they do blunt stress-induced responses. Ketamine is an NMDA antagonist and has been shown to be protective in animal models of ischaemia.[51] While the benzodiazepines decrease cerebral blood flow and cerebral metabolic rate, these effects are less impressive than with the intravenous anaesthetic agents. Despite occasional reports of neuroprotective benefit,[52] these drugs are not generally thought to be useful neuroprotective agents.

Inhalation anaesthetic agents

The primary mechanisms by which the inhalation agents, like the barbiturates, exert their cerebral protective effects may be their ability to suppress cortical electrical activity, and thus reduce the oxygen demands associated with synaptic transmission.[53,54,55] The reality of these effects is that they may be far more complex than once believed.[54,55] Halothane, not usually regarded as a cerebral protectant, provides a similar degree of protection to sevoflurane although it results in less metabolic suppression.[56,57] It appears that as inhalation agents only suppress cortical activity and not membrane/organelle function, the degree of suppression would only translate into a very short time of additional preserved organelle homoeostasis and would not provide a major clinical benefit.[55] However, the idea that inhalation agents provide cerebral protection is well established. Mechanisms by which these may occur are given in Box 3.1. Nitrous oxide is still used as part of a balanced technique for many procedures, without obvious adverse effect. However, it is unique amongst inhalation agents in that if any effect on neuronal protection, that effect may be detrimental to neuronal survival.[59]

NON-ANAESTHETIC AGENTS

Channel blockers

As enhanced calcium influx and accumulation is assumed to be a major cause of the pathophysiologic sequelae that arise during ischaemia, much interest has focused on drugs that reduce calcium influx through agonist-operated and voltage-sensitive calcium channels. The exact mechanism of cerebral protective action of these drugs has not been fully elucidated but it is presumed to be their ability to reduce calcium influx across plasma and mitochondrial membranes.[33] Only a few studies have, however, been performed that actually document alterations in regional brain Ca^{++} accumulation following CNS damage.[60]

Calcium channel antagonists have been successful in treating patients with subarachnoid haemorrhage and though they were thought to produce their effects by ameliorating vasospasm,[63] it now appears that direct cytoprotective effects may be important. However, despite some initial enthusiasm,[62] studies in traumatic brain injury and stroke have generally shown no clinical benefit. One possible explanation for these failures is that the calcium channel antagonists are only effective in blocking L-type channels, leaving T and N channels functional.[33] However, magnesium and cobalt are non-selective antagonists at all types of voltage-sensitive and NMDA-activated channels that are involved in calcium influx into neurones and this may account for their documented neuroprotective effect.[61] Other calcium antagonists have been reported to ameliorate ischaemic lesions, namely isradipine, S-emopamil and RS-87476 (a Na^+/Ca^+ channel modulator), but their neuroprotective efficacy and mechanisms of action are as yet not fully extablished.[28]

Sodium channel blockers have also been used as neuroprotective agents. Lignocaine-induced anaesthesia involves the selective blockade of Na channels in neuronal membranes, with resultant decrease in neuronal transmission. This reduces the $CMRO_2$ by that component of cellular metabolism responsible for synaptic transmission. In addition, it also reduces ionic leaks, i.e. Na^+ influx and K^+ efflux, and this reduces Na^+-K^+-ATPase pump energy requirements. While experimental studies are encouraging, human trials are awaited.[1,64] Other Na^+ channel blockers are the local anaesthetic agents QX-314 and QX-222 which have shown good *in vitro* results but again, human studies are awaited.[33] Enadoline is a new opioid with Na^+ channel-blocking properties under investigation.

The only ion channel blocker currently recommended for clinical use by the National Stroke Association in the USA is nimodipine in the setting of subarachnoid haemorrhage but recent papers have challenged even this use.[33,65] While nicardipine is reputed to cause less systemic hypotension than nimodipine and is marketed in the USA for similar clinical indications, no other channel blockers are currently available in the UK.

Excitatory amino acid antagonists

To date, approximately 19 agents that block EAA receptors have been shown to be effective in a variety of experimental brain injury models.[60] Non-competitive NMDA channel antagonists such as dizolcipine (MK-801) have a theoretical advantage over competitive agents such as CGS 19755, in that competitive antagonism may be overcome by the pathologically high concentrations of glutamate associated with cerebral ischaemia.[66] These two agents have proved particularly encouraging as neuroprotectants.[67–71] Again, as with so many neuroprotective agents, these seem to be more effective in focal ischaemia[72,73] than global ischaemia, although this may be open to debate.[74] One possible explanation for this is the occurrence of spontaneous depolarizations and repolarizations in the penumbral tissues of an infarct. These processes produce a heavy metabolic demand on the tissues and it may be here that NMDA antagonists act.[75] In global ischaemia no such processes occur and thus the antagonists may have no target on which to act. Unfortunately the non-selective blockers have been associated with the development of neuronal vacuolation in the posterior cingulate region in experimental models,[29] and have hence not been rapidly brought into clinical use.

Other NMDA antagonists have been shown to have experimental neuroprotective properties,[76] including agents which have been used in man. Ketamine has been shown to improve cognitive function[77,78,79] and dextromethorphan has been shown to improve neurologic motor function and decrease regional oedema formation[80,81,82] in experimental models. The degree of physiological blockade of the NMDA receptor by Mg_2+ ions may also be important and administration has been reported to be protective against cerebral ischaemia.[83,84]

AMPA receptor antagonists may well be more effective for both global and focal ischaemia,[85,86] and they appear not to have the same psychomimetic effects as the NMDA agents. Other agents that have been used in experimental neuroprotective research include felbamate (acting at glycine sites) and nitroso compounds, such as nitroprusside and glyceryl trinitrate, that act at redox modulator sites and prevent EAA-induced neuronal death in *in vitro* models.[66] Riluzole, a novel compound that inhibits presynaptic release of glutamate, has neuroprotective effects in rodent models.[87]

Free radical scavengers

The efficacy of the administration of protective enzymes or free radical scavengers in ameliorating neurologic injury after cerebral ischaemia is the subject of much investigation.[10] The beneficial effect depends on the involvement of free radicals in the pathological process, the biologic compatibility of the scavengers, appropriate dose selection and the ability to deliver the agent to the cellular site where the free radical is active. Pretreatment with α-tocopherol has been found to have beneficial effects in cerebral ischaemia,[88,89] subarachnoid haemorrhage,[90] spinal cord injury[91] and CNS trauma.[92,93] Other agents that have been tested include the iron chelator deferoxamine,[94] superoxide dismutase,[95,96] dimethyl superoxide,[97] superoxide dismutase conjugated to polyethylene glycol[98,99,100] and tirilazad mesylate.[101] Although all these agents have been shown to exhibit neuroprotective efficacy in animal models, there have been no successful clinical trials to date. Indeed, initial optimism regarding pegorgotein (PEG conjugated superoxide dismutase) and tirilazad mesylate has recently been proven to be unfounded.[29]

Free fatty acids and prostaglandin inhibitors

Calcium-induced phospholipase activation during ischaemia releases free fatty acids from membrane phospholipids. These FFAs can uncouple oxidative phosphorylation in mitochondria and cause efflux of Ca^2+ and K^+ into the cytosol and increases in levels of arachidonic acid, which is the rate-limiting substrate for prostanoid synthesis. Increase of arachidonic acid (the commonest FFA), during cerebral insults, results in increased concentrations of the endoperoxides PGG_2 and PGH_2, which are the precursors of prostacyclin (PC/PGI_2), and thromboxane A_2 made in vascular endothelial cells and platelets respectively. This results in inactivation of prostacyclin synthetase and relative overproduction of thromboxane A_2.[102,103] This relative imbalance between vasoconstrictor and vasodilator prostaglandins may contribute to postischaemic hypoperfusion. Arachidonic acid is also converted to leukotrienes which act as inflammatory mediators and may be associated with further free radical generation.[104] It is debatable at this stage whether inhibitors of the arachidonic cascade might be effective in ischaemia as although these compounds (indomethacin, ibuprofen) have been found to show variable neuroprotective efficacy in some studies of global ischaemia,[105,106] there were inconsistent effects on hypoperfusion and neurologic outcome.[107,108]

HYPOTHERMIA

Hypothermia treatment (mechanical cooling) was first described in 1943 and there have been sporadic attempts over the last 50 years to use it as a treatment modality.[60] Recent trials have suggested that it may be useful in patients with head injury.[109,110] The most recent trial[109] concludes that treatment with moderate hypothermia (33–34°C) for 24 h, initiated soon after head injury, significantly improved outcome at three and six months in those with a GCS of 5–7 (i.e. without flaccidity or decerebrate rigidity) and suggested improved outcome at 12 months. Mild hypothermia is not associated with the cardiovascular and metabolic derangements commonly observed at lower temperatures. However, the mechanisms by which hypothermia limits secondary brain injury are ill defined. Possible mechanisms are given in Box 3.2.

Hypothermia may be induced pharmacologically with chlorpromazine or other central nervous system cholinergic agonists.[111,112,113] Application of these methods requires further work. The question of whether hypothermia is clinically useful for stroke therapy remains unanswered. Zivin[114] suggests that physical considerations of heat transfer rates make it unlikely that pharmacological agents will be effective at reducing body temperature. The protective effects of the volatile agents may be as a result of the prevention of a cerebral hyperthermic response to ischaemia.[54,57] In studies where brain temperature has been increased compared with those with hypothermia, infarct size is increased. This highlights the importance of meticulous monitoring and control of cerebral temperature in studies of pharmacological neuroprotection.

CLINICAL PRACTICE[29]

The success of experimental neuroprotection is undeniable and new publications continue to explore novel and exciting therapeutic targets. However, the major challenge facing clinical neuroscientists is the general failure to translate these successes into positive results from outcome trials, possible reasons for which are listed in Box 3.3.

- Experimental demonstration of neuroprotection incomplete (functional endpoints?)
- Inappropriate agent: mechanism of action not relevant in humans
- Inappropriate dose of agent (plasma levels suboptimal either globally or in subgroups)
- Poor brain penetration by agent
- Efficacy limited by side effects that worsen outcome (e.g. hypotension)
- Inappropriate timing: mechanism of action not active at time of administration
- Inappropriate or inadequate duration of therapy
- Study population too sick to benefit
- Study population too heterogeneous: efficacy only in an unidentifiable subgroup
- Study cohort too small to remove effect of confounding factors
- Failure of randomization to evenly distribute confounding factors
- Insensitive, inadequate or poorly implemented outcome measures

Box 3.3   Possible causes of failure of trials of clinical neuroprotection.[29]

Two radically different approaches have been suggested to overcoming the problems inherent in patient heterogeneity and lack of sensitivity of outcome measures. The first of these is to accept that these problems are unavoidable and mount larger outcome trials of 10–20,000 patients which will address benefits of a magnitude less than the 10% improvement in outcome that most drug trials are designed to detect. The alternative strategy is to mount smaller but much more detailed studies in homogeneous subgroups of patients whose physiology is characterized by modern monitoring and imaging techniques. Repeated application of these techniques during the course of a trial can provide evidence of reversal of pathophysiology and hence mechanistic efficacy. Such surrogate endpoints could then be used to select drugs or combinations of drugs for larger outcome trials. It is likely that both approaches will find a place, depending on the setting.

REFERENCES

1. Verhaegen M, Warner DS. Brain protection and brain death. In: Van Aiken H, Jones RM, Aitkenhead AR, Foëx P (eds) Neuro-Anaesthetic Practice. BMJ Publishing Group, London, 1995, pp 267–293.

---

1. Reduction of rate of energy use for electrophysiological cortical activity and the homoeostatic functions required to maintain cellular integrity.
2. Reduction of extracellular concentrations of excitatory amino acids.
3. Suppressing the posttraumatic inflammatory response.
4. Attenuating free radical production.
5. Maintenance of high energy phosphate.

Box 3.2   Possible mechanisms for the neuroprotective effects of hypothermia.[55,100]

---

2. Graham D, Hume Adams J, Gennarelli TA et al. Pathology of brain damage in brain injury. In: Tindall G, Cooper R, Barrow D (eds) The practice of neurosurgery. Williams and Wilkins, Baltimore, 1996, pp 1385–1400.

3. Andrew K. Head injuries. In: Andrews K (ed) Essential neurosurgery. Churchill Livingstone, London, 1991, pp 59–80.

4. Alaich EF, Eisenberg HM. Diffuse brain injury. In: Tindall G, Cooper R, Barrow D (eds) The practice of neurosurgery. Williams and Wilkins, Baltimore, 1996, pp 1461–1490.

5. Povlishock JT, Christmas CW. The pathobiology of traumatically induced axonal injury in animals and humans: a review of current thoughts. J Neurotrauma, 1995: 12: 555–564.

6. Klauber MR, Marshall LF, Luerssen TG et al. Determinants of head injury mortality: importance of the low risk patient. Neurosurgery 1989; 24: 31–36.

7. Marshall LF, Toale BM, Bowers SA. The National Traumatic Coma Data Bank II. Patients who talk and deteriorate: implications for treatment. J. Neurosurg 1983; 59: 285–288.

8. Reilly PJ, Adams JH, Graham DI. Patients with head injury who talk and die. Lancet 1975; 2: 375–377.

9. Lian LM, Bergsneider M, Becker DP. Pathology and pathophysiology of head injury. In: Youmans JR (ed) Neurological surgery, 4th edn WB Saunders, Philadephia, 1996, pp 1549–1595.

10. Milde LN, Weglinski MR. Pathophysiology of metabolic brain injury. In: Cottrell JE, Smith DS (eds) Anaesthesia and neurosurgery, 3rd edn Mosby, St Louis, 1994, pp 59–92.

11. Vanhoutte PM. Calcium entry blockers, vascular smooth muscle and systemic hypertension. Am J Cardiol 1985; 55(suppl B): 17–23.

12. Albers GW Mechanisms of injury to the central nervous system. In: Andrews RJ (ed) Intraoperative neuroprotection. Williams and Wilkins, Baltimore, 1996, pp 7–19.

13. Benveniste H, Jorgensen M, Sandberg M et al. Ischaemic damage in hippocampal CA1 is dependent on glutamate release and intact innervation from CA3. J Cereb Blood Flow Metab 1989; 9: 629–639.

14. Drejer J, Benveniste H, Diemer NH, Schausboe A. Cellular origin of ischaemia–induced glutamate release from brain tissue in vivo and in vitro. J Neurochem 1985; 45: 145.

15. Munglani R, Hunt SP, Jones JG. The spinal cord and chronic pain. In: Kaufman L, Ginsburg R (eds) Anaesthesia review 12. Churchill Livingstone, London, 1995 pp 53–76.

16. Siësjo BK, Bengtsson F. Calcium fluxes, calcium antagonists, and calcium related pathology in brain ischaemia, hypoglycaemia, and spreading depression: a unifying hypothesis. J Cereb Blood Flow Metab 1989; 9: 127–140.

17. Ganong WF. Review of medical physiology. Endocrinology, metabolism and reproductive function, 16th edn. Appleton and Lange, New York, 1993, pp 253–286.

18. Siësjo BK. Cell damage in the brain. A speculative synthesis. J Cereb Blood Flow Metab 1981; 1: 155.

19. Siësjo BK, Siësjo P. Mechanisms of secondary brain injury. Eur Anaesthesiol 1996; 13: 247–268.

20. Lanier W, Stanglard K, Scheithauer BW et al. The effects of dextrose infusion and head position on neurologic outcome after complete cerebral ischaemia in primates. Examination of a model. Anesthesiology 1987; 66: 39–48.

21. Ganong WF. Review of medical physiology. The general and cellular basis of medical physiology, 16th edn. Appleton and Lange, New York 1993, pp 1–41.

22. Siesjo BK. Pathophysiology and treatment of focal cerebral ischaemia. Part I Pathophysiology. J Neurosurg 1992; 77: 169–182.

23. Fieschi C, Di Piero V, Lenzi GL et al. Pathophysiology of ischemic brain disease. Stroke 1990; 21(12): IV9–11.

24. Deshpande JK, Siesjo BK, Wieloch T. Calcium accumulation and neuronal damage in the rat hippocampus following cerebral ischaemia. J Cereb Blood Flow Metab 1987; 7: 89–95.

25. Cottrell JE. Possible mechanisms of pharmacological neuronal protection. Symposium article. J Neurosurg Anesthesiol 1995; 7(1): 31–37.

26. Alberts B, Bray D, Lewis J et al. Differentiated cells and the maintenance of tissues. In: Molecular biology of the cell, 3rd edn. Garland, New York, 1994, pp 1174–1175.

27. Stellar H. Mechanisms and genes of cellular suicide. Science 1995; 267: 1445–1449.

28. Siesjo BK Pathophysiology and treatment of focal cerebral ischaemia. Part II Mechanisms of damage and treatment. J Neurosurg 1992; 77: 337–354.

29. Menon DK, Summors A. Neuroprotection. Curr Opin Anaesthesiol 1998; 11: 485–496.

30. Gupta AK, Thiru S, Braley J, Marshall L, Menon DK. Delayed increases in adhesion molecule expression after traumatic brain injury in humans. J Cereb Blood Flow Metab 1995; 15(suppl 1): S33.

31. Chopp M, Zhang RL, Chen H, Jiang N, Rusche JR. Postischaemic administration of an anti-Mac-1 antibody reduces ischaemic cell damage after transient middle cerebral artery occlusion in rats. Stroke 1994; 25: 869–876.

32. Lindsberg PJ, Siren AL, Feuerstein GZ, Hallenbeck JM. Antagonism of neutrophil adherence in the deteriorating stroke model in rabbits. J Neurosurg 1995; 82: 269–277.

33. Hall R, Murdoch J. Brain protection physiological and pharmacological considerations. Part II: The pharmacology of brain protection. Can J Anaesth 1990; 37(7): 762–777.

34. Steen PA, Michenfelder JD. Mechanisms of barbiturate protection. Anesthesiology 1980; 53: 183–85.

35. Cuchiara RF, Michenfelder JD (eds). Clinical neuroanaesthesia Churchill Livingstone, New York, 1990, p 193.

36. Michenfelder J. The interdependency of cerebral function and metabolic effects following massive doses of thiopental in the dog. Anesthesiology 1974; 41: 231–236.

37. Abrahamson NF, Safar D, Detre KM. Randomised clinical study of thiopental loading in comatose survivors of cardiac arrest. N Engl J Med 1986; 314: 397–403.

38. Brain Resuscitation Trial. Randomised clinical study of thiopental loading in comatose survivors of cardiac arrest. N Engl J Med 1986; 314: 397–403.

39. Kuroiwa T, Bonnekoh P, Hossman KA. Therapeutic window of CA1 neuronal damage defined by an ultrashort-acting barbiturate after brain ischaemia in gerbils. Stroke 1990; 21: 1489–1493.

40. Warner DS, Zhou J, Ramani R, Todd MM. Reversible focal ischaemia in the rat: effects of halothane, isoflurane, and methohexital anaesthesia. J Cereb Blood Flow Metab 1991; 11: 794–802.

41. Vardesteene A, Tremport V, Engelna E et al. Effect of propofol on cerebral blood flow and metabolism in man. Anaesthesia 1988; 43: 42.

42. Varner PD, Vinik HR, Funderburg C. Survival during severe hypoxia and propofol or ketamine anaesthesia in mice. Anesthesiology 1988; 69: A571–1988.

43. Kocks E, Hoffman WE, Werner C et al. The effects of propofol on neurologic outcome from incomplete cerebral ischaemia in the rat. Anesthesiology 1990; 73: A718–1990.

44. Young Y, Menon DK, Tisaripat N et al. Propofol neuroprotection in a rat model of ischaemia reperfusion injury. Eur J Anesthesiol 1997; 14: 320–326.

45. Milde LN, Milde JH. Preservation of cerebral metabolites by etomidate during incomplete cerebral ischaemia in dogs. Anesthesiology 1985; 65: 272.

46. Tulleken CAF, Van Dieren A, Jonkman J et al. Clinical and experimental experience with etomidate as a brain protective agent, J Cereb Blood Flow Metab 1982; 2(suppl): 592.

47. Smith DS, Keykhah MM, O' Neill JJ et al. The effect of etomidate pretreatment on cerebral high energy metabolites, lactate and glucose during severe hypoxia in the rat. Anesthesiology 1989; 71: 438.

48. Baughman VL, Hoffman WE, Miletich DJ et al. Neurologic outcome following regional cerebral ischaemia with methohexital, midazolam, and etomidate (abstract). Anesthesiology 1987; 67: A582.

49. Drummond JC. Changing practices in neuroanaesthesia. Can J Anaesth 1990; 37: SLxxxix–Scvii.

50. Barber H, Hoyer S, Kreir C. The influence of etomidate upon cerebral metabolites after complete brain ischaemia in the rat. Eur J Anaesth 1991; 8: 233.

51. Hoffman WE, Pelligrino D, Werner C et al. Ketamine decreases plasma catecholeamines and improves outcome from incomplete cerebral ischaemia in rats. Anesthesiology 1992; 76: 755–762.

52. Nugent M, Artru AA, Michenfelder JD. Cerebral metabolic, vascular and protective effects of midazolam maleate. Anesthesiology 1982; 56: 172–176.

53. Drummond JC. Editorial. Brain protection during anaesthesia. Anesthesiology 1993; 79: 877–880.

54. Neuberg LA, Michenfelder JD. Cerebral protection by isoflurane during hypoxaemia or ischaemia. Anesthesiology 1983; 59: 29–35.

55. Todd M, Warner DS. A comfortable hypothesis re-evaluated. Cerebral metabolic depression and brain protection during ischaemia. Anesthesiology 1992; 76: 161–164.

56. Warner DS, Mc Farlane C, Todd MM, et al. Sevoflurane and halothane reduce focal ischaemic brain damage in the rat. Possible influence on thermoregulation. Anesthesiology 1993; 78: 985–992.

57. Rampil IJ. Cerebral protection, resuscitation and monitoring. A look into the future of neuroanaesthesia. Anaesthesiol Clin North Am 1992; 10(3): 683–718.

58. Larsen M, Heysted E, Berg-Johnsen J, Langmoen IA. Isoflurane increases the uptake of glutamate in synaptosomes from rat cerebral cortex. Br J Anaesth 1997; 78: 55–59.

59. Giffard RG, Jaffe RA. Anesthetic agents for neuroprotection. In: Andrews RJ (ed) Intraoperative neuroprotection. Williams and Wilkins, Baltimore, 1996, pp 23–36.

60. McIntosh TK, Smith DH, Garde E. Therapeutic approaches for the prevention of secondary brain injury. Eur J Anaesthesiol 1996; 13: 291–309.

61. Kaas IS, Cottrell JE, Chambers G. Magnesium and cobalt, not nimodipine protect neurones against anoxic damage in the rat hippocampal slice. Anesthesiology 1988; 69: 710–715.

62. Gelmans HJ, Garter K, De Weerdt CJ et al. Controlled trial of nimodipine in acute ischaemia stroke. N Engl J Med 1988; 318: 203–207.

63. Allen GS, Ahn HS, Preziosi TJ et al. Cerebral arterial spasm. A controlled trial of nimodipine in patients with subarachnoid haemorrhage. N Engl J Med 1983; 308: 619–624.

64. Astrap J, Sorensen PM, Sorensen HR Inhibition of Cerebral oxygen and glucose consumption in the dog by hypothermia pentobarbital and lidocaine. Anesthesiology 1981; 55: 263–268.

65. Mercier P, Alback, Rizk T et al. Are the calcium antagonists really useful in cerebral aneurysm surgery? A retrospective study. Neurosurgery 1004; 34: 30–37.

66. Hudspith MJ. Glutamate: a role in normal brain function, anaesthesia, analgesia and CNS injury. Review article. Br J Anaesth 1997; 78: 731–747.

67. Boast CA, Gerhardt SC, Pastor G et al. The N-methyl-D-aspartate antagonists CGS 19755 and CPP reduce

ischaemia brain damage in gerbils. Brain Res 1988; 442: 345.

68. Ozuart E, Graham D, Woodruff G, McCulloch J. Protective effect of the glutamate antagonist, MK-801 in focal cerebral ischaemia in the cat. J Cereb Blood Flow Metab 1988; 8: 134–143.

69. Church J, Zeman S, Lodge D. The neuroprotective action of ketamine and MK-801 after transient cerebral ischaemia in rats. Anesthesiology 1988; 69: 702–709.

70. Shapira Y, Yadid G, Cotev S et al. Protective effects of MK-801 in experimental brain injury. J Neurotrauma 1990; 7: 131–139.

71. Iversenn LL, Kemp JA. Non-competitive NMDA antagonists as drugs. In: Collingridge GL, Watkins JC, (eds) The NMDA receptor, 2nd edn Oxford University Press, Oxford, 1994 pp 469–486.

72. Lanier W, Perkins W, Karlson B et al. The effect of dizocilipine maleate (MK-801), an antagonist of the NMDA receptor, on neurologic recovery and histopathology following complete cerebral ischaemia in primates. J Cereb Blood Flow Metab 1990; 10: 252–261.

73. Nellgord B, Wieloch T. Post ischaemic blockade of AMPA but not NMDA receptors mitigates neuronal damage in the rat brain following transient severe cerebral ischaemia. J Cereb Blood Flow Metab 1992; 12: 2–11.

74. Meldrun BS, Chapman AG. Competitive NMDA antagonists as drugs. In: Collingridge GL, Watkins JC, (eds) The NMDA receptor, 2nd edn Oxford University Press, Oxford, 1994 pp 457–468.

75. Iijima T, Mies G, Hossman K. Repeated negative Dc deflections in rat cortex following middle cerebral artery occlusion are abolished by MK-801 – effect on volume of ischaemic injury. J Cereb Blood Flow Metab 1992; 12: 727–733.

76. Lipton SA. Prospects for clinically tolerated NMDA antagonists: open channel blockers and alternative redox states of nitric oxide. Trends Neurosci 1993; 16: 527–532.

77. Smith DH, Okiyama K, Geunarelli TA, McIntosh TK. Magnesium and ketamine attenuate cognitive dysfunction following experimental brain injury. Neurosci Lett 1993; 157: 211–214.

78. Lucas JH, Wolf A. In vitro studies of multiple impact injury in mammalian neurones: prevention of perikaryal damage by ketamine. Brain Res 1991; 543: 181–193.

79. Hoffman W, Pelligrino D, Werner C et al. Ketamine decreases plasma catecholamines and improves outcome from incomplete cerebral ischaemia in rats. Anesthesiology 1992; 76: 923–929.

80. Shohami E, Novikov M, Mechoulam R. A non-psychotropic cannabinoid, HU – 211, has cerebroprotective effects after closed head injury in the rat. J Neurotrauma 1993; 10: 109–119.

81. Choi DW. Dextrophan and dextromethorphan alternate glutamate neurotoxicity. Brain Res 1987; 403: 333–336.

82. Faden AI, Demedink P, Panter SS, Vink R. The role of excitatory amino acids and NMDA receptors in traumatic brain injury. Science 1989; 244: 798–800.

83. Goldman RS, Finkbeiner SM. Therapeutic uses of magnesium sulphate in selected cases of cerebral ischaemia and seizure N Engl J Med 1988; 319: 1224–1225.

84. Vacanti FX, Ames A. Mild hypothermia and Mg2+ protect against irreversible damage during CNS ischaemia. Stroke 1984; 15: 695–698.

85. Le Reille TE, Arvin B, Moucada C, Meldrum B. The non-NMDA antagonists, NBQX and GYKI52466, protect against cortical and striatal cell loss following transient global ischaemia in the rat. Brain Res 1992; 571: 115–120.

86. Gill R, Nordholm L, Lodge D. The neuroprotective actions of 2,3-dihydroxy-6-nitro-7-sulfamoyl-benzo (F) quinoxaline (NBQX) in a rat focal ischaemic model. Brain Res 1992; 580: 35–43.

87. McIntosh TK, Vaddi M, Smith DH, Stutzmann J-M. Ribuzole, a compound which interferes with glutamate neuro transmission, improves cognitive deficits following experimental brain injury in rats. J Neurotrauma 1995; 12: 379.

88. Abe K, Yuki S, Kogure K. Strong attenuation of ischaemic and post ischaemic brain edema in rats by a novel free radical scavenger. Stroke 1988; 19: 480–485.

89. Yamamato M, Shina T, Vozumi T et al. A possible role of lipid peroxidation in cellular damage caused by cerebral ischaemia and the protective effect of a-tocopherol administration. Stroke 1983; 14: 977–982.

90. Sakaki S, Ohta S, Wakamura H, Takeda S. Free radical reaction and biological defence mechanism in the pathogenesis and prolonged vasospasm in experimental subarachnoid haemorrhage. J Cereb Blood Flow Metab 1988; 8: 1–8.

91. Anderson D, Saunders R, Demedink P et al. Lipid hydrolysis and peroxidation in injured spinal cord: partial protection with methylprednisolone or vitamin E and selenium. J Neurotrauma 1985; 2: 257–267.

92. Clifton G, Lyeth BG, Jenkins LW et al. Effect of D1 α-tocopherol succinate and polyethylene glycol on performance tests after fluid percussion brain injury. J Neurotrauma 1989; 6: 71–81.

93. Hall ED, Youkers PA, Heron KL, Braughter JM. Correlation between attenuation of post-traumatic spinal cord ischaemia and preservation of tissue vitamin E by the 21-aminosteroid U74006F. J Neurotrauma 1992; 9: 169–176.

94. Panter SS, Braughter JM, Hall E. Dextron-coupled deferoxamine improves outcome in a murine model of head injury. J Neurotrauma 1992; 9: 47–53.

95. Lim KH, Connally M, Rose D et al. Prevention of the reperfusion injury of the ischaemic spinal cord: use of

recombinant superoxide dismutase. Ann Thorac Surg 1986; 42: 282–286.

96. Forsman M, Fleischer JE, Milde J, Steen P, Michenfelder J. Superoxide dismutase and catalase failed to improve neurologic outcome after complete cerebral ischaemia in the dog. Acta Anaesthesiol Scand 1988; 32: 152–155.

97. Coles JC, Ahmed SN, Mehta ITU, Kaufman JC. Role of radical scavenger in protection of spinal cord during ischemia. Ann Thorac Surg 1986; 41: 555–556.

98. Liu TH, Beckham JS, Freeman BA et al. Polyethylene-glycol-conjugated superoxide dismutase and catalase reduce ischemic brain injury. Am J Physiol 1989; 256: H589-H592.

99. Matsumiya N, Kochler RC, Kirsch JR, Traytsmon RJ. Conjugated superoxide dismutase reduced extent of caudate injury after transient focal ischemia in cats. Stroke 1991; 226: 1193–1200.

100. Muizelaar JP, Marmarou A, Young HF et al. Improving the outcome of severe head injury with the oxygen radical scavenger polyethylene glycol-conjugated super-oxide dismutase: a phase II trial. J Neurosurg 1993; 78: 375–382.

101. Andrews RJ, Giffard RG. Clinically useful nonanes-thetic agents. In: Andrews RJ (ed) Intraoperative neuro-protection. Williams and Wilkins, Baltimore, 1996, pp 37–63.

102. Egan RW, Paxton J, Kuehl FA. Mechanism for irre-versible self deactivation of prostaglandin synthetase. J Biol Chem 1976; 257: 7329.

103. Van Den Kerckhoff W, Hossman KA, Hossman V. No effect of prostacyclin on blood flow, regulation of blood flow and blood coagulation following global cerebral ischemia. Stroke 1983; 14: 724.

104. Hall ED, Wolf DC. A pharmacological analysis of the pathophysiological mechanisms of post-traumatic spinal cord ischemia. J Neurosurg 1986; 64: 951–961.

105. Dempsey RJ, Roy MW, Meyer KL et al. Indomethacin-mediated improvement following middle cerebral artery occlusion in cats. Effects of anaesthesia. J Neurosurg 1985; 62: 874.

106. Grice SC, Chappel ET, Drough DS et al. Ibuprofen improves cerebral blood flow after global cerebral ischaemia in dogs. Stroke 1987; 18: 787.

107. Boulu RG, Plotkine M, Gueniau C et al. Effect of indomethacin in experimental cerebral ischaemia. J Pathol Biol 1982; 30: 278.

108. Hallenbeck JM, Furlow TW. Prostaglandin I2 and indomethacin prevent impairment of post-ischemic brain reperfusion in the dog. Stroke 1979; 10: 629.

109. Marion DW, Penrod LE, Kelsey SF et al. Treatment of traumatic brain injury with moderate hypothermia. N Engl J Med 1997; 36(8): 540–546.

110. Shiozaki T, Sugimoto H, Taneda M et al. Effects of mild hypothermia on uncontrolled intracranial hypertension after severe head injury. J Neurosurg 1993; 79: 363–368.

111. Menon DK, Young Y. Pharmacologically induced hypothermia for cerebral protection in humans. Correspondence. Stroke 1994; 24(2): 522.

112. Hall ED, Andrus PK, Paroza KE. Protective efficacy of a hypothermic pharmacological agent in gerbil forebrain ischaemia. Stroke 1993; 24: 711–715.

113. Todd MM, Warner DS. A comfortable hypothesis re-evaluated. Cerebral metabolic depression and brain protection during ischaemia. Anesthesiology 1992; 76: 161–164.

114. Zivin JA. Correspondence. Stroke 1994; 24(2): 522–523.

4

INTRACRANIAL PRESSURE

John M. Turner

INTRODUCTION

The skull is a rigid, closed box and contains the brain, cerebrospinal fluid (CSF), arterial blood and venous blood. Brain function depends on the maintenance of the cerebral circulation within that closed space and arterial pressure forces blood into the skull with each heartbeat. CSF is being formed and absorbed and the result of these forces is a distinct pressure, the intracranial pressure (ICP). The difference between the mean arterial pressure (MAP) and the mean ICP is the pressure forcing blood through the brain, the cerebral perfusion pressure (CPP).

ICP is normal up to about 15 mmHg but it is not a static pressure and varies with arterial pulsation, with breathing and during coughing and straining. Each of the intracranial constituents occupies a certain volume and, being essentially liquid, is incompressible. In the closed box of the skull, if one of the intracranial constituents increases in size, then either one of the other constituents must decrease in size or the ICP will rise. Two of the constituents, CSF and venous blood, are contained in systems that connect to low-pressure spaces outside the skull, so displacement of these two constituents from the intracranial to the extracranial space may occur. This mechanism, then, compensates for a volume increase affecting any one of the intracranial constituents. The displacement of CSF is an important compensatory mechanism and is illustrated in the CT scan in Figure 4.1 where in response to the generalized development of cerebral oedema following head injury, the ventricles have been so compressed by the brain swelling that they are visible only as a slit. CSF absorption may increase as ICP rises and the CSF volume will be reduced.

The compensatory mechanism for intracranial space occupation obviously has limits. When the amount of CSF and venous blood that can be extruded from the skull has been exhausted the ICP becomes unstable and waves of pressure (plateau waves and B waves) develop.[1] As the process of space occupation continues, the ICP can rise to very high levels and the brain can become displaced from its normal position. High intracranial pressure can force the medulla out of the posterior fossa into the narrow confines of the foramen magnum, where compression of the vital centres is associated with bradycardia, hypertension and respiratory irregularity followed by apnoea.[2]

BRAIN

The brain weighs about 1400 g and occupies most of the intracranial space. The soft cerebral tissue is very susceptible to injury, although some protection is afforded by the skull and the CSF bathing the brain. Expanding mass lesions, such as a tumour, abscess or haematoma, increase the volume occupied by the brain. When such a space-occupying lesion develops, the brain can distort in a plastic fashion, allowing some compensation for the abnormal mass, but the distortion may produce neurological signs or CSF obstruction. Figure 4.2 shows a CT scan of patient with an extradural haematoma and also shows a considerable shift of the midline structures.

The symptoms and signs produced by a supratentorial tumour depend on its rate of growth and whether it is

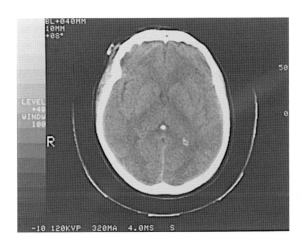

Figure 4.1   CT scan of a patient after head injury showing compression of the ventricles.

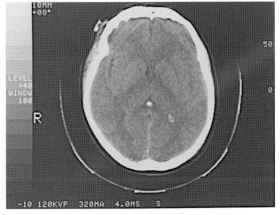

Figure 4.2   CT scan of a patient showing an extradural haematoma with considerable shift of the midline.

developing in a relatively silent area of the brain or in one of the eloquent areas, such as the motor cortex. A tumour developing in a silent area can achieve large size before presenting with symptoms and signs of raised ICP (Fig. 4.3). In this situation a major disruption of ICP dynamics may be present, with significant brain shift. A tumour may present rapidly if it is in an eloquent area, if it is a fast-growing tumour or if it causes CSF obstruction. Chapter 1 describes some of the common syndromes associated with tumour development.

Haematomas are usually fairly rapidly growing lesions and although they set in train the compensating mechanisms for intracranial space occupation, they will produce signs of raised ICP at an earlier stage.[3]

Space occupation in the posterior fossa has some characteristic features. The posterior fossa is a much smaller space than the anterior and middle cranial fossae and as tumours developing in the posterior fossa are growing in a more confined space, they tend not to grow to large size. The relatively small volume of the posterior fossa means that tumours tend to produce a rise in ICP early and this is accentuated by the fact that they frequently produce CSF obstruction. Distortion of the mid brain and compression of the lower cranial nerves may also be produced by posterior fossa tumours.

The bulk of the brain can also be increased by the development of cerebral oedema and frequently cerebral oedema is seen in association with a tumour (Fig. 4.4). The degree of space occupation produced by the oedema can be so great as to turn a relatively minor degree of space occupation from a small

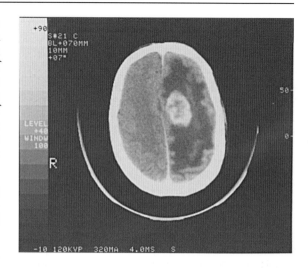

Figure 4.4   CT scan with contrast of a patient with a moderate sized glioma showing the extent of oedema formation.

tumour into a major problem requiring urgent treatment. Klatzo[4,5] provided a simple classification of cerebral oedema into two types: vasogenic and cytotoxic. In vasogenic brain oedema (VBO), the development of oedema results from damage to the blood–brain barrier, so that there is an increase in permeability of the cerebral capillaries and serum proteins leak into the brain parenchyma. The hydrostatic forces generated by the Starling balance at the capillary provide the impetus for the oedema fluid to spread through the brain; white matter, which has a less dense structure than grey, tends to offer less resistance. VBO may develop around neoplasms, haematomas and cerebral abcesses and in traumatized areas of the brain.

Once the primary lesion has allowed the initial formation of the protein-rich oedema fluid, several factors combine to spread the oedema and may be the result of arteriolar dilatation, increased systemic arterial pressure or a combination of both.[6] Increased intravascular pressure accelerates the rate of oedema spread. Eventually the fluid reaches the ependymal surface of the ventricles, where it passes into the CSF to be transported and absorbed by the mechanisms that regulate CSF outflow.[7] The production and maintenance of a low sagittal sinus venous pressure is important in allowing the resolution of cerebral oedema.

Cytotoxic brain oedema occurs after hypoxic or ischaemic episodes. The reduced state of oxygen delivery results in failure of the intracellular ATP-dependent sodium pump and therefore intracellular sodium accumulates followed by rapid increases in

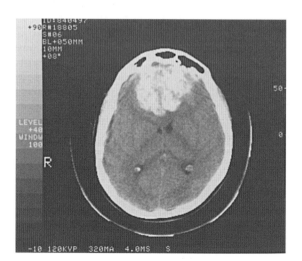

Figure 4.3   CT scan of a patient with a large, calcified frontal meningioma.

intracellular water. In a pure form of cytotoxic oedema, the blood–brain barrier remains intact.

Other workers describe other types of oedema including hydrostatic, interstitial and hypo-osmolar. Hydrostatic oedema[8] is due to an increase in the intravascular pressure transmitted to the capillary bed. The combination of cerebral arteriolar vasodilatation and raised arterial pressure may lead to an outpouring of water, even though the blood–brain barrier is not necessarily damaged. Hypo-osmolar oedema can occur when the serum osmolality is less than that in the brain. Clinically it may develop following excessive intravenous infusions of glucose-water solution with associated hyponatraemia. Glucose penetrates freely into the brain and an osmotic gradient may develop, leading to an increase in brain water content. Hypo-osmolar oedema may also be associated with inappropriate secretion of antidiuretic hormone. Interstitial oedema is seen in patients with obstructive high-pressure hydrocephalus, occurring when CSF seeps through the ependyma, increasing the water content of the periventricular structures. Shunting reduces the ventricular pressure and the water content returns to normal.[9]

The ability of the brain to distort in a plastic fashion allows some accommodation for intracranial space occupation and it is not uncommon to see shift of the midline structures due to a supratentorial lesion on angiography or CT scan. If unrelieved, this displacement can cause part of the cerebral hemisphere, usually the temporal lobe, to become impacted beneath the falx cerebri or the tentorial hiatus. Jefferson[10] described the tentorial pressure cone and though it is classically associated with an extradural temporal haematoma, due to haemorrhage from the middle meningeal artery, it may be produced by any expanding supratentorial lesion. The development of a pressure gradient across the tentorium allows downward impaction of the medial part of the temporal lobe, the uncus, into the tentorial hiatus. Compression of the cerebral peduncles and occulomotor nerve at first causes pupillary changes and a contralateral hemiparesis but at a later stage respiratory irregularity and apnoea may ensue. Upward herniation of the cerebellum into the tentorial hiatus may also take place and be due to an expanding lesion in the posterior fossa.[11]

The serious nature of the medullary pressure coning has been mentioned earlier (p. 000) and the Cushing response[2] described. The mechanism of the response appears to be generated by brainstem ischaemia and Doba and Reis[12] demonstrated the existence of a receptive area for the Cushing response in the lower brainstem.

CEREBROSPINAL FLUID

There is about 140 ml of CSF in the adult, half in the skull and half in the spinal subarachnoid space. CSF is formed at about 0.4 ml/min, so that an amount of CSF equal to the CSF volume is produced in 4 h.[13] This is an energy-dependent active process requiring carbonic anhydrase and a sodium-potassium activated ATPase. Cutler et al[14] showed that the rate of CSF production was constant in the face of a raised ICP up to 200 mmHg. After formation from the choroid plexus in the lateral ventricles, CSF flows through the third ventricle, along the aqueduct and into the fourth ventricle, where it reaches the subarachnoid space through the foramina of Luschka and Magendie. CSF is also formed by the passage of brain tissue water across the ependymal lining of the ventricles and along perivascular channels into the subarachnoid space, so that the composition of CSF changes as it circulates through the ventricular system. Shapira et al[15] studied the rate of CSF production during hypotension with either adenosine or haemorrhage. They found that adenosine-induced hypotension did not affect the rate of CSF production, whereas haemorrhage-induced hypotension reduced CSF production. Adenosine is a cerebral vasodilator and haemorrhage will constrict the vessels of the choroid plexus, so CSF production falls as the choroid plexus perfusion falls.

Reabsorption of CSF takes place through the arachnoid villi into the sagittal sinus and requires a pressure gradient between the CSF and the sagittal sinus venous pressure. If the venous pressure is raised, then CSF reabsorption is slowed.[16] Normally CSF production is in balance with reabsorption and the CSF system is at equilibrium as regards both pressure and volume. If ICP increases, the rate of absorption of CSF also increases and ultimately the new CSF volume at equilibrium will be smaller. The stiffness of the brain will also affect the plot of CSF pressure against CSF volume, because when the tissues around the CSF are stiff, the plot of CSF pressure against volume will be steep and the equilibrium volume of CSF small. A slack brain will be associated with a flat pressure/volume curve (see Fig. 4.5) and a larger CSF equilibrium volume.

The circulation of CSF may be obstructed in a number of ways and this may result in raised intracranial pressure. Aqueduct blockage may follow head injury or subarachnoid haemorrhage, producing hydrocephalus. Tumours and other mass lesions may also distort or compress CSF pathways and, by causing ventricular dilatation, will increase the degree of intracranial space occupation. The passage of CSF from the fourth

A

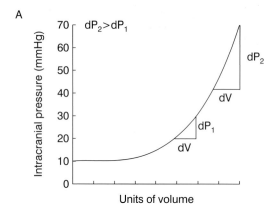

B

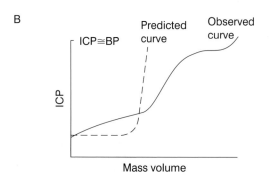

Figure 4.5   (A) Diagram of a volume/pressure curve. As the breakpoint is passed at 15 mmHg the curve becomes increasingly steep so that uniform increments of volume (dV) produce increasingly large rises in ICP (dp) (redrawn from reference[30], courtesy of the Editor). (B) ICP versus mass volume predicted by the Monroe–Kellie hypothesis for the curve observed during progressive epidural balloon inflation in animals. The observed curve is significantly different from the predicted curve in that its initial segment is not flat but increases slowly to a breakpoint. Beyond this breakpoint, the observed curve is not vertical but instead increases to a second plateau near the level of arterial blood pressure (redrawn from reference[55], courtesy of the Editor).

ventricle and through the foramen magnum may be impeded by congenital malformations.

Some elderly patients develop normal-pressure hydro-cephalus, in which they present with dementia and incontinence and CT scans show the appearance of hydrocephalus, though ICP measurement may be normal. Continuous measurement of ICP reveals periods of raised ICP, especially during sleep.[17] These patients often benefit from CSF shunting.

Reabsorption of CSF is reduced in benign intracranial hypertension,[18] resulting in a greatly increased

subarachnoid space. The condition tends to affect young women, particularly if they are obese. They present with headaches and the clinical picture includes marked papilloedema, which may be so marked as to affect vision. The ICP can reach very high values but without affecting consciousness. Once space occupation as a cause for the high ICP has been eliminated, lumbar puncture is safe.

ARTERIAL BLOOD VOLUME

The role of the arterial pulse in generating the ICP, along with the CSF, has been mentioned earlier (p. 000). Each arterial pulse produces a change in the level of ICP, with a rise in ICP during systole and a fall in diastole. Plum and Siesjö[13] suggested that CSF is able to absorb some of the energy in the arterial pulse wave because it transmits the pressure pulse out of the cranial cavity and into the more elastic spinal CSF space. Many workers have observed that as ICP rises, the pulse pressure of the ICP also increases.[19,20,21] Pickard and Czosnyka[20] suggest that two mechanisms may be active: first, the brain becomes stiffer (less compliant) as ICP rises and a given pulse volume load provokes a bigger pressure response; and second, the pulsatile component of cerebral blood flow (CBF) increases as the CPP is reduced.

The control of CBF is discussed in Chapter 00. If CBF rises, there will usually be an increase in ICP, produced by cerebral vasodilatation. Major changes in CBF and therefore ICP can be produced by $PaCO_2$ changes. There is a straight line relationship between CBF and $PaCO_2$: between the limits of 2.6 and 10.6 kPa (20–80 mmHg) $PaCO_2$, CBF changes 2 ml/100 g brain for every mmHg change in $PaCO_2$. The resultant change in cerebral blood volume (CBV) is 0.04 ml/100 g brain for every mmHg change in $PaCO_2$.[22]

When autoregulation is intact an increase in MAP will not normally be associated with an increase in CBF or ICP. If, however, the rise in MAP is so rapid or so great (as in the pressor response to intubation) as to exceed the capacity of the cerebral vessels to react, then an increase in CBF and ICP may occur. When autoregu-lation is impaired, as in diseased or damaged brain where local tissue acidosis produces local vasodi-latation, then any change in MAP will produce a change in CBF and therefore ICP.[23] The blood supply of a vascular tumour is not under autoregulatory control and the tumour blood flow and therefore the size of the tumour will alter passively with changes in blood pressure.

The cerebral vasodilatation produced by disease or injury may be associated with blood–brain barrier

(BBB) damage, so that local cerebral oedema results in and increases the tendency to raised ICP. In the experimental animal in which brain injury has been produced, arterial hypertension can cause cerebral oedema and tentorial herniation in a few minutes.[24]

VENOUS BLOOD VOLUME

The volume of venous blood in the skull offers one of the compensating mechanisms for abnormal intracranial space occupation, because the thin-walled cerebral veins can be compressed as the space occupation proceeds and blood therefore lost from the skull to the great veins in the chest. Obstruction of the cerebral venous drainage, then, not only removes one of the compensating mechanisms but will also tend to increase ICP by holding venous blood back in the skull, distending the cerebral veins. The volume of the venous compartment of the skull also increases when there is cerebral arterial dilatation, because of the increased intravascular hydrostatic pressure.

Cerebral venous obstruction also tends to promote oedema formation. The increase in ICP resulting from the venous obstruction therefore will not be completely corrected when the obstruction is relieved, because the oedema will not resolve immediately.

Cerebral venous obstruction may be caused in a number of ways, including the use of the supine or head-down position and an incorrectly set lung ventilator, as well as coughing, straining or incomplete muscle relaxation in a ventilated patient. The effects on ICP of intubating an incompletely relaxed patient are demonstrated by studies which show an increase in anterior fontanelle pressure resulting from awake intubation.[25] Millar and Bissonette[26] reported no change in cerebral blood flow velocity during awake intubation and conclude that the observed increase in anterior fontanelle pressure could be attributed to a reduction in the venous outflow from the cranium.

The effect of positive end-expired pressure (PEEP) on ICP appears to depend on the degree of intracranial compression. Aidinis et al[27] described two responses to PEEP in cats: one in which the ICP rose less than the amout of PEEP which was applied and another in which the ICP increase was greater than the PEEP applied. In patients, it has been shown that most of those with significant intracranial compression display increased ICP when PEEP is applied.[28] Continuous positive airway pressure (CPAP) has been investigated by Hörman et al[29] in volunteers demonstrating a mean increase of 4 mmHg when CPAP of 12 mmHg was applied. They suggest that the changes were of only minor clinical significance.

QUANTIFYING THE DEGREE OF INTRACRANIAL SPACE OCCUPATION

The choice of an anaesthetic technique is helped if the anaesthetist is able to make an estimate of the degree of intracranial space occupation. The symptoms and signs of raised ICP may coexist with those due to the lesion producing the raised ICP and with those resulting from brain shift and cerebral ischaemia. Headache, vomiting, papilloedema and drowsiness are said to be the signs produced by raised ICP,[30] whereas other signs such as pupillary changes, bradycardia and hypertension result from brainstem distortion or cerebral ischaemia.

The headache may be paroxysmal in nature, sometimes relieved by sitting and worsened on straining or coughing. Some patients find that the headache is worsened by flexion of the neck and they lie in a position of hyperextension.

Bilateral papilloedema is the one sign that appears to be directly related to raised ICP but it takes a little time to develop. Pickard and Czosnyka[20] point out that optic disc swelling was found in only 4% of head injury patients, even though 50% had raised ICP on monitoring. They comment that many of the later signs of raised ICP are the result of herniation and that monitoring of ICP should detect raised ICP at an earlier stage so that treatment is started before irreversible damage occurs.

VOLUME/PRESSURE RELATIONSHIP

The degree of intracranial space occupation can be difficult to estimate from the clinical history and examination and much work has been done to quantify the relationship between intracranial space occupation and ICP. The simplest understanding of the relationship arises from the Monroe–Kellie hypothesis that within the closed space of the skull, a change in the volume of one intracranial constituent will be balanced by a compensatory change in another, the four constituents being incompressible. As space occupation develops, ICP shows little tendency to increase as long as compensation for the space occupation is available. CSF, for example, may be moved into the spinal subarachnoid space and venous blood displaced towards the great veins in the chest. ICP will only rise when no further CSF or venous blood can be lost from the skull. When ICP does rise, CSF production will continue at its normal rate but reabsorption of CSF will be accelerated[31] and the CSF volume will be further reduced. As the space occupation develops further, then CSF pathways will become obstructed by the mass or by the brain shift it produces and distortion of veins, even collapse of veins around a mass, will begin to impede local venous drainage. Johnston and Rowan[32] showed that in such circumstances of high ICP, cerebral arteriolar dilatation occurs in an attempt to preserve CBF, adding to the already high ICP.

The exhaustion of the compensating mechanisms for intracranial space occupation implies that any further abnormal volume added to the tightly compressed intracranial state will produce a massive rise in ICP and clinically this may be associated with herniation of the brain through the tentorial hiatus or into the foramen magnum.

The process by which the intracranial space occupation gradually exhausts the compensating mechanisms is illustrated by the volume/pressure curve of the intracranial contents (Fig. 4.5).[21,33] At first the abnormal volume increase caused by a developing mass lesion produces little change in ICP. At a later stage, the same increase in volume produces a distinct rise in pressure. The steepest part of the curve represents the situation when the compensating mechanisms are virtually exhausted. The same volume increase at this point would produce a massive rise in ICP.

The addition of small volumes to the lateral ventricle while measuring ICP has been used to elucidate the patient's position on the volume/pressure response curve, the rise in pressure produced by the injected volume being called the volume/pressure response (VPR).[34,35] Leech and Miller[34,36] studied the relationship between the VPR and ICP in several conditions. At normal blood pressure they found that the VPR was unchanged by alterations in systemic arterial pressure but at raised arterial pressure, there was an increased VPR and a linear correlation between VPR and both arterial blood pressure and cerebral blood flow. They suggest that the clinical implication of this is that arterial hypertension in patients with raised ICP is likely to have a deleterious effect by increasing brain stiffness. They also studied the effect on the VPR of reducing ICP with hyperventilation or mannitol[37] and found that hyperventilation reduced ICP and VPR equally, whereas mannitol produced a greater reduction in VPR than ICP. They suggested that mannitol produced a more beneficial effect on intracranial compression than hyperventilation.

Measurement of the ICP, examination of the trace and measuring the VPR will yield useful information about the degree of intracranial space occupation but it is possible to obtain more information by infusion testing.[38] Pickard and Czosnyka[20] have suggested that close analysis of the ICP trace is able to reveal the mechanism responsible for the raised ICP and whether autoregulation remains intact.

Intracranial pressure waves

Episodes of very high ICP may occur when intracranial compression is advanced and the control of CBF has become unstable. These were first noted by Lundberg[1] who described A (or plateau waves), B and C waves occurring in patients in whom ventricular pressure was being continuously measured.

A waves represent considerable increases in ICP (up to 80 mmHg) and may persist for 15–20 min. Their appearance indicates the patient who is nearing the limits of compensation for intracranial space occupation. They are associated with cerebrovascular dilatation. During the plateau wave, the CPP may be greatly reduced, even though the systemic arterial pressure rises. In such periods of high ICP, the level of response may worsen with possible loss of control of the airway, exposing the patient to the further dangers of hypoxia and hypercarbia. A waves were observed in 18 out of 76 patients in one study of head-injured patients and 11 of the 18 died.[39] Tindall et al[40] showed that a transient rise in $PaCO_2$ often preceded the development of an A wave and Lassen and Christensen[41] suggested that painful stimulation could also produce an increase in CBF and initiate pressure waves. The increase in CBV[42] may in some cases be the result of inappropriate vasodilatation in response to a fall in CPP.

B waves are smaller in amplitude with an increase in ICP of 20–25 mmHg and a frequency of one per minute. They are of less serious import than A waves but do appear on occasion to be precursors of A waves. Cyclic variations in vascular resistance have been suggested as the cause of B waves[43] and transcranial Doppler (TCD) measurements of middle cerebral artery flow velocity have shown that MCA flow velocity increases during B waves.[44] The appearance of B waves during sleep in patients with normal-pressure hydrocephalus is said to be a helpful sign for a good outcome after shunting.[45] C waves occur six times per minute and are only just discernible on the pressure trace.

CT SCANS

CT scans give a valuable image revealing the size of a mass lesion and whether or not it is causing CSF obstruction, cerebral oedema or brain shift. Diffuse brain swelling can be evaluated by examining the size of both lateral and third ventricles and the perimesencephalic cisterns.

THE EFFECT OF RAISED ICP ON CEREBRAL BLOOD FLOW

Cerebral blood flow is controlled normally by cerebral metabolism. Autoregulation ensures that CBF remains constant even though the CPP may vary between 40 and 120 mmHg. Autoregulation is effective whatever the cause of the reduction in CPP, which can be either a reduction in the arterial pressure or an increase in ICP, or both. If CSF pressure is raised in experimental animals, CBF is maintained until CPP has been reduced to 30–40 mmHg; below this level, CBF falls rapidly.[46,47,48] Cortical electrical activity has been shown to remain normal in the face of experimentally induced intracranial hypertension to 40–50 mmHg.[49,50] The diseased or injured brain, where ischaemia may be part of the disease process, is less tolerant of high ICP.[51] There is frequently impairment of autoregulation, so that CBF becomes pressure dependent,[52] with the result that there may be a significant fall in CBF caused by a relatively small fall in CPP.

Other factors need to be taken into account. In the damaged brain there is frequently failure to observe an increase in cerebral perfusion despite an increase in CPP; that is, the hyperaemic brain may be suffering ischaemic damage. Langfitt et al[53] found that an induced rise in ICP produced arterial hypertension, followed by a secondary rise in ICP. Fitch et al,[54] studying the effects of expanding an artificial space-occupying lesion, showed that the arterial hypertension which was produced was not associated with any improvement in either CPP or CBF. Explanations include the fact that elevated blood pressure produces an increase in cerebral oedema which, by increasing tissue pressure, reduces perfusion at the capillary level.[55] In such circumstances, autoregulation is likely to be impaired or abolished and though an increase in CPP may not result in an improvement in cerebral perfusion, a fall in CPP will invariably cause a fall in CBF.[56]

DRUG EFFECTS

Anaesthetic agents alter cerebral function dramatically and it is possible to use some of their effects to benefit the patient undergoing neurosurgery. Some drugs have cerebral actions that may worsen the intracranial operating conditions, making the operation difficult or even impossible. The actions or side effects of drugs need always to be assessed in the light of the patient's clinical state. In the initial evaluation of Althesin, an intravenous anaesthetic, now withdrawn, which

reduced $CMRO_2$ and CBF, Turner et al[57] showed that the fall in ICP produced by althesin in a group of patients with intracranial space occupation was proportional to the initial height of the ICP. That is, the patients most at risk from the space occupation showed the greatest fall in ICP with althesin.

INDUCTION AGENTS

The effects of thiopentone on $CMRO_2$ and CBF are well studied. There is a dose-dependent fall in $CMRO_2$ and a parallel fall in CBF until the electroencephalogram (EEG) is isoelectric.[58] At this point the $CMRO_2$ is about 50% of control values and no further fall in $CMRO_2$ occurs if the thiopentone dosage is increased. ICP falls with the CBF.

Propofol has similar effects to thiopentone on $CMRO_2$ and CBF.[59,60] 1.5mg/kg propofol has been reported to produce a 32% fall in CSF pressure 2 min after induction of anaesthesia.[61]

VOLATILE AGENTS

To a variable extent, all volatile anaesthetic agents cause an increase in CBF and therefore ICP. The magnitude of the effect is important but so is the patient's position on the volume/pressure curve. If serious degrees of intracranial space occupation exist, then even a small increase in CBF may produce a significant rise in ICP.[62]

Isoflurane

Isoflurane is frequently used as part of a neurosurgical anaesthetic and has been extensively investigated.[63,64] Though it can cause an increase in CBF and therefore ICP,[65,66] the effect is not large and Muzzi et al[63] suggest that at 1 MAC isoflurane did not affect CSF pressure. The effect of higher concentrations on ICP can be modified by the use of hyperventilation; indeed, Jung et al[67] comment that when an increase in CSF pressure has been reported during isoflurane anaesthesia, it was in the presence of normocapnia or moderate hyperventilation in patients with major intracranial space occupation. Matta et al[68] produced in humans an isolectric EEG by infusion of propofol and then added first 0.5 MAC and then 1.5 MAC of either halothane, isoflurane or desflurane. They showed that all the agents have intrinsic, dose-related effects producing cerebral vasodilatation and that at 1.5 MAC, isoflurane and desflurane have a greater effect than halothane. They point out that these effects are normally modified by the metabolic suppression produced by the drug resulting in an indirectly caused cerebral vasoconstriction. When metabolic activity is minimal (here under the influence of the propofol infusion), the intrinsic vasodilatory action of the drug is revealed.

Desflurane

Desflurane has been shown to produce cerebral vasodilatation.[69] Clinical studies[68] have shown that the use of 1 MAC desflurane produced a rise in CSF pressure in patients with supratentorial mass lesions, whereas a group of patients receiving 1 MAC isoflurane showed no such rise. This last study showed that there was a gradual progressive increase in CSF pressure once desflurane was started and the authors suggested that the gradual increase in ICP could be due to either an increase in CSF production or a decrease in CSF reabsorption or a combination of both. Ornstein et al[70] measured CBF in patients with mass lesions, with both isoflurane and desflurane, and asserted that the two drugs are similar in terms of their effects on CBF.

Sevoflurane

Sevoflurane has been reported as causing an increase in ICP at high inspired concentrations, though the effect is much less at 0.5–1.0 MAC.[71] In a study[72] where 0.5, 1.0 and 1.5 MAC end-tidal concentrations of sevoflurane were compared with MAC-equivalent concentrations of enflurane and halothane, significant increases in ICP were found only with enflurane and halothane. Sevoflurane did not cause a rise in ICP but did produce a fall in MAP.

Enflurane[73,74]

Enflurane, like desflurane, appears to be associated with not only cerebral vasodilatation but also an increase in CSF production.

Nitrous oxide

The effect of nitrous oxide on CBF and ICP has been of interest for some time, not least because so many anaesthetics have been given for neurosurgery using nitrous oxide. As long ago as 1968, Theye and Michenfelder reported an increase in $CMRO_2$ with nitrous oxide[75] andHenriksen and Jørgensen[76] showed an increase in ICP when nitrous oxide was administered to normocarbic patients with intracranial tumours. More recently, Hansen et al[77] have demonstrated in rats that adding 0.5 MAC nitrous oxide to a background of 0.5 MAC halothane or isoflurane produced a greater rise in CBF than would be expected by increasing the concentration of the original agent to 1 MAC. Others have also shown a rise in CBF with nitrous oxide.[78]

ANALGESICS

The opioid analgesics have been extensively studied and some confusion exists. If ventilation is controlled, then morphine and pethidine have little effect on $CMRO_2$ and CBF.[79] Fentanyl used in combination with droperidol has been shown to have no significant effect on $CMRO_2$ and CBF[80] in man and, in a study measuring ICP in patients with space-occupying lesions, was shown either to have little effect on ICP or to produce a slight fall.[81] Other opioids seem to have different effects and there are many reports of opioid drugs increasing ICP.[82] Sufentanil was investigated in a study of brain-injured patients[83] in which great care was taken to analyse any ICP changes, relating them to changes in MAP. If there was a fall in MAP greater than 10 mmHg from baseline after sufentanil administration, then ICP was significantly increased. When MAP was constant, there was no increase in ICP. The authors suggest that sufentanil has no significant effect on ICP and that transient increases in ICP occur concomitantly with decreases in MAP, which they attribute to autoregulatory decreases in cerebral vascular resistance secondary to systemic hypotension. Sufentanil and fentanyl were compared in a similar study, which also showed no increase in ICP if MAP was controlled.[84] Alfentanil and remifentanil have been compared in hyperventilated patients with supratentorial space-occupying lesions receiving nitrous oxide and isoflurane; neither drug was associated with a significant increase in ICP, though both caused a fall in MAP.[85]

MUSCLE RELAXANTS

Non-depolarizing relaxants

The non-depolarizing relaxants generally have no effect on ICP (being highly polar molecules, they do not cross the blood–brain barrier) and this includes atracurium,[86,87] though it does have the potential to cause histamine release, and vecuronium.[88,89] The effects of rocuronium on ICP have been studied[90] because its relatively fast onset of action may be an advantage if a rapid-sequence induction is indicated. It was found to have no effect on ICP and not to cause histamine release. D-tubocurarine may increase ICP through its ganglion-blocking action[91] and also has the ability to cause histamine release.

Suxamethonium

Suxamethonium tends to cause an increase in ICP.[92,93] This is partly due to the muscle fasciculations which, by producing an increase in the intraabdominal and intrathoracic pressures, cause an increase in the cerebral venous pressure. Some workers[63,94] have suggested that the increased afferent neuronal traffic resulting from the fasciculations produces a cerebral activation and therefore a local increase in $CMRO_2$ and CBF, so that CBV is increased.

HYPOTENSIVE AGENTS

Labetalol is used during neuroanaesthesia[95] as an aid to the production of hypotension. It appears not to affect CBF or $CMRO_2$ or to impair autoregulation.[96,97] Trimetaphan has no major effect on ICP but if there is a serious degree of intracranial space occupation, the ganglionic blockade produced by trimetaphan will cause a minor rise in CBF and CBV, which may be associated with a significant rise in ICP.[98] Sodium nitroprusside, a direct-acting vasodilator, causes a rise in ICP,[78] especially if the reduction in MAP is only moderate; when MAP is reduced to less than 70% of the patient's normal MAP, the effect on ICP is hidden. Nitroglycerine has also been used for hypotension but does produce an increase in ICP.[99] In one series, in which dogs had an artificial intracranial space-occupying lesion implanted, starting the infusion of trinitroglycerine produced not only a further increase in ICP but also pupillary dilatation, suggesting the development of transtentorial pressure gradients and coning.[100]

CONCLUSION

Intracranial pressure is only the result of many factors. Although an understanding of the ways in which ICP can be altered and controlled is essential for neuroanaesthesia and intensive care, it is important to remember that the primary cause for a high ICP must be sought and treated. Outcome studies for any treatment are necessary to improve standards of patient care.

REFERENCES

1. Lundberg N. Continuous recording and control of ventricular fluid pressure in neurosurgical practice. Acta Psychiat Neurol Scand 1960; 36(suppl): 149.

2. Cushing H. Some experimental and clinical observations concerning states of increased intracranial pressure. Am J Med Sci 1902; 124: 375–400.

3. Fitch W, McDowall DG. Gradients of intracranial pressure produced by halothane in experimental space-occupying lesions. 1971. Br J Anaesth 1971; 40: 883.

4. Klatzo I. Neuropathological aspects of brain oedema. J Neuropath Exp Neurol 1967; 26: 1.

5. Klatzo, I. Brain oedema following brain ischaemia and the influence of therapy. Br J Anaesth 1985; 57: 18.

6. Hirano A, Becker NH, Zimmerman HM. The use of peroxidase as a tracer in studies of alteration of the blood brain barrier. J Neurol Sci 1970; 10: 205.

7. Reulen HJ, Tsoyumu M, Tack A, Fenske AR, Prioleau GR. Clearance of edema fluid into cerebrospinal fluid. J Neurosurg 1978; 48: 754.

8. Marshall WJS, Jackson JLF, Langfitt TW. Brain swelling caused by trauma and arterial hypertension. Arch Neurol Chicago 1969; 21: 545.

9. Granholm L. An explanation of the reversible memory defect in hydrocephalus. In: Beks JWF, Bosch DA, Brock M (eds) Intracranial Pressure III. Springer Verlag, Berlin, 1976; p. 173.

10. Jefferson G. The tentorial pressure cone. Arch Neurol Psychiat Lond 1938; 40: 857.

11. Jefferson G, Johnson RT. The cause of loss of consciousness in posterior fossa compressions. Folia Psychiat Neurol Neurochir Neerl 1950; 53: 306.

12. Doba N, Reis D. Localization within the lower brain stem of a receptive area mediating the pressor response to increased intracranial pressure (the Cushing response). Brain Res 1972; 47: 487–491.

13. Plum F, Siesjö BK. Recent advances in CSF physiology. Anesthesiology 1975; 42: 708.

14. Cutler RWP, Pale L, Galicich J, Watters GV. Formation and absorption of the cerebrospinal fluid in man. Brain 1968; 91: 707.

15. Shapira Y, Artrun A, Lam AM. Changes in the rate of formation and resistance to reabsorption of cerebrospinal fluid during deliberate hypotension induced with adenosine or hemorrhage. Anesthesiology 1992; 76: 432–439.

16. Potts DG, Gomez DG. Arachnoid villi and granulations. In: Lundberg N, Pontèn U, Brock M (eds) Intracranial pressure II. Springer Verlag, Berlin, 1975; p. 42.

17. Symon L, Dorsch NWC, Stephens RJ. Pressure waves in so-called low pressure hydrocephalus. Lancet 1972; 2: 1291–1292.

18. Johnston IH, Gilday DL, Paterson A, Hendrike EB. The definition of a reduced CSF absorption syndrome. Clinical and experimental studies. In: Lundberg N, Pontèn U, Brock M (eds) Intracranial pressure II. Springer Verlag, Berlin, 1975; p. 50.

19. Avezaat CJJ, Von Eijndhoven JHM, Wyper DJ. Cerebrospinal fluid pulse pressure and intracranial volume-pressure relationships. J Neurol Neurosurg Psychiat 1979; 42: 687–700.

20. Pickard JD, Czosnyka M. Management of raised intracranial pressure. J Neurol Neurosurg Psychiat 1993; 56: 845–858.

21. Turner JM, McDowall DG, Gibson RM, Khalili H. Computer analysis of intracranial pressure measurements: clinical value and nursing response. In: Beks JWF, Bosch DA, Brock M (eds) Intracranial Pressure III. Springer Verlag, Berlin, 1976; p. 293.

22. Grubb RL, Raichle ME, Eichling JD. The effects of changes in PaCO$_2$ on cerebral blood volume, blood flow and vascular mean transit time. Stroke 1974; 5: 630.

23. Alexander SC, Lassen NA. Cerebral circulatory response to acute brain disease. Anesthesiology 1970; 32: 60.

24. Schutta HE, Kassell NF, Langfitt TW. Brain swelling produced by injury and aggravated by arterial hypertension. Brain 1968; 91: 28.

25. Friesen RH, Honda AT, Thieme RE. Changes in anterior fontanelle pressure in pre-term neonates during tracheal intubation. Anesth Analg 1987; 66: 874–878.

26. Millar C, Bissonette J. Awake intubation increases intracranial pressure without affecting cerebral blood flow velocity in infants. Can J Anaesth 1994; 41: 281–287.

27. Aidinis SJ, Lafferty J, Shapiro HM. Intracranial responses to PEEP. Anesthesiology 1976; 45: 275.

28. Apuzzo MLJ, Weiss MH, Petersons V. Effect of positive end expiratory pressure ventilation on intracranial pressure in man. J Neurosurg 1977; 46: 227.

29. Hörman C, Mohsenipour I, Gottardis M, Benzer A. Response of cerebrospinal fluid pressure to continuous positive airway pressure in volunteers. Anesth Analg 1994; 78: 54–57.

30. Miller JD. Intracranial pressure monitoring. Br J Hosp Med 1978; 19: 497.

31. Heisey SR, Held D, Pappenheimer JR. Bulk flow and diffusion in the cerebrospinal fluid system of the goat. Am J Physiol 1962; 203: 775.

32. Johnston IH, Rowan JO. Raised intracranial pressure and cerebral blood flow. 3. Venous outflow tract pressure and vascular resistances in experimental intracranial hypertension. J Neurol Neurosurg Psychiat 1974; 37: 394.

33. Löfgren, J. The mechanical basis of the cerebrospinal fluid volume pressure curve. In: Lundberg N, Pontèn U, Brock M (eds) Intracranial pressure II. Springer Verlag, Berlin, 1975; p. 79.

34. Leech P, Miller JD. Intracranial volume/pressure relationships during experimental brain compression in primates. 1. Pressure response to change in ventricular volume. J Neurol Neurosurg Psychiat 1974; 37: 1093.

35. Miller JD, Garibi J. Intracranial volume pressure relationships during continuous monitoring of ventricular fluid pressure. In: Brock M, Dietz H (eds) Intracranial pressure I. Springer Verlag, Berlin, 1972; p. 27.

36. Leech P, Miller JD. Intracranial volume/pressure relationships during experimental brain compression in primates. 2. Effect of induced changes in systemic arterial pressure and cerebral blood flow. J Neurol Neurosurg Psychiat 1974; 37: 1099.

37. Leech P, Miller JD. Intracranial volume/pressure relationships during experimental brain compression in primates. 3. The effect of mannitol and hypocapnia. J Neurol Neurosurg Psychiat 1974; 37: 1105.

38. Miller JD, Garibi J, Pickard JD. Induced changes in cerebrospinal fluid volume. Effects during continuous monitoring of ventricular fluid pressure. Arch Neurol 1973; 28: 265–269.

39. Moss E, Gibson JS, McDowall DG, Gibson RM. Intensive management of severe head injuries. Anaesthesia, 1983; 38: 214.

40. Tindall GT, McGraw CP, Vanderveer RW, Iwata K. Cardiorespiratory changes associated with plateau waves in patients with head injury. In: Brock M, Dietz H (eds) Intracranial pressure I. Springer Verlag, Berlin, 1972, p. 397.

41. Lassen N, Christensen MS. The physiology of cerebral blood flow. Br J Anaesth 1976; 48: 719.

42. Rosner MJ, Becker DP. Origins and evolution of pleateau waves. Experimental observations and theoretical model. J Neurosurg 1984; 60: 312–324.

43. Sørensen SC, Gjerris F, Børgesen SE. Etiology of B-waves. In: Shulman K, Marmarou A, Miller JD, Becker DP, Hochwald GM, Brock M (eds) Intracranial pressure IV. Springer Verlag, Berlin, 1980, p. 123.

44. Newell DW, Aaslid R, Stooss R, Reulen HJ. The relationship of blood flow velocity fluctuations to intracranial pressure B waves. J Neurosurg 1992; 76: 415–421.

45. Pickard JD, Teasdale GM, Matheson M, Wyper DJ. Intracranial pressure waves – the best predictive test for shunting in normal pressure hydrocephalus. In: Shulman K, Marmarou A, Miller JD, Becker DP, Hochwald GM, Brock M (eds) Intracranial pressure IV. Springer Verlag, Berlin, 1980, 498–500.

46. Häggendahl E, Löfgren J, Nilsson NJ, Zwetnow NN. Effects of raised cerebrospinal fluid pressure on cerebral blood flow in dogs. Acta Physiol Scand1970; 79: 262.

47. Siesjö BK, Zwetnow NN. Effects of increased cerebrospinal fluid pressure upon adenine nucleotides and upon lactate and pyruvate in rat brain tissue. Acta Neurol Scand 1970; 46: 187.

48. Jennett WB, Harper AM, Miller JD, Rowan JO. Relation between cerebral blood flow and cerebral perfusion pressure. Br J Surg 1970; 57: 390

49. Grossman RG, Turner JW, Miller JD. The relationship between cortical electrical activity, cerebral perfusion pressure and cerebral blood flow during increased intracranial pressure. In: Langfitt TW, McHenry LC, Reivich M (eds) Cerebral circulation and metabolism. Springer Verlag, Berlin, 1975, p. 232.

50. Teasdale G, Rowan JO,Turner JW. Cerebral perfusion failure and cortical electrical activity. In: Cerebral function, metabolism and circulation (supplement). Ingvar DH and Lassen NA (eds). Acta Neurol Scand 1977; 56(suppl 64): 430.

51. Miller JD. Head injury and brain ischaemia – implications for therapy. Br J Anaesth 1985; 45: 486.

52. Miller JD, Stanek AE, Langfitt TW. Concepts of cerebral perfusion pressure and vascular compression during intracranial hypertension. Prog Brain Res 1972; 35: 411.

53. Langfitt TW, Kassell NF, Weinstein JD. Cerebral blood flow with intracranial hypertension. Neurology (Minneap), 1965: 15: 761.

54. Fitch WL, McDowall DG, Keaney NP, Pickerodt VWA. Systemic vascular responses to increased intracranial pressure. J Neurol Neurosurg Psychiat 1977; 40: 843.

55. Miller JD, Sullivan HG. Severe intracranial hypertension. In: Trubovich RB (ed) Management of acute intracranial disasters. Int Anesth Clin 1979; 17: 19.

56. Reilly PL, Farrrar JK, Miller JD. Apparent autoregulation in damaged brain. In: Harper AM, Jennett WB, Miller JD (eds) Blood flow and metabolism in the brain. Churchill Livingstone, Edinburgh, 1975, p. 621.

57. Turner JM, Coroneos N, Gibson RM, Powell D, Ness MA, McDowall DG. The effect of Althesin on intracranial pressure in man. Br J Anaesth 1973; 45: 168.

58. Michenfelder JD The interdependency of cerebral function and and metabolic effects following maximum doses of thiopentone in the dog. Anesthesiology 1974; 41: 231.

59. Newman MF, Murkin JM, Roach G et al. Cerebral physiologic effects of burst suppression doses of propofol during nonpulsatile cardiopulmonary bypass. Anesth Analg 1995; 81: 452–457.

60. Stephan S, Sonntag H, Schenk HD, Kohlhausen S. Effect of Disoprivan (propofol) on the circulation and oxygen consumption of the brain and CO_2 reactivity of brain vessels in the human. Anaesthetist 1987; 36: 60–65.

61. Ravussin P, Guinard JP, Ralley F, Thorin D. Effect of propofol on cerebrospinal fluid pressure and cerebral perfusion pressure in patients undergoing craniotomy. Anaesthesia 1988; 43(suppl): 32.

62. Grosslight K, Foster R, Colchan AR Bedford RF. Isoflurane for neuroanaesthesia; risk factors for increases in intracranial pressure. Anesthesiology 1985; 63: 533–536.

63. Muzzi DA, Losasso TJ, Dietz NM, Faust RJ, Cucchiara RF, Milde LN. The effect of desflurane and isoflurane on cerebrospinal fluid pressure in humans with mass lesions. Anesthesiology 1992; 76: 720–724.

64. Adams RW, Cucchiara RF, Gronert GA, Messick JM, Michenfelder JD. Isoflurane and cerebrospinal fluid pressure in neurosurgical patients. Anesthesiology 1981; 54: 97–99.

65. Newberg LA, Milde JH, Michenfelder JD. The cerebral metabolic effects of isoflurane at and above concentrations that suppress cortical electrical activity. Anesthesiology 1983; 59: 23–28.

66. Newberg LA, Milde JH, Michenfelder JD. Systemic and cerebral effects of hypotension induced with isoflurane in dogs. Anesthesiology 1984; 60: 541–546.

67. Jung R, Reisel R, Marx W, Galicich J, Bedford RF Isoflurane and nitrous oxide: comparative impact on cerebrospinal fluid pressure in patients with brain tumours. Anesth Analg 1992; 75: 724–728.

68. Matta BF, Mayberg TS, Lam AM. Direct cerebrovasodilatory effects of halothane, isoflurane and desflurane during propofol induced isoelectric electroencephalogram in humans. Anesthesiology 1995; 83: 980–985.

69. Lutz LJ, Milde JH, Milde LN. The cerebral functional, metabolic and hemodynamic effects of desflurane in dogs. Anesthesiology 1990; 75: 125–131.

70. Ornstein E, Young WL, Fleischer LH, Ostapkovich N. Desflurane and isoflurane have similar effects on cerebral blood flow in patients with intracranial mass lesions. Anesthesiology 1993; 79: 498–502.

71. Scheller MS, Teteishi A, Drummond JC, Zornow MH. The effects of sevoflurane on cerebral blood flow, cerebral metabolic rate for oxygen, intracranial pressure, and the electroencephalogram are similar to those of isoflurane in the rabbit. Anesthesiology 1988; 68: 548–551.

72. Takahashi H, Murata K, Ikeda K. Sevoflurane does not increase intracranial pressure in hyperventilated dogs. Br J Anaesth 1993; 71: 551–555.

73. Artru AA, Nugent M, Michenfelder JD. Enflurane causes a prolonged and reversible increase in the rate of CSF production in the dog. Anesthesiology 1982; 57: 255–260.

74. Artru AA. Effects of enflurane and isoflurane on resistance to reabsorption of cerebrospinal fluid in dogs. Anesthesiology 1984; 61: 529–533.

75. Theye RA, Michenfelder JD. The effect of nitrous oxide on canine cerebral metabolism. Anesthesiology, 1968; 29: 1119.

76. Henriksen HT, Jørgensen PB. The effect of nitrous oxide on intracranial pressure in patients with intracranial disorders. Br J Anaesth 1973; 45: 486–491.

77. Hansen TD, Warner DS, Todd MM. Nitrous oxide is a more potent vasodilator than either halothane or isoflurane. Anesthesiology 1988; 69: A537.

78. Field LM, Dorrance DE, Krzeminska EK, Barsaum LZ. Effect of nitrous oxide on cerebral blood flow in normal humans. Br J Anaesth 1993; 70: 154–159.

79. Jobes DR, Kennell E, Bitner R, Swenson E, Wollman H. Effects of morphine-nitrous oxide anaesthesia on cerebral autoregulation. Anesthesiology 1975; 42: 30.

80. Sari A, Okuda Y, Takeshita H. The effects of thalamonal on cerebral circulation and oxygen consumption in man. Br J Anaesth 1972; 44: 330.

81. Fitch W, Barker J, Jennett WB, McDowall DG. The influence of neuroleptanalgesic drugs on cerebrospinal fluid pressure. Br J Anaesth 1969; 41: 800.

82. Sperry RJ, Bailey PL, Reichman MV, Peterson JC, Peterson PB, Pace NL. Fentanyl and sufentanil increase intracranial pressure in head trauma patients. Anesthesiology 1992; 77: 416–420.

83. Werner C, Kochs E, Bause H, Hoffman WE, Schulte am Esch, J. Effects of sufentanil on cerebral hemodynamics and intracranial pressure in patients with brain injury. Anesthesiology 1995; 83: 721–726.

84. Jamali S, Ravussin P, Archer D, Goutallier D, Parker F, Ecoffey C. The effects of bolus administration of opioids on cerebrospinal fluid pressure in patients with supratentorial lesions. Anesth Analg 1996; 82: 600–606.

85. Warner DS, Hindman BJ, Todd MM et al. Intracranial pressure and hemodynamic effects of remifentanil versus alfentanil in patients undergoing supratentorial craniotomy. Anesth Analg 1996; 83: 348–353.

86. Minton MD, Stirt JA, Bedford RF, Haworth C. Intracranial pressure after atracurium in neurosurgical patients. Anesth Analg 1985; 64: 1113–1116.

87. Rosa G, Orfei P, Sanfilippo M, Vilardi V, Gasparetto A. The effects of atracurium besylate (Tracrium) on intracranial pressure and cerebral perfusion pressure. Anesth Analg 1986; 65: 381–384.

88. Rosa G, Sanfilippo M, Vilardi V, Orfei P, Gasparetto A. Effects of vecuronium bromide on intracranial pressure and cerebral perfusion pressure. A preliminary report. Br J Anaesth 1986; 58: 437–440.

89. Stirt JA, Maggio W, Haworth C, Minton MD, Bedford RF. Vecuronium: effect on intracranial pressure and hemodynamics in neurosurgical patients. Anesthesiology 1987; 67: 570–573.

90. Schramm WM, Strasser K, Bartunek A, Spiss CK. Effects of rocuronium and vecuronium on intracranial pressure, mean arterial pressure and heart rate in neurosurgical patients. Br J Anaesth 1996; 77: 607–611.

91. Tarkkanen L, Laitinen L, Johanssohn G. Effects of d-tubocurarine on intracranial pressure and thalamic electrical impedance. Anesthesiology 1974; 40: 247.

92. Lanier WL, Milde JH, Michenfelder JD. Cerebral stimulation following succinylcholine in dogs. Anesthesiology, 1986; 64: 551–559.

93. Ducey JP, Deppe SA, Foley KT. A comparison of the effects of suxamethonium, atracurium and vecuronium on intracranial hemodynamics in swine. Anaesth Intens Care 1989; 17: 448–455.

94. Cottrell JE, Hartung J, Giffin JP, Shwiny B. Intracranial and hemodynamic changes after succinylcholine administration in cats. Anesth Analg 1983; 62: 1006–1009.

95. O'Mahony BJ, Bolsin SNC. Anaesthesia for closed embolisation of cerebral arterial malformations. Anaesth Intens Care 1988; 16: 318–323.

96. Olsen KS, Svendsen LB, Larsen FS, Pulson OB. Effect of labetalol on cerebral blood flow, oxygen metabolism and autoregulation in healthy humans. Br J Anaesth 1995; 75: 51–54.

97. Schroeder T, Schierbeck J, Howardy P, Knudsen L, Skafte-Holm P, Gefke E. Effect of labetalol on cerebral blood flow and middle cerebral arterial flow velocity in healthy volunteers. Neurol Res 1991; 13: 10–12.

98. Turner JM, Powell D, Gibson RM, McDowall DG. Intracranial pressure changes in neurosurgical patients during hypotension induced with sodium nitroprusside or trimetaphan. Br J Anaesth 1977; 49: 419.

99. Morris PJ, Todd M, Philbin D. Changes in canine intracranial pressure in response to infusion of sodium nitroprusside and trinitroglycerin. Br J Anaesth 1982; 54: 991.

100. Burt DER, Verniquet AJW, Homi J. The response of canine intracranial pressure to hypotension induced with nitroglycerin. Br J Anaesth 1982; 54: 665.

SECTION 2

MONITORING THE CENTRAL NERVOUS SYSTEM

5

ELECTROPHYSIOLOGICAL MONITORING OF THE CENTRAL NERVOUS SYSTEM

Brian McNamara & Simon J. Boniface

INTRODUCTION

The techniques of clinical neurophysiology provide a non-invasive and inexpensive means of assessing brain function. The EEG and evoked potentials respond rapidly to changes in cerebral physiology and are therefore a useful means of monitoring cerebral function during surgery and in the postoperative period.

PHYSIOLOGY

The electroencephalogram represents the electrical activity of the brain as recorded from the scalp surface. Most of the activity recorded from the scalp surface is generated by cortical neurones. Pyramidal neurones are particularly important in generating the EEG as they are vertically orientated with regard to the cortex. Potentials arising in subcortical nucleii or in cells orientated horizontal to the cortex contribute little to the EEG.[1,2] The scalp potentials recorded during EEG are probably due to the summation of excitatory or inhibitory postsynaptic potentials from many pyramidal neurones.[3,4] The generation of the rhythmicity of the EEG is not well understood but is believed to be due to a combination of the inherent rhythmicity of some pyramidal neurones and the effect of pacemaker nucleii, with the reticular thalamus and thalamus thought to be particularly important in this respect.[5,6]

Evoked potentials (EPs) are the potentials elicited by physiological stimulation of receptors or electrical stimulation of peripheral nerves. EPs are generated in the cerebral cortex, subcortical nucleii, brainstem and spinal cord.[7] The potential recorded from the scalp is probably due to the summation of excitatory postsynaptic potentials from many neurones. Visual evoked potentials (VEP) are the cortical response to visual stimulation with either a flashing light or reversing checkerboard pattern. Brainstem auditory evoked potentials (BAEP) are the potentials produced by brainstem structures in response to an auditory stimulus. Somatosensory evoked potentials (SEP) are the response from the brain or spinal cord in response to electrical stimulation of a peripheral sensory nerve.[7]

PRACTICAL ASPECTS

The EEG is normally recorded from the scalp surface using metal disc electrodes (usually silver) attached using a viscous conductive paste, usually containing silver chloride.[8] The electrodes are arranged on the scalp surface using an internationally recognized system of electrode placement; most EEG laboratories use the 10: 20 electrode placement system[9] (Fig. 5.1). The recorded signal is amplified and filtered to remove unwanted electrical activity. Most modern EEG machines can record from eight to 24 channels of electrical activity. These channels record the distribution of electrical potential on the scalp surface by interconnecting the electrodes in two different ways. The potential difference between pairs of electrodes can be recorded (the *bipolar derivation*) or the potential difference between each electrode and a common reference point can be recorded (the *referential derivation*). Using the bipolar montage, the EEG can be recorded from chains of electrodes which run from anterior to posterior or transversely along the scalp surface. The electrical signal is then recorded over time using either a pen and paper system or digitally converted and the EEG stored and reviewed using a personal computer.[8]

Evoked potentials are quite small when compared with background EEG activity. To eliminate background EEG and allow the evoked potentials to be studied in greater detail, the evoked potential is averaged by recording the response to successive sensory or electrical stimuli. The degree of averaging depends on the modality of the evoked potential: for VEPs, 100 stimuli are normally sufficient; for brainstem responses over 1000 stimuli may be required.[7]

THE EEG IN NORMAL PATIENTS

The EEG is normally interpreted according to the following criteria.

- *Frequency* of the background rhythm. For convenience, the rhythm is classified into one of the following frequency bands: δ 1–4 Hz, θ 4–7 Hz, α 8–13 Hz and β <13 Hz.

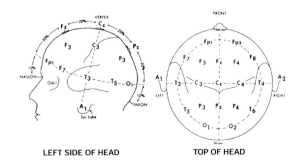

Figure 5.1   The international 10: 20 system of electrode placement.

- *Amplitude* of the EEG. Most normal EEG activity is between 20 and 200 μV.
- *Paroxysmal activity*. This refers to any bursts of transient activity.
- *Location*. Some indication of the source of EEG or evoked potentials can be gained by studying the distribution of the electrical activity over the scalp surface.[10]

The EEG in normal patients depends on the age and state of arousal. In normal awake adults, the dominant rhythm has a frequency of about 9 Hz (α rhythm), is symmetrical, is located in the posterior two quadrants, is inhibited by eye opening and has an amplitude of 50–100 μV (Fig. 5.2). In young adults, an α frequency rhythm known as a μ-rhythm may be seen over central and parietal regions. Sharp transients called λ waves may be seen over occipital regions when subjects have their eyes open. As subjects become drowsy the α rhythm becomes intermittent and the

amount of θ and δ activity increases. In light sleep the α rhythm disappears. In stage 2 sleep sharp transients known as vertex sharp waves are seen over the vertex in the midline. In addition, complex waveforms known as K-complexes appear (Fig. 5.3). Bursts of rhythmical activity known as sleep spindles may also be seen. In stage 3 and stage 4 sleep the K-complexes and spindles become less evident and the EEG becomes dominated by high-amplitude θ and δ activity. REM sleep is usually associated with a mixed frequency recording containing variable amounts of β, α, θ and α activity.[11]

The EEG evolves considerably during childhood. At one year of age the dominant rhythm has a frequency of 5–6 Hz, increasing to 8 Hz at three years and reaching adult frequency by 15 years. In addition, a varying amount of θ and δ activity may be seen over the frontocentral and occipital regions as the child matures (Fig. 5.4).[12]

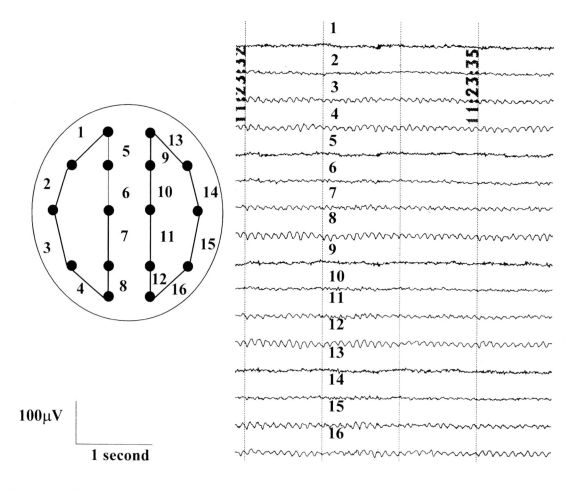

100μV

1 second

Figure 5.2   EEG from a normal awake adult. The EEG is dominated by an α rhythm (approximately 10Hz) located in the posterior quadrants–channels 4,8,12 and 16.

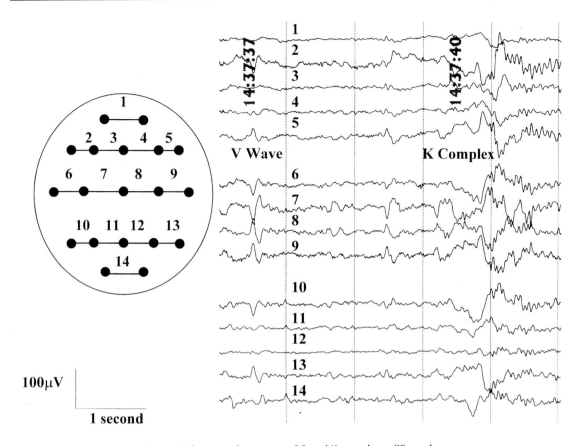

Figure 5.3   EEG in stage 2 sleep. Both vertex sharp waves (V) and K-complexes (K) can be seen.

EVOKED POTENTIALS IN NORMAL SUBJECTS

Evoked potential waveforms are named according to whether they are positive (designated P) or negative (designated N) with reference to a reference zero voltage and according to the latency with which they are generated after application of the sensory stimulus (normally indicated by a subscript). For example, the positive waveform seen approximately 100ms after application of the visual stimulus in VEP testing is called the P100.

SEPs are produced by electrical stimulation of a peripheral nerve. The electrical stimulus used activates fast-conducting group Ia and group II sensory afferents. The different components of the SEP are generated by sequential activation of neural generators by the ascending volley. An example of the SEP recorded from the scalp surface is shown in Figure 5.5. The first component (N9 or P9 with median nerve stimulation, P18 with posterior tibial nerve stimulation) is produced by the volley of action potentials reaching the brachial or sacral plexus. The next component (with a latency of about 12ms following median nerve stimulation) is produced by the sensory volley passing through the dorsal column. A slightly later wave can sometimes be detected due to the activation of the dorsal grey matter of the spinal cord. These early spinal components are most easily recorded by electrodes placed over the neck or thoracolumbar spine. The later components are for the most part cortically generated and are recorded best at the scalp surface. The most important of these is the N20/P22 complex (N38/P38 complex after posterior tibial nerve stimulation). These are generated by the somatosensory cortex (N20 and N38/P38) and motor and premotor cortex (P22). There are also later components (P27, N30, P45 and N60). The P27 is generated by the parietal cortex, the N30 is generated by the supplementary motor area and the exact source of the P45 and N60 has not been clearly described.[13]

BAEPs are produced by applying a simple auditory stimulus, which is normally a click. A typical BAEP is shown in Figure 5.6. Wave I originates from the

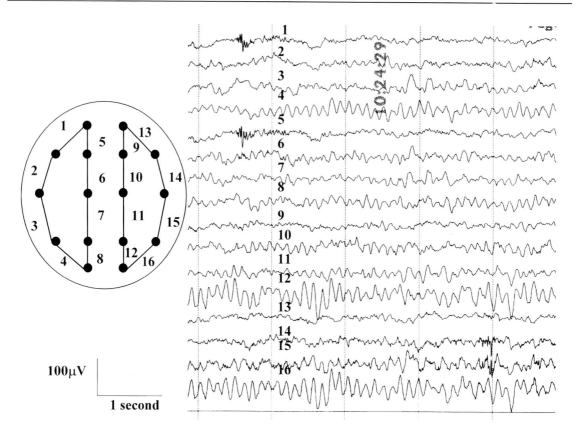

Figure 5.4   EEG from a normal six-year-old. As in the adult, there is an α rhythm located in the posterior quadrants. However, there is also underlying θ and δ activity in the frontal and central regions.

peripheral portion of the cochlear nerve. Wave II represents stimulation of the proximal portion of the cochlear nerve and postsynaptic responses from cochlear nucleus cells. Wave III is generated by the pontine portion of the auditory pathway. The source of wave IV is not clearly established but it is probably due to propagation of action potentials in the lateral lemniscus. Wave V is probably generated by a combination of the action potentials in the lateral lemniscus and postsynaptic responses in the midbrain auditory nucleii.[14]

Most VEP paradigms used in clinical practice employ a checkerboard with alternating black and white squares as a stimulus. The VEP waveform contains three peaks: N75, P100 and N145. The most consistent of these is P100, which is generated in the visual cortex.[15]

PROCESSING OF THE EEG

The routine EEG results in a large amount of data requiring specialist interpretation. To facilitate the

continuous EEG monitoring, a number of techniques have been developed to simplify and summarize the data. The most commonly used methods are based on analysis of the frequency of the EEG signal over time or amplitude over time.

One of the most commonly used frequency-based methods is power spectral analysis. A fixed period or epoch of EEG signal is digitized and mathematically manipulated using a fast Fourier transform. The distribution of EEG frequencies in each epoch is then plotted in a spectral array. An EEG with a normal α rhythm would therefore be summarized as a single plot with a peak at 9–10 Hz. To simplify the data even further, the frequency spectrum can be presented as a single number which summarizes the distribution of frequencies in that spectrum. Two descriptors commonly used in clinical practice are the spectral edge frequency (SEF) and the median frequency (MF). The spectral edge frequency is defined as the frequency below which 95% of the power in the EEG lies (SEF_{95}). The median frequency is the frequency below which 50% of the power in the EEG spectrum is

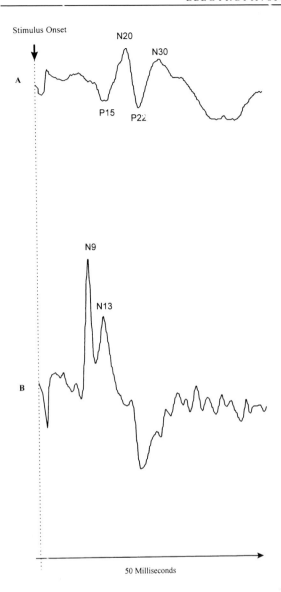

Figure 5.5 An example of the SEP (following left median nerve stimulation) recorded from left Erb's point (B) and right central region (A). Components generated by the brachial plexus (N9), spinal cord (N13) and cerebral cortex (N20, P22 and N30) can be clearly seen with left median nerve stimulation.

found. Each time period or epoch analysed in this way generates a spectrum and spectra for succeeding epochs can be stacked on top of one another to show how the distribution of frequencies varies with time in a montage termed a *compressed spectral array*.[16]

Aperiodic analysis is utilized by commercially available monitors. It maps each waveform in terms of its frequency amplitude and time of occurrence. The EEG signal is subdivided into three components: 1–8 Hz, 9–30 Hz and a composite signal which can detect spikes. The computer can then display a summary of wave amplitude and frequency on a graphical display.[17]

One of the simplest methods of processing the EEG is the cerebral function monitor (CFM) first developed by Maynard et al.[18] This processes only one channel of EEG data, normally from a pair of parietal electrodes. This signal is filtered, compressed and rectified to produce a single trace which is dependent on both the amplitude and frequency of the underlying EEG (Fig. 5.7). Although a great deal of information is lost in summarizing complex data in this manner, this single trace on the CFM monitor trace can be easily interpreted with a minimum of training. A more sophisticated version of the CFM monitor is the cerebral function analysing monitor (CFAM) which displays three amplitude traces, showing the 10th centile, mean and 90th centile of the amplitude of the processed EEG signal. There is also a frequency display which shows the percentage of EEG power in each of the four major frequency bands.[19]

THE EEG AND GENERAL ANAESTHETICS

As a general rule, the EEG alters in a predictable manner as the depth of anaesthesia increases. The initial phase is dominated by the appearance of β activity over the frontal regions, followed by gradual disappearance of the α rhythm. As anaesthesia deepens, the amount of δ and θ activity increases. Eventually a burst suppression pattern is attained consisting of periods where the EEG is isoelectric or of low voltage alternating with periods of high-amplitude activity (Fig. 5.8).[20] Some anaesthetic agents can alter the amplitude and latency of evoked potentials.

INHALED AGENTS

Nitrous Oxide

Nitrous oxide can produce characteristic fast (34Hz) oscillatory activity in humans. It can also reduce the amplitude of auditory and visual evoked potentials without affecting the latency.

Halothane

Halothane produces a progressive slowing of the EEG frequency. It also decreases SEP amplitude in a dose-dependent fashion. It also increases VEP latency and reduces amplitude.

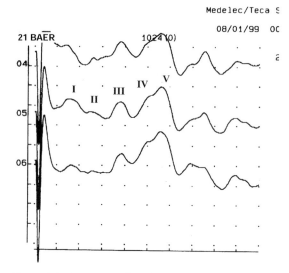

Figure 5.6   BAEP recording showing waves I–V.

Enflurane

Enflurane causes progressive slowing of the EEG and eventual burst suppression. It can also reduce SEP amplitude with slight effects on latency.

Isoflurane

This initially produces fast activity, followed at higher levels of anaesthesia by an increasing amount of high-amplitude δ activity, eventually culminating in burst suppression at approximately 2 MAC. Isoflurane decreases SEP amplitude and high concentrations can completely suppress the scalp SEP.[21]

INTRAVENOUS AGENTS

Barbiturates at low doses cause an increase in β activity while higher doses successively produce EEG slowing and burst suppression and very high doses cause elec-

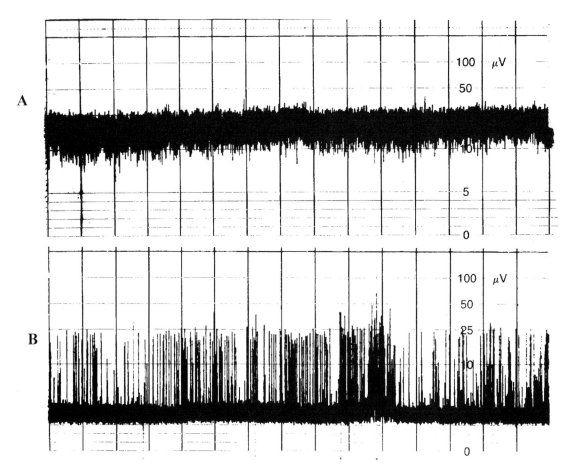

Figure 5.7   CFM tracing. The EEG data from a single channel is summarized as a tracing which is dependent on the frequency and amplitude of the EEG signal. The top tracing (A) was obtained from a patient post-head injury. The bottom tracing was obtained in the same patient after barbiturate established burst suppression.

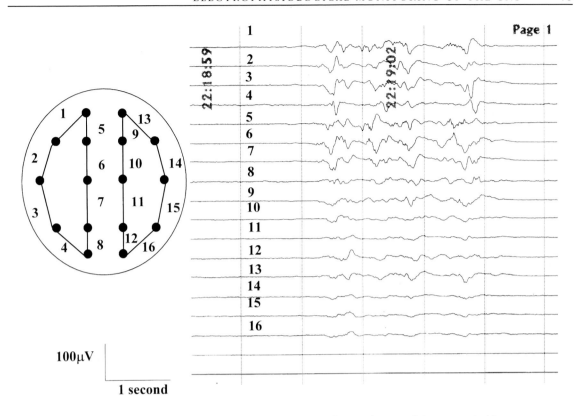

Figure 5.8   EEG obtained from a patient in deep barbiturate anaesthesia. The record shows a typical burst-suppression pattern with high-amplitude activity interrupted by episodes when the EEG is almost isoelectric.

trocortical silence. Thiopentone causes a dose-dependent increase in SEP latency with moderate amplitude decrease. Etomidate is known to produce myoclonic movements but this is not associated with any increase in epileptogenic activity on the EEG. Etomidate increases θ wave amplitude and slows the α rhythm at increasing doses. Methohexitone causes similar changes to barbiturates and has also been reported to increase epileptiform activity on the EEG of patients known to have epilepsy. Propofol produces a gradual increase in δ activity as the depth of anaesthesia increases. Like methohexitone, propofol can increase epileptiform activity in patients known to have seizures. Opioids produce gradual slowing of the EEG with increasing concentrations but, even at high doses, cannot elicit burst suppression. They can also cause a slight increase in the SEP latency without increasing the amplitude.[21]

PREOPERATIVE ASSESSMENT IN EPILEPSY SURGERY

Probably the most important area where neurophysiology is used in the preoperative assessment of patients is in epilepsy surgery. EEG is essential to identify the epileptogenic zone, to confirm that the seizures originate from the part of the brain to be resected at surgery and to exclude non-epileptic attacks or psychogenic seizures. In almost all cases the routine interictal EEG is supplemented with 24-h video telemetry which allows simultaneous video and EEG recording of the patient's seizures. It may also be necessary to improve localization of the epileptogenic zone by recording from sphenoidal or foramen ovale electrodes.

In most cases a Wada test is performed before surgery to determine hemispheric language dominance before surgery. This is performed by injecting 100–200mg of sodium amytal into the internal carotid and rendering the ipsilateral hemisphere non-functional. Neuropsychological testing can demonstrate impairment of speech, verbal memory and non-verbal memory. The test is performed using EEG monitoring which shows a build-up of high-amplitude δ over the impaired hemisphere. Electrocorticographic recording (i.e. an EEG over the exposed cortex) may be performed intraoperatively for seizures for which no standard *en bloc* resection procedure exists. This is particularly true for surgery with multiple subpial resections.[22]

NEUROPHYSIOLOGICAL MONITORING AND INTRAOPERATIVE CARE

The primary role of neurophysiological monitoring during surgery is to detect and remedy brain or spinal cord damage. EEG and evoked potential monitors are non-invasive and respond rapidly to alterations in brain or spinal cord function and are therefore particularly suited to intraoperative monitoring.

MONITORING THE DEPTH OF ANAESTHESIA

Because there is a consistent evolution of the EEG as the depth of anaesthesia increases, the EEG could theoretically be used to perform surgery at a constant level of anaesthesia. The spectral edge frequency correlates with the depth of anaesthesia so this simply interpreted EEG variable could be used to assess the level of anaesthesia.[23] The CFAM also shows easily recognized changes as the depth of anaesthesia increases.[24] Evoked potentials also show changes in amplitude and latency as the depth of anaesthesia increases.[25,26]

Neurophysiological monitoring has yet to gain widespread acceptance as a means of assessing the depth of anaesthesia because the changes in EEG and evoked potentials are agent specific and show a great deal of variation between patients. However, when performing intraoperative monitoring it is important to remember that alterations in EEG may be caused by changes in the level of anaesthesia. Consequently, it is best to start monitoring before induction of anaesthesia, to monitor before and after surgical positioning and maintain a constant level of anaesthetic agents during monitoring where possible.

The bispectral index (BIS)

One major criticism of the above techniques of EEG analysis is that they tend to ignore the phase information in the EEG and also the phase relationships between different EEG frequencies. It has been suggested that since the different frequencies in the EEG are closely related and influenced by common inputs, such phase relationships may provide important information.[88] Such phase relationships are quantified as the EEG *bispectrum*, which is normalized as a percentage of the maximal achievable phase coupling (measured as the *real triple product*) to produce a percentage variable that accounts for changes in amplitude and is termed the *bicoherence index*. The *bispectral index (BIS)* is a multivariate measure containing features that include the EEG bicoherence, bispectrum and real triple product, along with time domain features such as the burst suppression ratio.[88] The BIS provides a single number that is a measure of CNS depression but is probably incapable of distinguishing different causes of such depression (e.g. natural sleep vs anaesthesia). The BIS in awake subjects is reported at 95 and varies between 50 and 70 during sedation/anaesthesia. A given BIS value may provide an assessment of the probability that an anaesthetized subject is unaware and unlikely to retain postoperative memories of intraoperative events.[89] Recent articles provide an excellent review of the basis of bispectral analysis.[90,91]

NEUROPHYSIOLOGICAL MONITORING AND CAROTID ENDARTERECTOMY

Carotid endarterectomy has a morbidity of approximately 2% and about half of the complications occur during the intraoperative period.[27] During carotid surgery, ischaemia can occur for a number of reasons. When the carotid artery clamp is applied, ischaemia can result if the collateral circulation is not adequate or if embolization occurs from the operative site. Placement of an intraoperative shunt can also cause increased morbidity as a result of increased operating time or embolism from two sites of artery puncture.

The most effective surgical strategy would therefore appear to be selective shunting guided by monitoring. The EEG has many theoretical advantages as a monitoring modality for this purpose. It responds rapidly to developing ischaemia, it is sensitive and will show significant alterations when the blood flow falls below 15ml/100g/min and it is relatively inexpensive.[27,28] Unfortunately, there are no controlled trials of EEG monitoring during carotid surgery; in particular, there are no trials looking at the reduction in morbidity produced by monitoring. While most evidence is based on historical controls, a significant correlation between ischaemic EEG events and postoperative neurological deficit has been found in a number of series.[29,30] There appears to be some dispute about the sensitivity of EEG monitoring and some series claim that all perioperative strokes were predicted by the EEG (i.e. 100% sensitivity)[30] while others have found a significant number of false negatives (as high as 50% in one series).[31] EEG monitoring has also been shown to result in a significant fall in perioperative strokes when the monitored groups are compared with historical controls.[32]

A similar correlation has been found between SEP amplitude and cerebral blood flow. SEP monitoring can be easier to maintain as monitoring SEP amplitude produces only a single number which is more easily interpreted than the complex waveform seen with EEG. Metaanalysis of a number of series of SEP monitoring during surgery shows that SEP has a sensitivity of about 96%.[33]

A number of centres monitor some index of cerebral blood flow as opposed to neurophysiological monitoring. Two of the more commonly applied methods are carotid stump pressure and transcranial Doppler. There are no controlled trials directly comparing outcome between neurophysiological monitoring and transcranial Doppler. EEG would appear to be at least as sensitive though possibly less specific than transcranial Doppler.[34] Comparison of stump pressure monitoring with EEG in the same patients would suggest that stump pressure monitoring is possibly more sensitive with similar specificity.[31]

SPINAL SURGERY

Operations which compromise the spinal cord or its blood flow can also be monitored using evoked potentials. Examples of such surgery include removal of spinal cord tumours and vascular malformations. There is also a small but significant risk of spinal cord damage associated with the surgical management of scoliosis. This occurs particularly with sublaminar wiring. The integrity of the spinal cord can be assessed by continuous monitoring of the SEP throughout the surgery. This can be done by recording the cortical SEP or spinal SEP with epidural electrodes. Monitoring of the spinal SEP has the advantage of being more robust and resistant to changes in anaesthetic concentration and blood pressure.

There is no direct evidence from controlled clinical trials that monitoring reduces the incidence of complications. However, the occurrence and degree of preoperative changes correlate with the postoperative deficit and the risk of postoperative deficit is reduced if the electrophysiological changes can be reversed.[35,33] A multicentre survey has shown a lower incidence of complications in those centres where scoliosis surgery is performed with spinal monitoring performed by experienced staff.[36]

OTHER PROCEDURES

In many neurosurgical procedures neurophysiological monitoring may be useful in minimizing the surgical morbidity. In pituitary gland surgery VEPs may be useful in monitoring for optic chiasm damage.[37] SEP and BAEP are useful means of monitoring brainstem function during surgery in posterior cranial fossa.[38,39] SEP and EEG monitoring allow detection of developing cerebral ischaemia in aneurysm surgery.[40,41]

ELECTROPHYSIOLOGICAL MONITORING IN THE INTENSIVE CARE UNIT

The techniques of neurophysiology provide a useful extension of clinical examination in the assessment of patients in the intensive care unit. In particular, there are four areas where neurophysiological methods are beneficial:

1. making specific diagnoses;
2. continuous EEG or evoked potential monitoring of critically ill patients;
3. management of status epilepticus;
4. using EEG and evoked potentials to predict outcome.

EEG AND SPECIFIC DIAGNOSES

While many neurological conditions are associated with changes on the EEG, the number of conditions with specific diagnostic EEG changes is limited.[42] Examples of these include herpes simplex encephalitis, post measles encephalitis and Creutzfeldt–Jakob disease (Fig. 5.9). There is also a subgroup of patients who may not be able to have an MRI scan for clinical reasons, in whom the EEG may point towards lateralized pathology such as ischaemia or space-occupying lesions before changes appear on CT scanning.

CONTINUOUS MONITORING

The possibility of continuous EEG monitoring is very attractive. The goal of such monitoring would be to allow the clinician to detect cerebral dysfunction before it has become irreversible. In particular, the EEG demonstrates cerebral ischaemia, which may not be immediately obvious in the sedated patient, and subclinical seizures[43]. While the EEG reflects changes in intracranial pressure, this may not be relevant in centres with continuous intracranial pressure monitoring.

However, there are considerable difficulties involved in establishing continuous EEG monitoring in the ICU setting. First, it is technically difficult to maintain a continuous low-noise, low-impedance connection between the patient and the EEG machine. To maintain a continuous connection therefore requires

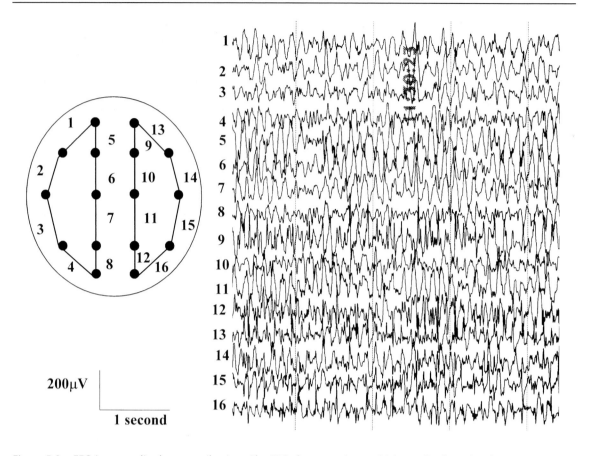

Figure 5.9   EEG in generalized status epilepticus. The EEG shows continuous high-amplitude epileptiform activity.

special training of the nursing staff and several daily visits by the technician. Monitoring is also impeded by multiple generators of artefact in the ICU setting. High-frequency electrical noise is generated by other computerized equipment in the ICU. Mechanical ventilators generate both mechanical and electrical rhythmical artefact. Nursing procedures and chest physiotherapy can generate a large amount of mechanical artefact that is in the frequency range of the EEG.[44] Because of the large amount of data generated by continuous monitoring, the EEG is often supplemented by some form of automated EEG processing (Lifescan, CFAM or compressed spectral array).

Given the considerable investment of time and resources required for continuous EEG monitoring in the ICU, it is pertinent to question the benefits of continuous monitoring. One study of patients with a variety of different neurological diagnoses showed that the EEG had a significant impact on patient management in 50% of cases.[45] In a study of 18 patients with carotid stenosis the EEG showed alteration when the patients were subjected to hypotensive or hypertensive stress and this information was a factor in considering patients for surgery.[46] Recent studies in acute stroke have shown that certain EEG patterns are predictive of a poor outcome and allow diagnosis of cerebral infarction before changes are seen on CT scanning.[47] Further, continuous monitoring allows detection of cerebral ischaemia and vasospasm in patients with subarachnoid haemorrhage, allowing treatment to begin earlier.[48] In one study alterations in the processed EEG predicted vasospasm before transcranial Doppler in 70% of cases.[49] In severe head trauma and postneurosurgical patients continuous EEG monitoring allows the immediate diagnosis and treatment of non-convulsive status epilepticus. Unfortunately, there are no controlled trials assessing the objective benefit to morbidity and mortality of continuous EEG. The indirect evidence that continuous EEG monitoring allows the detection of subclinical seizures and ischaemia suggests that when available, EEG monitoring is a useful adjunct to other forms of CNS monitoring in the management of the unconscious patient.

THE EEG IN STATUS EPILEPTICUS

The EEG is an important tool in the management of both convulsive status epilepticus and non-convulsive status epilepticus (Fig. 5.10). While status epilepticus is a medical emergency and treatment should not be delayed if an EEG is not available, clinical examination alone may result in misdiagnosis of status epilepticus for two reasons. First psychogenic status is a common cause of diagnostic confusion. In one study 20% of patients presenting to an accident and emergency department of a tertiary referral centre with intractable convulsive movements had psychogenic seizures.[49] Second non-convulsive status is underrecognized and patients with non-convulsive status are often mislabelled as being confused or postictal.[43]

Once treatment for convulsive status is established, the role for the EEG is not clear. Certainly in sedated patients treated with general anaesthesia, continuous EEG monitoring allows immediate recognition and treatment of seizures. Seizure activity increases cerebral metabolic rate of oxygen and causes excito-toxic cell damage.[50,51] Continuous EEG monitoring facilitates adequate seizure control without overtreatment in status epilepticus and reduces this risk of excitotoxic cell damage. While there are no controlled trials to support this conclusion, there is some indirect evidence. Mortality in status epilepticus increases with the duration of seizures.[52] It is therefore reasonable to assume that early detection of subclinical seizures in the ICU reduces mortality and mortality.

Where continuous EEG monitoring is not available it is reasonable to obtain an EEG daily while the patient remains unconscious and to consider performing an

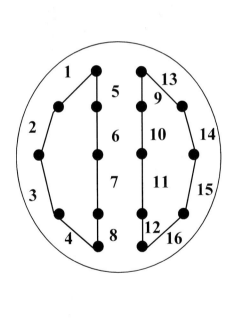

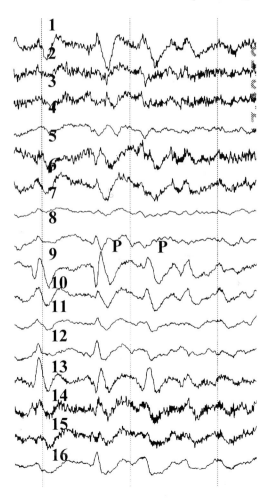

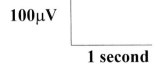

Figure 5.10   EEG in Creutzfeldt–Jakob disease. The EEG shows a characteristic pattern of periodic positive sharp wave complexes.

EEG before making significant alterations to therapy.

NEUROPHYSIOLOGY AND PREDICTING OUTCOME

There is a great need to develop reliable techniques for predicting outcome in both traumatic and non-traumatic coma. Early prediction of outcome is important for a number of reasons, including clinical decision making, the allocation of resources and counselling of relatives. Of the many sources of predictive information available, the most commonly utilized is the Glasgow Coma Scale (GCS). The GCS is a clinical assessment based upon eye opening, best verbal and best motor response.[53] Other scales use patients' age, injury severity score, pupil score and the presence or absence of haematoma on CT scan.[54] However, an accurate clinical assessment of patients in the ICU is frequently obscured by sedative medication, intubation, peripheral injuries, facial injuries, hypoxia, behavioural fluctuation and the subjective interpretation of the observer.[55] As a result workers have begun to explore the use of objective laboratory investigations to supplement clinical observations such as the GCS.

To be an effective prognostic test, the laboratory investigation should fulfil four criteria:

1. it should be useful in predicting the outcome in the majority of patients who enter the ICU and therefore be universally applicable;
2. it should be accurate;
3. it should have quantifiable sensitivity, specificity and predictive value;
4. it should be safe, inexpensive and reproducible.

Among the many objective laboratory investigations that fulfil such criteria, those of neurophysiology have received considerable interest. Neurophysiological assessments provide non-invasive objective measurements of brain activity, which are relatively inexpensive and can easily be performed in the intensive care environment without moving the patient.

THE ELECTROENCEPHALOGRAM (EEG)

There appears a good argument for the use of the EEG in predicting outcome from coma. In essence, the EEG is a non-invasive assessment of cortical function which, by definition, should provide important indices for studying coma. Indeed, early work documented numerous EEG patterns in coma, with several patterns associated with poor outcome.[56] However, initial clinical utility was marred by the lack of a clear distinction between the EEG patterns associated with good and poor outcome. More recently, workers have attempted to remedy this failing by devising objective grading systems which attempt to group EEG patterns with a similar prognosis together.

The two grading systems that are commonly used are summarized in Boxes 5.1 and 5.2.[56,57] In addition, there are more complex rating scales which involve scoring the EEG according to the presence or absence of specific EEG waveforms.[58] Other techniques have also been proposed, including those looking for EEG reactivity to external stimuli, variability in the EEG and sleep-related activity.[59–62]

There have been a number of studies considering the accuracy of one or several of the grading systems. One retrospective study is that of Synek,[63] testing the prognostic validity of his own grading system in traumatic coma.

The results (summarized in Table 5.1) are promising. Patients having a 'malignant' pattern on EEG would appear to have a high probability of a poor outcome. However, EEG patterns regarded as 'uncertain' provide no prognostic information. Indeed, approxi-

Benign	Normal α
	Θ dominant
	Frontal rhythmic δ
Uncertain	Diffuse δ
	Epileptiform changes
Malignant	Low-amplitude δ–non reactive
	Burst suppression
	α coma
	Isoelectric

Box 5.1   EEG grading scale

Grade I	Dominant α, reactive
Grade II	Dominant Θ–δ reactive
Grade III	Dominant δ–Θ, no α
Grade IV	Burst suppression
	Low-voltage δ, unreactive
	periodic general phenomena
Grade V	Very low voltage EEG
	Isoelectric EEG

Box 5.2   EEG grading scale

Table 5.1	Prognostic validity of Synek's grading system[63]	
EEG pattern	Survived	Died
Benign	15.9%	1.6%
Uncertain	14.3%	13.2%
Malignant	0	55%

mately half of the 'uncertain' group died. Since about 30% of patients fell into this category, the grading system fails to fulfil the criteria of being a universally applicable prognostic test. In essence, it only provides prognostic information for 70% of the patient group studied.

A convenient model for studying non-traumatic coma is that of coma following cardiac arrest in hospital. In this patient group the onset of coma is clearly documented and the timing of the EEG can be easily controlled. Four recently published studies adopting this model are summarized in Table 5.2.[64–67] In essence, they confirm the trend seen in the retrospective studies: an EEG pattern regarded as 'malignant' is a useful predictor of poor outcome but patterns regarded as 'benign' or 'uncertain' do not appear to predict a good outcome.

Furthermore, a prospective study in traumatic coma,[68] although difficult to compare with the findings in non-traumatic coma (the data are presented as a correlation between EEG score and Glasgow Outcome Score), found a correlation between EEG score and outcome. However, the EEG did not add any further information to that provided by clinical assessment alone. The EEG is therefore a useful extension of clinical examination and is particularly helpful when clinical assessment is impeded. However, it is not always possible to make an accurate prediction of outcome on the basis of the EEG alone.

THE SOMATOSENSORY EVOKED POTENTIAL (SEP)

The SEP has several advantages over the EEG in assessing outcome. In the EEG there are many patterns which have to be subjectively graded whereas the SEP is either present or absent, delayed or not delayed, with a normal or abnormal waveform. Many studies have looked at using the SEP to predict outcome in both traumatic and hypoxic coma. These are summarized in Table 5.3.[64–66,69–74] To compare studies, we divided SEP findings into three groups:

1. normal SEP where the latency and the waveform of the SEP were within acceptable limits;
2. unilaterally abnormal SEP where the SEP is either delayed, absent from one hemisphere or has an abnormal waveform;
3. bilaterally absent SEP.

As with the EEG, the SEP accurately identifies a group of patients who do badly. Patients with bilaterally absent SEP will invariably have a bad outcome. These findings are supported by a systematic review of prediction of poor outcome in anoxic ischaemic coma. Pooled data from 11 studies showed that a bilaterally absent SEP is the most accurate predictor of a poor outcome.[75] However, if the SEP is present patients may still do badly, so in this group of patients the SEP does not provide any additional prognostic information. Unlike the EEG, which is generated by the brain alone, the SEP may be influenced by injuries

Table 5.2	Summary of four prospective studies looking at EEG grade and outcome in hypoxic/ischaemic coma (from references[64–67])				
Authors	No. of patients	No. with benign, uncertain or grades I–III	No. with good outcome (GOS 3–5)	No. with malignant or grades IV or V	No. with bad outcome Death or PVS
Chen et al	34	12	5	22	20
Rothstein et al	40	29	14	11	11
Scollo et al	26	12	5	14	12
Bassetti et al	60	40	12	20	20
Total	160	93	36	66	61

Table 5.3 Using SEP to predict outcome in coma (from references[64-66,69-74])

Author	No. of patients	Normal SEP	No. with good outcome	Abnormal SEP	No. with good outcome	Absent SEP	No. with good outcome
Cant et al	40(T)	21	17	5	3	14	2
Judson et al	100(T)	38	33	26	19	36	3
Bassetti et al	60(H)	20	10	12	1	23	0
Brunko et al	50(H)	20	5	Not given	Not given	30	0
Chen et al	34(H)	16	7	6	2	12	0
Goldie et al	36(T)	16	9	8	2	12	6
Rothstein et al	40(H)	14	11	7	3	19	0
Goldberg	24(H+T)	4	4	15	9	5	0
Goodwin	37(H+T)	8	6	2	0	29	0

H = hypoxic/ischaemic coma
T = traumatic coma

elsewhere in the nervous system, including the peripheral nerves and spinal cord. There are a number of studies where the SEP grade or central conduction time is correlated with final outcome or disability score, in all of which the SEP was more effective than clinical examination alone.[58,76,77]

BRAINSTEM AUDITORY EVOKED POTENTIAL (BAEP)

The BAEP has a number of theoretical advantages over the SEP for assessing prognosis. It is less likely to be influenced by injury elsewhere in the nervous system. It would appear logical to assume that the brainstem is the most critical point in determining survival so assessing brainstem function should give a good guide as to prognosis. Again, the value of BAEP in assessing prognosis has been investigated in a number of studies.[60,78,79] Some of these are reviewed in Table 5.4. A significant relationship between interpeak latency and mortality has also been shown.[80]

An abnormal BAEP does not always imply a poor outcome and in three of the four studies reviewed, a significant number of survivors had an abnormal BAEP. BAEP would appear to be less useful than the SEP in prediction of outcome.

EVENT-RELATED POTENTIALS

These are scalp potentials produced in response to a simple discrimination task and are probably the electrophysiological representation of cognitive processing. They are probably generated by subcortical/cortical and cortico/cortical circuits and therefore have a potential theoretical application in predicting coma outcome since they depend on an extensive network of connections. One such potential, the P300, was used to predict outcome in a group of 20 patients[81] in non-traumatic coma. The relationship to outcome in this study is summarized in Table 5.5.

The P300 is useful to identify a subgroup of patients who will improve but unfortunately does not identify those patients who will do badly. Another auditory event-related potential is the mismatch negativity (MMN) in oddball paradigms of AEP recording. The relationship of MMN to outcome was examined in a group of head-injured patients[82] and is summarized in Table 5.6.

The other interesting finding in this study was the role of MMN in predicting awakening. They found a subgroup of 13 patients in whom the MMN was initially absent but later returned. The return of the MMN always preceded clinical awakening (by 24 h to 21 days).

ROLE OF FUNCTIONAL IMAGING

Functional imaging techniques such as positron emission tomography (PET), single photon emission computed tomography (SPECT) and functional magnetic resonance imaging (fMRI) allow an accurate determination of regional cerebral blood flow and metabolism. Studies with SPECT in acutely brain-injured patients can potentially be used to estimate the severity of brain injury and to predict clinical outcome.[83,84,85] In addition, early studies have shown a strong correlation between alteration in the EEG and changes in cerebral blood flow elucidated with PET.[86]

Table 5.4 Summary of studies looking at outcome and BAEP (from references[60,78,79])					
Author	No. of patients	No. with normal BAEP	No. of survivors	No. with abnormal BAEP	No. of dead or PVS
Cant et al	40	32	19	8	7
Karnaze et al	26	19	17	7	4
Karnaze et al	45	29	28	16	8
Goldberg	32	16	16	16	5

Studies which combine functional imaging with EEG and evoked potentials will allow a greater insight into the changes in cerebral blood flow and metabolism which underlie the changes which are seen on the EEG in acute brain injury. This knowledge may allow EEG to be even more widely applied in determining the severity of brain injury and predicting clinical outcome.

CONCLUSION

There are significant correlations between parameters measured by many of the neurophysiological techniques and outcome. However, none of the techniques listed above is sufficiently accurate to predict outcome in all cases. Can the accuracy of these neurophysiological techniques be improved? A number of studies have examined the predictive value of combinations of either EEG and SEP [63,65] or SEP and BAEP.[87] As the EEG or BAEP is less effective at predicting outcome than SEP, the combinations are not much more effective than SEP alone. However, a combination of bilateral SEP and EEG is easily obtained and interpreted. The EEG may give other useful information such as the detection of epileptiform activity or burst suppression. Using these techniques, a group of patients in whom there is a high probability of a bad outcome can be identified. More specialized techniques such as event-related potentials may have a role in patients with prolonged coma, particularly in predicting awakening. In the future it is predicted that

functional imaging in combination with neurophysiology will widen the scope for the clinical assessment of brain-injured patients.

SUMMARY

EEG, nerve conduction studies and evoked potentials provide a safe and inexpensive means of monitoring brain function in the operating theatre and the intensive care unit. We hope that the newer techniques will shed light on the causes of the evolution in the EEG that occurs in anaesthesia and cerebral injury. An increasing understanding of the alterations in cerebral physiology which underlie electrophysiological changes in unconscious patients is likely to improve our ability to draw firm clinical conclusions based on the EEG.

Acknowledgements

We would like to thank Mr Nicholas Carvill, Dr Julian Ray and Mr Martin Coleman for their assistance in the preparation of this manuscript.

Table 5.6 MMN and outcome in traumatic coma (from reference[82])		
	Alive	Dead
MMN present	35	1
MMN absent	4	14

Table 5.5 P300 and outcome in non-traumatic coma (from reference[81])		
	Awake	No awakening
P300 present	5	1
P300 absent	4	10

REFERENCES

1. Creutzfeldt OD, Watanabe S, Lux HD. Relations between EEG phenomena and potentials of single cortical cells. Spontaneous and convulsoid activity. Electroencephalogr Clin Neurophysiol 1966; 20: 19–37.

2. Thatcher R, John ER. Foundations of cognitive processes. 1977, Wiley, New York.

3. Creutzfeldt OD. The neural generation of the EEG. In: Redmond A (ed) ECN handbook, vol. 2, part C, 1974, Elsevier, Amsterdam.

4. Li CL, Jasper HH. Microelectrode studies of the cerebral cortex of the cat. J Physiol 1953; 121: 117–140.

5. Burns BD. Some properties of the cat's isolated cortex. J Physiol 1950; 111: 50–68.

6. Jasper H. Diffuse projection system: the integrative action of the thalamic reticular system. Electroencephalogr Clin Neurophysiol 1949; 1: 405–409.

7. Maugiere F. Evoked potentials. In: Osselton JW (ed) Clinical neurophysiology, Butterworth-Heinemann, Oxford, 1995, pp 323–334.

8. Hughes JR. The EEG in clinical practice, 1994. Butterworth-Heinemann, Boston.

9. Jasper HH. The ten-twenty electrode system of the international federation. Electroencephalogr Clin Neurophysiol 1958; 10: 371–375.

10. Aminoff MJ. Electroencephalography: general principles and clinical applications. In: Aminoff MJ (Ed) Electrodiagnosis in clinical neurology. Churchill Livingstone, New York, 1986, pp 21–76.

11. Blume WT, Kaibara M. Atlas of adult electroencephalography. 1995, Raven Press, New York.

12. Blume WT. Atlas of paediatric electroencephalography. 1982, Raven Press, New York.

13. Aminoff MJ, Eisen AA. AAEM mimeograph 19: somatosensory evoked potentials. Muscle Nerve 1998; 21: 277–290.

14. McPherson D, Starr A. Auditory evoked potentials in the clinic. In: Haliday AM (ed) Evoked potentials and clinical testing, 2nd edn. Churchill Livingstone, London, 1993, pp 383–420.

15. Halliday AM. The visual evoked potential in healthy subjects. In: Haliday AM (ed) Evoked potentials and clinical testing, 2nd edn. Churchill Livingstone, London, 1993, pp 358–379.

16. Bickford RG. Newer methods of recording and analysing EEG. In: Klass DW, Daly DD (eds) Current practice of clinical electroencephalography. 1979, Raven Press, New York.

17. Gregory TK, Pettus, DC. An electroencephalographic processing algorithm specifically intended for analysis of cerebral electrical activity. J Clin Monit 1986; 2: 190–197.

18. Maynard DE, Prior PF, Scott DF. Device for monitoring of cerebral activity in resuscitated patients. BMJ 1969; 4: 545–546.

19. Sebel PS, Maynard DE, Major E, Frank, M. The cerebral function analysing monitor (CFAM). Br J Anaesth 1983; 55: 1265–1270.

20. Bauer G, Bauer R. EEG drug effects and central nervous system poisoning. In: Niedermyer E, Lopes Da Silva F (eds) Electroencephalography 4th edn. Williams and Wilkins, Baltimore, 1998, pp 671–691.

21. McPherson RW. Neuroanaesthesia and intraoperative monitoring. In: Niedermyer E, Lopes Da Silva F (eds) Electroencephalography 4th edn. Williams and Wilkins, Baltimore, 1998, pp 1092–1106.

22. Niedermyer E. Neurosurgical treatment of the epilepsies. In: Niedermyer E (ed) The epilepsies. Urban and Schwarzenberg, Munich, 1990, pp 342–368.

23. Rampil IJ, Mateo RS. Spectral edge frequency – a new correlation of anaesthetic depth. Anaesthesiology 1987; 50: S12.

24. Yate PM, Maynard DE, Major E. Anaesthesia with ICI 35 868 monitored by the cerebral function analysing monitor. Eur J Anaesth 1986; 3: 159–166.

25. Samra SK, Vandezant, CW, Domer PA, Sackellares JC. Differential effects of isoflurane on human median nerve somatosensory evoked potentials. Anaesthesiology 1987; 66: 29–35.

26. Sebel PS, Flynn PJ, Ingram DA. Effect of nitrous oxide on visual, auditory and somatosensory evoked potentials. Br J Anaesth 1984; 54: 1403–1407.

27. Sundt TM, Sharborough FW, Piepgras DG, Kearns TP, Messick JM, O'Fallon WM. Correlation of cerebral blood flow with electroencephalographic changes during carotid endarterectomy. Mayo Clin Proc 1981; 56: 533–543.

28. Igvar DH, Sjolund B, Ardo A. Correlation between dominant EEG frequency and cerebral oxygen uptake and blood flow. Clin Neurophysiol 1976; 41: 268–276.

29. Rampil IJ, Holzer JA, Quest DO, Rosenbaum SH, Correll JW. Prognostic value of computerised EEG during carotid endarterectomy. Anaesth Analg 1983; 62: 186–192.

30. Ballotta E, Dagiau G, Saladini M et al. Results of electroencephalographic monitoring of 369 revascularisations. Eur Neurol 1997; 37: 43–47.

31. McCarthy WJ, Park AE, Koushanpour E, Pearce WH, Yao JS. Carotid enarterectomy. Lessons from intraoperative monitoring – a decade of experience. Ann Surg 1996; 224: 297–305.

32. Fisher RS, Raudzens P, Nunemacher M. Efficacy of intraoperative neurophysiological monitoring. J Clin Neurophysiol 1995; 12: 97–109.

33. Plestis KA, Loubser P, Mizrahi EM, Kantis G, Jiang ZD, Howell, JF. Continuous electroencephalographic monitoring and selective shunting reduces the neurologic morbidity rates in carotid endarterectomy. J Vasc Surg 1997; 25: 620–628.

34. Arnold M, Sturzenegger M, Schaffler L, Seiler RW. Continuous intraoperative monitoring of middle cerebral artery blood flow velocities and electroencephalography during carotid endarterectomy. A comparison of the two methods to detect cerebral ischaemia. Stroke 1997; 28: 1345–1350.

35. May DM, Jones SJ, Crockard HA. Somatosensory evoked potential monitoring in cervical surgery: identification of pre- and intraoperative risk factors associated with deterioration. J Neurosurg 1996; 85: 566–573.

36. Nuwer MR, Dawson EG, Carlson LG, Kanim LEA, Sherman JE. Somatosensory evoked potential spinal cord monitoring reduces neurological defecits after scoliosis surgery: results of a large multicentre survey. Electroencephalogr Clin Neurophysiol 1985; 96: 6–11.

37. e Costa Silva I, Wang AD, Symon L. The application of flash visual evoked potentials during operations on the anterior visual pathways. Neurol Res 1985; 7: 11–16.

38. Grudy BL, Janetta PJ, Lina A, Procopio PT, Boston JR, Doyle, E. Intraoperative monitoring of brainstem auditory evoked potentials. J Neurosurg 1982; 57: 674–681.

39. Grundy BL, Lina A, Doyle E, Procopio P. Somatosensory cortical evoked potential monitoring neurosurgical operations. Anaesth Analg 1982; 55: 462–466.

40. Little JR, Lesser RP, Luders H. Electrophysiological monitoring during basilar aneurysm operations. Neurosurgery 1987; 20: 421–427.

41. Symon L, Wang AD, Costa e Silva IE, Gentili F. Perioperative use of somatosensory evoked potential monitoring in aneurysm surgery. J Neurosurg 1984; 60: 269–270.

42. Niedermyer E. Abnormal EEG patterns (epileptic and paroxysmal). In: Niedermyer E, Lopes Da Silva F (Eds) Electroencephalography 4th edn. Williams and Wilkins, Baltimore, 1998, pp 235–261

43. Jordan, KG. Neurophysiologic monitoring in the neuroscience intensive care unit. Neurol Clin North Am 1995; 13: 579–626.

44. Chiappa KH, Hoch DB. Electrophysiological monitoring In: Roper A (ed) Neurological and neurosurgical intensive care, 3rd edn. Raven Press, New York, 1993, pp 147–183.

45. Jordan KG. Continuous EEG monitoring (CEEG) in the neuroscience intensive care unit. Neurology 1990; 40(suppl 1): 180.

46. Suzuki A, Yoshioka K, Yasui N. Clinical applications of EEG topography in cerebral ischaemia: detection of functional reversibility and haemodynamics. Brain Topogr 1990; 3: 167–174.

47. Jordan KG. Regional attenuation without delta (RAWOD): a distinctive early EEG pattern in acute cerebral infarction. Neurology 1998; 50(suppl 1): A243.

48. Vespa PM, Nuwer MR, Juhasz C. Early detection of vasospasm after acute subarachnoid haemorrhage using continuous EEG ICU monitoring. Electroencephalogr Clin Neurophysiol 1997; 103: 607–615.

49. Luther JS, McNamara JO, Carwile S. Pseudo-epileptic seizures: methods and video analysis to aid diagnosis. Ann Neurol 1982; 12: 458–461.

50. Meldrum, BS, Brierly JM. Prolonged epileptic seizures in primates: ischaemic cell changes and its relationship to ictal physiologic events. Arch Neurol 1993; 28:10–15.

51. Nevander G, Ingvar M, Auer R. Status epilepticus in well oxygenated rats causes neuronal necrosis. Ann Neurol 1985; 18: 281.

52. Young GB, Jordan KG, Doig GS. An assessment of nonconvulsive seizures in the intensive care unit using continuous EEG monitoring: an investigation of variables associated with mortality. Neurology 1996; 47: 83–89.

53. Teasdale G, Jennett, B. Assessment of outcome and impairment of consciousness. A practical scale. Lancet 1974; 2(7872): 81–84.

54. Signorini DF, Andrews PJD, Jones PA, Wardlaw JM, Miller JD. Predicting survival using simple clinical variables: a case study in traumatic brain injury. J Neurol Neurosurg Psychiatry 1999; 66: 20–25.

55. Becker DP, Miller JD, Greenberg RP. Prognosis after head injury. In: Youmans JR (Ed) Neurological surgery. WB Saunders, Philadelphia 1982, pp 2137–2174.

56. Hokaday JM, Potts F, Epstein E, Bonazzi A, Schwabb RS. EEG changes in acute cerebral anoxia from cardiac or respiratory arrest. Electroencephalogr Clin Neurophysiol 1965; 18: 575–586.

57. Synek VM. Value of a revised EEG coma scale for prognosis after cerebral anoxia and diffuse head injury. Clin Electroencephalogr 1990; 21(1): 25–30.

58. Rae-Grant AD, Barbour PJ, Reed J. Development of an EEG rating scale for head injury using dichotomous variables. Electroencephalogr Clin Neurophysiol 1991; 79: 349–357.

59. Evans BM, Bartlett JR. Prediction of outcome in severe head injury based on recognition of sleep related activity in the polygraphic electroencephalogram. J Neurol Neurosurg Psychiatry 1995; 59(1): 17–25.

60. Karnaze DS, Marshall LF, Bickford RG. EEG monitoring of clinical coma: the compressed spectral array. Neurology 1982; 32(3): 289–292.

61. Gutling E, Gonser A, Imhof HG, Landis T. EEG reactivity in the prognosis of severe head injury. Neurology. 1995; 45(5): 915–918.

62. Hulihan JF Jr, Syna DR. Electroencephalographic sleep patterns in post-anoxic stupor and coma. Neurology 1994; 44(4): 758–760.

63. Synek VM. Validity of a revised EEG coma scale for predicting survival in anoxic encephalopathy. Clin Exper Neurol 1989; 26: 119–127.

64. Chen R, Bolton CF, Young B. Prediction of outcome in patients with anoxic coma: a clinical and electrophysiologic study. Crit Care Med 1996; 24: 672–678.

65. Scollo-Lavizzari G, Bassetti C. Prognostic value of EEG in post-anoxic coma after cardiac arrest. Eur Neurol. 1987; 26(3): 161–170.

66. Bassetti C, Bomio F, Mathis J, Hess CW. Early prognosis in coma after cardiac arrest: a prospective clinical, electrophysiological, and biochemical study of 60 patients. J Neurol Neurosurg Psychiatry 1996; 61(6): 610–615.

67. Rothstein TL, Thomas EM, Sumi SM. Predicting outcome in hypoxic-ischemic coma. A prospective clinical and electrophysiologic study. Electroencephalogr Clin Neurophysiol 1991; 79(2): 101–107.

68. Rae Grant AD, Eckert N, Barbour PJ et al. Outcome of severe brain injury: a multi-modality neurophysiologic study. J Trauma 1996; 40(3): 401–406.

69. Cant BR, Hume AL, Judson JA, Shaw NA. The assessment of severe head injury by short-latency somatosensory and brain-stem auditory evoked potentials. Electroencephalogr Clin Neurophysiol 1986; 65(3): 188–195.

70. Brunko E, Zegers-de-Beyl D. Prognostic value of early cortical somatosensory evoked potentials after resuscitation from cardiac arrest. Electroencephalogr Clin Neurophysiol 1987; 66(1): 15–24.

71. Goodwin SR, Friedman WA, Bellefleur, M. Is it time to use evoked potentials to predict outcome in comatose children and adults? Crit Care Med 1991; 19(4): 518–524.

72. Goldberg G, Karazim E. Application of evoked potentials to the prediction of discharge status in minimally responsive patients: a pilot study. J Head Trauma Rehab 1998; 13(1): 51–68.

73. Judson JA, Cant BR, Shaw NA. Early prediction of outcome from cerebral trauma by somatosensory evoked potentials. Crit Care Med 1990; 18: 363–368.

74. Goldie WD, Chiappa KH, Young RR, Brooks ER. Brainstem auditory and short latency somatosensory evoked responses in brain death. Neurology 1981; 31: 248–256.

75. Zandbergen EJG, De Haan RJ, Stoutenbeek CP, Koelmen HTM, Hijdra A. Systematic review of early prediction of poor outcome in anoxic-ischaemic coma. Lancet 1998; 352: 1808–1812.

76. Houlden DA, Li C, Schwartz ML, Katic M. Median nerve somatosensory evoked potentials and the Glasgow Coma Scale as predictors of outcome in comatose patients with head injuries. Neurosurgery 1990; 27(5): 701–707.

77. Lindsay K, Pasaoglu A, Hirst D, Allardyce G, Kennedy I, Teasdale G. Somatosensory and auditory brain stem conduction after head injury: a comparison with clinical features in prediction of outcome. Neurosurgery 1990; 26(2): 278–285.

78. Karnaze DS, Weiner JM, Marshall LF. Auditory evoked potentials in coma after closed head injury: a clinical-neurophysiologic coma scale for predicting outcome. Neurology 1985; 35(8): 1122–1126.

79. Karnaze DS, Marshall LF, McCarthy CS, Klauber MR, Bickford RG. Localizing and prognostic value of auditory evoked responses in coma after closed head injury. Neurology 1982; 32(3): 299–302.

80. Facco E, Martini A, Zuccarello M, Agnoletto M, Giron GP. Is the auditory brain stem response effective in the assessment of post traumatic coma? Electroencephalogr Clin Neurophysiol 1985; 62: 332–337.

81. De Giorgio CM, Rabinowicz AL, Gott PS. Predictive value of P300 event related potentials compared with EEG and somatosensory evoked potentials in non-traumatic coma. Acta Neurol Scand 1993; 87: 423–424.

82. Kane NM, Curry SH, Rowlands CA et al. Event-related potentials – neurophysiological tools for predicting emergence and early outcome from traumatic coma. Intens Care Med 1996; 22(1): 39–46.

83. Kao CH, Wang PY, Wang YL, Chang L, Wang SJ, Yeh SH. A new prognostic index – leucocyte infiltration – in human cerebral infarcts by 99Tcm-HMPAO-labelled white blood cell brain SPECT. Nuclear Med Comm 1991; 12: 1007–1012.

84. Roper SN, Mena I, King et al. An analysis of cerebral blood flow in acute closed head injury using technetium 99m-HMPAO SPECT and computerised tomography. J Nuclear Med 1991; 32: 1684–1691.

85. Jacobs A, Put E, Ingels M, Bossuyt A. Prospective evaluation of technetium-99m HMPAO SPECT in mild to moderate traumatic brain injury. J Nuclear Med 1994; 35: 942–947.

86. Jansen HML, Van Der Naalt J, Van Zomeren AH et al. Cobalt 50 positron emission tomography in traumatic brain injury: a pilot study. J Neurol Neurosurg Psychiatry 1996; 60: 221–224.

87. Haupt WF, Pawlik G. Contribution of initial median-nerve somatosensory evoked potentials and brainstem auditory evoked potentials to prediction of clinical outcome in cerebrovascular critical care patients: a statistical evaluation. J Clin Neurophysiol 1985; 15(2): 154–158.

88. Sigl JC, Chamoun NG. An introduction to bispectral analysis for the electroencephalogram. J Clin Monit 1994; 10: 392–404.

89. Glass PS, Bloom M, Kearse L, Rosow C, Sebel P, Manberg P. Bispectral analysis measures sedation and memory effects of propofol, midazolam, isoflurane, and alfentanil in healthy volunteers. Anesthesiology 1997; 86: 836–847.

90. Rampil IJ. A primer for EEG signal processing in anesthesia. Anesthesiology 1998; 89: 980–1002.

91. Todd-MM. EEGs, EEG processing, and the bispectral index. Anesthesiology 1998; 89: 815–817.

6

BEDSIDE MEASUREMENTS OF CEREBRAL BLOOD FLOW

Sarah Walsh & Basil F. Matta

INTRODUCTION

Although alterations in cerebral blood flow (CBF) often accompany brain injury and exacerbate secondary neuronal injury,[1-3] the management of neurologically critically ill patients does not routinely involve the monitoring of CBF.[4] This, in part at least, is due to the lack of non-invasive, easy-to-use, reliable equipment that can measure CBF with well-defined thresholds.

However, the benefits of monitoring CBF in the brain-injured patient are becoming more apparent. In addition to avoiding the dangers of transferring critically ill patients for 'single time point' measurements in the CT or PET scanner, continuous bedside monitoring may detect transient ischaemic events. Furthermore, continuous assessment of CBF permits rapid diagnoses and early therapeutic interventions, which may improve outcome. Unfortunately, many of the techniques available for the bedside measurement of CBF are either cumbersome, have a large interobserver bias or depend on various assumptions for calculating CBF and hence are indirect or open to criticism. This chapter will outline the methods most commonly employed for the measurement of CBF in theatre and intensive care.

KETY–SCHMIDT METHOD

The first practical quantitative method of measuring cerebral blood flow, now regarded as the gold standard, is the technique described by Kety and Schmidt in 1945.[5,6] All CBF measurement techniques in use today are either derived from this method or have been validated against it. This method, adapted from the original technique for the measurement of pulmonary blood flow, is based on the Fick principle. Briefly, this states that the amount of a substance taken up or eliminated by an organ is equal to the difference between the amount in the arterial blood and the amount in the venous blood supplying that organ, in the same time period.

Thus for the brain:

$$QBt = QAt - QVt \qquad (i)$$

where QBt is the quantity of tracer taken up by the brain in time t, QAt is the quantity of tracer delivered to the brain by arterial blood in time t and QVt is the amount of tracer removed by cerebral venous blood in time t.

For the measurement of CBF using N_2O, the subject inhales 10% nitrous oxide (N_2O) in air for 10 min

during which time arterial and jugular bulb blood samples are taken and analysed for N_2O content. The initial difference between the arterial and venous concentrations of N_2O decreases as the tracer is taken up by the brain. The brain tissue is fully saturated when jugular bulb and arterial blood concentrations of N_2O are almost equal.

The amount of N_2O delivered to or removed by the brain thus equals CBF multiplied by the arterial or venous concentrations respectively. As the arterial and venous concentrations of N_2O vary with time, the equation can be rearranged:

$$QBt = TF. \int (A - V)\, dt \qquad (ii)$$

where TF is cerebral blood flow (ml/min), A is arterial N_2O concentration (ml/l) and V is venous N_2O concentration. Thus:

$$TF = \frac{QBt}{\int (A - V)\, dt} \qquad (iii)$$

CBF per gram weight of brain is then:

$$CBF = \frac{QBt/W}{\int (A - V)\, dt} \qquad (iv)$$

where W is the brain weight in grams (g).

It is not easy to measure the brain concentration of N_2O (QB) clinically. However, if enough time is allowed for equilibration to occur, then the brain N_2O concentration will equal the partition coefficient of N_2O (the amount of gas dissolved in the blood

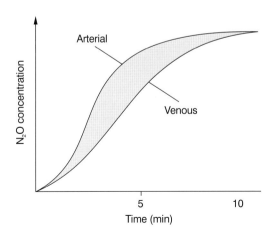

Figure 6.1   The Kety–Schmidt technique for measuring cerebral blood flow using the freely diffusible tracer N_2O. After 10 min of N_2O inhalation, the brain is theoretically saturated with the arterial and venous concentrations of N_2O almost equal. The shaded area between the two curves is proportional to hemispheric blood flow.

relative to brain) multiplied by the cerebral venous concentration:[7]

$$QBt = \frac{\lambda . Vt}{W} \qquad (v)$$

where λ is the partition coefficient, 1.06 in the case of nitrous oxide, and Vt is the cerebral venous concentration of nitrous oxide at equilibrium. This yields the final expression:

$$CBF = \frac{\lambda . Vt}{\int (A-V) \, dt} \qquad (vi)$$

It is then possible to calculate CBF once the arterial and cerebral venous concentrations of N_2O are measured.

Once CBF is determined, additional values such as cerebral metabolic requirement for oxygen and vascular resistance may be derived. N_2O offers significant advantages over other agents used for the measurement of CBF in that it is safe, stable, cheap, readily available and, most importantly, has a partition coefficient unaffected by varying levels of lipid and water and hence is unlikely to change with age or cerebral oedema.[8,9] However, the original Kety–Schmidt technique for measuring CBF has a number of limitations.[10–12] Timely arterial and jugular bulb blood samples are required. In order to reduce extracranial contamination, the position of the jugular bulb catheter must be confirmed radiographically with the tip at the level of and just medial to the mastoid bone. The Van Slyke manometric technique for measuring N_2O concentration in blood, used in the original experiments, required large volumes of blood and an experienced operator has now been replaced by more efficient, less operator-dependent methods for measuring N_2O concentration. These include gas chromatography and infrared spectroscopy.[13,14]

Finally, CBF calculated by this technique represents the mean blood flow from the area of the brain (plus some extracranial tissues) draining into the particular jugular venous bulb being sampled: the ipsilateral cerebral hemisphere. Therefore, the Kety–Schmidt method of CBF measurement is unable to discriminate between grey and white matter and is insensitive to regional changes in flow.[15]

RADIOACTIVE TRACER CLEARANCE TECHNIQUES

As an extension to Kety's work, the introduction of radioisotope techniques for the measurement of CBF allowed the progression from global CBF measure-

ments to two-dimensional maps of cortical blood flow.[2,16,17] The radioactive isotope (initially [85]krypton, now replaced with [133]xenon) dissolved in saline is injected into the internal carotid artery and the radioactivity is measured using a number of scintillation counters placed externally over the scalp.[18] By using tracers which are relatively insoluble in blood and so are eliminated in one passage through the lungs, the arterial concentration is zero during the period of measurement. The ^{133}Xe is taken up into the brain and, like nitrous oxide, this radioactive inert gas enters and leaves depending on its physical properties (diffusion and solubility). Hence, following injection, it will distribute and rapidly equilibrate throughout the brain tissue. After completion of injection, CBF can then be measured by the exponential pattern of clearance of the gas from the brain and hence from the body. Scintillation crystals placed externally over the scalp, so that each counter looks at a defined volume of brain, record the γ-emissions of [133]Xe. The signals from the crystals are fed through pulse height analysers and clearance curves are created. Mean blood flow through the volume of brain 'seen' by each crystal is thus:

$$Flow \ (ml/g/min) = \frac{\lambda . (Hmax - H10)}{A}$$

where λ = brain-blood partition coefficient, Hmax = maximal height of the clearance curve, H10 = height at 10 min, A = area under clearance curve.

In humans, when clearance curves are plotted on a semilogarithmic scale, two rates of exponential decay representing flow through grey and white matter are

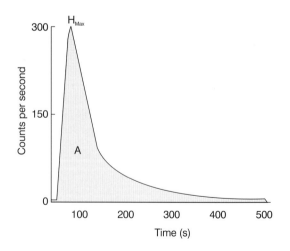

Figure 6.2   Measurement of CBF using intracarotid injection of [133]Xe. Blood flow is calculated from the maximal height (H_{max}) and integration of the area under the curve (A).

identified. Using a process termed 'exponential stripping', it is possible to identify the individual components of blood flow.

The inert gas clearance method can be applied quite easily to the bedside measurement of CBF and portable units are available. The technique is relatively simple and is reliable and reproducible. Patient and operator radiation exposure is low, enabling repeated studies on a patient, and since ^{133}Xe has a low solubility in blood and hence is rapidly cleared from it, further studies can be performed within approximately 30 min.[18] An obvious advantage of this method over the Kety–Schmidt technique is the absence of repeated blood sampling. Other advantages include the ability to calculate either the 'mean' flow value from height/area under the curve analysis or more specific regional flow rates by exponential stripping. The accuracy and specificity of this method depend on the number and size of externally placed detectors.[19] With a larger number of detectors (up to 254 detectors have been used), it is possible to measure flow in discrete lesions and detection of even small changes in blood flow associated with functional brain activation is possible.

Disadvantages of the clearance technique for bedside CBF measurement include the necessity for carotid artery puncture, potential inaccuracies from variations in the partition coefficient of ^{133}Xe in normal or abnormal brain tissue,[20–22] and the 'look-through' artefact phenomenon,[23] where the external detectors pick up highly perfused brain tissue but not ischaemic areas.

The inert gas clearance techniques have been modified over the years to reduce the disadvantages and enhance their applicability in the bedside measurement of CBF. The radioactive isotope commonly used is ^{133}Xe because of its short half-life and its γ-emissions, which are easily detected by scintillation counters. The method of administration of the radioactive isotope has also been altered to either the less hazardous intravenous route[24] or the non-invasive inhalation route.[25] Both approaches use the same external detectors as with the intraarterial approach, applying the same principles and theory. These routes of administration of xenon have reduced morbidity over the intraarterial route and certainly the inhalation technique is relatively non-invasive. In addition, with the advance of technology, the reduction in size of apparatus and microprocessor-based computers, equipment has become far more portable and user friendly for application in the intensive care unit or the ward.

However, the non-invasive techniques are not without their disadvantages. As well as exposing the whole body to radiation, inhalation of radioactive xenon distorts the clearance curves because of isotope recirculation. This necessitates the measurement of end-tidal ^{133}Xe and performing a correction computation which accounts for this recirculation. The presence of radioactive isotope in the scalp and extracranial tissues requires a further correction before accurate estimations of CBF are possible.

JUGULAR VENOUS BULB OXIMETRY

Jugular venous bulb oximetry, first described in 1927 and frequently used in the intensive care of patients with brain injury,[26] can also be utilized as a bedside tool to estimate CBF.[27–29] Cerebral blood flow and metabolism are closely coupled. Therefore, during periods of constant cerebral metabolism, CBF can be determined from the arteriovenous oxygen content difference across the cerebral circulation $(AVDO_2)$.[30,31] The $AVDO_2$ can be measured using a Co-oximeter or it can be calculated using the equation:

$$AVDO_2 = CaO_2 - CjvO_2 = [Hb \times 1.39 \times SaO_2 + (.003 \times PaO_2)] - [Hb \times 1.39 \times SjvO_2 + (.003 \times PjvO_2)]$$

where CaO_2 is the arterial oxygen content, $CjvO_2$ the jugular venous content, Hb the haemoglobin concentration, SaO_2 the arterial oxygen saturation, PaO_2 the arterial partial pressure of oxygen, $SjvO_2$ the jugular venous oxygen saturation and $PjvO_2$ the jugular venous partial pressure of oxygen.

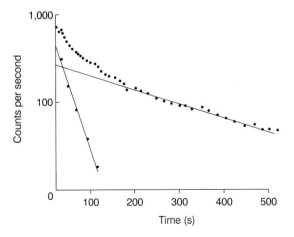

Figure 6.3   Compartmental analysis of CBF using a semilogarithmic plot. The curve shows flow through grey and white matter or fast and slow components respectively.

Although this simple, relatively non-invasive method for estimating CBF can act as an 'early warning device' for cerebral ischaemia, particularly in head-injured patients undergoing mechanical ventilation, the technique has several limitations. $AVDO_2$ is a global measure that cannot reliably detect regional ischaemia. Although sampling from the right jugular bulb has been commonly assumed to provide the best estimate of hemispheric blood flow (the cortex is preferentially drained via the right jugular bulb),[32] this may not apply in all patients or conditions. For example, significant differences in oxygen content between the left and right jugular bulb blood have been demonstrated in head-injured patients.[33] Other factors that can affect the accuracy of CBF estimation using jugular bulb oximetry include contamination of jugular bulb blood with extracerebral blood, malpositioning of the catheter tip, speed of blood withdrawal from the catheter and the position of the patient's head.[34–39] Therefore, for best results, radiographic confirmation of catheter tip position (at the level of and just medial to the mastoid bone), withdrawal of blood at a rate < 2 ml/min and careful attention to head position are mandatory.

JUGULAR THERMODILUTION TECHNIQUE

This technique, first used to measure coronary sinus flow by Ganz et al,[40] has been successfully adapted to measure CBF with reasonable accuracy.[41–43] A catheter is placed in the jugular bulb and the position of its tip confirmed radiographically. Cold fluid is then injected at a constant rate and the resulting change in temperature measured a short distance downstream with a built-in thermistor.

Jugular venous flow, and hence CBF, are then calculated using the equation:

$$(Tb - Tm) \times Vb \times \lambda b \times \rho b =$$
$$(Tm - Ti) \times Vi \times \lambda i \times \rho i$$

(heat lost by blood) = (heat lost by indicator)

where Tb, Ti and Tm are the temperature of blood, indicator and mixture of blood and indicator respectively, Vb and Vi the volumes (ml) of blood and indicator, λb and λi the specific heat of blood and indicator, and ρb and ρi the density of blood and indicator.

If time is brought into the equation, the volumes become flows and:

$$Fb = Fi \times \frac{(\lambda i \times \rho i) \times (Tm - Ti)}{(\lambda b \times \rho b) \times (Tb - Tm)}$$

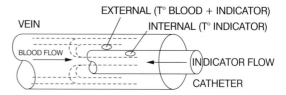

THERMISTORS

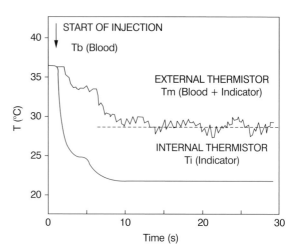

Figure 6.4   (Top trace) Diagrammatic representation of a thermodilution catheter using two thermistors which can be inserted in the jugular bulb for the measurement of CBF. (Bottom trace) This shows temperatures recorded by internal and external thermistors over a period of 30 min (Redrawn with permission from reference[43]).

If saline is used as the indicator:

$$\frac{\lambda i \times \rho I}{\lambda b \times \rho} = \frac{1.005 \times 0.997}{1.045 \times 0.87} = 1.10$$

When a preset pump determines the rate of saline infused, flow can be calculated.

This technique is simple, safe, reproducible and easy to apply at the bedside. Measurements can be repeated at frequent intervals and as the 'indicator' is non-cumulative, there is no associated morbidity for the patient or clinician.

In addition to the limitations of jugular bulb catheters for the measurement of CBF, adequate mixing of the blood and injectate at the thermistor, accurate injectate temperature recording and heat loss from the system may also affect the accurate measurement of CBF.

LASER DOPPLER FLOWMETRY

Laser Doppler flowmetry (LDF) is a relatively new technique for the measurement of local microcirculatory cerebral and spinal blood flow. The flow estimate by this technique, first described by Williams et al in 1980,[44] is based on the assessment of the Doppler shift of low-power laser light, which is scattered by the moving red blood cells (RBCs).[45,46]

Briefly, monochromatic laser light, with a wavelength above maximal absorption of haemoglobin and below maximal absorption of water (600–780 nm), is delivered to and detected from a 1mm³ volume of brain tissue by a flexible fibreoptic light guide. The laser light is scattered randomly by both static structures and moving tissue particles, mainly RBCs. Laser light reflected from stationary tissues remains unchanged in frequency, whereas light reflected by moving particles is both scattered and undergoes a frequency shift. Multiple scattering at various angles of incidence complicates and precludes the exact measurement of velocity of the moving RBCs. However, as the bandwidth of the Doppler shift frequencies increases linearly in proportion to the RBCs' velocities when tissue geometry remains constant, the mean frequency shift and the power are directly proportional to the velocity and the number of moving RBCs respectively.

As the blood cell flux is equal to the velocity of the cells multiplied by their concentration, if the concentration of the RBCs remains constant, the power of the frequency-weighted Doppler spectrum is proportional to the RBC flux through the capillary bed and, hence, CBF.[47]

The Doppler shift back-scattered light is sampled by the detecting probe, which is present in the same flexible tubing. The signal is then amplified, frequency analysed, squared, integrated and directed as a voltage signal. The laser Doppler flowmeter produces a continuous, real-time flow output which is linearly related to CBF.[48–50] Currently available instruments cannot accurately quantify absolute CBF and so relative changes are more meaningful.

Although LDF is a fast, continuous, non-radioactive bedside monitoring of CBF that can detect changes at the cellular level, there are still many practical as well as theoretical limitations to overcome. The device is invasive, requiring insertion at operation or via a burr hole. Changes in tissue perfusion are often accompanied by changes in the tissue geometry and may affect flow measurements.

Tissue density and geometry may also be altered after brain injury. Therefore, site selection is critical to the measurements due to the high degree of spatial and temporal resolution. The probes are designed to

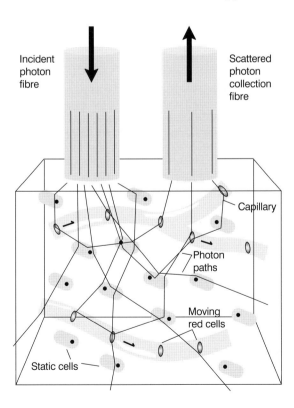

Figure 6.5   A graphic depiction of the principle of laser Doppler flowmetry (Redrawn with permission from reference[55]).

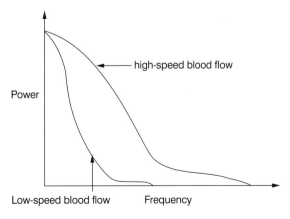

Figure 6.6   The theory behind laser Doppler flowmetry for the measurement of CBF. Doppler frequency and power depend on the speed of RBCs. Bandwidth broadens as RBC speed increases but amplitude and shape remain constant.

measure capillary blood flow and so macroscopic vessels will strongly bias readings. Similarly, as the probes will measure flow within approximately 1.5mm of the tips, the measurement area is extremely precise and localized. Therefore, caution must be exercised in making assumptions about global cerebral blood flow. Other limitations to the technique include the problems of movement artefacts: those of the patient, the probe relative to the tissue and also the individual optical fibres themselves. A further source of false readings is the presence of arterioles and venules which elevate LDF signals, so overrepresenting microvascular blood flow.[51–55]

THERMAL CLEARANCE

Thermal diffusion flowmetry is used to estimate cortical blood flow by measuring changes in a temperature gradient which exists between two gold plates within a probe applied to the cortex,[56,57] Although there are several systems available, the basic measurement technique relies on detection of the temperature gradient between the large plate generating heat and the second smaller detector plate. The difference in temperature between the two plates is inversely proportional to the thermal conductivity of the brain tissue. The temperature gradient decreases as the flow increases so that:

$$CBF = K (1/V - 1/V_0)$$

where CBF is cortical blood flow, K is a constant, V is the voltage difference between the two plates at time of measurement and V_0 is the voltage difference at no flow.[58]

The thermal diffusion CBF technique has been used to assess changes in cortical perfusion in many situations.[57,59–61] It has many advantages in that it is simple, continuous and does not use ionizing radiation. However, in common with LDF, this technique also suffers many limitations. Commercial devices available at present are not reliable enough for clinical use. Measurement of absolute flow is not possible, as voltage difference at no flow cannot be determined in the clinical setting.

NEAR INFRARED SPECTROSCOPY

Near infrared spectroscopy (NIRS) is a non-invasive method of estimating cerebral oxygenation. In common with pulse oximetry, NIRS takes advantage of the relatively translucent nature of tissue and bone

to light in the near infrared (NIR) region of the spectrum (700–1000 nm). When NIR light enters a tissue it is both scattered and absorbed. Provided the geometry of the tissue remains constant (and there is little evidence to suggest that this is the case in many situations where NIRS may be useful), the absorption of NIR light is proportional to the concentration of the chromophores (oxyhaemoglobin (HbO_2), deoxyhaemoglobin (Hb) and oxidized cytochrome aa3 ($CytO_2$)), according to the modified Beer–Lambert Law which describes optical attenuation in a highly scattering medium. 'Transmission spectroscopy', although possible in neonates, is not feasible in adults because of the large head and thick skull. By placing the optodes a few centimetres apart on the same side of the head, it is possible to measure changes in cerebral oxygenation in adults using 'reflectance spectroscopy'.[62] Despite the initial enthusiasm for this promising technology, there remain many practical as well as theoretical limitations to overcome. It is important to understand both the assumptions on which NIRS is based and the limitations of this technology in order to interpret the results correctly.

NIRS has been used as a non-invasive method of measuring changes in CBF and cerebral blood volume (CBV). Detailed explanation of the principles involved have been described elsewhere (Ch. 9). Briefly, CBF can be measured using a modification of the Fick principle. A sudden increase in SaO_2 produces a bolus of HbO_2, which acts as an arterial tracer, which is measured in the arterial system by the pulse oximeter and in the brain by NIRS. Similarly, CBV can be calculated by inducing small but slow changes in SaO_2 and measuring changes in HbO_2 and Hb by NIRS. The potential advantages of being able to measure CBF and CBV non-invasively are obvious but 30% of the data are rejected because of variations in the baseline NIR signal, MAP or end-tidal CO_2. Furthermore, data published by Owen-Reece et al suggest that the technique considerably underestimates CBF because of the optical effects of extracranial tissue.[63] Hence further validation of these techniques is required before they can be adopted as part of normal clinical practice.

TRANSCRANIAL DOPPLER ULTRASONOGRAPHY

The transcranial Doppler ultrasonography (TCD) is a non-invasive monitor which calculates red blood cells (FV) in the large vessels at the base of the brain using the Doppler shift principle.[64] The most commonly insonated vessel is the middle cerebral artery (MCA) which carries about 75–80% of the ipsilateral carotid artery blood flow and thus is representative of hemispheric CBF. TCD measures velocity and not flow and therefore, changes in FV only represent true changes in CBF when both the angle of insonation and the diameter of the vessel insonated remain constant. The angle of insonation can be kept constant by fixing the probe in position using a head strap or frame. There is also ample evidence suggesting that the diameter of the MCA does not change significantly with changes in arterial pressure, carbon dioxide partial pressure or the use of anaesthetic or vasoactive agents.[65–70] Hence, it is generally accepted that during steady-state anaesthesia, changes in FV reflect corresponding changes in cortical CBF.

TCD is covered elsewhere in this book (Ch. 8), so the details will not be repeated. TCD can be used with ease at the bedside to monitor changes in FV safely, noninvasively and without detriment to the patient or clinician. It has no associated morbidity and is a reliable, real-time monitor. However, it must be remembered that CBF indices are derived from measurements made on velocity, so that TCD findings should not be used in isolation, as with any clinical measurement, but more to complement other monitoring available in neurointensive care.

REFERENCES

1. Bouma GJ, Muizelaar JP, Choi SC et al. Cerebral circulation and metabolism after severe traumatic brain injury: the elusive role of ischemia. J Neurosurg 1991; 75: 685–693.

2. Langfitt TW, Obrist WD. Cerebral blood flow and metabolism after intracranial trauma. Prog Neurol Surg 1981; 10: 14.

3. Graham DI, Adams JH. Ischaemic brain damage in fatal head injuries. Lancet 1971; 1: 265–266.

4. Matta BF, Menon DK. Severe head injury in the United Kingdom and Ireland: a survey of practice and implications for management. Crit Care Med 1996;24: 1743–1748.

5. Kety SS, Schmidt CF. The determination of cerebral blood flow in man by the use of nitrous oxide in low concentrations. Am J Physiol 1945; 143: 53–55.

6. Kety SS, Schmidt CF. The nitrous oxide method for the quantitative determination of cerebral blood flow in man: theory, procedure and normal values. J Clin Invest 1948; 27: 476–483.

7. Kety SS, Harmel MH, Brommell HT et al. The solubility of nitrous oxide in blood and brain. J Biol Chem 1948; 173: 487–496.

8. Mapleson WW, Evans DE, Flook V. The variability of partition coefficients for nitrous oxide and cyclopropane in the rabbit. Br J Anaesth 1970; 42: 1033–1041.

9. Kozam RL, Landau SM, Cubina JM, Lukas DS. Solubility of nitrous oxide in biologic fluid and myocardium. J Appl Physiol 1970; 29: 593–597.

10. Sharples PM, Stuart AG, Aynsley-Green A et al. A practical method of serial bedside measurements of cerebral blood flow and metabolism during neurointensive care. Arch Dis Child 1991; 66: 1326–1332.

11. Gibbs EL, Lennox WG, Gibbs FA. Bilateral internal jugular blood. Comparison of A-V differences, oxygendextrose ratios and respiratory quotients. Am J Psychiatry 1945; 102: 184–190.

12. Kirsch JR, Traystman RJ, Rogers MC. Cerebral blood flow measurement techniques in infants and children. Pediatrics 1985; 75; 887–895.

13. Lawther PJ, Bates DV. A method for the determination of nitrous oxide in blood. Clin Sci 1952; 12: 91–95.

14. Swedlow DB, Lewis LE. Measurement of cerebral blood flow in children. Anesthesiology 1980; 53: S160.

15. Stocchetti N, Paparella A, Bridelli F et al. Cerebral venous oxygenation studied with bilateral samples in the internal jugular veins. Neurosurgery 1994; 34: 38–44.

16. Lassen NA, Ingvar DH. The blood flow of the cortex determined by radioactive krypton. Experientia 1961; 17: 42.

17. Ingvar DH, Lassen NA. Quantitative determination of cerebral blood flow in man. Lancet 1961; 2: 806–807.

18. Anderson RE. Cerebral blood flow Xenon-133. Neurosurg Clin North Am 1996; 7(4): 703–708.

19. Paulson OB, Cronqvist S, Risberg J et al. Regional cerebral blood flow: comparison of 8-detector and 16-detector instrumentation. J Nucl Med 1968; 10: 164–173.

20. Waltz AG, Wanek AR, Anderson RE. Comparison of analytic methods for calculation of cerebral blood flow after intracarotid injection of Xenon-133. J Nucl Med 1972; 13: 66–72.

21. Veall N, Mallett BL. The partition of trace amount of Xenon between human blood and trace tissues at 37°C. Phys Med Biol 1965; 10: 375–380.

22. Halsey JH Jr, Nakai K, Wariyar B. Sensitivity of rCBF to focal lesions. Stroke 1981; 12: 631–635.

23. Donley RF, Sundt TM Jr, Anderson RE et al. Blood flow measurements and the 'look-through' artifact in focal cerebral ischemia. Stroke 1975; 6: 121–131.

24. Obrist WD, Wilkinson WE. Regional cerebral blood flow measurements in humans by Xenon-133. Cerebrovasc Brain Metab Rev 1990; 2: 283–327.

25. Obrist WD, Thompson HK, King CH et al. Determination of regional cerebral blood flow by inhalation of Xenon-133. Circ Res 1967; 20: 124–135.

26. Meyerson A, Halloran RD, Hirsh HL. Technique for obtaining blood from the internal jugular vein and carotid artery. Arch Neurol Psychiat 1927; 17: 807–809.

27. Cruz J. Combined continuous monitoring of systemic and cerebral oxygenation in acute brain injury: preliminary observations. Crit Care Med 1993; 21: 1225–1232.

28. Robertson C, Narayan R, Gokaslan Z et al. Cerebral arteriovenous oxygen difference as an estimate of cerebral blood flow in comatose patients. J Neurosurg 1989; 70: 222–230.

29. Schneider GH, Von Helden A, Lanksch WR, Unterberg A. Continuous monitoring of jugular bulb oxygen saturation in comatose patients – therapeutic implications. Acta Neurochir 1995; 134(1–2): 71–75.

30. Baron JC, Rougemont D, Soussaline F et al. Local interrelationships of cerebral oxygen consumption and glucose utilization in normal subjects and in ischemic stroke patients: a positron-emission tomography study. J Cereb Blood Flow Metab 1984; 4: 140–149.

31. Mayberg T, Lam A. Jugular bulb oximetry for the monitoring of cerebral blood flow and metabolism. Neurosurg Clin North Am 1996; 7(4): 755–765.

32. Gibbs EL, Gibbs FA. The cross section areas of the vessels that form the torcular and the manner in which blood is distributed to the right and the left lateral sinus. Anat Rec 1934; 54: 419–426.

33. Stocchetti N, Paparella A, Bridelli F et al. Cerebral venous oxygen saturation studied with bilateral samples in the internal jugular veins. Neurosurgery 1994; 34: 38–44.

34. Andrews PJD, Dearden NM, Miller JD. Jugular bulb cannulation: description of a cannulation technique and validation of a new continuous monitor. Br J Anaesth 1991; 67: 553–558.

35. Cruz J. Contamination of jugular bulb venous oxygen measurements. J Neurosurg 1992; 77: 975–976.

36. Dearden NM, Midgeley S. Technical considerations in continuous jugular venous oxygen saturation measurement. Acta Neurochir (Wien) 1993; 59(suppl): 91–97.

37. Sheinberg M, Kanter MJ, Robertson CS et al. Continuous monitoring of jugular venous oxygen saturation in head injured patients. J Neurosurg 1992; 76: 212–217.

38. Gunn H, Matta BF, Lam AM, Mayberg TS. Accuracy of continuous jugular bulb venous oximetry during intracranial surgery. J Neurosurg Anesthesiol 1995; 7: 174–177.

39. Matta BF, Lam AM. The speed of blood withdrawal affects the accuracy of jugular venous bulb oxygen saturation measurements. Anesthesiology 1996; 86: 806–808.

40. Ganz W, Tamura K, Marcus HS et al. Measurement of coronary sinus blood flow by continuous thermodilution in man. Circulation 1971; 44: 181–195.

41. Wilson EM, Halsey JH Jr. Bilateral jugular venous blood flow by thermal dilution. Stroke 1970; 1: 348–355.

42. Van Der Linden J, Wesslen O, Ekroth R et al. Transcranial doppler-estimated versus thermodilution-estimated cerebral blood flow during cardiac operations. Influence of temperature and arterial carbon dioxide tension. J Thorac Cardiovasc Surg 1991; 102: 95–102.

43. Melot C, Berre J, Moraine JJ, Kahn RJ. Estimation of cerebral blood flow at bedside by continuous jugular thermodilution. J Cereb Blood Flow Metab 1996; 16(6): 1263–1270.

44. Williams PC, Stern MD, Bowen PD et al. Mapping of cerebral cortical strokes in Rhesus monkeys by laser Doppler spectroscopy. Med Res Eng 1980; 13: 1–4.

45. Bonner R, Nossal R. Model for laser Doppler measurements of blood flow in tissue. Appl Opt 1981; 20: 2097–2107.

46. Bonner R, Nosser R, Havlin S, Weiss GH. Model for photon migration in turbid biological media. J Opt Soc Am A 1987; 4: 423–432.

47. Shepherd AP, Oberg PA (eds). Laser-Doppler flowmetry. Kluwer Academic, Amsterdam, 1990.

48. Meyerson BA, Gunaskera L, Linderoth B et al. Bedside monitoring of regional cortical blood flow in comatose patients using laser Doppler flowmetry. Neurosurgery 1991; 29: 750–755.

49. Borgos J. Laser Doppler monitoring of cerebral blood flow. Neurol Res 1996; 18: 251–255.

50. Kirkpatrick PJ, Czosynka M, Smielewski P et al. Continuous monitoring of cortical perfusion using laser Doppler flowmetry in ventilated head injured patients. J Neurol Neurosurg Psychiatry 1994; 57: 1382–1388.

51. Rosenblaum BR, Bonner RF, Oldfield EH. Intraoperative measurement of cortical blood flow adjacent to cerebral AVM using laser Doppler velocimetry. J Neurosurg 1987; 66: 396–399.

52. Bologneses P, Miller J, Heger IM, Milhorat TH. Laser-Doppler flowmetry in neurosurgery. J Neurosurg Anesthesiol 1993; 5(3): 151–158.

53. Arbit E, DiResta GR, Bedford RF et al. Intraoperative measurement of cerebral tumour blood flow with laser Doppler flowmetry. Neurosurgery 1989; 24: 166–170.

54. Richards HK, Czosnyka M, Kirkpatrick P, Pickard JD. Estimation of laser Doppler flux biological zero using basilar artery flow velocity in the rabbit. Am J Physiol 1995; 268: 213–217.

55. Arbit E, DiResta GR. Application of laser Doppler flowmetry in neurosurgery. Neurosurg Clin North Am 1996; 7(4): 741–748.

56. Carter LP, Atkinson JR. Cortical blood flow in controlled hypotension as measured by thermal diffusion. J Neurol Neurosurg Psychiatry 1973; 36: 906–913.

57. Carter LP, White WL, Atkinson JR. Regional cortical blood flow at craniotomy. Neurosurgery 1978; 2: 223–229.

58. Carter LP, Erspamer R, Bro WJ. Cortical blood flow: thermal diffusion versus isotope clearance. Stroke 1981; 12: 513–518.

59. Sioutos P, Carter LP, Hamilton AJ et al. Intraoperative measurement of peritumoral regional cortical cerebral blood flow. Oncol Reports 1996; 3: 593–596.

60. Sioutos PJ, Orozco JA, Carter LP et al. Continuous regional cerebral cortical blood flow monitoring in head-injured patients. Neurosurgery 1995; 36: 943–950.

61. Weinand ME, Carter LP, Patton DD et al. Long-term surface cortical cerebral blood flow monitoring in temporal lobe epilepsy. Neurosurgery 1994; 35: 657–664.

62. Elwell CE, Owen-Reece H, Cope M et al. Measurement of adult cerebral haemodynamics using near infrared spectroscopy Acta Neurochir 1993; 599(suppl): 74–80.

63. Owen-Reece H, Elwell CE, Harkness W et al. Use of near infrared spectroscopy to estimate cerebral blood flow in conscious and anaesthetised patients. Br J Anaesth 1996; 76: 43–48.

64. Aaslid R (ed). Transcranial doppler sonography. Springer-Verlag, New York, 1986.

65. Giller CA, Bowman G, Dyer H et al. Cerebral arterial diameters during changes in blood pressure and carbon dioxide during craniotomy. Neurosurgery 1993; 32: 737–741.

66. Kirkham FJ, Padayachee TS, Parsons S et al. Transcranial measurements of blood flow velocities in the basal arteries using pulsed Doppler ultrasound: velocity as an index of flow. Ultrasound Med Biol 1986; 12: 15–21.

67. Newell WD, Aaslid R, Lam AM et al. Comparison of flow and velocity during dynamic autoregulation testing in humans. Stroke 1994; 25: 793–797.

68. Huber P, Handa J. Effects of contrast material, hypercapnia, hyperventilation, hypertonic glucose and papaverine on the diameter of the cerebral arteries – angiographic determination in man. Invest Radiol 1967; 2: 17–32.

69. Matta BF, Lam AM. Isoflurane and desflurane do not dilate the middle cerebral artery appreciably. Br J Anaesth 1995; 74: 486P–487P.

70. Matta BF, Mayberg TS, Lam AM. The effect of halothane, isoflurane, and desflurane on cerebral blood flow velocity during propofol-induced isoelectric electroencephalogram. Anesthesiology 1995; 83: 980–985.

7

MONITORING INTRACRANIAL PRESSURE

Marek Czosnyka

INTRODUCTION

Intracranial pressure (ICP) monitoring is now widely accepted as central to the management of patients with head trauma because cerebral perfusion pressure (CPP) targeted therapy improves outcome after brain injury.[1] ICP measurements are used to estimate CPP using the formula:

Mean CPP = mean arterial blood pressure (MAP) – Mean ICP

CPP represents the pressure gradient acting across the cerebrovascular bed and is a factor in the regulation of cerebral blood flow (CBF).[2,3] In order to avoid overestimation of CPP, the arterial pressure transducer should be positioned at the level of the external auditory meatus and not at the level of the heart, particularly when the patient's head is elevated.

MEASUREMENT TECHNIQUES

In adults, the normal ICP under resting conditions is between 0 and 10 mmHg, with 15 mmHg being the upper limit of normal. Active treatment is instituted if ICP exceeds 25 mmHg for more than 5 min, although a treatment threshold 15 mmHg has been suggested to improve outcome.[5]

The gold standard of ICP monitoring remains the measurement of intraventricular fluid pressure either directly or via a CSF reservoir, with the opportunity to exclude zero drift.[6] Subdural and epidural fluid-filled catheters are less accurate when ICP exceeds 30 mmHg, but are associated with a lower risk of infection, epilepsy and haemorrhage than ventricular catheters.[7,8] The more recently introduced micro-transducers are either silicon chips with diffused pressure-sensitive resistors forming a bridge or are dependent on fibreoptic technology.[9] These transducers, which include the Camino OLM ICP Monitor (Heyer-Schulte Neuro Care), the Codman Microsensor ICP Transducer (Codman and Shurtlef Inc., USA) and the Ventrix ICP Monitoring Catheter Kit (Heyer-Schulte Neuro Care), can be placed in the ventricle, brain parenchyma, subarachnoid and epidural spaces and have been shown to be comparable to fluid-filled catheters for the measurement of ICP.[10,11] In addition to the very low zero drift over long periods of monitoring, very good frequency response and stable linearity, microtransducers are associated with a lower risk of infection.[12–16] Because of its superior performance in terms of zero and temperature drift, ICP waveform analysis and ease of integration into other bedside monitoring devices, the Codman Microsensor ICP Transducer is preferred in our unit.

DETERMINANTS OF ICP

The mechanisms responsible for ICP within the skull vault are complex.[4] The components that make up the intracranial contents are: the brain bulk (80%), blood volume (5%) and the cerebrospinal fluid (CSF) (15%). As the skull is a rigid box, any increase in volume in any of the components will lead to a rise in the intracranial pressure. This pressure–volume relationship is commonly referred to as the intracranial compliance curve.[20,22,23] Small increases in intracranial volume can be partially compensated for by translocation of CSF into the spinal subarachnoid space and compression of the venous blood volume, but this compensatory mechanism is easily exhausted and further increases in intracranial content will lead to a rise in ICP and, hence, concomitant reductions in CPP. When rises in ICP are sustained, secondary neuronal injury ensues.

Although intracranial pressure is often assumed to be uniform within the skull, pressure gradients, which may be clinically significant, may exit between different parts of the injured brain. Furthermore, changes in intracranial compliance affect not only the mean value of ICP but also the frequency response for the intracranial cavity, defined as the intracranial transfer factor. Therefore, the presence of mass lesions or increased ICP changes the response of the ICP waveform to a given arterial pressure waveform input.[19,38]

ICP MONITORING

INTERPRETATION OF RAW DATA

In the absence of disease, ICP may rise by 50 mmHg during coughing or sneezing without noticeable neurologic impairment. Therefore, it is the interaction of raised ICP with other intracranial pathology which produces the pathologic consequences, as opposed to the rise in ICP *per se*. Different ICP patterns are associated with different pathologic processes. These include patterns describing tends in mean ICP over minutes (Lundberg waves A, B and C),[17] and changes in ICP waveforms. The patterns of ICP most commonly observed are described below.

Low and stable pressure

This pattern is characterized by low ICP (mean value 15 mmHg) and low pulse amplitude with a relatively stable mean ICP value over time (Fig. 7.1). This pattern

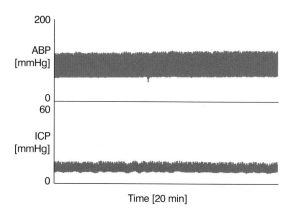

Figure 7.1   Example of recording of intracranial pressure (ICP) and arterial blood pressure (ABP) in patient following head injury with low and well-stabilized ICP.

is commonly seen in the first 6–8 h after head injury in those with CT scan showing no space-occupying lesions with little or no swelling and is usually associated with good outcome.

Elevated and stable pressure

Mean ICP >20 mmHg that is stable with very limited expression of the slow vasogenic waves are the hallmarks of this pattern (Fig. 7.2). The presence of this pattern after head injury may be indicative of posttraumatic acute hydrocephalus (moderate amplitude of pulse waveform of specific triangle shape; Fig. 7.2A) or generalized brain swelling (in this case a pulse wave is usually lower with a rather blunt peak; Fig. 7.2B).

CSF pressure waves

Lundberg described three types of cyclic CSF pressure waves: A, B and C.[17] Cyclical relatively regular waves with frequency from 20 s to 2 min are often classified as 'B' waves. These waves of limited amplitude (up to 3 mmHg) can be seen in normal subjects. When the amplitude increases above 5–8 mmHg they clearly manifest intracranial pathology, either diffused or focal, reducing pressure–volume compensatory reserve[15] Systems exhibiting dominant fast vasogenic waves are undoubtedly unstable. Pulse amplitude of ICP increases on the tops of these waves (Fig. 7.3).

The most famous 'A' wave, or what has been known as the plateau wave, is a slow vasogenic wave which may produce gross intracranial hypertension above 40–80 mmHg, dramatically reducing CPP and causing cerebral ischaemic insults in a matter of minutes (Fig. 7.4). These waves may be the result of a 'vasodilatory cascade' initiated by a reduction in CPP.[18,19] The initial reduction in CPP is the result of spontaneous decrease in arterial blood pressure which leads to cerebral vasodilatation and an increase in cerebral blood volume, ICP and a further decrease in CPP. The cascade then continues to produce more vasodilatation and reduction in CPP until maximal cerebral vasodilatation with an ICP plateau. This positive feedback may be reversed by increasing arterial blood pressure, leading to cerebral vasoconstriction, reduction in cerebral blood volume and a decrease in ICP. However, despite the attractiveness of this theory, these so-called 'spontaneous' reductions in arterial blood pressure are not always easy to detect (see

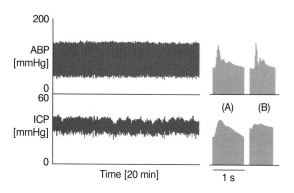

Figure 7.2   Example of recording of intracranial pressure (ICP) and arterial blood pressure (ABP) in patient who had predominantly well-stabilized ICP with increased mean value (35 mmHg). (Right) Two patterns of ICP pulse waveform: triangle shape, specific for acute hydrocephalus (A); blunt top, specific for brain swelling or space-occupying lesion (B).

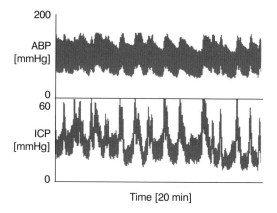

Figure 7.3   Example of fast (period around 1 min) and very deep (amplitude 35 mmHg) vasogenic waves recorded in Intracranial Pressure (ICP). The same frequency and similar amplitude of waves can be seen in recording of arterial blood pressure (ABP). Waves in both signals are obviously phase shifted.

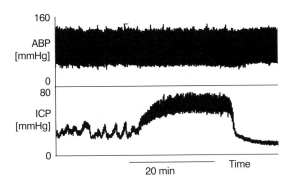

Figure 7.4 Example of plateau wave of intracranial pressure (ICP). Note fast vasogenic waves (as in Fig. 7.3 but of smaller amplitude) preceding the plateau increase in ICP.

example on Fig. 7.4). Nevertheless, regardless of the underlying mechanism, plateau waves result in severe intracranial hypertension which increases secondary ischaemic insults. Plateau waves can last several minutes (or even hours) with pulse amplitude usually rising steeply in line with an increase in mean ICP.

Refractory intracranial hypertension

This uncontrollable increase in ICP often results in structural brain shifts and herniation within the cranium. Mean ICP may increase to well above 80 mmHg as a result of rapid brain swelling over a period of few hours. This increase in ICP is commonly accompanied by a reduction in pulse amplitude and a gradual increase in arterial blood pressure (Cushing's response). The moment of brainstem herniation is commonly marked by a rapid decrease in arterial blood

pressure, a rise in a heart rate and a terminal decrease in CPP to negative values (Fig. 7.5).

C waves occur at the rate of 4–5 per min with the ICP and systemic variations completely in sync, with minimal variations in CPP with these waves. These waves are of limited duration and amplitude and therefore are probably of limited clinical importance.

ANALYSIS OF PULSE WAVEFORMS

In 1953, Ryder et al reported that an increase in ICP pulse waveform accompanied elevations in mean ICP.[20,21] Based on these observations, Langfitt et al, Lofgren et al[22] and Marmarou et al[23] introduced the monoexponential model of cerebrospinal pressure–volume relationship (the pressure–volume curve). Briefly, this model predicts that the intracranial pressure change in response to an increase in cerebral blood volume as a result of one heart contraction is dependent on the resting ICP, with higher resting ICP producing greater pressure increases for a given volume of blood. In other words, the intracranial compliance is reduced as the resting ICP increases. Although this model, modified slightly in 1986 by Van Eijndhoven and Avezaat,[24] has been widely adopted, it remains unclear which variable should be expressed on the x-axis of the pressure–volume curve: net intracranial volume, its absolute change in intracranial volume, as Lofgren et al[22] and Marmarouet al[23] suggested, or the volume of one selected compartment.

The intracranial amplitude–pressure relationship is further complicated when the Monro–Kellie doctrine is considered.[25] Briefly, this hypothesis states that changes in any of the three components of the intracranial space – brain, CSF or blood – will necessitate compensatory

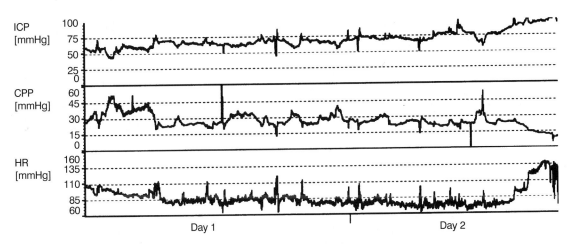

Figure 7.5 Example of two-day monitoring of patient who had a course of refractory intracranial hypertension. Patient died on day 2. This was marked by a final decrease in CPP below 30 mmHg and an increase in heart rate (HR).

changes in the volume of one or more of the other compartments if the ICP is to remain constant. This would imply that each pulsatile increase in cerebral arterial blood volume be compensated for by a reciprocal change in CSF volume or brain tissue. The mean time for such a change to be accomplished ranges from a few to over 30 min, depending on whether this involves simple translocation of CSF or extra- or intracellular brain tissue change.[19,26] Limited compensatory reserve is provided by the pulsatile CSF flow through the foramen magnum to the more compliant lumbar subarachnoid space. However, when this pathway is obstructed, in patients suffering from non-communicating hydrocephalus or head injuries with compressed ventricles, it is interesting that this only alters the gradient and not the linear character of the amplitude–pressure relationship.[26] Therefore, the rapid, pulse-related inflow of the arterial blood can be compensated for by an equivalent outflow of the venous blood.[25] Because of the different time profiles of arterial pulsatile inflow and the venous outflow, the temporal increase in total blood volume produces the pressure response observed as the amplitude of the ICP pulse waves. Therefore, delays in venous outflow produce rises in intracerebral blood volume, thus increasing the amplitude of ICP pulse waves. These findings have been reaffirmed by Chan et al[27] and Nelson et al[28] who reported increases in the amplitude of pulsatile blood inflow as the CPP decreases.

Therefore, the exponential shape of the pressure–volume relationship is not the only factor influencing the magnitude of ICP pulse waves in head injured patients.[29] The four simultaneously acting mechanisms are:

1. the gradient of the pressure–volume curve equivalent to the brain elasticity, which increases with mean ICP;
2. the pulsatile inflow of arterial blood that increases with falling CPP or changing arterial pulse pressure;
3. the delay between arterial inflow and venous outflow profiles that varies with ICP;
4. the delay between arterial blood inflow and CSF outflow through the foramen magnum to the lumbar CSF space.

In order to examine the short-term relationship between mean ICP and pulse amplitude (AMP), we developed a computer program which linearly correlates the mean ICP and AMP.[30,31] The linear correlation coefficient RAP (R=symbol of correlation, A=amplitude, P=pressure) describes the relationship between pulse amplitude of ICP and mean ICP value over short periods of time (1–3 min).[30] When RAP is

positive, changes in AMP are in the same direction as changes in mean ICP. When the RAP is negative, the change in AMP is reciprocal to those in mean ICP value. Lack of synchronization between fast changes in amplitude and mean ICP is depicted by a RAP of 0.

There are several advantages to using this method to describe the relationship between amplitude and mean value of ICP. The coefficient has a normalized value from −1 to +1 so comparison between patients is straightforward. Because the RAP coefficient is calculated using the fundamental harmonic of ICP pulse wave, a wide bandwidth pressure transducer is not necessary and a relatively inexpensive subdural catheter connected to an external membrane transducer can be used.

Another potential application of this model is in predicting outcome after severe head injury. When RAP is examined in individual patients, it can be clearly seen that as the mean ICP increases, the linear correlation between AMP and mean ICP becomes distorted by an upper breakpoint, as seen in Figure 7.6. This breakpoint is always associated with a decrease in RAP coefficient from around +1 to negative values.

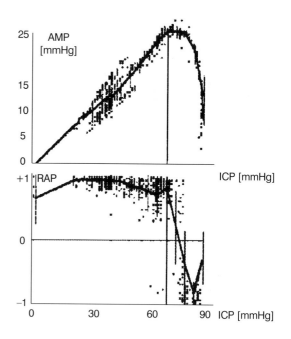

Figure 7.6   Pulse amplitude of ICP (AMP=fundamental harmonic component) increases with mean ICP until critical threshold is reached, above which it starts to decrease (upper graph). The correlation coefficient between AMP and ICP (RAP – bottom graph) marks this threshold by decreasing from positive to negative values. (Redrawn from reference[31] with permission.)

A similar relationship between AMP and ICP has been demonstrated in a group of severely head-injured patients.[31] In patients who had a favourable outcome, AMP usually increased when ICP increased from 5 to 25 mmHg (Fig. 7.7A), above which the AMP increased even faster with increases in ICP. In patients with poor outcome (dead or in persistent vegetative state), AMP also increased when ICP increased from 5 to 30 mmHg, but further increase in ICP >40 mmHg resulted in no more increase or a fall in AMP (Fig. 7.7B).

Another interesting relationship is delineated when RAP is plotted against ICP in this group of patients. In those patients with good and moderate outcome, the RAP is usually low with a tendency to increase towards +1 when ICP increases >10 mmHg (Fig. 7.8A). In patients who died, the RAP reached a maximum at ICP about 20 mmHg and then decreased rapidly,

reaching a negative value as the ICP increased towards 50 mmHg (Fig. 7.8B). Furthermore, in all patients who died after a course of gross intracranial hypertension, RAP either decreased from around +1 to 0 or negative values before brainstem herniation (Fig. 7.9A) or was permanently low in spite of ICP >20 mmHg (Fig. 7.9B).

The correlation between the amplitude of the pulse wave and mean ICP is a time-dependent phenomenon and an inverse correlation is almost always seen on top of plateau waves.[30,32,33] This has been suggested as the point of maximal vasodilatation. Rosner and Coley[19] postulated that plateau waves were the result of maximal vasodilatation by the so-called 'vasodilatory cascade'. However, it is not always possible to detect this phenomenon by plotting an amplitude versus mean ICP curve. During plateau waves, when cerebral vasodilatation is responsible for the rise in ICP,[21] the upper breakpoint of the AMP–ICP curve is hardly detectable as ICP rises only up to the level of maximal vasodilatation but never crosses this threshold.

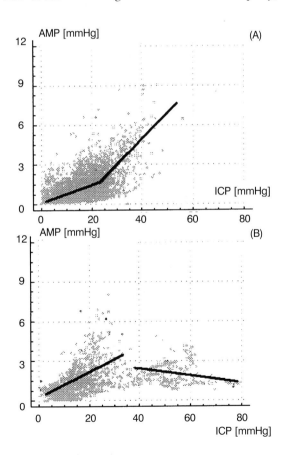

Figure 7.7   Scatterplots of AMP versus ICP from 52 head-injured patients studied in reference[31]. Straight lines show sections of consistent linear model. (A) Patients with good/moderate outcome. (B) Patients with fatal outcome (dead or persistently vegetative) (Reproduced from reference[31] with permission.)

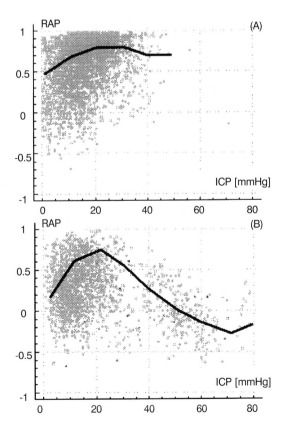

Figure 7.8   Scatterplots of RAP versus ICP. Dark lines show empirical regression curve. (A) Patients with good/moderate outcome. (B) Patients with fatal outcome (Reproduced from reference[31] with permission.)

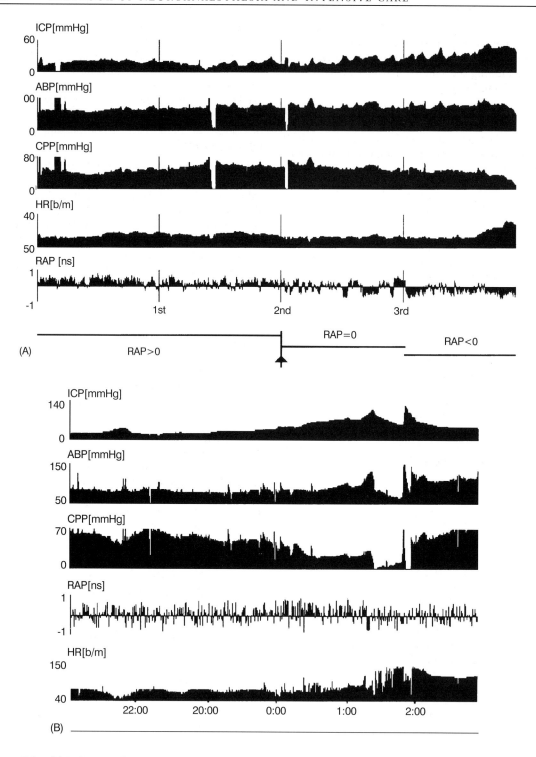

Figure 7.9   (A) Patient aged 18. Time average RAP decreased towards 0 on the second day after injury, despite mean CPP >65 mmHg. On the third day ICP increased, demonstrating strong vasogenic waves (plateau). Time average RAP became negative. Brainstem herniation was confirmed on day 4 after injury. (B) Boy aged 15, Glasgow Coma Scale 3 on admission. The RAP coefficient was oscillating around 0 from the very beginning of monitoring, despite gross intracranial hypertension. Patient died around 1.00 am (Reproduced from reference[31] with permission.)

Therefore, the amplitude of ICP seldom starts to decrease significantly at the plateau of the wave. In contrast, RAP always decreases significantly at this point, indicating the state of maximal vasodilatation (see Figs 7.6 and 7.9).

Therefore, in conclusion, when ICP increases to very high values, the decrease in RAP from +1 to zero or negative often precedes the final decrease in ICP pulse amplitude and is a sign of impending brainstem herniation.

ANALYSIS OF VARIATION OF ICP CAUSED BY CENTRAL VASOCYCLING

Arterial blood pressure fluctuations are frequently transmitted to the intracranial pressure.[34,35,36] However, the time relationship between blood pressure and ICP waves is complex and influenced by compliance of the arterial walls, muscular basal tone and cerebrovascular resistance.[37,38]

Cerebrovascular pressure reactivity describes the ability of the cerebral circulation to change the basal tone of smooth muscle in arterial walls in response to changes in transmural pressure. This mechanism is responsible for cerebral autoregulation. When cerebral autoregulatory reserve is exhausted and cerebral blood flow is no longer stable, vessels may continue to react to further reductions in perfusion pressure.[39,40] Hence, vascular pressure reactivity may extend beyond the range of the normal cerebral blood flow autoregulatory range.[41]

Vascular pressure reactivity can be derived continuously by analysing the transmission of the heart pulse from the arterial blood pressure to the ICP waveform.[14,38] Because the time constant of the autoregulatory response is much longer than a heart cycle, very precise signal processing is necessary if this is to be achieved in clinical practice.[3] Deriving this information from transmission of the respiratory wave, almost always present in the arterial blood pressure signal in ventilated patients, is very complex since both arterial and venous factors contribute to the respiratory wave seen in ICP. Slow fluctuations lasting from 30 s to a few minutes are almost always present in arterial blood pressure[36,37,41] and their rate of change is usually sufficiently long to provoke a noticeable vasomotor response. Hypothetically, providing the cerebrovascular pressure reactivity is intact, an increase in arterial blood pressure should produce vasoconstriction, a decrease in cerebral blood volume and, if brain compliance is limited, a decrease in ICP.[42] If reactivity is disturbed an increase in arterial blood pressure would passively increase the cerebral blood volume and subsequently ICP. A detailed description

of the methodology and its clinical utility has been given elsewhere.[34,35,43] System analysis using a cross-correlation function, which characterizes the time sequence between coherent slow waves in blood pressure and ICP, has recently been proposed.[44] We used the simplified Pressure Reactivity Index (PRx) to investigate time responses to intracranial hypertension or changes in mean arterial blood pressure in head-injured patients.[45]

Pearson's moving correlation coefficients between 40 consecutive past samples of averaged (over 6 s periods) values of ICP and ABP can be computed. Positive PRx signifies a positive gradient of the regression line between the slow components of ABP and ICP, which we hypothesize to be associated with passive behaviour of a non-reactive vascular bed (Fig. 7.10A). A negative value of PRx reflects a normally reactive vascular bed, as blood pressure waves provoke inversely correlated waves in ICP (Fig. 7.10B). As the correlation coefficient has a standardized value (range from −1 to +1), PRx becomes a convenient index which is more suitable for comparison between patients than the gradients of the ICP–blood pressure regression lines would be. The PRx may be presented and analysed as a time-dependent variable, responding to dynamic events such as ICP plateau waves or incidents of arterial hypo- and hypertension.

During ICP plateau waves, PRx consistently increased from negative or near-zero values to positive values, which were maximal at the top of the plateau waves (Fig. 7.11A). During episodes of arterial hypotension, PRx similarly increases to positive values (Fig. 7.11B). During arterial hypertension, increases in mean ABP >110 mmHg provoked increases in PRx to positive values.

Disturbed pressure reactivity (i.e. positive PRx) correlated with lower admission GCS, poorer outcome, greater ICP and disturbed TCD-derived index of autoregulation.[44] ANOVA plots of PRx versus mean ICP and CPP presented in Figure 7.12 indicated that critical mean value of CPP for cerebrovascular pressure reactivity was around 60 mmHg in our patients. Below this breakpoint, the mean value of PRx started to increase rapidly when CPP decreased. PRx did not show any significant breakpoint versus ICP. It increased from the baseline to positive values when ICP increased above 20 mmHg.

Analysis of variance for PRx versus time following head injury demonstrated a non-specific time profile of changes in the cerebrovascular pressure reactivity in patients with favourable outcome (Fig. 7.13). By contrast, in patients with unfavourable outcome, PRx demonstrated a significantly non-uniform time

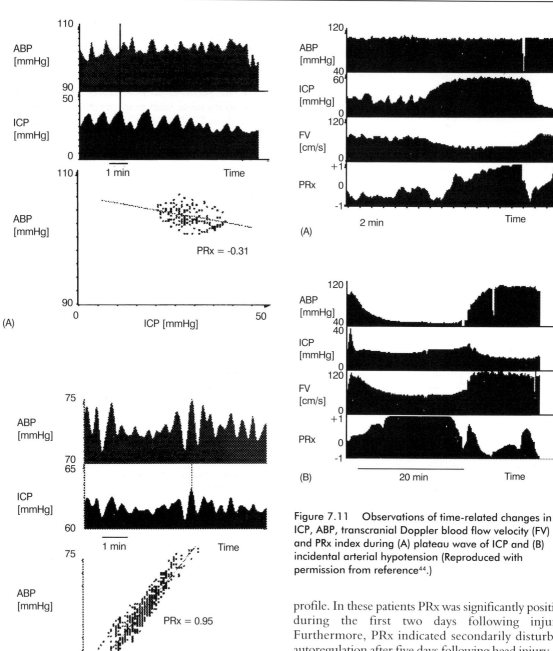

Figure 7.11   Observations of time-related changes in ICP, ABP, transcranial Doppler blood flow velocity (FV) and PRx index during (A) plateau wave of ICP and (B) incidental arterial hypotension (Reproduced with permission from reference[44].)

Figure 7.10   PRx index is calculated as linear correlation coefficient between averaged (over 6 s periods) ABP and ICP from the time window of the length of 3–4 min. Good cerebrovascular reactivity is associated with negative PRx (A), poor reactivity with positive PRx (B) (Reproduced from reference[44] with permission.)

profile. In these patients PRx was significantly positive during the first two days following injury. Furthermore, PRx indicated secondarily disturbed autoregulation after five days following head injury.

ICP AND OUTCOME FOLLOWING HEAD INJURY

Reports from almost all centres involved in head injury clinical research confirm that mean intracranial pressure correlates with outcome following head injury. The critical threshold is, by consensus, regarded as 25 mmHg. CPP was demonstrated to have an important contribution to overall outcome in the late 1980s.[4] CPP-

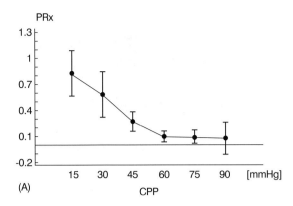

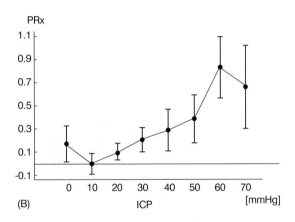

Figure 7.12   (A) Statistical relationship between PRx and CPP. (B) ICP measured in group of 82 head-injured patients (Reproduced from reference[44] with permission.)

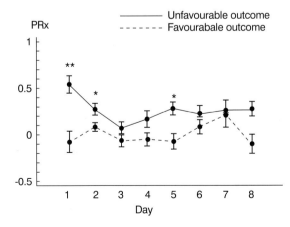

Figure 7.13   Statistical presentation of distribution of PRx in time following head injury in patients with favourable (dashed line) and unfavourable (solid line) outcome. Stars denote statistically significant positive value of PRx, seen only in patients with unfavourable outcome.

oriented therapy was introduced and popularized with a target to keep mean CPP above 70 mmHg. In recent published series,[45,46] CPP does not correlate with a poor outcome, which is a measure of success in reaching this target rather than an overall improvement in neurointensive care. ICP-derived indices such as PRx and RAP proved to correlate with outcome much better than mean ICP or CPP. This reflects an important role of additional ICP analysis in assessment of the efficacy of neurointensive care (Fig. 7.14 on p110).

REFERENCES

1. Rosner MJ, Rosner SD, Johnson AH. Cerebral perfusion pressure: management protocol and clinical results. J Neurosurg 1995; 83: 949–962.

2. Harper AM. Autoregulation of cerebral blood flow: influence of arterial blood pressure on blood flow through the cerebral cortex. J Neurol Neurosurg Psychiatry 1966; 29: 398–403.

3. Paulson OB, Strandgaard S, Edvinsson L. Cerebral autoregulation. Cerebrovasc Brain Metab Rev 1990; 2: 161–192.

4. Pickard JD, Czosnyka M. Management of raised intracranial pressure. J Neurol Neurosurg Psychiatry 1993; 56: 845–858.

5. Saul TG, Ducker TB. Effects of intracranial pressure monitoring and aggressive treatment on mortality in severe head injury. J Neurosurg 1982; 56: 498–503.

6. Marmarou A, Anderson RL, Ward JD et al. Impact of ICP instability and hypotension in patients with severe head trauma. J Neurosurg 1991; 75: 859–866.

7. Gaab MR, Heissler HE, Ehrhardt K. Physical characteristics of various methods for measuring ICP. In: Hoff JT, Betz AL (eds) Intracranial pressure VII. Springer Verlag, Berlin, 1989, pp 16–21.

8. Raabe A, Totzauer R, Meyer O, Stockel R, Hohrein D, Schoeche J. Reliability of extradural pressure measurement in clinical practice. Behavior of three modern sensors during simultaneous ipsilateral intraventricular or intraparenchymal pressure measurement. Neurosurgery 1998; 43: 306–311.

9. Ostrup RC, Luerssen TG, Marshall LF, Zornow MH. Continuous monitoring of intracranial pressure with miniaturized fiberoptic device. J Neurosurg 1987; 67: 206–209.

10. Marmarou A, Tsuji O, Dunbar JG. Experimental evaluation of a new solid state ICP monitor. In: Nagai H, Kemiya K, Ishii S (eds) Intracranial pressure IX. Springer Verlag, Berlin, 1994, pp 15–19.

11. Statham P, Midgley S, Dearden NM, McIntosh C, Miller JD. A clinical evaluation of intraparenchymal intracranial pressure transducer. In: Avezaat CJJ, Van Eijndhoven JHM, Maas AIR, Tans JTJ (eds) Intracranial pressure VIII. Springer Verlag, Berlin, 1993, pp 7–10.

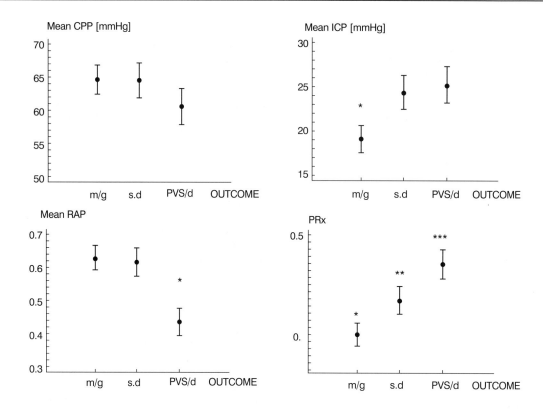

Figure 7.14   Mean values and 95% confidence limit bars of mean ICP, CPP, calculated coefficients RAP and PRx in 96 head-injured patients treated in the Addenbrooke's Hospital, Cambridge. Stars denote statistical difference (p<0.05) between outcome groups.

12. Czosnyka M, Czosnyka Z, Pickard JD. Laboratory testing of three intracranial pressure microtransducers: technical report. Neurosurgery 1996; 38: 219–224.

13. Robertson CS, Narayan RK, Contant CF et al. Clinical experience with a continuous monitor of intracranial compliance. J Neurosurg 1989; 71: 673–680.

14. Portnoy HD, Chopp M, Branch C, Shannon M. Cerebrospinal fluid pulse waveform as an indicator of cerebral autoregulation. J Neurosurg 1982; 56: 666–678.

15. Gopinath SP, Robertson CS, Narayan RK, Grossman RG. Evaluation of a microsensor intracranial pressure transducer. In: Nagai H, Kemiya K, Ishii S (eds) Intracranial pressure IX. Springer Verlag, Berlin, 1994, pp 2–5.

16. Luerssen TG, Shields PF, Vos HR, Marshall LF. Clinical experience with fiber optic brain parenchymal pressure monitor. In: Hoff JT, Betz AL (eds) Intracranial pressure VII. Springer Verlag, Berlin, 1989, pp 35–37.

17. Lundberg N. Continuous recording and monitoring of ventricular fluid pressure in neurosurgical practice. Acta Psychiat Neurol Scand 1960; 140(suppl): 36.

18. Rosner M. Pathophysiology and management of increased intracranial pressure. In: Andrews BT (ed) Neurosurgical intensive care. McGraw-Hill, New York, 1993.

19. Rosner MJ, Coley I. Cerebral perfusion pressure: a hemodynamic mechanism of mannitol and the post-mannitol hemogram. Neurosurgery 1987; 21: 147–156.

20. Ryder HW, Epsey FP, Kimbell FD. The mechanism of the change in cerebrospinal fluid pressure following an induced change in the volume of the fluid space. J Lab Clin Med 1953; 41: 428–435.

21. Langfitt TW, Weinstein JD, Kassell NF. Cerebral vaso-motor paralysis produced by intracranial pressure. Neurology (Minneap) 1965; 15: 622–641.

22. Lofgren J, Von Essen C, Zwetnow NN. The pressure–volume curve of the cerebrospinal fluid space in dogs. Acta Neurol Scand 1973; 49: 557–574.

23. Marmarou A, Shulman K, LaMorgese J. Compartmental analysis of compliance and outflow resistance of the cerebrospinal fluid system. J Neurosurg 1975; 43: 523–534.

24. Van Eijndhoven JHM, Avezaat CJJ. Cerebrospinal fluid pulse pressure and the pulsatile variation in cerebral blood volume: an experimental study in dogs. Neurosurgery 1986; 19: 507–522.

25. Avezaat CJJ, Van Eijndhoven JHM. Thesis. Jongbloed and Zoon Publishers, The Hague, 1984.

26. Czosnyka M, Batorski L, Roszkowski M et al. Cerebrospinal compensation in hydrocephalic children. Childs Nerv Syst 1993; 9: 17–22.

27. Chan KH, Miller DJ, Dearden M, Andrews PJD, Midgley S. The effect of changes in cerebral perfusion pressure upon middle cerebral artery blood flow velocity and jugular bulb venous oxygen saturation after severe brain trauma. J Neurosurg 1992; 77: 55–61.

28. Nelson RJ, Czosnyka M, Pickard JD et al. Experimental aspects of cerebrospinal haemodynamics: the relationship between blood flow velocity waveform and cerebral autoregulation. Neurosurgery 1992; 31: 705–710.

29. Nornes H, Aaslid R, Lindegaard KF. Intracranial pulse pressure dynamics in patients with intracranial hypertension. Acta Neurochir 1977; 38: 177–186.

30. Czosnyka M, Price JD, Williamson M. Monitoring of cerebrospinal dynamics using continuous analysis of intracranial pressure and cerebral perfusion pressure in head injury. Acta Neurochir 1994; 126: 113–119.

31. Czosnyka M, Guazzo E, Whitehouse H et al. Significance of intracranial pressure waveform analysis after head injury. Acta Neurochir (Wien) 1996; 138: 531–542.

32. Brawanski A, Meixensberger J, Zophel R, Ulrich W. The PA/ICP relationship in head injured patients: is there only one relationship? In: Hoff JT, Betz AL (eds) Intracranial pressure VII. Springer Verlag, Berlin, 1989, pp 634–636.

33. Price JD, Czosnyka M, Williamson M. Attempts to continuously monitor autoregulation and compensatory reserve in severe head injuries. In: Avezaat CJJ, Van Eijndhoven JHM, Maas AIR, Tans JTJ (eds) Intracranial pressure VIII, Springer Verlag, Berlin, 1993, pp 61–66.

34. Lang EW, Chesnut RM. Intracranial pressure and cerebral perfusion pressure after severe head injury. New Horizons 1995; 3: 400–409.

35. Muizelaar JP, Ward JD, Marmarou A, Newlon PG, Wachi A. Cerebral blood flow and metabolism in severely head-injured children. Autoregulation. J Neurosurg 1989; 71: 72–76.

36. Newell DW, Aaslid R, Stooss R, Reulen HJ. The relationship of blood flow velocity fluctuations to intracranial pressure B waves. J Neurosurg 1992; 76: 415–421.

37. Deley ML, Psupathy H, Griffith M, Robertson JT, Leffler CW. Detection of loss of cerebral vascular tone by correlation of arterial and intracranial pressure signals. IEEE Trans Biomed Eng 1995; 42: 420–424.

38. Piper I, Miller JD, Dearden M, Leggate JRS, Robertson I. System analysis of cerebrovascular pressure transmission: an observational study in head injured patients. J Neurosurg 1990; 73: 871–880.

39. Cold GE, Jensen FT. Cerebral autoregulation in unconscious patients with brain injury. Acta Anaesth Scand 1978; 22: 270–280.

40. Enevoldsen EM, Jensen FT. Autoregulation and CO_2 responses of cerebral blood flow in patients with acute severe head injury. J Neurosurg 1978; 48: 689–703.

41. Jones SC, Williams JL, Shea M, Easley KA, Wei D. Cortical cerebral blood flow cycling: anaesthesia and arterial blood pressure. Am J Phys 1995; 268: H569–H575.

42. Rosner MJ, Rosner SD, Johnson AH. Cerebral perfusion pressure: management protocol and clinical results. J Neurosurg 1995; 83: 949–962.

43. Turner JM, Powell D, Gibson RM, McDowall DG. Intracranial pressure changes in neurosurgical patients during hypotension induced with sodium nitroprusside or trimatephan. Br J Anaesth 1977; 49: 419–425.

44. Steinmaier R, Bauhuf C, Bondar I, Fahlbusch R. Relationship of spontaneous ICP fluctuations to cerebral blood flow and metabolism in comatose patients (abstract). J Neurotrauma 1995; 12: 403.

45. Czosnyka M, Smielewski P, Kirkpatrick P, Laing RJ, Menon D, Pickard JD. Continuous assessment of the cerebral vasomotor reactivity in head injury. Neurosurgery 1997; 41: 11–19.

46. Czosnyka M, Smielewski P, Kirkpatrick P, Menon DK, Pickard JD. Monitoring of cerebral autoregulation in head-injured patients. Stroke 1996; 27: 829–834.

8

TRANSCRANIAL DOPPLER ULTRASONOGRAPHY

Mayesh Prabhu & Basil F. Matta

INTRODUCTION

Transcranial Doppler ultrasonography (TCD), introduced in 1982 by Aaslid et al, has become one of the most useful methods of non-invasively examining cerebral haemodynamics.[1] Providing the limitations of this technology are recognized, it is possible to obtain information about the cerebral circulation which can be used in the perioperative and intensive care of the brain-injured patient (head injury) and in those at risk of cerebral ischaemia (carotid endarterectomy).

PRINCIPLES OF TCD

Transcranial Doppler ultrasonography calculates the velocity of red blood cells (FV) flowing through the large vessels at the base of the brain using the Doppler principle. This principle, first described by Christian Doppler in 1843, relates the shift in the frequency of a sound wave when either the transmitter or the receiver is moving with respect to the wave-propagating medium. The change in the frequency perceived depends on the velocity of the red blood cells and is described by the formulae:

$$f_1 = f_0 (1 + FV/c)$$
$$f_2 = f_0 (1 + 2 . FV/c)$$

where f_1 is the frequency encountered, f_0 is the transmitted frequency, c is the propagation velocity of ultrasound, f_2 is the frequency received by the stationary transducer and FV is the velocity of the reflector or the moving red cells. In order to penetrate the skull, a pulsed Doppler instrument is used with the same transducer both transmitting and receiving wave energy at regular intervals. By convention, the shift in Doppler frequency is expressed in cm/s as this allows the comparison of readings from instruments which operate at different emission frequencies. The frequency best suited for transcranial Doppler applications is in the order of 2 MHz.[2]

A constant vessel diameter and constant angle of insonation are the two main assumptions that govern the use of TCD as an indirect measure of cerebral blood flow (CBF). The velocity detected by the TCD probe as a fraction of the real velocity is dependent on the cosine of the angle of red cell insonation (TCD-measured velocity = real velocity × cosine of angle of incidence). Therefore, at 0° the TCD-calculated and true red cell velocities are equal (cosine of 0 = 1), while at 90° TCD-calculated velocity is zero irrespective of true velocity. Fortunately, the anatomic limitations of transtemporal insonation of the middle cerebral artery (MCA) are such that signal capture is only possible at narrow angles (<30°). Thus, the detected velocity is a very close approximation of the true velocity (87–100%). Furthermore, as long as the angle of insonation is kept constant by fixing the probe in position, changes in the detected velocity closely reflect changes in the true velocity.

The volume passing through a particular segment of a vessel depends on the velocity of red cells and the diameter of the vessel. Therefore, for FV to be a true reflection of CBF, the diameter of the vessel insonated must not change significantly during the measurement period. Arterial carbon dioxide tension ($PaCO_2$), blood pressure (BP), anaesthetic agents and vasoactive drugs may affect the diameter of vessel insonated. However, the basal cerebral arteries are conductance vessels and thus do not dilate or constrict as the vascular resistance changes. It has been shown angiographically that change in $PaCO_2$, one of the most important determinants of cerebrovascular resistance, has no effect on the diameter of the basal arteries.[3] Moreover, CO_2 reactivity studies using TCD have demonstrated similar values to those obtained with conventional CBF measurements.[4-6] Similarly, changes in BP have negligible influence on the diameter of the proximal segments of the basal arteries.[6,7] The effect of vasoactive drugs on cerebral conductance vessels is variable. While sodium nitroprusside and phenylephrine do not significantly affect the proximal segments of the MCA,[8,9] significant vasodilatation occurs when nitroglycerine is administered to healthy volunteers.[10]

The effect of anaesthetic agents on the diameter of the basal vessels remains controversial. The intravenous agents are devoid of direct cerebral vascular effects and it is generally accepted that these agents do not affect the diameter of the conductance vessels.[11] However, most but not all the evidence available suggests that the inhaled anaesthetics have negligible effects on the basal arteries.[12-15] Nevertheless, it is generally accepted that during steady-state anaesthesia, changes in FV reflect corresponding changes in cortical CBF.[16-20]

Intracranial pathology may affect the reliability of TCD as a measure of CBF. Cerebral vasospasm, space-occupying lesions and increases in intracranial pressure (ICP) may affect the accuracy of FV measurements.[20,21]

TCD IN CLINICAL PRACTICE

CLINICAL EXAMINATION

A complete diagnostic examination of the cerebral circulation will usually utilize the transtemporal approach through the thin bone above the zygomatic

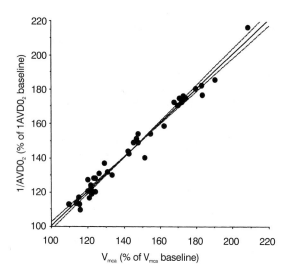

Figure 8.1   A plot of the % increase in flow velocity in the middle cerebral artery (V_{mca}) versus the % increase in cerebral blood flow equivalent (CBFE = $1/AVDO_2$, = $AVDO_2$ = arteriovenous oxygen content difference across the cerebral circulation) in 21 anaesthetized patients. Data were pooled and then subjected to linear correlation analysis. The best-fit line and 95% confidence limits are shown. (Redrawn with permission from reference[15].)

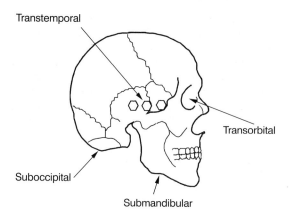

Figure 8.2   Skull ultrasonic windows: the transtemporal approach through the thin bone above the zygomatic arch to the anterior, middle and posterior cerebral arteries, the transorbital (and submandibular) approach to the carotid siphon and the suboccipital route to the basilar and vertebral arteries.

arch to the anterior, middle and posterior cerebral arteries, the transorbital approach to the carotid siphon and the suboccipital route to the basilar and vertebral arteries. However, because the probe can be easily secured in position once a signal is obtained, intraoperative monitoring usually utilizes the transtemporal route. In expert hands it is possible to transtemporally insonate the proximal segment (M1) of the MCA in over 90% of people.[2,22–24] The MCA carries about 75% of the ipsilateral carotid artery blood flow and thus is representative of hemispheric CBF. However, as the successful transmission of ultrasound through the skull is dependent on the thickness of the skull, which varies with gender, race and age, the failure rate can be as high as 20–30% in elderly black females.[25–27] The incidence of failure can be decreased by increasing the power and, in some instances, by the use of 1 MHz probes.[28] The theoretical risk of eye damage limits the use of the transorbital route and the lack of suitable means to secure the probe in position makes the suboccipital route impractical.

Transtemporal insonation will allow examination of the middle (MCA), anterior (ACA) and posterior (PCA) cerebral arteries. In each patient, the same insonation window should be used throughout the entire study period. This could be accomplished by putting a small marker at the patient's temporal region. The Doppler examination begins with the identification of the bifurcation of the intracranial portion of the internal carotid artery into the MCA and ACA according to the method described by Aaslid.[2] This bifurcation can usually be identified at a depth of 60–65 mm. The typical Doppler signal from the carotid bifurcation, which consists of images above and below the zero line of reference, represents the flow directions towards and away from the ultrasound probe of the MCA and ACA respectively. The depth of insonation is then reduced to follow the upward deflection image of the MCA flow velocity as the vessel runs towards the skull. The MCA can usually be traced up to a depth of 30 mm, which is beyond the bifurcation of the MCA into the peripheral branches. The proximal portion of the main trunk of the MCA (the M1 segment) can be located at a depth of around 45–55 mm. The depth which gives the highest velocity is usually chosen for measurement. In children, this depth is usually 10 mm less than that of adults, but the same principles apply. This method of obtaining the MCA signal eliminates the possibility of mistaking the PCA for the MCA because the PCA signal cannot be obtained at a depth less than 55 mm for anatomical reasons.

After the MCA signal is obtained, the depth of insonation is increased so that the image of the carotid bifurcation can be seen again; the depth is increased further with the probe directed slightly anteriorly so that the ACA image can be found. The first part of the ACA (the A1 segment) is recognized by a direction of flow that is away from the probe. With the identification of the ACA, the depth of insonation is decreased until the carotid bifurcation signal is obtained. The probe is then angled slightly posteriorly until the signal of the PCA is seen. The PCA can be distinguished from the MCA signal by a lower flow velocity and failure to obtain the PCA signal when the depth of insonation is decreased below 55 mm. A more detailed description of the TCD examination can be found in a standard textbook.[24]

DATA COLLECTION AND ANALYSIS

Velocity measurements

Because the volume of blood flowing through a vessel depends on the velocity of the moving cells and the diameter of vessel concerned, for a given blood flow, the velocity increases with decreases in diameter. Although CBF in ml/min per 100g of brain tissue is relatively constant, FV in the MCA ranges from 35 to 90 cm/s in the awake resting state, reflecting the variations in vessel diameter and angles of insonation between individuals examined.[2] This probably accounts for the poor correlation between absolute FV and CBF in any given population. However, during steady states, relative changes in FV accurately reflect variations in CBF.[5–19]

FV varies with age. MCA red cell velocity is lowest at birth (24 cm/s), peaks at the age of 4–6 years (100 cm/s),[25,26] and thereafter decreases steadily to about 40 cm/s during the seventh decade of life.[1,22,29] This reduction is partly due to the increase in the diameter of basal arteries which occurs with age,[30] but is mostly due to the genuine decrease in hemispheric CBF with age.[31,32]

A reduction in haematocrit has been shown to increase CBF in a linear fashion and probably accounts for the increased velocities reported in haemodilutional states.[33–35] When used in isolation, the increased FV observed in haemodilutional states may be mistaken for vessel narrowing in patients with potential arterial stenotic lesions, such as subarachnoid haemorrhage.

Hemispheric CBF and FV are 3–5% higher in females.[35,36] Although a convincing explanation for these differences in CBF and FV has not yet been found, a lower haematocrit and slightly higher arterial CO_2 tension found in premenopausal women may partly explain these increases.[29,37]

The weighted mean velocity (FV_{mean}) takes into consideration the different velocities of the formed elements in the blood vessel insonated and hence is the most physiological correlate with actual CBF. However, because of the higher signal-to-noise ratio, the maximal flow velocity (FV_{max} as depicted by the spectral outline) is generally used. Furthermore, because the flow is usually laminar as in the basal cerebral arteries, there is good correlation between the FV_{max} and FV_{mean}. The time-mean FV, displayed in most commercially available instruments, usually refers to the mean velocity of FV_{max}. The time-averaged FV_{max} is determined from the area under the spectral curve or approximated by the equation:

$$mean\ FV_{max} = [(FV_{sys} - FV_{dias})/3] + FV_{dias}$$
$$where\ FV_{sys} = systolic\ blood\ velocity,$$
$$V_{dias} = diastolic\ blood\ velocity.$$

Waveform pulsatility

Pulsatility describes the shape of the envelope (maximal shift) of the Doppler spectrum from peak systolic to end diastolic with each cardiac cycle.[38] Arterial blood pressure waveform, the viscoelastic properties of the cerebral vascular bed and blood rheology determine the FV waveform. Thus, in the absence of vessel stenosis or vasospasm and changes in arterial blood pressure and blood rheology, the pulsatility reflects the distal cerebrovascular resistance.[38,39] This resistance has been quantified by two indices: the Pulsatility Index (PI or Gosling Index) = $(FV_{sys} - FV_{dias})/ FV_{mean}$;[39] and the Resistance Index (RI or Pourcelot Index) = $(FV_{sys} - FV_{dias})/FV_{sys}$.[40] In a highly pulsatile spectrum, FV_{sys} is peaked and much greater than end FV_{dias}, while FV_{dias} greater than 50% of FV_{sys} gives a 'damped' waveform. Normal PI ranges from 0.6 to 1.1 with no significant side-to-side or cerebral interarterial differences.[41]

Although in general both PI and RI can provide information about cerebral vascular resistance, neither index provides meaningful information regarding the cause of the change, e.g. increase in PI can be due to cerebral vasoconstriction (intrinsic, as in hyperventilation), or high intracranial pressure (extrinsic from obstruction). Furthermore, PI is very sensitive to changes in heart rate and is best compared during periods of similar heart rates. The main advantage of PI is that it is dimensionless and therefore is not affected by the angle of insonation because the equation used to calculate PI has the cosine of the angle of incidence in both the numerator and denominator.

Cerebral vascular reactivity

The effect of $PaCO_2$

Cerebral vascular reactivity to CO_2 describes the near linear relationship between arterial CO_2 tension and CBF. This can be tested by observing the change in CBF in response to a change in $PaCO_2$. TCD is particularly suitable for such investigations since multiple paired measurements are taken and linear regression lines can be constructed more accurately than with a limited number of conventional blood flow measurements.[4,44,46] Moreover, both the absolute and the relative FV-$PaCO_2$ (% change in FV from baseline) relationships can be examined. The absolute CO_2 reactivity will depend on the baseline FV. Therefore, when the baseline FV is low, such as during intravenous anaesthesia, the change per kPa change in $PaCO_2$ is similarly reduced. However, when this is normalized to a FV at $PaCO_2$ of 5.3 kPa, the relative slope expressed in percentage approximates the awake value.[44] Compared to the absolute change, the percentage change in FV with change in $PaCO_2$ shows less dependence on baseline value and is therefore a more valid indicator of CO_2 reactivity and a more appropriate variable for comparison between experimental conditions.[43–46]

In normal individuals CBF (or FV) changes by approximately 20% for every kPa change in $PaCO_2$. TCD can therefore be used in many clinical situations to assess cerebral vascular reserve such as in those patients with carotid artery stenosis and after head injury. The effect of anaesthetics and vasoactive drugs on CO_2 reactivity can also be easily examined using TCD.[5,9,44,46,47]

Cerebral vasoreactivity to CO_2 can also be examined using carbonic anhydrase inhibitors. Intravenous administration of 1g of acetazolamide produces an increase in CO_2 tension and therefore should result in a concomitant increase in FV. Although this method obviates the need for hyperventilation in those patients with cardiac and respiratory disease, it only provides a unidirectional crude estimate of the cerebral vasomotor reactivity. Increasing and decreasing CO_2 tension tests both the vasodilatory and vasoconstrictive capabilities of the cerebral circulation and thus is a more 'complete' test of CO_2 reactivity.

The effect of perfusion pressure

Cerebral autoregulation, a sensitive mechanism impaired by pathologic process and inhalational anaesthesia, minimizes deviations in CBF when cerebral perfusion pressure (CPP) changes between 50 and 170 mmHg.[48–54] Cerebral autoregulation has been traditionally assessed by repeated static measurements of CBF during a period of hypotension or hypertension. In addition to the bulky equipment and/or radioactive material necessary for these measurements, the process is labour intensive and assumes that cerebral autoregulation is a uniform and slow-acting process. Furthermore, drugs used to induce hypertension or hypotension may influence autoregulation.[49]

It is now generally accepted that cerebral autoregulation is a complex process composed of at least two mechanisms operating at different rates: a rapid response sensitive to pressure pulsations followed by a slow response to changes in mean pressure.[55,56]

Conventional CBF measurement techniques, with the inability to record instantaneous changes, probably would miss these initial fast components and therefore at best can be characterized as an incomplete assessment of the cerebral autoregulatory response. Hence, TCD allows continuous measurement of the autoregulatory response and can provide insight into both the rapid and delayed components of cerebral autoregulatory mechanisms. Many methods for the assessment of cerebral autoregulation have been described and the methods most commonly employed are outlined below.

Static autoregulation

As already mentioned above, cerebral autoregulation has traditionally been assessed by repeated static measurements of CBF during a period of hypotension or hypertension. Static autoregulation can be easily tested using TCD by inducing an approximately 20 mmHg increase in mean BP (MBP) using a 0.01% phenylephrine infusion and simultaneously recording the FV. The FV and MBP recorded are then used for subsequent calculation of the estimated cerebral vascular resistance (CVRe = MBP/FV). The static rate of autoregulation or the index of autoregulation (IOR) is the ratio of percentage change in estimated CVRe to percentage change in MBP.[44] Theoretically, no change in the FV would occur if the percentage change in CVRe was equal to the percentage change in MBP. Thus, an IOR of one implies perfect autoregulation and an IOR of zero complete disruption of autoregulation. When intracranial pressure is available, cerebral perfusion pressure is substituted for MBP. Static autoregulation describes the 'slow response' in cerebral vascular resistance to changes in mean pressure.

Dynamic autoregulation

Dynamic autoregulation is tested by measuring the recovery in FV after a rapid transient decrease in MBP induced by deflation of large thigh cuffs. These large blood pressure cuffs modified with larger tubings are placed around one or both thighs and inflated to 50 mmHg above systolic pressure for 3 min, then deflated to produce an approximately 20 mmHg drop in MBP. By using an algorithm previously validated,[56,57] the FV response to the drop in blood pressure is fitted to a series of curves to determine the rate of dynamic cerebral autoregulation (dRoR). These curves are generated by a computer model of cerebral autoregulation that predicts the autoregulatory response on the

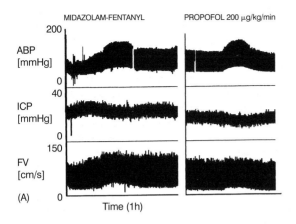

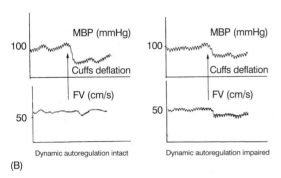

Figure 8.3   (A) Testing static autoregulation during midazolam/fentanyl sedation and propofol anaesthesia in a head-injured patient receiving intensive care. (Top tracing) Mean arterial pressure (ABP) in mmHg. (Middle tracing) Intracranial pressure (ICP in mmHg). (Bottom tracing) Blood velocity (FV) in cm/s. There is no change in FV despite the increase in ABP as a result of 0.01% phenylephrine infusion during propofol anaesthesia (right trace) autoregulation intact. The increase in ABP during midazolam-fentanyl sedation is accompanied by a similar increase in FV and ICP, indicating impaired autoregulation. (B) The recovery in blood velocity (FV cm/s) after thigh cuff deflation is 'steeper' in patients with intact (left) dynamic autoregulation (dROR). In contrast, the FV remains depressed after cuff deflation in those with impaired autoregulation during desflurane anaesthesia (right trace).

basis of the continuous blood pressure record and compares its predictions with the measured response.[55] The dRoR describes the rate of restoration of FV (%/s) with respect to the drop in MBP: in other words, the rate of change in cerebral vascular resistance or 'the fast process'.

The normal dRoR is 20%/s (i.e. process is complete within approximately 5 s).[56] The time for autoregulation to normalize FV during normocapnia occurs

well within the period of hypotension achieved with cuff deflation before the MAP returns to baseline (10–20 s).[56,57] Collection of autoregulation data in the first 10 s avoids the influence of CO_2-rich blood from the legs following thigh cuff deflation. Hypercapnia increases CBF by vasodilatation of cerebral blood vessels and reduces autoregulatory capacity.[23]

Transient hyperaemic response test

This test is performed by compressing the common carotid artery for a period of 5–8 s and observing the change in FV in the ipsilateral circle of Willis. When the carotid artery is compressed, FV decreases and the distal cerebrovascular bed dilates in response to the drop in perfusion pressure. When the compression is released, an increase in FV_{mca} is observed as a result of this dilatation, which persists until the distal cerebrovascular bed constricts to its former diameter. The compression results in this 'transient hyperaemia' only when autoregulation is intact. When autoregulation is impaired, no dilatation of the distal cerebral vascular beds occurs in response to the compression and hence, no transient hyperaemia is detected.

Although this test is reproducible and easily performed, the results depend heavily on the compression technique. The magnitude of FV drop during compression and the hyperaemia following release are dependent on the degree of occlusion and the patency of the collateral circulation at the circle of Willis.[58–60] Furthermore, in patients with carotid disease there are theoretical risks associated with the

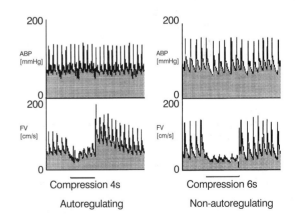

Figure 8.4   Autoregulation testing using the transient hyperaemic response test in two patients receiving intensive care. Transient hyperaemia of the MCA FV following a short-term compression of the common carotid artery indicates intact autoregulation (left) and the lack of response suggests impaired autoregulation (right). (Figure courtesy of M Czosnyka.)

manoeuvre, including the possibility of dislodging atheroma. Nevertheless, preliminary results indicate that the test may be useful in the assessment of outcome after head injury.[60]

Estimation of cerebral perfusion pressure

FV flow pattern is highly dependent on cerebral perfusion pressure. When intracranial pressure increases and cerebral perfusion pressure correspondingly decreases, a highly pulsatile FV pattern is seen. As the intracranial resistance to flow continues to increase, a progressive loss of diastolic flow to systolic spike and eventually to an oscillating flow pattern is observed. This oscillating flow pattern signifies the onset of intracranial circulatory arrest and, if not reversed, is terminal.[61-64]

The Pulsatility Index (defined either as Gosling PI (GPI), i.e. peak-to-peak amplitude of FV pulsations divided by time average FV, or 'spectral' PI (SPI), i.e. first harmonic component of FV pulsations divided by mean FV) is inversely proportional to reductions in CPP.[65,66] This inverse relationship between CPP and PI has been used to non-invasively estimate CPP.[67] By relating the first harmonic component of arterial blood pressure pulse waveform to SPI, Aaslid et al demonstrated the ability to estimate CPP ± 27 mmHg from arterial blood pressure and TCD recording.[67] An improved method of estimating CPP using mean arterial pressure, diastolic and mean blood velocities was recently published from our institution.[68] We were able to estimate CPP non-invasively with errors of estimation <10 mmHg in over 71% of the measurements compared with 52% using the formula proposed by Aaslid et al.[67,68] The accuracy of this method has been further improved with better signal acquisition (prototype tests, unpublished data, BFM). Furthermore, when used as a continuous monitor, it was able to detect real-time changes in 'true' CPP. Bilateral monitoring may also provide useful information about side-to-side variations in perfusion that in turn may allow clinical decisions to be made earlier.

There are obvious advantages in being able to estimate CPP non-invasively. This form of monitoring is particularly useful in centres where ICP monitoring is not routinely used or in patients in whom ICP monitoring is deemed not indicated and yet the patient may have decreased intracranial compliance (e.g. after a concussion or mild closed head injury). Patients awaiting transfer to a neurosurgical centre from the referring district general hospital may also benefit from the availability of this device. The role of TCD in non-invasively estimating cerebral perfusion is promising.

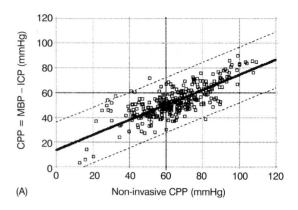

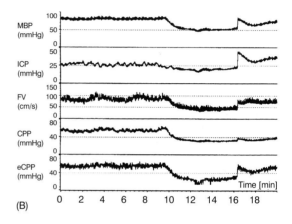

Figure 8.5   (A) Relationship between our estimation of CPP (non-invasive CPP) and measured CPP (ABP-ICP). Non-invasive CPP = ABP * FV_{dia}s/ FV_{mean}. Dashed lines are 95% confidence limits. (B) A representative trace of arterial blood pressure (ABP), ICP, FV and eCPP during an episode of hypotension in a head-injured patient. ABP = mean arterial blood pressure (mmHg); ICP = intracranial pressure (mmHg); FV = flow velocity in the middle cerebral artery (cm/s); eCPP = non-invasive cerebral perfusion pressure.

TCD as a component in multimodality monitoring

TCD is an integral component of multimodality monitoring.[69] When it is used in conjunction with intracranial pressure measurement, jugular venous bulb oximetry (SjO_2), near infrared spectroscopy, laser Doppler flowmetry (LDF) and brain microelectrodes, important minute-by-minute information can be obtained in the brain-injured patient. Multimodal data are captured and examined at the bedside or subsequently in the light of available clinical information. The effect of interventions or pathological processes on cerebral haemodynamics can be viewed from several angles. The main factor controlling the ability to process such information is data acquisition. Up to 50% of data collected are often discarded because of poor quality (unpublished data, BFM). Nevertheless, time trends of multiple parameters get us one step closer to observing the 'whole picture' of secondary ischaemic brain insults. More detailed information on multimodality monitoring can be found in Chapter 11.

TCD IN ANAESTHESIA AND INTENSIVE CARE

CAROTID ARTERY DISEASE

Carotid endarterectomy (CEA) can only be justified if the risk of perioperative stroke does not exceed the risk of stroke from the disease process. Therefore, maximum benefit of this procedure can only be realized if perioperative cerebral perfusion is optimized and embolic phenomena are minimized. Although the majority of perioperative strokes are embolic, hypoperfusion and or hyperperfusion may be responsible for over 40% of perioperative strokes.[70,71] Because it is continuous and non-invasive and the transducer can be fixed in position without impinging on the surgical field, TCD has become one of the most important monitors of cerebral perfusion during crossclamping of the carotid artery. TCD is also an important tool in the preoperative assessment and postoperative care of patients with carotid disease because it allows assessment of cerebral vascular reserve by examining CO_2 reactivity, the detection of pre- and postoperative emboli and testing cerebral autoregulation.[70–89]

Cerebral ischaemia during clamping of the internal carotid artery (ICA) is considered absent if FV_{mca} is >40%, mild if 16–40% and severe if 0–15% of the preclamping value.[78] This correlates well with subsequent ischaemic electroencephalographic (EEG) changes and may be used as an indication for shunt placement.[73–78] An intravascular shunt used to bypass the clamped ICA is effective in restoring blood flow but does carry its own inherent problems: potential dislodgement of embolus from the distal ICA, traumatic dissection of the vessel wall resulting in an occluding intimal flap and a technically more difficult endarterectomy. Furthermore, there is some evidence to suggest that the placement of shunts in patients with post-ICA clamping velocities >40% of preclamping value increases the risk of embolic stroke.[78] Although there is no universal consensus on the magnitude of FV_{mca} change that necessitates shunt placement, a reduction in FV_{mca} to <40% of baseline prior to clamping is the most commonly accepted indication. Unnecessary shunting is best avoided. TCD can also instantly detect malfunctioning shunts due to kinking or thrombosis.[80]

Emboli are detected on TCD as short-duration, high-intensity 'chirps' and waveform analysis can help differentiate air from particulate emboli.[90] Nevertheless, there are currently no automatic detection systems that have the required sensitivity and specificity for clinical use.[91] Emboli can occur throughout the operation but are more frequent during dissection of the carotid arteries, upon release of ICA crossclamp and during wound closure.[81,82,92] Although the clinical significance of TCD-detected emboli is not yet fully understood, they probably represent adverse embolic events during surgery.[81,86,91,93] The rate of microembolus generation can indicate incipient carotid artery thrombosis and has been related to intraoperative infarcts and correlated to postoperative neuropsychological morbidity.[82,86,93]

At operation, emboli are clearly audible and, interestingly, surgeons will tend to adapt their operative technique to minimize embolus generation. Following the introduction of intraoperative TCD monitoring, some centres have reported a reduction in operative stroke rates.[71,77] While it is tempting to attribute this reduction to the introduction of TCD monitoring, many other factors have also changed over this period of time.

Following closure of the arteriotomy and release of carotid clamps, FV will typically increases immediately to levels above baseline and gradually correct back to the preclamping baseline over the course of a few minutes.[86] This hyperaemic response is to be expected as the dilated vascular bed vasoconstricts in autoregulatory response to an increased perfusion pressure. However, approximately 10% of patients are at increased risk of cerebral oedema or haemorrhage because of gross hyperaemia with velocities 230% of baseline value lasting from several hours to days.[83–85,88,94] This persistent postoperative hyperaemia, most likely in patients with high-grade stenosis, is probably the result of defective autoregulation in the ipsilateral hemisphere as a reduction in blood pressure is effective in normalizing FV and alleviating the symptoms.[87] TCD provides the means of early detection and effective treatment of this potentially fatal complication.

Finally, the development of sudden postoperative symptoms should prompt an immediate TCD examination with reexploration of the endarterectomy if there is a progressive fall in velocity to below preclamping values indicating postoperative occlusion of the ipsilateral carotid artery.[88]

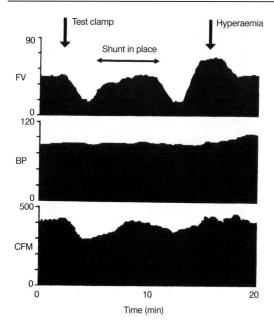

Figure 8.6   Monitoring during carotid endarterectomy. When a *test clamp* was performed, there was a rapid fall in blood velocity (FV cm/s) which was accompanied by a sustained fall in the cerebral function monitor (CFM μV). Signals recovered with the insertion of an intravascular shunt (*shunt in place*), with a second fall seen during shunt removal. *Hyperaemia* is observed when the crossclamp is released at end of procedure. Fv = blood velocity in middle cerebral artery (cm/s); BP = mean arterial blood pressure (mmHg); CFM = cerebral function monitor (μV).

INTRACRANIAL VASCULAR DISEASE

Subarachnoid haemorrhage

Cerebral vasospasm is the leading cause of morbidity and mortality in patients who survive a subarachnoid haemorrhage (SAH). Although radiological evidence of vasospasm has been reported in up to 70% of angiograms performed within the first week of aneurysmal rupture, the incidence of clinically significant vasospasm approximates 20%.[95,96] The aetiology remains uncertain but appears to be related to the amount and distribution of blood in the subarachnoid space. Recent work suggests that nitric oxide (NO) levels are reduced by extravascular oxyhaemoglobin and/or the presence of the potent vasoconstrictor endothelin.[97] In the patient with SAH, the appearance of new focal neurological signs or a decrease in the level of consciousness may be an early sign of vasospasm. This is normally confirmed by CT scan and angiography. Wardlaw et al showed, in a prospective observational study, that routine TCD examinations made a positive contribution to the diag-

nosis of ischaemic neurological deficits in 72% of patients with this complication and led to altered management for the benefit of the patient in 43%. More importantly, TCD results did not have any adverse influence on management or outcome.[98]

Although TCD is unreliable as a measure of CBF in patients with SAH because of vasospasm-associated changes in vessel diameter, it has become valuable for diagnosing vasospasm non-invasively prior to the onset of clinical symptoms. As the vessel diameter is reduced, for a given blood flow, FV increases. Hence, cerebral vasospasm is considered present when FV_{mca} >120 cm/s or the ratio between the FV_{mca} and the FV in the ICA exceeds 3.[99,100] In the sedated patient, the diagnosis of cerebral vasospasm relies on gross neurological signs, CT scan, cerebral angiography and TCD. Cerebral angiography and CT scan can only be performed intermittently, leaving TCD as the only way of diagnosing, judging the severity and the efficacy of treatment of cerebral vasospasm. The ratio of FV in the MCA to ICA should decrease with effective treatment. Needless to say, in order to rule out cerebral vasospasm by TCD, a thorough examination of the basal arteries is mandatory. Unfortunately, it is not possible to detect 'small' vessel spasm. Our policy is to perform daily TCD examination in all patients with SAH. Initial impressions suggest that the incidence of TCD-diagnosed vasospasm is much higher than clinically significant vasospasm and therefore we rarely escalate therapy purely on TCD findings.

In addition to the detection and treatment of vasospasm, TCD has been successfully used in the perioperative management of patients with cerebral aneurysms in a variety of other situations. Eng et al reported the advantages of TCD monitoring for the perioperative management of a patient in whom the aneurysm ruptured before dural incision.[101] Giller et al recently highlighted the relatively rare but very important incidence of embolic cerebral ischaemia after aneurysm surgery. Over a two-year period, nine out of 11 patients observed to have emboli on TCD after aneurysm surgery developed low-density areas on their CT scans, with credible sources of emboli identified in all patients studied.[102] The advantages of detecting embolic sources are self-evident.

The treatment of giant aneurysms and certain vascular masses often necessitates ligation of the carotid artery. The ability to predict tolerance to carotid artery occlusion is therefore of benefit when planning such procedures. Although a trial angiographic balloon occlusion of the carotid artery, when awake, with concurrent blood flow studies is an accepted method for testing tolerance, it is invasive and cannot be performed at the bedside. TCD has been used to observe change in Vmca during manual compression of the ICA at the bedside. When the fall in FVmca does not exceed 65% of baseline value, ICA occlusion is generally well tolerated. However, when the FVmca falls below 65% of baseline, focal neurologic deficit can be expected in over 85% of patients tested.[103] The use of TCD for extracranial-intracranial bypass surgery is further discussed in Chapter 15.

Arteriovenous malformations

Arteries leading to an arteriovenous malformation (AVM) shunt blood to the venous side with flow rates out of proportion to the low metabolism within this abnormal vascular network. These 'feeder' vessels are characterized by high blood velocity, low pulsatility, low perfusion pressure and decreased CO_2 reactivity.[104–109] It is possible to diagnose AVMs from characteristic findings of blood velocity, waveform pulsatility and CO_2 reactivity.[106] Embolization or resection of AVMs results in normalization of FV, pulsatility and CO_2 reactivity.[110–113] Provided the feeding vessel can be monitored, intraoperative TCD can be used for estimating the completeness of AVM resection and for the diagnosis and treatment of the hyperperfusion syndrome.[114,115] The difference in velocity and pulsatility of the feeding vessel and the contralateral non-feeding vessel should decrease as the AVM is resected or embolized.

CLOSED HEAD INJURY

Although many factors affect outcome after head injury, episodes of hypoxaemia, hypotension and reduced cerebral perfusion due to high ICP are predictive of poor outcome.[116,117] As they may only last a few minutes, the reliable detection and quantification of such episodes requires real-time measurement. The recent increase in the availability of multimodal monitoring (ICP, CPP, SjO_2 and TCD) has made the detection of such pathophysiological episodes possible. Furthermore, as more of the 'picture' is seen with several monitors observing the changes at the same time, appropriate therapeutic interventions are made early. For example, Kirkpatrick et al were able to demonstrate that it is possible to distinguish between rises in ICP as a result of low CPP and those that result from hyperaemia by using TCD as part of a multimodal set-up (see Ch. 8 for more detail).[118]

TCD monitoring can be used to observe changes in FV and waveform pulsatility as well as for testing cerebral vascular reserve. Cerebral autoregulation is often impaired after head injury with an increased susceptibility to secondary ischaemic insults and possible correlation with poor outcome.[116,119–121] The transient hyperaemic response test,[60] cuff deflation-induced drop in MBP (dynamic tests) and vasopressor-induced increase in MBP (static tests) have all been used to test autoregulation after head injury.[120–123] However, the most non-invasive and most continuous assessment of autoregulation relies on correlating the spontaneous fluctuations in FV_{mca} waveform and CPP. When autoregulation is present, little change is observed in FV_{mca} during changes in CPP. Conversely, in those with impaired autoregulation, a positive linear correlation between FV_{mca} and CPP is observed.[122] In addition, by continuously recording the FV_{mca}, the autoregulatory 'threshold' or breakpoint, the CPP at which autoregulation fails, can be easily detected, thus providing a target CPP value for treatment.

Czosnyka et al have recently published a sophisticated way of estimating cerebral autoregulatory reserve by the continuous assessment of the FV wave profile.[122] As CPP falls, increases in pulse amplitude and PI are seen as a result of the divergence of systolic and diastolic FV. Thus, a decline in FV_{dias} with a concomitant increase in PI gives an early warning of impending autoregulatory failure. If FV_{sys} also falls with the drop in CPP, then all components of the FV waveform have reached the autoregulatory threshold, indicating severely depleted cerebrovascular reserve and worse outcome.

Cerebral vasospasm causing ischaemia or non-contusion related infarction remains an important cause of morbidity and mortality after head injury.[124–126] The appearance of new focal neurological signs or a decrease in the level of consciousness after head injury may be an early sign of vasospasm. TCD can be used to diagnose and treat cerebral vasospasm using the same criteria as for patients with SAH. Increased FV in combination with high SjO_2 values and MCA/ICA ratio <2 indicates hyperaemia, while high FV in the presence of low or normal SjO_2 values and an MCA/ICA ratio >3 suggests cerebral vasospasm.[124–126]

Although clinical decisions on outcome after head injury cannot be based solely on TCD findings, the information obtained may provide guidance for further therapy and likely outcome. Cerebral autoregulation and CO_2 vasoreactivity can be repeatedly tested in the intensive care unit. The loss of these hallmarks of a normal cerebral vasculature suggests poor prognosis.[122,128] Similarly, the oscillating FV pattern typically seen prior to complete circulatory arrest can be used to confirm the diagnosis of brain death.[129,130] The use of TCD for non-invasively estimating CPP has already been addressed.

STROKE

As well as helping to identify the source of emboli in acute ischaemic stroke, TCD can be used to identify cerebral arterial occlusion,[130] recanalization[132–134] and the risk of haemorrhagic transformations of large-volume ischaemic lesions.[135] It is possible to identify those patients at risk for further ischaemic episodes by repeated TCD examinations within 6, at 24 and 48 h after admission with acute stroke.[136] Furthermore, the effect of anticoagulation on reperfusion, recanalization and outcome can also be evaluated.[137] Unilateral emboli most commonly originate from the carotid arteries, while bilateral emboli most commonly arise from cardiac sites.

NON-NEUROSURGICAL APPLICATIONS

Because it is non-invasive, TCD has found many applications outside neurosurgery and neurointensive care, mainly in those patients at risk of brain injury secondary to primary pathology outside the central nervous system.

Cardiac surgery

Detection of microemboli and the estimation of cerebral perfusion during cardiac surgery are probably the most important applications outside neurosurgery and neurointensive care. While the incidence of stroke after cardiac surgery is estimated at 5%, subtler cognitive dysfunction has been reported in over 60% of patients.[138] Although it may not always be a reliable monitor of CBF during cardiopulmonary bypass (CPB),[139,140] TCD has been successfully used for emboli detection during and after cardiopulmonary bypass,[141–145,147,148] for testing cerebral autoregulation and CO_2 reactivity,[146] for comparing the effects of different techniques of blood gas management,[147] and for detecting hyperperfusion during cardiac surgery.[148] Furthermore, with the increase in minimally invasive cardiac surgery, TCD has been used to ensure correct positioning of the endovascular aortic balloon clamp.[149]

Miscellaneous uses

Alterations in CBF are implicated in the aetiology of portosystemic encephalopathy, a major complication of acute and chronic liver disease, with possible cerebral vasodilatation resulting in cerebral oedema and reduced CPP.[150]

TCD has been used to assess CO_2 reactivity and cerebral autoregulation in patients with liver failure. Although cerebral autoregulation is often impaired in acute hepatic failure and may be restored by hypocapnic hyperventilation, CO_2 reactivity remains unaffected.[151,152] Early indications suggest that by using TCD waveform analysis (as described for head-injured patients), it is possible to non-invasively estimate CPP in patients with liver failure (unpublished data, BFM). The advantages of not inserting ICP measuring devices into patients who are often coagulopathic are self-evident.

TCD has been used to measure FV in normal pregnancy and in mothers with preeclampsia. Up to 70% of abnormal pregnancies were associated with elevated FV when compared to normal pregnancies.[153] Furthermore, the degree of toxaemia correlated with the increase in FV, with progressive increases in FV often preceding neurologic symptoms.[153,154] Although the significance of cerebral vasospasm in preeclampsia remains controversial, the cause of this increase in FV requires further investigation.

TCD has been used to detect intraoperative microemboli during major head and neck surgery.[155] It has been used as a simple bedside test for assessment of shunt function and also for early identification of potential organ transplant donors.[156,157]

CONCLUSION

Transcranial Doppler ultrasonography is a useful non-invasive monitor of cerebral haemodynamics, benefits of which have been demonstrated in many specific instances. This 'window' on the brain has been severely disadvantaged by the inability to fix the probe in position. The majority of fixation devices require constant adjustment and often interfere with the surgical field or the intensive care of the patient. Although the 'Lam Frames', holders that attach to the ear canals and the bridge of the nose, seem to provide the most reliable intraoperative recordings (DWL, Sipplingen, Germany), ear plugs do not allow proper patient care and therefore make these frames unsuitable for long-term monitoring in intensive care. Recently, various non-invasive, neuromonitoring parameters including TCD robotic probes, near infrared spectroscopy and 'active electrodes ' for measuring bioelectric neural activity have been integrated in a helmet construction for recording and processing over longer periods.[158,159] As manufacturers and clinicians continue to address the problem, more successful solutions will increase the use of this exciting technology, thereby improving our understanding of cerebral pathophysiology and, hence, patient care.

REFERENCES

1. Aaslid R, Markwalder TM, Nornes H. Non-invasive transcranial Doppler ultrasound recording of flow velocity in basal cerebral arteries. J Neurosurg 1982; 57: 769.

2. Aaslid R. Transcranial Doppler examination techniques. In: Aaslid R (ed.) Transcranial Doppler sonography. Springer-Verlag, New York, 1986, p39.

3. Huber P, Handa J. Effect of contrast material, hypercapnia, hyperventilation, hypertonic glucose and papaverine on the diameter of the cerebral arteries – angiographic determination in man. Invest Radiol 1967; 2: 17.

4. Markwalder TM, Grolimund P, Seiler RW et al. Dependency of blood flow velocity in the middle cerebral artery on end-tidal carbon dioxide partial pressure – a transcranial ultrasound Doppler study. J Cereb Blood Flow Metab 1984; 4: 368.

5. Eng CC, Lam AM, Mayberg TS, Mathisen TL. Influence of propofol and propofol-nitrous oxide anesthesia on cerebral blood flow velocity and carbon dioxide reactivity in humans. Anesthesiology 1992; 77: 872.

6. Newell WD, Aaslid R, Lam AM et al. Comparison of flow and velocity during dynamic autoregulation testing in humans. Stroke 1994; 25: 793.

7. Giller CA, Bowman G, Dyer H et al. Cerebral arterial diameters during changes in blood pressure and carbon dioxide during craniotomy. Neurosurgery 1993; 32: 737.

8. Strebel SP, Kindler C, Bissonnette B et al. The impact of systemic vasoconstrictors on the cerebral circulation of anesthetized patients. Anesthesiology 1998; 89: 67.

9. Matta BF, Lam AM, Mayberg TS et al. The cerebrovascular response to carbon dioxide during sodium nitroprusside- and isoflurane-induced hypotension. Br J Anaesth 1995; 74: 296.

10. Dahl A, Russell D, Nyberg-Hansen R, Rootwelt K. Effect of nitroglycerin on cerebral circulation measured by transcranial Doppler and SPECT. Stroke 1989; 20: 1733.

11. Schregel W, Schafermeyer H, Muller C et al. The effect of halothane, alfentanil and propofol on blood flow velocity, blood vessel cross section and blood volume flow in the middle cerebral artery. Anaesthesist 1992; 41: 21.

12. Kochs E, Hoffman WE, Werner C et al. Cerebral blood flow velocity in relation to cerebral blood flow, cerebral metabolic rate for oxygen, and electroencephalogram analysis during isoflurane anesthesia in dogs. Anesth Analg 1993; 76: 1222.

13. Matta BF, Lam AM. Isoflurane and desflurane do not dilate the middle cerebral artery appreciably. Br J Anaesth 1995; 74: 486P.

14. Schregel W, Schafermeyer H, Muller C et al. The effect of halothane, alfentanil and propofol on blood flow velocity, blood vessel cross section and blood volume flow in the middle cerebral artery. Anaesthesist 1992; 41: 21.

15. Matta BF, Mayberg TS, Lam AM. Direct cerebrovasodilatory effects of halothane, isoflurane and desflurane during propofol-induced isoelectric encephalogram in humans. Anesthesiology 1995; 83: 980.

16. Schregel W, Schaefermeyer H, Sihle-Wissel M, Klein R. Transcranial Doppler sonography during isoflurane/N$_2$O anesthesia and surgery: flow velocity, 'vessel area' and 'volume flow'. Can J Anaesth 1994; 41: 607.

17. Werner C, Kochs E, Reimer R et al. The effect of postural changes on cerebral hemodynamics during general anesthesia. Anaesthesist 1990; 39: 429.

18. Bissonnette B, Leon JE. Cerebrovascular stability during isoflurane anaesthesia in children. Can J Anaesth 1992; 39: 128–134.

19. Lam AM, Mayberg TS, Cooper JO et al. Nitrous oxide is a more potent cerebrovasodilator than isoflurane in humans. Anesth Analg 1994; 78: 462.

20. Kontos HA. Validity of cerebral arterial blood calculations from velocity measurements. Stroke 1989; 20: 1.

21. Brauer P, Kochs E, Werner C et al. Correlation of transcranial Doppler sonography mean flow velocity with cerebral blood flow in patients with intracranial pathology. J Neurosurg Anesthesiol 1998; 10: 80.

22. Harders A. Neurosurgical applications of transcranial Doppler sonography. Springer Verlag, Vienna, 1986, pp 28.

23. Harders A, Gilsbach J. Transcranial Doppler sonography ad its application in extracranial-intracranial bypass surgery. Neurol Res 1985; 7: 129.

24. Newell DW, Aaslid R. Transcranial Doppler. Raven Press, New York, 1992.

25. Bode H, Wais U. Age dependence of flow velocity in basal cerebral arteries. Arch Dis Child 1988; 63: 606.

26. Adams RJ, Nichols FT, Stephens S. Transcranial Doppler: the influence of age and hematocrit in normal children. J Cardiovasc Ultrasound 1988; 7: 201.

27. Arnolds BJ, Von Reuten GM. Transcranial Doppler sonography. Examination technique and normal reference values. Ultrasound Med Biol 1986; 12: 115.

28. Klotzsch C, Popescu O, Berlit P. A new 1 NHz probe for transcranial Doppler sonography in patients with inadequate temporal bone windows. Ultrasound Med Biol 1998; 24: 101.

29. Grolimund P, Seiler RW. Age dependence of the flow velocity in the basal cerebral arteries – a transcranial Doppler ultrasound study. Ultrasound Med Biol 1988; 14: 191.

30. Gabrielsen TO, Greitz T. Normal size of the internal carotid, middle cerebral and anterior cerebral arteries. Acta Radiol 1970; 10: 1.

31. Kennedy C, Sokoloff L. An adaptation of nitrous oxide method to the study of the cerebral circulation in

children: normal values for cerebral blood flow and metabolic rate in childhood. J Clin Invest 1957; 36: 1130.

32. Leenders KL, Perani D, Lammertsma AA et al. Cerebral blood flow, blood volume and oxygen utilisation. Normal values and effect of age. Brain 1990; 113: 27.

33. Heyman A, Patterson JL, Duke TW. Cerebral circulation and metabolism in sickle cell and other chronic anemias, with observations on the effects of oxygen inhalation. J Clin Invest 1952; 31: 824.

34. Brass L, Pavlakis S, DeVivo D et al. Transcranial Doppler measurements of the middle cerebral artery: effect of hematocrit. Stroke 1988; 19: 1466.

35. Thomas DJ, Marshall J, Ross Russell RW et al. Effects of hematocrit on cerebral blood flow in man. Lancet 1987; 2: 941.

36. Vriens EM, Kraier V, Musbach M et al. Transcranial pulsed Doppler measurements of blood velocity in the middle cerebral artery: reference values at rest and during hyperventilation in healthy volunteers in relation to age and sex. Ultrasound Med Biol 1989; 15: 1.

37. Brouwers P, Vriens EM, Musbach M et al. Transcranial pulsed Doppler measurements of blood velocity in the middle cerebral artery: reference values at rest and during hyperventilation in healthy children and adolescents in relation to age and sex. Ultrasound Med Biol 1990; 16: 1.

38. Czosnyka M, Guazzo E, Iyer V et al. Testing of cerebral autoregulation by waveform analysis of blood flow velocity and cerebral perfusion pressure. Acta Neurochir 1994; 60: 468.

39. Gosling RG, King DH. Arterial assessment by Doppler shift ultrasound. Proc Roy Soc Med 1974; 67: 447.

40. Planiol T, Purcelot L, Itti R. La circulation carotidienne et cerebrale. Progres realises dans l'etude par les methodes physiques sexternes. Nouv Presse Med 1973; 37: 2451.

41. Sorteberg W, Langmoen IA, Lindergaard KF, Nornes H. Side to side differences and day to day variations of transcranial Doppler parameters in normal subjects. J Ultrasound Med 1990; 9: 403–409.

42. Hirst RP, Slee TA, Lam AM. Changes in cerebral blood flow velocity after release of intraoperative tourniquets in humans: a transcranial Doppler study. Anesth Analg 1990; 71: 503.

43. Kirkham FJ, Padayachee TS, Parsons S et al. Transcranial measurements of blood flow velocities in the basal arteries using pulsed Doppler ultrasound: velocity as an index of flow. Ultrasound Med Biol 1986; 12: 15–21.

44. Matta BF, Lam AM, Strebel S, Mayberg TS. Cerebral pressure autoregulation and CO_2-reactivity during propofol-induced EEG suppression. Br J Anaesth 1995; 74: 159.

45. Kaiser L. Adjusting for baseline: change or % change? Statistics Med 1989; 8: 1183.

46. Strebel S, Kaufmann M, Guardiola P-M et al. Cerebral vasomotor responsiveness to carbon dioxide is preserved during propofol and midazolam anesthesia in humans. Anesth Analg 1994; 78: 884.

47. Cho S, Fujigaki T, Uchiyama Y et al. Effects of sevoflurane with and without nitrous oxide on human cerebral circulation. Anesthesiology 1996; 85: 755.

48. Paulson OB, Strandgaard S, Edvinsson L. Cerebral autoregulation. Cerebrovasc Brain Metab Rev 1990; 2: 161.

49. Strandgaard S, Paulson OB: Cerebral autoregulation. Stroke 1984; 15: 413.

50. Lassen NA. Cerebral blood flow and oxygen consumption in man. Physiol Rev 1959; 39: 183.

51. Harper AM. Autoregulation of cerebral blood flow: influence of arterial blood pressure on the blood flow through the cerebral cortex. J Neurol Neurosurg Psychiatry 1966; 29: 398.

52. Agnoli A, Fieschi C, Bozzao L et al. Autoregulation of cerebral blood flow: studies during drug-induced hypertension in normal subjects and in patients with cerebral vascular diseases. Circulation 1968; 38: 800.

53. Smith AL, Neigh JL, Hoffman JC et al. Effects of general anesthesia on autoregulation of cerebral blood flow in man. J Appl Physiol 1970; 29: 665.

54. Miletich DJ, Ivankovich AD, Albrecht RF et al. Absence of autoregulation of cerebral blood flow during halothane and enflurane anesthesia. Anesth Analg 1976; 55: 100.

55. Held K, Niedermayer W, Gottstein U. Reactivity of cerebral blood flow to variations of transmural pressure. Circulation 1971; 43/44: 11.

56. Aaslid R, Lindegaard KF, Sorteberg W, Nornes H. Cerebral autoregulation in humans. Stroke 1989; 20: 45.

57. Aaslid R, Newell DW, Stooss R et al. Assessment of cerebral autoregulation dynamics from simultaneous arterial and venous transcranial Doppler recordings in humans. Stroke 1991; 22: 1148.

58. Giller CA. A bedside test for cerebral autoregulation using transcranial Doppler ultrasound. Acta Neurochir 1991; 108: 7.

59. Smielewski P, Czosnyka M, Kirkpatrick P et al. Assessment of cerebral autoregulation using carotid artery compression. Stroke 1996; 27: 2197.

60. Smielewski P, Czosnyka M, Kirkpatrick PJ et al. Validation of the computerised transient hyperemic response test as a method of testing autoregulation in severely head injured patients. J Neurotrauma 1995; 12: 420.

61. Hassler W, Steinmetz H, Gawlowske J. Transcranial Doppler ultrasonography in raised intracranial pressure and in intracranial circulatory arrest. J Neurosurg 1988; 68: 745.

62. Hassler W, Steinmetz H, Pirschel J. Transcranial Doppler study of intracranial circulatory arrest. J Neurosurg 1989; 71: 195.

63. Homburg AM, Jakobsen M, Enevoldsen E. Transcranial Doppler recordings in raised intracranial pressure. Acta Neurol Scand 1993; 87: 488.

64. Sanker P, Richard KE, Weigl HC et al. Transcranial Doppler sonography and intracranial pressure monitoring in children and juveniles with acute brain injuries or hydrocephalus. Childs Nerv Syst 1991; 7: 391.

65. Chan KH, Miller DJ, Dearden M et al. The effect of changes in cerebral perfusion pressure upon middle cerebral artery blood flow velocity and jugular bulb venous oxygen saturation after severe brain trauma. J Neurosurg 1992; 77: 55.

66. Czosnyka M, Richards HK, Whitehouse H et al. Relationship between transcranial Doppler-determined pulsatility index and cerebrovascular resistance: an experimental study. J Neurosurg 1996; 84: 79.

67. Aaslid R, Lundar T, Lindergaard KF et al. Estimation of cerebral perfusion pressure from arterial blood pressure and transcranial Doppler recordings. In: Miller JD, Teasdale GM, Rowan JO et al (eds) Intracranial pressure VI. Springer-Verlag, Berlin, 1986, p 226.

68. Czosnyka M, Matta BF, Smielewski P et al. Cerebral perfusion pressure in head injured patients: a non invasive assessment using transcranial Doppler ultrasonography. J Neurosurg 1998; 88: 802.

69. Czosnyka M, Kirkpatrick E, Guazzo H et al. Assessment of the autoregulatory reserve using continuous CPP and TCD blood flow velocity measurement in head injury. In: Nagai H, Kamiya K, Ishii S (eds) Intracranial pressure IX. Springer-Verlag, Berlin, 1994, p 593.

70. Krul JMJ, Van Gijn J, Ackerstaff RGA et al. Site and pathogenesis of infarcts associated with carotid endarterectomy. Stroke 1989; 20: 324.

71. Spencer MP. Transcranial Doppler monitoring and causes of stroke from carotid endarterectomy. Stroke 1997; 28: 685.

72. Halsey JH, McDowell HA, Gelman S et al. Blood velocity in the middle cerebral artery and regional cerebral blood flow during carotid endarterectomy. Stroke 1989; 20: 53.

73. Jorgensen LG, Schroeder TV. Transcranial Doppler for detection of cerebral ischemia during carotid endarterectomy. Eur J Vasc Surg 1992; 6: 142.

74. Powers AD, Smith RR, Graeber MC. Transcranial Doppler monitoring of cerebral flow velocities during surgical occlusion of the carotid artery. Neurosurgery 1989; 25: 383.

75. Spencer MP, Thomas GI, Moehring MA. Relationship between middle cerebral artery blood flow velocity and stump pressure during carotid endarterectomy. Stroke 1992; 23: 1439.

76. Steiger HJ, Schaffler L, Boll J et al. Results of microsurgical carotid endarterectomy: a prospective study with transcranial Doppler sonography and EEG monitoring and elective shunting. Acta Neurochir 1989; 100: 31.

77. Jansen C, Vriens EM, Eikelboom BC et al. Carotid endarterectomy with transcranial Doppler and electroencephalographic monitoring. A prospective study in 130 operations. Stroke 1993; 24: 665.

78. Halsey JH Jr. Risks and benefits of shunting in carotid endarterectomy. The International Transcranial Doppler Collaborators. Stroke 1992; 23: 1583.

79. Kalra M, Al-Khaffaf H, Farrell A et al. Comparison of measurement of stump pressure and transcranial measurement of flow velocity in the middle cerebral artery in carotid surgery. Ann Vasc Surg 1994; 8: 225.

80. Naylor AR, Wildsmith JA, McClure J et al. Transcranial Doppler monitoring during carotid endarterectomy. Br J Surg 1991; 78: 1264.

81. Spencer MP, Thomas GL, Nicholls SC et al. Detection of middle cerebral artery emboli during carotid endarterectomy using transcranial Doppler ultrasonography. Stroke 1990; 21: 415.

82. Jansen C, Ramos LM, Van Heesewijk JP et al. Impact of microembolism and hemodynamic changes in the brain during carotid endarterectomy. Stroke 1994; 25: 992.

83. Piepgras DG, Morgan MK, Sundt TM et al. Intracerebral hemorrhage after carotid endarterectomy. J Neurosurg 1988; 68: 532.

84. Sbarigia E, Speziale F, Giannoni MF et al. Post-carotid endarterectomy hyperperfusion syndrome: preliminary observations for identifying at risk patients by transcranial Doppler sonography and the acetazolamide test. Eur J Vasc Surg 1993; 7: 252.

85. Powers AD, Smith RR. Hyperperfusion syndrome after carotid endarterectomy: a transcranial Doppler evaluation. Neurosurgery 1990; 26: 56.

86. Naylor AR, Whyman M, Wildsmith JAW et al. Immediate effects of carotid clamp release on middle cerebral artery blood flow velocity during carotid endarterectomy. Eur J Vasc Surg 1993; 7: 308.

87. Jorgensen LG, Schroeder TV. Defective cerebrovascular autoregulation after carotid endarterectomy. Eur J Vasc Surg 1993; 7: 370.

88. Jansen C, Sprengers AM, Moll FL et al. Prediction of intracerebral haemorrhage after carotid endarterectomy by clinical criteria and intraoperative transcranial Doppler monitoring. Eur J Vasc Surg 1994; 8: 303.

89. Gaunt ME, Ratliff DA, Martin PJ et al. On-table diagnosis of incipient carotid artery thrombosis during carotid endarterectomy by transcranial Doppler scanning. J Vasc Surg 1994; 20: 104.

90. Marcus HS, Tegeler CH. Experimental aspects of high intensity transient signals in the detection of emboli. J Clin Ultrasound 1995; 23: 81.

91. Ringelstein EB, Droste DW, Babikian VL et al. Consensus on microembolus detection by TCD. International consensus group on microemboli detection. Stroke 1998; 29: 725.

92. Gravilescu T, Babikian VL, Cantelmo NL et al. Cerebral microembolism during carotid endarterectomy. Am J Surg 1995; 170: 159.

93. Gaunt ME, Martin PJ, Smith JJ et al. Clinical relevance of intraoperative embolisation detected by transcranial Doppler ultrasonography during carotid endarterectomy: a prospective study of 100 patients. Br J Surg 1994; 81: 1435.

94. Schroeder T, Sillesen H, Sorensen O et al. Cerebral hyperperfusion syndrome following carotid endarterectomy. J Neurosurg 1987; 28: 824.

95. Weir B, Grace M, Hansen J et al. Time course of vasospasm in man. J Neurosurg 1978; 48: 173.

96. Kassell NF, Torner JC, Jane JA et al. The International Co-operative Study on the Timing of Aneurysm Surgery, part 1: overall management results. J Neurosurg 1990; 73: 18.

97. Macdonald RL, Weir BKA. A review of hemoglobin and the pathogenesis of cerebral vasospasm. Stroke 1991; 22: 971.

98. Wardlaw JM, Offin R, Teasdale GM, Teasdale, EM. Is routine transcranial Doppler ultrasound monitoring useful in the management of subarachnoid hemorrhage? J Neurosurg 1998; 88(2): 272–276.

99. Aaslid R, Huber P, Nornes H. Evaluation of cerebrovascular spasm with transcranial Doppler ultrasound. J Neurosurg 1984; 60: 37.

100. Lindegaard KF, Nornes H, Bakke SJ et al. Cerebral vasospasm after subarachnoid hemorrhage investigated by means of transcranial Doppler ultrasound. Acta Neurochir 1988; 24: 81.

101. Eng CC, Lam AM, Byrd S et al. The diagnosis and management of a perianesthetic cerebral aneurysmal rupture aided with transcranial Doppler ultrasonography. Anesthesiology 1993; 78: 191.

102. Giller CA, Giller AM, Landreneau F. Detection of emboli after surgery for intracerebral aneurysms. Neurosurgery 1998; 42: 490.

103. Giller CA, Mathews D, Walker B et al. Prediction of tolerance to carotid artery occlusion using transcranial Doppler ultrasound. J Neurosurg 1994; 81: 15.

104. Hassler W, Steinmetz H. Cerebral hemodynamics in angioma patients: an intraoperative study. J Neurosurg 1987; 67: 822.

105. Fleischer LH, Young WL, Pile-Spellman J et al. Relationship of transcranial Doppler flow velocities and arteriovenous malformation feeding artery pressures. Stroke 1993; 24: 1897.

106. Lindegaard KF, Grolimund P, Aaslid R et al. Evaluation of cerebral arteriovenous malformations using transcranial Doppler ultrasound. J Neurosurg 1986; 65: 335.

107. Massaro AR, Young WL, Kader A et al. Characterisation of arteriovenous malformation feeding vessels by carbon dioxide reactivity. Am J Neuroradiol 1994; 15: 55.

108. Diehl RR, Henkes H, Nahser HC et al. Blood flow velocity and vasomotor reactivity in patients with arteriovenous malformations. A transcranial Doppler study. Stroke 1994; 25: 1574.

109. De Salles AA, Manchola I. CO2 reactivity in arteriovenous malformations of the brain: a transcranial Doppler ultrasound study. J Neurosurg 1994; 80: 624.

110. Chioffi F, Pasqualin A, Beltramello A et al. Hemodynamic effects of preoperative embolization in cerebral arteriovenous malformations: evaluation with transcranial Doppler sonography. Neurosurgery 1992; 31: 877.

111. Petty GW, Massaro AR, Tatemichi TK et al. Transcranial Doppler ultrasonographic changes after treatment for arteriovenous malformations. Stroke 1990; 21: 260.

112. Kader A, Young WL, Massaro AR et al. Transcranial Doppler changes during staged surgical resection of cerebral arteriovenous malformations: a report of three cases. Surg Neurol 1993; 39: 392.

113. Pasqualin A, Barone G, Cioffi F et al. The relevance of anatomic and hemodynamic factors to a classification of cerebral arteriovenous malformations. Neurosurgery 1991; 28: 370.

114. Spetzler RF, Wilson CB, Weinstein P. Normal perfusion pressure breakthrough theory. Clin Neurosurg 1978; 25: 651.

115. Matta BF, Lam AM, Winn HR. The intraoperative use of transcranial Doppler ultrasonography during resection of arteriovenous malformations. Br J Anaesth 1995; 75: 242P.

116. Marmarou A, Anderson RL, Ward JD et al. Impact of ICP instability and hypotension on outcome in patients with severe head trauma. J Neurosurg 1991; 75: S59.

117. Andrews PJD. What is the optimal cerebral perfusion pressure after brain injury? A review of the evidence with an emphasis on arterial pressure. Acta Anaesthesiol Scand 1995; 39: 112.

118. Kirkpatrick PJ, Czosnyka M, Pickard JD. Multimodality monitoring in intensive care. J Neurol Neurosurg Psychiatry 1996; 60: 131.

119. Miller JD. Head injury and brain ischemia. Implications for therapy. Br J Anaesth 1985; 57: 120.

120. Junger EC, Newell DW, Grant GA et al. Cerebral autoregulation after minor head injury. J Neurosurg 1997; 86: 425.

121. Strebel S, Lam AM, Matta BF et al. Impaired cerebral autoregulation after mild brain injury. Surg Neurol 1997; 47: 128.

122. Czosnyka M, Smielewski P, Kirkpatrick P et al. Monitoring of cerebral autoregulation in head injured patients. Stroke 1996; 27: 1829.

123. Matta BF, Risdall J, Menon DK et al. The effect of propofol on cerebral autoregulation after head injury: a preliminary report. Br J Anaesth 1997; 78: A237.

124. Chan KH, Dearden NM, Miller JD. The significance of posttraumatic increase in cerebral blood flow velocity: a transcranial Doppler ultrasound study. Neurosurgery 1992; 30: 697.

125. Martin NA, Patwardhan RV, Alexander MJ et al. Characterisation of cerebral hemodynamic phases following severe head trauma: hypoperfusion, hyperemia, and vasospasm. J Neurosurg 1997; 87: 9.

126. Lee JH, Martin NA, Alsinda G et al. Hemodynamically significant cerebral vasospasm and outcome after head injury. J Neurosurg 1997; 87: 221.

127. Rommer B, Bellner J, Kongstad P et al. Elevated transcranial Doppler flow velocities after severe head injury: cerebral vasospasm or hyperemia? J Neurosurg 1996; 85: 90.

128. Schal'en W, Messeter K, Nordstrom CH. Cerebral vasoreactivity and the prediction of outcome in severe traumatic brain lesions. Acta Anaesthesiol Scand 1991; 35: 113.

129. Werner C, Kochs E, Rau M et al. Transcranial Doppler sonography as a supplement in the detection of cerebral circulatory arrest. J Neurosurg Anesthesiol 1990; 2: 159.

130. Feri M, Ralli L, Felici M et al. Transcranial Doppler and brain death diagnosis. Crit Care Med 1994; 22: 1120.

131. Zanette EM, Fieschi C, Bozzao L et al. Comparison of cerebral angiography and transcranial Doppler sonography in acute stroke. Stroke 1989; 20: 899.

132. Toni D, Fiorelli M, Zanette EM et al. Early spontaneous improvement and deterioration of ischemic stroke patients. A serial study with transcranial Doppler ultrasonography. Stroke 1998; 29: 1144.

133. Fieschi C, Argentino C, Lenzi GL et al. Clinical and instrumental evaluation of patients with ischemic stroke within 6 hours. J Neurol Sci 1989; 91: 311.

134. Zanette EM, Roberti C, Mancini G et al. Spontaneous middle cerebral artery reperfusion in ischemic stroke. A follow up study with transcranial Doppler. Stroke 1995; 26: 430.

135. Alexandrov AV, Black SE, Ehrlich LE et al. Prediction of hemorrhagic transformation occurring spontaneously and on anticoagulants in patients with acute ischemic stroke. Stroke 1997; 28: 1198.

136. Sliwa U, Lingnau A, Stohlman WD et al. Prevalence and time course of microembolic signals in patients with acute stroke: a prospective study. Stroke 1997; 28: 358.

137. Yasada M, O'Keefe GJ, Chambers BR et al. Streptokinase in acute stroke: effect on reperfusion and recanalization. Australian Streptokinase Trial Study Group. Neurology 1998; 50: 626.

138. Murkin JM. Anesthesia, the brain, and cardiopulmonary bypass. Ann Thorac Surg 1993; 56: 1461.

139. Van Der Linden J, Wesslen O, Ekroth R et al. Transcranial Doppler-estimated versus thermodilution-estimated cerebral blood flow during cardiac operations. J Thorac Cardiovasc Surg 1991; 102: 95.

140. Grocott HP, Amory DW, Lowry E et al. Transcranial Doppler blood flow velocity versus 133Xe clearance cerebral blood flow during mild hypothermic cardiopulmonary bypass. J Clin Monit Comput 1998; 14: 35.

141. Van Der Linden J, Casmir-Ahn H. When do cerebral emboli appear during open heart operations? A transcranial Doppler study. Ann Thorac Surg 1991; 51: 237.

142. Clarke RE, Brillman J, Davis DA et al. Microemboli during coronary artery bypass grafting – genesis and effect on outcome. J Thorac Cardiovasc Surg 1995; 109: 249.

143. Grocott HP, Croughwell ND, Amory DW et al. Cerebral emboli and serum S100beta during cardiac operations. Ann Thorac Surg 1998; 65: 1645.

144. Sliwka U, Georgiadis D. Clinical correlation of Doppler microembolic signals in patients with prosthetic cardiac valves: analysis of 580 cases. Stroke 1998; 29(1): 140–143.

145. Nabavi DG, Arato S, Droste DW et al. Microembolic load in asymptomatic patients with cardiac aneurysm, severe ventricular dysfunction, and atrial fibrillation. Clinical and hemorheological correlates. Cerebrovasc Dis 1998; 8(4): 214–221.

146. Lundar T, Lindegaard KF, Froysaker T et al. Dissociation between cerebral autoregulation and carbon dioxide reactivity during non pulsatile cardiopulmonary bypass. Ann Thorac Surg 1985; 40: 582.

147. Venn GE. Patel RL, Chambers DJ. Cardiopulmonary bypass: perioperative cerebral blood flow and postoperative cognitive deficit. Ann Thorac Surg 1995; 59: 1331.

148. Briliman J, Davis D, Clark RE et al. Increased middle cerebral artery flow velocity during the initial phase of cardiopulmonary bypass may cause neurological dysfunction. J Neuroimag 1995; 5: 135.

149. Grocott HP, Smith MS, Glower DD et al. Endovascular aortic balloon clamp malposition during minimally invasive cardiac surgery: detection by transcranial Doppler monitoring. Anesthesiology 1998; 88: 1396.

150. Gitlin N, Lewis DC, Hinckley L. The diagnosis and prevalence of subclinical hepatic encephalopathy in apparently healthy, ambulant, nonshunted patients with cirrhosis. J Hepatol 1986; 3: 75.

151. Katz JJ, Mandell MS, House RM et al. Cerebral blood flow velocity in patients with subclinical portal-systemic encephalopathy. Anesth Analg 1998; 86: 1005.

152. Strauss G, Hansen BA, Knudsen GM et al. Hyperventilation restores cerebral blood flow autoregulation in patients with acute liver failure. J Hepatol 1998; 28: 199.

154. Hansen WF, Burnham SJ, Svendsen TO et al. Transcranial Doppler findings of cerebral vasospasm in pre-eclampsia. J Matern Fetal Med 1996; 5: 194.

155. Nosan DK, Gomez CR, Boyd JH et al. Intraoperative transcranial Doppler ultrasound in head and neck surgery: a preliminary report. Am J Otolaryngol 1998; 19(4): 223.

156. Jindal A, Mahapatra AK. Correlation of ventricular size and TCD findings before and after ventriculo-peritoneal shunt in patients with hydrocephalus:

prospective study of 35 patients. J Neurol Neurosurg Psychiatry 1998; 65(2): 269.

157. Valentin A, Karnik R, Winkler WB et al. Trnscranial Doppler for early identification of potential organ transplant donors. Wien Klin Wochenschr 1997; 109(21): 836.

158. Litscher GA. Multifunctional helmet for non invasive monitoring. J Neurosurg Anesthesiol 1998; 10: 116–119.

159. Bazzochi M, Quaia E, Zucani C, Mosoldo M. Transcranial Doppler: state of the art. Eur J Radiol 1998; 2: S141–S148.

9

CEREBRAL OXIMETRY

Arun K. Gupta & Basil F. Matta

The potential advantages of monitoring cerebral oxygenation in patients at risk for cerebral ischaemia are self-evident. The most acceptable and reliable method so far has been jugular venous bulb oximetry. The search for non-invasive methods of detecting cerebral desaturation has increased interest in near infrared spectroscopy (NIRS). In highly specialized centres, multiparameter probes are frequently used for detecting changes in brain tissue and cerebrospinal fluid PO_2, PCO_2 and pH.

JUGULAR BULB OXIMETRY

ANATOMY

The jugular bulb, a dilatation in the upper end of the internal jugular vein, is the final common pathway for venous blood draining from the cerebral hemispheres, cerebellum and brainstem. Therefore, jugular bulb oxygen saturation (SJO_2) reflects the balance between brain supply and consumption of oxygen.

The veins draining blood from the brain join to form six major cranial sinuses (superior and inferior sagittal, the straight, occipital, right and left transverse). These venous channels, located between the dura mater and the periosteum lining the cranium, have no valves or muscle in their walls. The final common pathway for the majority of blood returning from the brain is through the right and left sigmoid sinuses, which curve down through the posterior fossa, over the mastoid portion of the temporal bone and then run forward to form the right and left internal jugular veins in the posterior part of the jugular foramen. Exceptions to this are the inferior petrosal sinus which joins the internal jugular vein directly and the occipital sinus which communicates with the internal vertebral venous plexus.[1]

The internal jugular vein (IJV) begins at the jugular foramen and runs down through the neck in the carotid sheath to form the brachiocephalic vein by joining the subclavian vein behind the medial end of the clavicle. Within the carotid sheath, the vein is lateral to the vagus nerve and the carotid artery. The vein is related anterolaterally to the superficial cervical fascia, the platysma, the transverse cutaneous nerve, the deep cervical fascia and the sternocleidomastoid muscle. Posterior to the vein lies the transverse processes of the cervical vertebrae, cervical plexus, phrenic nerve, vertebral vein, the first part of the subclavian artery and, on the left side, the thoracic duct. The lower end of the IJV dilates to form the inferior jugular bulb, above which is a bicuspid valve.

INSERTION TECHNIQUE

Jugular venous bulb catheters can be placed in a matter of minutes, with a complication rate similar to that seen with the placement of antegrade jugular venous lines.[6] As with any form of invasive monitoring, maximum benefit can only be realized when complications of the technique are minimized. Therefore, catheters are best avoided in those with coagulation abnormalities, sepsis or local neck trauma.

SJO_2 monitoring accurately reflects global and hemispheric cerebral oxygenation only when the dominant jugular bulb is cannulated.[24] However, selecting the optimal side for monitoring remains difficult. Cortical blood from the sagittal sinus flows into the right lateral sinus while subcortical blood from the straight sinus usually goes to the left lateral sinus. Overall, flow is greater to the right jugular venous bulb[2,3] but up to 15% difference between right and left SJO_2 has been

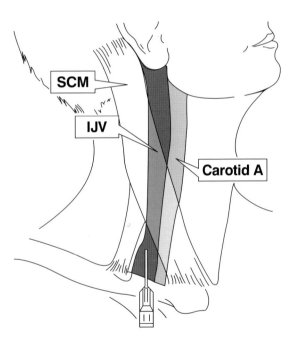

Figure 9.1   The technique used in our unit for inserting jugular bulb catheters. The junction between the sternal and clavicular heads of the sternocleidomastoid muscle is localized and the skin is punctured with a 16 gauge 5.25 inch Angiocath catheter (Becton and Dickinson) mounted with a 5 ml syringe. During gentle aspiration, the needle is passed in a cranial direction for 1–2 cm, at an angle of 15–20° in the sagittal plane. Once the vein is entered, the catheter is advanced over the needle until a slight elastic resistance is felt or until the tip of the catheter is estimated to be just behind the mastoid process. SCM = sternocleidomastoid muscle; IJV = internal jugular vein; carotid A = carotid artery.

demonstrated in patients with head trauma.[4] It is possible to determine the dominant side of venous drainage by sequential temporary manual occlusion of the right and then left IJV and observing the resultant rise in intracranial pressure (ICP).[5] Compressing the dominant jugular vein will lead to venous obstruction and a greater increase in ICP. Therefore, SJO_2 should be monitored on the side producing the largest rise in ICP when the IJV is manually compressed. When the rise in ICP is similar during right and left IJV compression, the side with the greatest degree of pathology as determined by computed tomographic scan is used or in the case of diffuse injury, the right side is used.[6] In our unit, right-sided jugular venous oximetry is used almost exclusively.

There are two main approaches for retrograde cannulation of the IJV. The vessel can be located by inserting the needle lateral to the carotid artery at the level of the inferior border of the thyroid cartilage, aiming towards the external auditory meatus.[5] We prefer to locate the vessel at the junction of the sternal and clavicular heads of the sternocleidomastoid muscle.

Once the site is selected, it is prepared with antiseptic solution, draped with sterile towels and infiltrated with local anaesthetic. The patient is then placed in the horizontal position, with the neck in the neutral position or slightly turned to the contralateral side. The junction between the sternal and clavicular heads of the sternocleidomastoid muscle is localized and the skin is punctured with a 16 gauge 5.25 inch Angiocath catheter (Becton and Dickinson) mounted with a 5 ml syringe. During gentle aspiration, the needle is passed in a cranial direction for 1–2 cm, at an angle of 15–20° in the sagittal plane. Once the vein is entered, the catheter is advanced over the needle until a slight elastic resistance is felt or until the tip of the catheter is estimated to be just behind the mastoid process. If difficulty in localizing the vein is encountered, the patient is tilted 15° head down until the vein is located, after which the head is elevated. A guidewire (Seldinger technique) is used when difficulty in passing the catheter is encountered despite a head-down tilt. If a central venous line is also required, it is possible to use the same side as the SJO_2 catheter.

The Seldinger technique is used to insert the antegrade line and after placement of the guidewire, the retrograde catheter is inserted as described above. The central venous catheter is then threaded over the guidewire. This sequence prevents the accidental shearing of the central venous catheter when the SJO_2 catheter is inserted. The area is then covered by a sterile dressing, the catheter is connected to a three-

way stopcock and a slow continuous infusion of 0.9% saline is started to prevent catheter blockage.

When a continuous catheter is required, the Seldinger technique is used to insert the 16 gauge cannula through which the fibreoptic catheter is threaded and then secured. A pressurized heparanized flush system is used to maintain patency of the catheter and reduce the incidence of wall artefacts.[7]

The position of the catheter should be confirmed by lateral cervical spine X-ray or an anteroposterior chest X-ray that includes a view of the neck.[10] The end of the catheter should lie at the level of and just medial to the mastoid bone above the lower border of C1.

SJO_2 can be measured intermittently by sampling blood or continuously using a fibreoptic oximetry. Serial sampling is cheaper and allows calculation of arteriovenous content difference in oxygen ($AVDO_2$), glucose and lactate. The early problems encountered with the use of fibreoptic oximetric catheters seem to have been reduced by the development of new, 'stiffer' catheters, less prone to kinking and curling back, and by careful positioning and calibration of the catheter. This has been recently confirmed by Gunn et al[7] during intracranial surgery and Souter et al[8] and Coplin et al[26] in the intensive care setting. Nonetheless, suspected jugular bulb desaturation should be verified by cooximetry before taking therapeutic actions.

Two catheters are currently available for jugular bulb oximetry: the Oximetrix (Abbott Laboratories, North Chicago, Illinois, USA) and the Edslab II (Baxter Healthcare Corporation, Irvine, California, USA).[14] Both are size 4 French gauge double-lumen catheters.

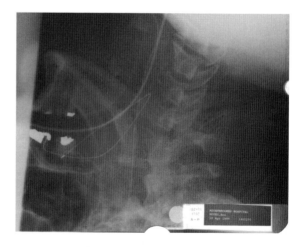

Figure 9.2 A lateral cervical spine X-ray following the insertion of a jugular bulb catheter. The arrow points to the tip of the catheter at the level of the mastoid bone.

The distal lumen is used to aspirate blood for in vivo calibration while the other lumen contains two optical fibres, one to transmit and the other to receive light transmitted to and then returned from the jugular bulb. The Oximetrix catheter has three light-emitting diodes while the Edslab II has two. These diodes send red and near infra-red light, at 1 ms intervals to blood passing through the jugular bulb where it is absorbed, reflected and refracted. The reflected light from haemoglobin is detected by a photoelectric sensor and averaged for the previous 5 s to calculate haemoglobin oxygen saturation, which is then updated every second. If the light source at the catheter tip abuts the vessel wall a low light intensity or signal quality alarm is displayed. The Edslab II system requires the insertion of the patient's haemoglobin concentration for in vivo calibration, which may cast doubt on its accuracy in situations where the haemoglobin concentration is unstable, such as with rapid large blood loss. This and any other comparison of the two different systems are difficult to make as no clinical data comparing the two have been published.

Continuous fibreoptic oximetric catheters can be calibrated prior to (in vitro) or after insertion (in vivo). In vivo calibration is more accurate and subject to less drift.[5,7,11] Drift can be further reduced by recalibration at 12-hourly intervals. The sampling port of the catheter should be continuously flushed with heparinized saline (1 IU/ml) at a rate of 2–4 ml/h to maintain its patency. Contamination of jugular bulb blood with extracranial blood depends on the speed of blood withdrawal from the catheter, with up to 25% higher jugular venous oxygen saturation (SJO$_2$) values seen with faster rates of blood withdrawal(>2 ml/min).[9]

Complications from jugular bulb catheterization are similar to those seen during the placement of ante-grade internal jugular venous lines and are dependent on the experience of the operator.[6,12] The commonest are carotid artery puncture and haematoma formation which occur in about 1–4% of insertions and are self-limiting. Other complications, which include damage to adjacent structures such as the carotid artery, vagus and phrenic nerves and the thoracic duct, are rare. Pneumothorax, venous air embolism and venous thrombosis are also infrequent. There is an increased risk of local and systemic infection with long-term placement.

CLINICAL APPLICATIONS

The first measurements of SJO$_2$ in humans were made in the 1920s by Myerson et al.[15] They sampled the jugular bulb directly with a needle placed near the base of the skull just below and anterior to the tip of the mastoid process. In 1953, Seldinger described the insertion of a wire into an artery via a needle, followed by the insertion of a catheter over the wire. This led the way to intermittent indirect sampling of the jugular bulb via catheters inserted into the proximal IJV and then passed distally up into the jugular bulb. In the late 1980s, fibreoptic catheters which could continuously measure oxygen saturation of haemoglobin were introduced into clinical practice.[16]

Cerebral oxygenation

Normal SJO$_2$ ranges between 55% and 85%. Levels below 55% suggest cerebral hypoperfusion with oxygen demand exceeding supply, while levels above 85% indicate relative hyperaemia. SJO$_2$ is a global hemispheric measurement with obvious limitations in that regional ischaemia cannot be detected. This is exemplified by the case reported by Chieregato et al, where jugular bulb oximetry without intracranial pressure monitoring was suboptimal for managing a patient with subarachnoid haemorrhage and raised intracranial pressure.[18] Nevertheless, while a normal SJO$_2$ does not rule out regional ischaemia, a low SJO$_2$ indicates that there is an increase in oxygen extraction or a reduction in oxygen delivery which may be an early warning sign of ischaemia.[27]

Episodes of cerebral venous oxygen desaturation are common in comatose patients as a result of head trauma or subarachnoid haemorrhage even when receiving intensive care with invasive haemodynamic and intracranial pressure monitoring.[17,19,32] The observation that these patients have a higher mortality than those without such episodes (SJO$_2$ <50% for more than 15 min) highlights the potential benefit of detecting and treating cerebral venous oxygen desaturation.[17] Many of these episodes can be attributed to

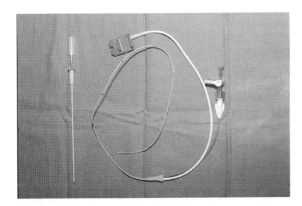

Figure 9.3 A single-use Angiocath catheter (Becton and Dickinson) and a continuous fibreoptic jugular bulb catheter (the Edslab II by Baxter Healthcare Corporation, Irvine, California, USA).

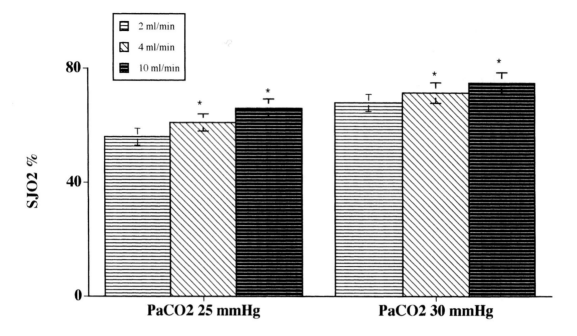

Figure 9.4   The speed of blood withdrawal from jugular bulb catheters affects accuracy of reading. SJO_2 values are higher with faster rates of blood withdrawal due to contamination with extracranial blood. Optimal rate appears to be 2 ml/min.

High SjO_2	Abnormal autoregulation	Hyperaemia
	Increased oxygen supply	Polycythaemia
	Decreased oxygen consumption	Hypothermia
		Sedative drugs
		Anaesthetic drugs
		Cerebral infarction
	Extracerebral blood	
Low SjO_2	Abnormal autoregulation	
	Decreased oxygen supply	Hypoxia
		Hypotension
		Intracranial hypertension
		Hyperventilation
		Low cardiac output
		Anaemia
	Increased oxygen consumption	Hyperthermia
		Seizures
		Sepsis

hyperventilation (even moderate), reduced cerebral perfusion pressure or cerebral arterial vasospasm.

Analysis of very early jugular bulb oximetry data from severely head-injured patients revealed a high incidence of disturbed and inadequate cerebral perfusion in the first hours after the injury.[25] These findings have important implications for the emergency management of such patients, as outcome may be improved by better management in the early hours after traumatic brain injury.

Matta et al demonstrated a 50% incidence of jugular venous desaturation in patients undergoing neurosurgical procedures, although the incidence of severe desaturation (SJO_2 <45%) was much lower at 17%.[6] These desaturations could not have been predicted by the $PaCO_2$ level alone. In other words, without this monitor many of the episodes would have gone unnoticed.

Moss et al studied the effects of changing mean arterial pressure (MAP) on SJO_2 and lactate oxygen index (LOI) in 26 patients undergoing anaesthesia for clipping of cerebral aneurysm.[20] When considering an SJO_2 value less than 54% indicative of cerebral hypoperfusion, they were able to identify a critical MAP of between 80 and 110 mmHg in nine patients. Patients with an LOI <0.08 at any time during the procedure had a worse clinical outcome within the first day. Although an increase in MAP resulted in a similar increase in SJO_2 in 19 of the patients studied, this was not always accompanied by an improved LOI. The study further highlights the benefits of jugular bulb cannulation to assess cerebral hypoperfusion during the intra- and postoperative management of patient with subarachnoid haemorrhage.

Jugular bulb oxygen desaturations have also been correlated with poor outcome in patients undergoing cardiac surgery. Croughwell et al used jugular bulb oximetry to calculate $AVDO_2$ in 255 patients undergoing cardiopulmonary bypass.[21] They found that cerebral venous desaturations (SJO_2 <50%) occurred in up to 23% of the patients and correlated with worse postoperative cognitive function.[21] The desaturations observed were the result of inadequate cerebral blood flow (CBF) in proportion to oxygen consumption, as indicated by a decreased CBF to $AVDO_2$ ratio. Other suggested causes include microembolic events and disturbances in cerebral autoregulation. The episodes of desaturation were observed during both normothermic and hypothermic cardiopulmonary bypass. In a follow-up study, the same group highlighted the importance of continuously monitoring cerebral oxygenation during cardiac surgery as neither mixed venous oximetry nor systemic pump venous saturation

is able to detect the adequacy of cerebral perfusion in these patients.[22]

Takasu et al continuously monitored systemic and jugular venous oxygenation during the 24 h after resuscitation from cardiac arrest in eight patients.[23] The three patients that survived had significantly lower jugular venous oxygen saturation (67%) than non-survivors (80%), whereas mixed venous saturations were higher in the survivors than in the non-survivors (74% and 64% respectively). The authors suggest that damaged neurons are unable to utilize oxygen adequately, resulting in the high SJO_2 value and the poor neurologic outcome in resuscitated patients after cardiac arrest. Unfortunately, because normal SJO_2 values vary between 55% and 85%, it is unlikely that this information will be of benefit in the immediate management of these patients.

Cerebral blood flow and metabolism

Jugular bulb oximetry has evolved from a combination of old and new technology. The first measurements taken from the jugular bulb were used to calculate cerebral blood flow (CBF) using the Fick principle.[13] Cerebral metabolic rate for oxygen ($CMRO_2$) can be calculated from the CBF and the difference between the arteriovenous oxygen content difference ($AVDO_2$) using the equation:

$$CMRO_2 = CBF \times (\text{arterial oxygen content} - \text{jugular venous bulb oxygen content})$$

The oxygen content can be determined using co-oximetry or calculated using the equations:

$$\text{Arterial oxygen content} = [(Hb \times 1.34 \times SaO_2) + (PaO_2 \times 0.0031)]$$

$$\text{Jugular venous oxygen content} = [(Hb \times 1.34 \times SJO_2) + (PvO_2 \times 0.0031)]$$

where Hb = haemoglobin in g/dl, SaO_2 = arterial saturation, SJO_2 = jugular venous bulb saturation, PaO_2 = oxygen partial pressure in arterial blood in mmHg, and PvO_2 = oxygen partial pressure in venous blood in mmHg.

As the haemoglobin concentration is the same in arterial and venous blood and the amount of dissolved oxygen is minimal, cerebral metabolic rate for oxygen can be estimated from CBF and the difference in the arteriojugular bulb oxygen saturation.

$$CMRO_2 = CBF \times (SaO_2 - SjO_2)$$

Therefore, the arteriovenous oxygen content (or saturation) difference can be used to relate changes in metabolism to alterations in CBF. Ischaemia results in an increased $AVDO_2$, while hyperaemia will lead to a reduction in the $AVDO_2$. The same principle can be applied to other metabolites such as glucose and lactate.

Defining critical thresholds

Over the last 10 years the use of jugular bulb oximetry has moved from being a research tool to a standard of care in many units. In a survey of the intensive care management of severe head injuries in the United Kingdom published in 1996, 12% of the units questioned used a jugular bulb catheter for routine monitoring in more than 50% of their patients with a traumatic brain injury.[28]

Although prolonged marked hyperventilation is associated with poor neurological outcome after head injury, acute hyperventilation may be life saving.[33] Hypocapnia induces cerebral vasoconstriction and although the resultant decrease in CBF and ICP may improve cerebral perfusion. However, excessive cerebral vasoconstriction has been shown to cause cerebral ischaemia. In addition, hyperventilation shifts the oxygen-haemoglobin dissociation curve to the left, thus reducing the amount of oxygen released from haemoglobin to brain tissue. Therefore, hyperventilation must be used with great care and should not be used to lower intracranial pressure without some measure of cerebral oxygenation.[29,30] If hyperoxia can be used as a temporary measure to improve cerebral oxygen delivery during marked hyperventilation.[34,35] SJO_2 monitoring allows fine tuning of ventilation so that optimal brain oxygenation is achieved.

Brain injury is often associated with impaired cerebral pressure autoregulation. The critical perfusion threshold can be established by close examination of changes in SJO_2 in response to changes in perfusion pressure. Lewis et al were able to demonstrate that a critically low level of SJO_2 is a late indicator of failed autoregulation and, when used in combination with transcranial Doppler, may be useful in determining the level of cerebral perfusion pressure at which therapy should be aimed in the early resuscitation of head trauma.[31]

NEAR INFRARED SPECTROSCOPY

Near infrared spectroscopy (NIRS) is an application of a technology that has been available for a number of years. It can be used to provide information about changes in regional cerebral oxygenation, cerebral blood flow and volume and oxygen utilization in the brain.

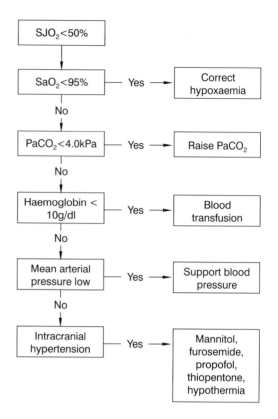

Figure 9.5   Suggested algorithm for treatment of jugular venous desaturation.

PRINCIPLES

The principle behind NIRS is based upon the fact that light in the near infrared range (700–1000 nm) can pass through the skin, bone and other tissues relatively easily. When a beam of light is passed through brain tissue, it is both scattered and absorbed. The absorption of near infrared light is proportional to the concentration of certain chromophores, notably iron in haemoglobin and copper in cytochrome aa_3. Oxygenated (HbO_2) and deoxygenated haemoglobin (Hb) and cytochrome aa_3 have different absorption spectra, depending on the substances' oxygenation status. The isobestic point of oxygenated and deoxygenated haemoglobin is at about 810 nm. Oxyhaemoglobin has a greater light absorption above this wavelength and deoxyhaemoglobin has greater light absorption below 810 nm. The maximum oxidation/reduction proportion for cytochrome oxidase or cytochrome aa_3, which is the terminal member of the mitochondrial respiratory chain, is at 830 nm. This allows for the measurement of oxidation status.

Changes of concentration of the near infrared light as it passes through these compounds can be quantified using a modified Beer–Lambert Law which describes optical attenuation. It is expressed as:

$$\text{Attenuation (OD)} = \text{Log}\,\frac{Ia}{I} = \alpha\ C\ LB + G$$

OD = optical densities
Ia = incident light intensity
I = detected light intensity
α = absorption coefficient of chromophore ($mM^{-1}\ cm^{-1}$)
C = concentration of chromophore (mM)
L = physical distance between the points where light enters and leaves the tissue (cm)
B = pathlength factor
G = factor related to the measurement geometry and type of tissue.

In this way, changes in concentration of each of the chromophores (HbO_2, Hb $Cyto_2$) can be determined and thus the regional cerebral oxygenation obtained.[36]

'Transmission spectroscopy', although possible in neonates, is not feasible in adults because of the large head and thick skull. By placing the optodes a few centimeters apart on the same side of the head, it is possible to measure changes in cerebral oxygenation in adults using 'reflectance spectroscopy'.

Near infrared instruments are made for clinical use by a number of manufacturers. They generally consist of small optical probes connected to a monitoring device by a wire bundle. This enables the monitor to be placed at a distance from the patient which will facilitate its use in intensive care and during surgery. The rubber optical probes contain light sources consisting of small tungsten light filaments of less than 3 watts and two photo diodes filtered at 760 nm and 850 nm. The light sources are recessed so as to prevent direct skin contact. A photodiode detector converts the reflected light to a current and then to a voltage for amplification and signal detection.

The probes illuminate up to a volume of 10 ml of hemispherical tissue. The radial depth will depend on the interoptode distance. The optodes are placed on one side of the forehead away from the midline, cerebral venous sinuses and temporalis muscle and at an acute angle to each other with an interrupted spacing of 4–7 cm.

Using a derived algorithm, the measured changes in attenuation at each wavelength (for each chromophore) can be converted into equivalent changes in the concentration of HbO_2, Hb and cytochrome aa_3. All measurements are expressed as absolute concentration changes from an arbitrary zero at the start of the measurement period. Normal values of HbO_2 are reported to be 60–80% and the ischaemic threshold is estimated to be 47% saturation.[37]

CLINICAL APPLICATIONS

Near infrared spectroscopy was first used to monitor cerebral and myocardial insufficiency by Jobsis in 1977.[38] Since then, it has been used to measure cerebral oxygenation particularly in the paediatric population to detect changes in secondary brain injury due to hypoxaemia and during deep hypothermic cardiopulmonary bypass.[39]

One of the major problems with NIRS is the inability to reliably distinguish between extracranial and intracranial changes in blood flow and oxygenation which may affect its rehability as a monitor of brain oxygenation in clinical practice.[40–43] This is highly dependent on where the optodes are placed and on the distance between them. The amount of extracranial contamination decreases with increased optode separation, but is still noticeable at 7 cm separation.[43] It is now accepted that optode separation less than 4 cm predominantly reflects extracranial tissue changes.[44]

More recently, NIRS has been used in adults to monitor patients with head injury and intracranial haemorrhage and those undergoing carotid endarterectomy. Kirkpatrick et al[45] used the NIRO 500 cerebral oximeter (Hamamatsu Photonics, Japan) to monitor cerebral saturations (ScO_2) in patients undergoing carotid endarterectomy under general anaesthesia. A transcranial Doppler ultrasound to measure middle cerebral artery flow velocity (Vmca) and cerebral function analysing monitor were also used. The NIRS was able to detect rapid changes in cerebral oxygenation without significant contamination from extracranial vessels. The authors were able to identify three categories of NIRS response during carotid endarterectomy:

1. no change in HbO_2 on internal carotid clamping;
2. decrease in HbO_2 that recovers during clamping;
3. decrease in HbO_2 that only recovered with the release of the clamp.

In those patients in whom spontaneous recovery of the signal did not occur, a hyperaemic response with an increase in HbO_2 and Vmca above baseline was observed.

By using bilateral cerebral oximetry, Samra et al were able to demonstrate a significant but variable drop in the ipsilateral ScO_2 without neurologic dysfunction in patients undergoing carotid endarterectomy under regional anaesthesia. However, they were unable to identify the critical ScO_2 or change in ScO_2 that requires the insertion of a shunt.[46]

In patients with head injury, changes in HbO_2 correlate well with changes in jugular bulb oximetry, transcranial Doppler and laser Doppler flowmetry.[47,48] However, there were instances where observed changes in Hb and HbO_2 were not matched by similar changes in SJO_2.[47] Although the significance of these findings is not clear, it may be that mixing of venous blood draining from the sinuses reduces the sensitivity of SJO_2 monitoring. In contrast, the positioning of the NIRS probe in the frontal region allows monitoring of oxygenation in a small region of the cortex. Whatever the case, these discrepancies require further investigation.

Although NIRS has been used to examine changes in cerebral saturation in patients undergoing cardiac surgery,[49–51] because we do not fully understand how extracorporeal circulation affects the assumptions upon which NIRS technology is based, it is not yet possible to say with certainty how useful NIRS will be in patients undergoing cardiac surgery.

By using a modification of the Fick principle, NIRS can detect changes in CBF and cerebral blood volume (CBV).[52–54] A sudden increase in SaO_2 produces a bolus of HbO_2, which acts as an arterial tracer which is measured in the arterial system by the pulse oximeter and in the brain by NIRS. Similarly, CBV can be calculated by inducing small but slow changes in SaO_2 and measuring changes in HbO_2 and Hb by NIRS. Gupta et al reported that CBV reactivities in volunteers ranged between 1.25 and 1.05 ml/100 g/kPa of CO_2.[53]

The potential advantages of being able to measure CBF and CBV non-invasively are obvious but, 30% of the data are rejected because of variations in the baseline NIRS signal, MAP or end-tidal CO_2. Furthermore, recently published data by Owen-Reece et al suggest that the technique considerably underestimates CBF because of the optical effects of extracranial tissue.[55] Hence further validation of these techniques is required before they can be adopted as part of normal clinical practice.

Regardless of these problems NIRS is able to monitor trends in oxygenation in the individual patient and may be useful as an adjunct to the multimodal monitoring system described elsewhere.

TISSUE OXYGEN MEASUREMENT

The ability to measure oxygen tension in tissue was first reported by Clark in 1956. Polarographic multiwire surface and depth electrodes have since been used to measure oxygenation and various experiments have been performed to assess brain tissue PO_2 and its regulatory mechanisms.[56–67] There are now a number of reports on in vivo measurements of tissue PO_2 in human brain cortex.[56,61] At present, two commercially available sensors are used for measuring brain tissue oxygenation. One is the Licox sensor (GMS, Germany), which measures brain tissue oxygen only, and the other is the Neurotrend sensor (Diametrics Medical, High Wycombe, UK), which measures brain tissue oxygen, carbon dioxide and pH. Both devices can be used to measure brain temperature. The increased interest in the use of these sensors has come from the inability of jugular bulb oximetry to accurately detect regional ischaemia and the contamination of the NIRS signal with extracranial blood.

BRAIN TISSUE OXYGEN MONITORING (LICOX)

This consists of a polarographic electrochemical microsensor and a thermocouple which measure oxygen and temperature respectively. The polarographic cell, 0.47 mm and 200–300 mm in length depending on the type of probe is contained in a closed flexible polythene tube. The PO_2 sensor is 4.5 mm long and lies 7 mm from the tip. The probe is usually inserted into the brain via a single or triple-lumen bolt fixed into the skull. The probe requires a 20-min period of stabilization. Oxygen diffuses from the tissue through the polyethylene wall of the catheter into its inner electrolyte chamber. A current is generated by the transformation of oxygen by the polarographic cathode, a negatively polarized precious metal electrode, to hydroxide ions, which is then displayed as PO_2 and temperature values. The sensor is calibrated prior to insertion into the tissue either by inserting the catheter in an O_2 free nitrogen solution and subsequently in room air, which takes approximately 1 h and has the potential risk of compromising sterility, or by using the manufacturer's catheter-specific calibration settings on the monitor.

Clinical application

The Licox sensor has been used to measure PO_2 in a variety of tissues that include skeletal muscle, liver, cutaneous tissue, myocardium and brain. Data available suggest that, at least in animals, arterial PO_2 and PCO_2 exert a major influence on CSF PO_2 which ranges from 61 to 64 mm Hg. Not surprisingly, CSF PO_2 values are also dependent on changes in cerebral perfusion, intracranial and mean arterial pressures.[68] In an experimental model of cerebral ischaemia, in addition to confirming the relationship between arterial PO_2 and CSF PO_2, Mass et al were able to demonstrate that during reperfusion, brain tissue PO_2 may remain low or even decrease further despite increases in CSF PO_2.[69]

Although normal brain tissue PO_2 values in humans are similar to those in animals (25–30 mmHg), some investigators have reported higher levels in patients with brain tumours, especially in the peritumoural tissue.[56,61] Increases in intracranial pressure and brain swelling decrease brain tissue PO_2, with levels as low as 5 mmHg preceding the clinical manifestation of cerebral herniation leading to brain death.[69,70] Meixensberger et al demonstrated that changes in arterial PO_2 correlate with changes in normal but not abnormal brain tissue PO_2.[70] Hypoventilation, however, leads to a reduction in both normal and abnormal brain tissue PO_2.[70]

The effects of reducing cerebral perfusion pressure on CSF and brain tissue PO_2 are demonstrated in Figure 9.5.

Brain tissue PO_2 values < 20 mmHg have been reported in the first 24 h after head injury.[71] Levels below 6 mmHg after brain trauma are associated with increased risk of death.[83]

The Licox sensor uderestimates brain tissue PO_2 by up to 8.5% especially in the first four days of monitoring.[72] Overall, both the sensitivity drift (-8.5%) and the zero drift (1.5 mmHg) are found to be acceptable in clinical practice. Despite its highly invasive nature, early reports suggest this type of monitoring is safe, with no increased incidence of infection and only a very small risk of haematoma formation.[72]

MULTIPARAMETER MONITORING OF BRAIN TISSUE (NEUROTREND)

Measurement of brain tissue PO_2, PCO_2, pH and temperature was first performed using a Paratrend 7 sensor soon after the introduction of the Licox probe as a brain tissue PO_2 sensor. The sensor was originally designed for continuous intra-arterial blood gas monitoring and has been recently adapted for continuous intracerebral monitoring (renamed Neurotrend[TM]).

The pH sensor is a 175 μm polymethyl methacrolate fibre with three radial holes drilled in it using a laser. A stainless steel mirror is encapsulated in the end of the fibre. This arrangement represents a miniature spectrophotometer. Into the holes is placed polyacrylamide gel containing immobilized phenol red dye. The dye changes colour in response to the concentration of hydrogen ions. The change is reversible so that both increases and decreases in pH can be detected by irra-

diating the dye cell with green light. By measuring the absorbence of green light by the phenol red dye, a measurement of the pH can be made.[73]

The PCO_2 sensor is similar to the pH fibre but has a gas-permeable membrane enclosing the holes in the fibre. The membranes and the holes in the fibre are filled with a bicarbonate solution containing phenol red dye as indicator. Carbon dioxide is diffused through the membrane into the reservoir and changes the pH of the solution.

The oxygen sensor in the recently introduced Neurotrend sensor is based on fluorescent technology and contains entrapped ruthenium-based dye, which absorbs the blue light at 450–470 nm passed down the fibre. The dye then emits a proportion of the energy it has absorbed as light of another wavelength (620 nm). The difference between the two wavelengths, the absorption and emission, is called the *Stoke's shift*. Oxygen reduces the amount of fluorescent light, so-called 'oxygen quenching'. The amount of quenching is proportional to the concentration of oxygen and thus, changes in fluorescent light are used to estimate PO_2. Preliminary data from using this probe are promising.

The thermocouple is constructed by the welding of copper and constantan wires into a ball weld of 0.0036 inches. The weld is then potted in silicone rubber to prevent corrosion. The four sensors are place inside a polyethylene sheath, the front region of which is microporous and covers the sensing ends of the sensors. The microporous region is filled with polyacrylamide gel which contains phenol red. The outer surface of the sensor is coated with a covalently bonded polyethylene. The outer diameter of the whole sensor is approximately 0.5 mm. In order to achieve this compact configuration, the individual sensing elements are staggered from the tip. The probe is packaged with the sensor sealed within a tonometer containing buffer solution, through which standard precision gases are bubbled for calibration of the sensor. It is supplied as a sterile, single-use, disposable device designed to be inserted through an 18 or 20 gauge arterial cannula.

Prior to insertion, the sensor is calibrated with the three precision gases supplied. The first gas contains 2% CO_2, 15% O_2 and a balance of nitrogen; the second gas comprises 5% CO_2, 15% O_2 and a balance of nitrogen; the third gas is 10% CO_2, 15% O_2 and a balance of nitrogen. Each gas is bubbled into the calibrating solution for 10 min. The oxygen calibration curve is constructed using an electric zero and 15% oxygen gas, assuming linear properties of the electrode. The CO_2 and pH calibration curves are constructed within the range 10–80 mmHg using the three CO_2 gas concentrations: 2%, 14 mmHg (pH 7.83); 5%, 36 mmHg (pH 7.43); and 10%, 71 mmHg (pH 7.13). The range of 95 % confidence limits for each sensor has been determined by in vitro testing.[73]

These sensors have been mainly evaluated for continuous intra-arterial use,[73–75] continuous monitoring of gastrointestinal mucosal PCO_2[76] and are increasingly being implanted into brain tissue to continuously monitor tissue CO_2, pH, PO_2 and temperature.[77,78] The effects of temporary focal ischaemia, hypoventilation and anaesthetic drugs on brain parenchyma PO_2 PCO_2 and pH are being evaluated. Initial reports suggest the changes to be reliable and reproducible.[79,80] Reported brain tissue PO_2 values in patients who have suffered a severe head injury are similar to those obtained using the Licox sensor. Furthermore, it appears that focal changes in oxygenation may not be always reflected by global measurements such as SJO_2.[81,82,84]

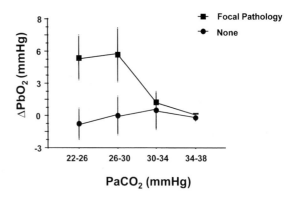

Figure 9.7   The effect of hyperventilation on brain tissue oxygenation in areas of focal pathology and with no focal pathology (reproduced with permission from reference[83]).

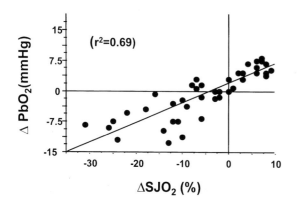

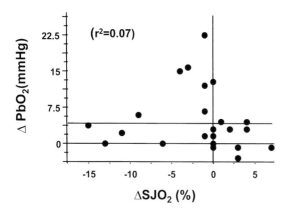

Figure 9.6   Demonstration that the correlation between changes in jugular venous oxygen saturation (∂SJO_2) and brain tissue PO_2 (∂PbO_2) is dependent on the position of the sensor. Good correlation when the sensor is in normal brain tissue (A) and poor correlation when the sensor is in an area of focal pathology (B) (reproduced with permission from referemce[83]).

A variety of bolts for inserting brain tissue sensors into brain tissue are currently available. Although there have been no reports of adverse effects associated with the insertion of these sensors, the true risks associated with the use of brain tissue probes will only become apparent once a large number of sensors have been used. Furthermore, as these measurements have not been correlated against a 'gold standard' of brain oxygenation such as positron emission tomography, further studies are required to confirm the reliability and accuracy of these sensors as estimates of brain tissue PO_2, PCO_2 and pH.

CONCLUSION

By providing an indication of cerebral ischaemia, cerebral oximetry may allow appropriate therapy to be given before neurologic damage becomes permanent. There is no 'gold standard' for measuring cerebral oxygenation. Jugular venous bulb oximetry is a global hemispheric measure with low sensitivity for detecting regional ischaemia. Although the non-invasive NIRS is promising, the assumption that NIRS always reflect cerebral changes is unwarranted at present. The microprobe electrode is highly sensitive but, because of its highly invasive nature, is unlikely to be widely used outside specialized neurosurgical units. At present, none of the methods available is sufficiently reliable or well tested to enable us to influence the clinical management of neurologically injured patient with absolute certainty. However, further research and improvement in technology and the ability to incorporate these methods into multimodal monitoring may allow early interventions with an improvement in outcome.

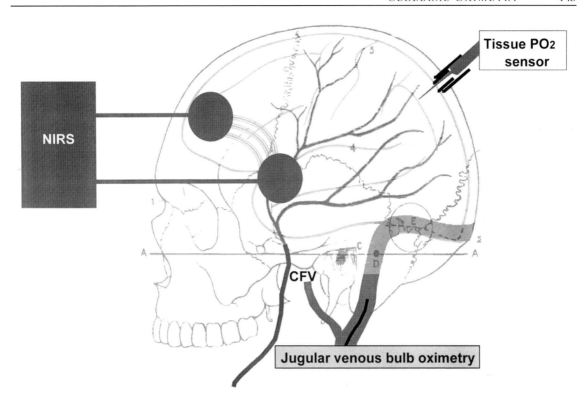

Figure 9.8   A summary diagram showing the currently available methods for cerebral oximetry. NIRS = near infrared spectroscopy.

REFERENCES

1. Epstein HM, Linde HM, Crampton AR. The vertebral venous plexus as a major cerebral venous outflow tract. Anaesthesiology 1970; 132: 332–338.

2. Gibbs EL, Gibbs FA. The cross sectional areas of the vessels that form the torcular and the manner in which blood is distributed to the right and to the left lateral sinus. Anat Rec 1934; 54: 419.

3. Gibbs EL, Lennox WG, Giggs FA. Bilateral internal jugular blood, comparison of A-V differences, oxygen-dextrose ratios and respiratory quotients. Am J Psychiat 1945; 102: 184–190.

4. Stocchetti N, Paparella A, Brindelli F, Bacchi M, Piazza P, Zuccoli P. Cerebral venous oxygen saturation studied with bilateral samples in the internal jugular veins. Neurosurgery 1994; 34: 38–44.

5. Andrews PJD, Dearden NM, Miller JD. Jugular bulb cannulation: description of a cannulation technique and a validation of a new continuous monitor. Br J Anaesth 1991; 67: 553–558.

6. Matta BF, Lam AM, Mayberg TS, Shapira Y, Winn HR. A critique of the intraoperative use of jugular venous bulb catheters during neurosurgical procedures. Anesth Analg 1994; 79: 745–750.

7. Gunn HC, Matta BF, Lam AM, Mayberg TS. Accuracy of continuous jugular bulb venous oximetry during intracranial surgery. J Neurosurg anesthesiol 1995; 7: 174–177.

8. Souter MJ, Andrews PJD. Validation of the Edslab dual lumen oximetry catheter for continuous monitoring of jugular bulb oxygen saturation after severe head injury. Br J Anaesth 1996; 76: 744–746.

9. Matta BF, Lam AM. The speed of blood withdrawal affects the accuracy of jugular venous bulb oxygen saturation measurements. Anesthesiology 1996; 86: 806–808.

10. Bankier AA, Fleischmann D, Windiscch A et al. Position of jugular oxygen saturation catheter in patients with head trauma: assessment by use of plain films. Am J Radiol 1995; 164: 437–441.

11. Lewis SB, Myburgh JA, Reilly PL. Detection of cerebral venous desaturation by continuous jugular bulb oximetry following acute neurotrauma. Anaesth Intens Care 1995; 23: 307–314.

12. Goetting MG, Preston G. Jugular bulb catheterization: experience with 123 patients. Crit Care Med 1990; 18: 1220–1223.

13. Ketty SS, Schmidt CF. The nitrous oxide method for the quantitative determination of cerebral blood flow in

man: theory, procedure and normal values. J Clin Invest 1948; 27: 476–483.

14. De Deyne C, Decruyenaere J, Colardyn F. How to interpret jugular bulb oximetry? In: Vincent JL, (ed) Yearbook of intensive care and emergency medicine. Springer-Verlag, Berlin, 1996; pp 731–741.

15. Myerson A, Halloran RD, Hirsch HL. Technique for obtaining blood from the internal jugular vein and internal carotid artery. Arch Neurol Psychiat 1927; 17: 807.

16. Cruz J, Miner ME. Modulating cerebral oxygen delivery and extractions in acute traumatic coma. In: Miner ME, Wagner KA (eds) Neurotrauma, rehabilitation, and related issues. Butterworths, Boston 1986; pp 55–72.

17. Schneider GH, Helden AV, Lanksch WR, Untergberg A. Continuous monitoring of jugular bulb oxygen saturation in comatose patients–therapeutic implications. Acta Neurochir (wien) 1995; 134: 71–75.

18. Chieregato A, Targa L, Zatelli R. Limitations of jugular bulb oxyhemogobin saturation without intracranial pressure monitoring in subarachnoid hemorrhage. J Neurosurg Anesthesiol 1996; 8: 21–25.

19. Sheinberg GM, Kanter MJ, Robertson CS et al. Continuous monitoring of jugular venous oxygen saturation in head-injured patients. J Neurosurg 1992; 76: 212–217.

20. Moss E, Dearden NM, Berridge JC. Effects of changes in mean arterial pressure on SjO2 during cerebral aneurysm surgery. Br J Anaesth 1995; 75: 527–530.

21. Croughwell ND, Newman MF, Blumenthal JA et al. Jugular bulb saturation and cognitive dysfunction after cardiopulmonary bypass. Ann Thorac Surg 1994; 58: 1702–1708.

22. Croughwell ND, White WD, Smith LR et al. Jugular bulb saturation and mixed venous saturation during cardiopulmonary bypass. J Card Surg 1995; 10: 503–508.

23. Takasu A, Yagi K, Ishihara S, Okada Y. Combined continuous monitoring of systemic and cerebral oxygen metabolism after cardiac arrest. Resuscitation 1995; 29: 189–194.

24. Lam JM, Chan MS, Poon WS. Cerebral venous oxygen saturation monitoring: is dominant jugular bulb cannulation good enough? Br J Neurosurg 1996; 10(4): 357–364.

25. De Deyne C, Decruyenaere J, Calle P et al. Analysis of very early jugular bulb oximetry data after severe head injury: implications for the emergency management? Eur J Emerg Med 1996; 3(2): 69–72.

26. Coplin WM, O'Keefe GE, Grady MS et al. Accuracy of continuous jugular bulb oximetry in the intensive care unit. Neurosurgery 1998; 42(3): 533–539.

27. Gupta AK, Hutchinson PJ, Al-Rawi P et al. Measuring brain tissue oxygenation compared with jugular venous oxygen saturation for monitoring cerebral oxygenation after traumatic brain injury. Anesth Analg 1999; 88: 549–553.

28. Matta B, Menon D. Severe head injury in the United Kingdom and Ireland: a survey of practice and implications for management. Crit Care Med 1996; 24: 1743–1748.

29. Schneider GH, Helden AV, Lanksch WR, Utergerg A. Continuous monitoring of jugular bulb oxygen saturation in comatose patients – therapeutic implications. Acta Neurochir 1995; 134: 71–75.

30. Sheinberg M, Kanter MJ, Rogertson CS. Continuous monitoring of jugular venous oxygen saturation in head-injured patients. J Neurosurg 1992; 76: 212–217.

31. Lewis S, Wong M, Myburgh J, Reilly P. Determining cerebral perfusion pressure thresholds in severe head trauma Acta Neurochir (Wien) 1998; 71(suppl): 174–176.

32. Gopinath SP, Rogertson CS, Constant CF et al. Jugular venous desaturation and outcome after head injury. J Neurol Neurosurg Psychiat 1994; 57: 717–723.

33. Muizelaar JP, Marmarou A, Ward JD et al. Adverse effects of prolonged hyperventilation in patients with severe head injury: a randomised clinical trial. J Neurosurg 1991; 75: 731–739.

34. Matta BF, Lam AM, Mayberg TS. The influence of arterial hyperoxygenation on cerebral venous oxygen content during hyperventilation. Can J Anaesth 1994; 41: 1041–1046.

35. Thiagarajan A, Goverdhan P, Chari P, Somasunderam K. The effect of hyperventilation and hyperoxia on cerebral venous oxygen saturation in patients with traumatic brain injury. Anesth Analg 1998; 87: 850–853.

36. Elwell CE, Owen-Reece H, Cope M et al. Measurement of adult cerebral haemodynamics using near infrared spectroscopy. Acta Neurochir 1993; 59(suppl): 74–80.

37. Levy WJ, Levin S, Chance B. Near infrared measurement of cerebral oxygenation, correlation with electroencephalographic ischaemia during ventricular fibrillation. Anesthesiology 1995; 83: 738–746.

38. Jobsis FF. Infrared monitoring of cerebral and myocardial oxygen sufficiency and cirulatory parameter Science 1977; 198: 1264–1267.

39. Kurth CD, Steven JM, Nicholson SC. Cerebral oxygenation during paediatric cardiac surgery using deep hypothermic circulatory arrest. Anesthesiology 1995; 82: 74–82.

40. Germon TJ, Kane NM, Manara AR, Nelson RJ. Near-infrared spectroscopy in adults: effects of extracranial ischaemia and intracranial hypoxia on estimation of cerebral oxygenation. Br J Anaesth 1994; 73: 503–506.

41. Germon TJ, Young AER, Manara AR, Nelson RJ. Extracerebral absorption of near infrared light influences the detection of increased oxygenation monitored by near infrared spectroscopy. J Neurol Neurosurg Psychiat 1995; 58: 477–479.

42. Harris DNF, Bailey SM. Near infrared spectroscopy in adults: Does the Invos 3100 really measure intracerebral oxygenation? Anaesthesia 1993; 48: 694–696.

43. Harris DN, Cowans FM, Wertheim DA, Hamid S. NIR in adults–effect of increasing optode separation. Adv Exp Med biol 1994; 345: 837–840.

44. Duncan A, Meek JH, Clemence M et al. Optical path-length measurement on adult head, calf, forearm and the head of the newborn infant using phase resolved optical spectroscopy. Physiol Med Biol 1995; 40: 295–304.

45. Kirkpatrick PJ, Smielewski P, Whitfield PC, Czosnyka M, Menon D, Pickard JD. An observational study of near infrared spectroscopy during carotid endarterectomy. J Neurosurg 1995; 82: 756–763.

46. Samra SK, Dorje P, Zelenock GB, Stanley JC. Cerebral oximetry in patients undergoing carotid endarterectomy under regional anaesthesia. Stroke 1996; 27: 49–55.

47. Kirkpatrick PJ, Smielewski P, Czosnyka M, Menon DK, Pickard JD. Near infrared spectroscopy use in patients with head injury. J Neurosurg 1995; 83: 963–970.

48. Tateishi A, Maekawa T, Soejima Y. Qualitative comparison of carbon dioxide-induced changes in cerebral near-infrared spectroscopy versus jugular venous oxygen saturation in adults with acute brain disease. Crit Care Med 1995; 23: 1734–1738.

49. Liem KD, Hopman JCW, Oeseburg B, Haan AFJ, Festen C, Kollee LAA. Cerebral oxygenation and haemodynamics during induction of extracorporeal membrane oxygenation as investigated by near infrared spectroscopy. Paediatrics 1995; 95: 555–561.

50. Kurth CD, Steven JM, Nicholson SC. Cerebral oxygenation during pediatric surgery using deep hypothermic circulatory arrest. Anesthesiology 1995; 82: 74–82.

51. Du Pleissis AJ, Newburger J, Jonas SA et al. Cerebral oxygen supply and utilization during infant cardiac surgery. Ann Neurol 1995; 37: 488–497.

52. Elwell CE, Owen-Reece H, Cope M et al. Measurement of adult cerebral haemodynamics using near infrared spectroscopy. Acta Neurochir 1993; 59(suppl): 74–80.

53. Gupta AK, Menon DK, Czosnyka M, Smielewski P, Kirkpatrick PJ, Jones JG. Non-invasive measurement of cerebral blood volume in volunteers. Br J Anaesth 1997; 78: 39–43.

54. Wyatt JS, Cope M, Delpy DT et al. Quantification of cerebral blood volume in newborn infants by near infrared spectroscopy. J Appl Physiol 1990; 68: 1086–1091.

55. Owen-Reece H, Elwell CE, Harkness W et al. Use of near infrared spectroscopy to estimate cerebral blood flow in conscious and anesthetized patients. Br J Anaesth 1996; 76: 43–48.

56. Assad F, Schultheiss R, Leniger-Follert E, Wullenweber R. Measurement of local oxygen partial pressure (PO2) of the brain cortex in cases of brain tumors. Adv Neurosurg 1984; 12: 263–266.

57. Bicher HI, Bruley D, Reneau DD, Knisely M. Regulatory mechanisms of brain oxygen supply. In: Kessler M et al (eds) Oxygen supply. Theoretical and practical aspects of oxygen supply and microcirculation of tissue. Urban and Schwarzenberg, Munich, 1973; pp 180–185.

58. Fleckenstein W, Maas AIR, Nollert G, De Jong DA. Oxygen pressure in cerebrospinal fluid. In: Ehrly AM et al (eds) Clinical oxygen pressure measurement II. Blackwell Ucberreuter Wissenschaft, Berlin, 1990; pp 368–395.

59. Ingvar DH, Lubbers DW, Siesjo B. Measurement of oxygen tension on the surface of the cerebral cortex of cat during hyperoxia and hypoxia. Acta Physiol Scand 48: 1960; 373–381.

60. Jamieson D, Vanden Brenk HAS. Measurement of oxygen tensions in cerebral tissues in rats exposed to high pressure of oxygen. J Appl Physiol 1963; 18: 869–876.

61. Kayama T, Yoshimoto T, Fujimoto S, Sakurai Y. Intratumoral oxygen pressure in malignant brain tumor. J Neurosurg 1991; 74: 55–59.

62. Leniger-Follert E. Direct determination of local oxygen consumption of the brain cortex in vivo. Adv Exp Med Biol 1977; 94: 325–330.

63. Leniger-Follert E, Lubbers DW, Wrabctz W. Regulation of local tissue PO2 of the brain cortex at different arterial O2 pressues. Pflugers Arch 1975; 359: 81–95.

64. Nair P, Whalen WJ, Burck D. PO2 of cat cerebral cortex: response to breathing N2 and 100% O2. Microvasc Res 1975; 9: 158–165.

65. Silver JA. Brain oxygen tension and cellular activity. In: Kessler M et al (eds) Oxygen supply. Theoretical and practical aspects of oxygen supply and microcirculation of tissue. Urban and Schwarzenberg, Munich, 1973; pp 186–188.

66. Smith RH, Guibeau EJ, Reneau DD. The oxygen tension field within a discrete volume of cerebral cortex. Microvasc Res 1977; 13: 233–240.

67. Whalen WJ, Ganfield R, Nair P. Effects of breathing O2 or O2 + CO2 and of the injection of neurotumors on the PO2 of cat cerebral cortex. Stroke 1970; 1: 194–200.

68. Fleckenstein W, Nowack G, Kehler U et al. Oxygen pressure measurement in cerebral spinal fluid. Medizin Technik 1990; 110 (2): 44 -53.

69. Maas AIR, Fleckenstein W, De Jong DA, Van Santbrink H. Monitoring cerebral oxygenation: experimental studies and preliminary clinical results of continuous monitoring of cerebral spinal fluid and brain tissue oxygen tension. Acta Neurochir 1993; 59(suppl): 50–57.

70. Meixenberger J, Dings J, Kuhnigk H, Roosen K. Studies of tissue PO2 in normal and pathological human brain cortex. Acta Neurochir 1993; 59(suppl): 58–63.

71. Santbrink H, Maas AIR, Avezaat CJJ. Continuous monitoring of partial pressure of brain tissue oxygen in patients with severe head injury. Neurosurgery 1996; 38: 21–31.

72. Dings J, Meixensberger J, Roosen K. Brain tissue PO2 monitoring: catheter stability and complications. Neurol Res 1997; 19: 241–245.

73. Venkatesh V, Clutton-Brock TH, Hendry SP. Continuous measurement of blood gases using a combined electro chemical spectrophotometric sensor. J Med Eng Technol 1994; 18(5): 165–168.

74. Venkatesh V, Clutton-Brock TH, Hendry SP. Multiparameter sensor for continuous infra arterial blood gas monitoring: a prospective evaluation. Crit Care Med 1994; 22: 588–594.

75. Clutton-Brock TH, Fink S, Luthra AJ, Hendry SP. The evaluation of a new intravascular blood gas monitoring system in the pig. J Clin Monit 1994; 10: 387–391.

76. Knichwitz G, Rotker J, Brussel T, Kuhmann M, Mertes N, Mollhoff T. A new method of continuous intra mucosal PCO₂ measurement in the gastro intestinal tract. Anesth Analg 1996; 83: 6–11.

77. McKinley BA, Morris WP, Parmley CL, Butler BD. Brain parenchyma PO₂ PCO₂ and pH during and after hypoxic ischaemic brain insult in dogs. Crit Care Med 1996; 24: 1858–1868.

78. Zauner A, Bullock R, Di X, Young HF. Brain oxygen CO₂ pH and temperature monitoring: evaluation in the feline brain. J Neurosurg 1995; 37: 1168–1177.

79. Hoffman WE, Charbel FT, Edelman G, Hannigan K, Ausman JI. Brain tissue oxygen pressure, carbon dioxide pressue and pH during ischaemia. Neurol Res 1996; 18: 54–56.

80. Hoffman WE, Charbel FT, Edelman G. Brain tissue oxygen, carbon dioxide and pH in neurosurgical patients at risk from ischaemia. Anesth Analg 1996; 82: 582–586.

81. Gupta AK, Gupta S, Swart M, Al Rawi P, Hutchinson P, Kirkpatrick P. Comparison of brain tissue oxygenation during hyperventilation in severely head injured patients measured by a new multi-parameter sensor. J Neurosurg Anaesthesiol 1997; 8: 325.

82. Heath K, Gupta A, Matta B. Brain microprobe electrodes: a case for monitoring regional cerebral oxygenation in the severely head injured patient. J Neurosurg Anaesthesiol 1998; 1: 22–24.

83. Valdaka AB, Gopinath SP, Constant CF, Usura M, Robertson CS. Relationship of brain tissue PO2 to outcome after severe head injury. Crit Care Med 1998; 26: 1576–1581.

84. Gupta AK, Hutchinson PJ, Al-Rawi P et al. Measuring brain tissue oxygenation compared with jugular venous oxygen saturation for monitoring cerebral oxygenation after traumatic brain injury. Anesth Analg 1999; 88: 549–553.

10

MONITORING BRAIN CHEMISTRY

Peter J. A. Hutchinson & Mark T. O'Connell

INTRODUCTION

The cellular mechanisms which accompany injury to the brain following ischaemia or trauma are complex and poorly understood. They include direct damage as a result of the mechanical event, chemical damage mediated by neurotransmitters, damage resulting from abnormal fluxes of ions across membranes, free radical-induced damage and various inflammatory responses.[1-4] These events do not occur in isolation but interact to form a cascade which ultimately results in cell death (see Ch. 4). Attempts to block these mechanisms have progressed to clinical trials in head injury.[5-6] However, despite success in pre clinical research studies, experimental therapies have not been proven in human head injury and stroke.

The ability to investigate the chemistry at a cellular level is likely to assist in the understanding of the pathophysiology following brain injury. Several methods exist to monitor brain metabolism including imaging techniques such as positron emission tomography (PET), magnetic resonance spectroscopy (MRS) and analysis of the venous blood from the jugular bulb and CSF sampling from ventricular drains and lumbar puncture. However, the ability to directly measure the chemistry continuously in the brain following injury has only recently become possible using the technique of microdialysis.

MONITORING BRAIN CHEMISTRY

The methods available for measuring substances in the brain can be divided into imaging techniques and direct sampling procedures.

IMAGING TECHNIQUES

Imaging techniques enable cerebral chemistry to be investigated non-invasively and provide global images of the whole brain. PET measures the local rates of chemical processes in humans *in vivo* using similar principles to quantitative autoradiography in animals.[7-9] Tissue take-up of radiolabel from a labelled compound circulating in the blood is imaged. PET can measure cerebral blood flow, local oxygen consumption, local glucose utilization and protein synthesis.

Brain chemistry can also be investigated using MRS, the application of magnetic resonance imaging (MRI) to assess the metabolism of tissues.[10-13] Conventional MRI assesses the concentration of water in molar terms. MRS provides information on brain chemistry

by focusing on metabolites, e.g. N-acetyl-aspartate, choline, creatinine, lactate and glutamate, in milli- and micromolar terms.

Imaging techniques have the advantage of assessing substance concentration non-invasively, enabling regional and global measurements of metabolism. However, the number of substances that can be measured compared to focal invasive techniques such as microdialysis is limited and continuous monitoring over hours and days is not possible. Imaging techniques also do not typically differentiate between the intra- and extracellular components of the tissue. They therefore provide measures of activity within tissues but do not measure the concentration of substances in the interstitial fluid where interactions between cells occur.

DIRECT SAMPLING TECHNIQUES

The application of fine probes to monitor neurosurgical patients is well established. Fibreoptic sensors and pressure transducers are routinely used to measure intracranial pressure.[14-16] Laser Doppler probes have been used to measure local cerebral blood flow.[17-18] More recently, modified Clark electrodes have been developed to measure brain tissue oxygen. Miniature spectrophotometers measure the tissue concentration of carbon dioxide and hydrogen ions.[19-23] These techniques are described in Chapter 9.

Measurement of substrate and metabolite concentration of the brain as opposed to physiological parameters such as pressure and tissue gas concentration is now possible using microdialysis.[24-27] Pioneered by Ungerstedt in animal studies, this technique has now been applied to monitor the biochemistry of the human brain.[28-32]

PRINCIPLES OF MICRODIALYSIS

The principle of microdialysis is based on the passive transfer of substances across a dialysis membrane (Fig. 10.1). A fine concentric catheter lined with dialysis membrane is placed within the tissue, for example cerebral parenchyma, and perfused continuously with a physiological solution such as normal saline or Ringer's solution at very low flow rates (typically 0.5–1.5 ml/day) using a precision pump. Ions, metabolite/substrates (e.g. glucose, lactate, pyruvate), amino acids, neurotransmitters and drugs are able to cross the dialysis membrane, which typically has a molecular weight cut-off of 20kD, into the dialysate. Membranes with higher molecular weight cut-offs, e.g. 100kD, can be used to monitor polypeptides and

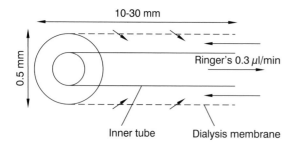

Figure 10.1   Diagram of concentric microdialysis catheter. The catheter consists of two tubes. The outer tube consists of dialysis membrane. Physiological solution is pumped through the space between the dialysis membrane and the inner tube. Molecules diffuse across the membrane from the extracellular fluid into the physiological solution which, on reaching the tip of the catheter, passes up the inner tube into collecting vials for analysis.

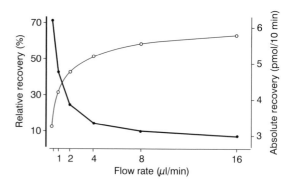

Figure 10.2   Schematic representation of the effect of changing flow rate on relative and absolute recovery of an analyte for a standard concentric microdialysis catheter.

proteins such as cytokines. The dialysate is collected from the catheter into vials which are changed as required, for example every 10–60 min, for analysis using a bedside spectrophotometry analyser or liquid chromatography system.

The level of substance detected in the dialysis fluid does not equate with the true extracellular fluid concentration.[27–28] The term 'recovery' is applied to the proportion of substance in the extracellular fluid that is detected in the dialysate. It depends on the length of the dialysis membrane, the rate of flow of the perfusion liquid, the speed of diffusion of the substance and the properties of the membrane. The ability of the microdialysis catheter to extract substances from the extracellular fluid can be described in two ways. *Relative* (concentration) recovery is defined as the ratio of the concentration of the substance in the dialysate to that in the medium surrounding the probe and is expressed as a percentage (Fig. 10.2). It approaches 100% when flow rate approaches zero. *Absolute* (mass) recovery is defined as the amount of substance in the dialysate output during a defined time period, usually the sampling period. It approaches a maximum value at higher flow rates because the concentration gradients between the environment and the perfusate/dialysate are then maximal. In practice, long membranes (4–30mm) and slow flow rates (0.3–2 μl/min) are used to increase recovery rates. However, long membranes are more difficult to implant and may monitor heterogeneous brain areas, while slow flow rates cause greater delay in sample analysis and produce lower volumes.

Although *in vitro* recovery studies can be useful in defining the performance of a microdialysis catheter, these data cannot be used to calculate the true extracellular *in vivo* concentration of a substance due to site-to-site variation in mass transfer properties, such as the contribution of active processes from local blood vessels.[33–35]

A number of models have been proposed to enable *in vivo* calibration to be performed. These include the extrapolation to zero flow model, no net flux model and dialysable reference model.[36] The application of probes to monitor brain metabolism is associated with a number of potential complications which require critical appraisal. Concern that probe insertion causes cellular injury has been investigated in animal studies. Early studies conducted in animals reported evidence of reversible uncoupling of local cerebral blood flow from glucose metabolism following probe insertion.[25,37] However, this was probably a consequence of the damage caused using the relatively large devices available at the time. After several days reticular formation and gliosis were commonly observed in these early studies.[38] This is almost certainly a consequence of a lack of sterility of the catheter. Histological studies show only occasional microhaemorrhages.[38] Increasing experience in human cerebral microdialysis has demonstrated that the technique can be applied safely. Substance recovery rates may take longer to stabilize than in animal studies which may be related to membrane length. However, probe performance is maintained without loss of recovery rates for several days. Postmortem studies of sheep and human brain have revealed no or minimal disruption of the cerebral parenchyma as a result of microdialysis catheter implantation.[39–40]

The diffusion properties of substances in simple solution *in vitro* differ from those of the complex environment of the brain.[31] *In vivo* calibration studies as described above are therefore required to determine the true extracellular concentration of substances. The expansion of the extracellular space in vasogenic oedema will potentially lead to a greater volume of distribution of substances and a higher diffusion coefficient than in normal brain. The extent to which this potential problem applies to clinical cerebral microdialysis monitoring is unknown.

The differentiation between the detection of true synaptic neurotransmitter release and non-specific overflow from synaptic and non-synaptic sources is also unclear.[27] Currently the smallest catheters available are about 200 μm external diameter. The synaptic cleft is approximately 0.02 μm across. Consequently, it is not possible to monitor neurotransmitter release in this region. However, considerable evidence suggests that many systems function via overflow mechanisms as well as classic vesicular release from the presynaptic membrane, diffusion across the synaptic cleft and binding to postsynaptic membrane receptors. For many neurotransmitter systems (e.g. noradrenaline, dopamine, serotonin, glutamate), reuptake mechanisms ensure termination of effect by removal of the transmitter from the synaptic cleft.

Despite these concerns, clinical cerebral microdialysis has been successfully introduced into several neurosurgical units.

CLINICAL APPLICATIONS OF CEREBRAL MICRODIALYSIS

Clinical microdialysis has been applied in the ward, in intensive care, in the operating theatre and to ambulatory patients. Microdialysis catheters may be secured in position by tunnelling and suturing to the scalp or inserted via a fixation bolt in combination with other monitoring probes such as intracranial pressure transducers and brain oxygen sensors.[22,41,42] In addition to cerebral monitoring, the technique has been used in other sites including skin,[43] subcutaneous adipose tissue,[44,45] myocardium and skeletal muscle.[46] Peripheral microdialysis has been used to measure subcutaneous glucose concentrations in diabetic patients[47] and to monitor the metabolism of flaps in plastic surgery.[48]

Glucose, lactate, the lactate:pyruvate (LP) ratio, glutamate and glycerol have been identified as useful markers of disturbances in brain energy metabolism. The level of glucose indicates the amount of glucose available to the cells, the lactate and LP ratio indicate the amount of oxygen and glucose used by the cells, the level of glutamate indicates the extent of possible cytotoxic damage to the cells and the level of glycerol indicates the extent of cell membrane disintegration.

The first report of human intracerebral microdialysis investigated biochemical changes during thalamotomy for Parkinson's disease.[49] Subsequent studies have focused on ischaemia/trauma, epilepsy and tumours.

ISCHAEMIA/TRAUMA

The application of microdialysis for monitoring patients on neurosurgical intensive care was pioneered in Uppsala, Sweden. Changes in the microdialysis concentration of lactate, pyruvate and glutamate in four patients corresponded with clinical events such as periods of raised intracranial pressure.[50] Further studies by the same group demonstrated correlation between levels of excitatory amino acids and outcome in subarachnoid haemorrhage[51] and increased levels in energy-related metabolites in areas of ischaemia as defined by PET.[52] Glycerol was recognized as a marker of cell membrane breakdown in ischaemia.[53]

In Richmond, Virginia, Bullock and Marmarou have investigated in detail patterns of excitatory amino acid release following severe head injury in a series of 80 patients, demonstrating that in patients without secondary brain injury, excitatory amino acid release is a transient phenomenon but in patients with secondary insults and particularly patients with contusions, very high levels of glutamate are detected.[54-55] Glutamate release has also been shown to relate to intracranial hypertension, seizure activity[56] and outcome. Other investigators have shown a relationship between lactate levels and outcome following head injury and increased lactate levels in response to periods of physiological deterioration.[57-59] Figure 10.3 shows improving metabolism in a patient following severe head injury.

In addition to monitoring patients on the intensive care unit, peroperative microdialysis has been applied to monitor metabolism during cerebrovascular surgery. The effects of ischaemia during aneurysm surgery have been related to low levels of glucose and raised levels of ascorbic acid, glutathione, lactate, glutamate and glial fibrillary acidic protein.[60-65] We have demonstrated increases in the LP ratio and decreases in glucose in association with reduced brain tissue oxygen during and following aneurysm surgery (Fig. 10.4).[66]

EPILEPSY

Evidence that glutamate is implicated in the pathogenesis of epileptic seizures has prompted studies of

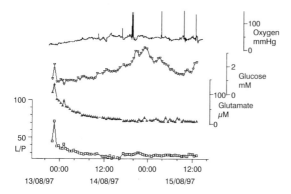

Figure 10.3   Cerebral hemisphere microdialysis and oxygen levels in a patient with a brainstem haemorrhage showing decrease in lactate:pyruvate ratio and glutamate concentration and fluctuation in glucose concentration. Spikes in the oxygen tracing represent periods of bagging with 100% oxygen.

microdialysis during epilepsy surgery.[67–69] Bilateral hippocampal microdialysis has been performed to test the hypothesis that an increase in extracellular glutamate may trigger spontaneous seizures.[70] Immediately prior to seizure activity, high concentrations of glutamate were measured in the epileptogenic hippocampus.[67] During seizure activity, rises in glutamate concentrations to potentially neurotoxic concentrations were documented. Rises in aspartate, lactate, adenosine, glycine, serine, alanine and phosphoethanolamine have also been reported in epileptic foci.[68,69,71–73]

TUMOURS

In comparison to the investigation of patients with head injury, subarachnoid haemorrhage and epilepsy, tumour chemistry has not been extensively investi-

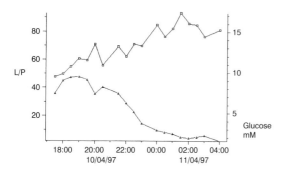

Figure 10.4   Cerebral microdialysis monitoring in patient with cerebral ischaemia following subarachnoid haemorrhage showing increase in lactate : pyruvate ratio and decrease in glucose.

gated. However, microdialysis has been used to administer exogenous substances to the brain. L-2,4 diaminobutyric acid, an amino acid with potent anti-tumour activity delivered using microdialysis into gliomas, has demonstrated tumour necrosis.[74]

SUMMARY

Microdialysis is an *in vivo* sampling technique which measures the level of extracellular molecules. It is based on the transfer of molecules across a dialysis membrane and enables the biochemical monitoring of metabolic events. It can be performed in many types of tissue. Human cerebral microdialysis has been used to determine the metabolic state of the brain in patients with head injury and subarachnoid haemorrhage. Studies to determine whether microdialysis has a role in assisting in therapeutic decision making are currently in progress.

REFERENCES

1. Siesjo BK. Pathophysiology and treatment of focal cerebral ischaemia. Part I: pathophysiology. J Neurosurg 1992; 77: 169–184.

2. Siesjo BK. Pathophysiology and treatment of focal cerebral ischaemia. Part II: mechanisms of damage and treatment. J Neurosurg 1992; 77: 337–354.

3. Teasdale GM, Graham DI. Craniocerebral trauma: protection and retrieval of the neuronal population after injury. Neurosurgery 1998; 43: 723–738.

4. Lynch DR, Dawson TM. Secondary mechanisms in neuronal trauma. Curr Opin Neurol 1994; 7: 510–516.

5. Doppenberg EM, Bullock R. Clinical neuro-protection trials in severe traumatic brain injury: lessons from previous studies. J Neurotrauma 1997; 14: 71–80.

6. Doppenberg EM, Choi SC, Bullock R. Clinical trials in traumatic brain injury. What can we learn from previous studies? Ann NY Acad Sci 1997; 825: 305–322.

7. Prichard JW, Brass LM. New anatomical and functional imaging methods. Ann Neurol 1992; 32: 395–400.

8. Frackowiak RS, Lenzi GL, Jones T, Heather JD. Quantitative measurement of regional cerebral blood flow and oxygen metabolism in man using 15O and positron emission tomography: theory, procedure, and normal values. J Comput Assist Tomogr 1980; 4: 727–736.

9. Phelps ME, Mazziotta JC. Positron emission tomography: human brain function and biochemistry. Science 1985; 228: 799–809.

10. Ross B, Kreis R, Ernst T. Clinical tools for the 90s: magnetic resonance spectroscopy and metabolite imaging. Eur J Radiol 1992; 14: 128–140.

11. Prichard JW. Magnetic resonance spectroscopy of the brain. Clin Chim Acta 1992; 206: 115–123.

12. Miller BL. A review of chemical issues issues in 1H NMR spectroscopy: N-acetyl-L-aspartate, creatine and choline. NMR Biomed 1991; 4: 47–52.

13. Duncan JS. Magnetic resonance spectroscopy. Epilepsia 1996; 37: 598–605.

14. Gopinath SP, Robertson CS, Narayan RG et al. Evaluation of a microsensor intracranial pressure transducer. In: Nagai H et al (eds.) Intracranial pressure IX. Springer Verlag, Berlin, 1994, pp 2–5.

15. Marmarou A, Tsuji O, Dunbar JG. Experimental evaluation of a new solid state ICP monitor. In: Nagai H et al, (eds.) Intracranial pressure IX. Spinger Verlag, Berlin, 1994, pp 15–19.

16. Czosnyka M, Czosnyka Z, Pickard JD. Laboratory testing of three intracranial pressure microtransducers – a technical report. Neurosurgery 1996; 38: 219–224.

17. Kirkpatrick PJ, Smielewski P, Czosnyka M, Pickard JD. Continuous monitoring of cortical perfusion by laser doppler flowmetry in ventilated patients with head injury. J Neurol Neurosurg Psychiatry 1994; 57: 1382–1388.

18. Haberl RL, Villringer A, Dirnagl U. Applicability of laser-doppler flowmetry for cerebral blood flow monitoring in neurological intensive care. Acta Neurochir 1993; 59: 64–68.

19. Zauner A, Bullock R, Di X, Young HF. Brain oxygen, CO2, pH, and temperature monitoring: evaluation in the feline brain. Neurosurgery 1995; 37: 1168–1176.

20. Van Santbrink HV, Maas AIR, Avezaat CJJ. Continuous monitoring of partial pressure of brain tissue oxygen in patients with severe head injury. Neurosurgery 1996; 38: 21–31.

21. Charbel FT, Hoffman WE, Misra M, Hannigan K, Ausman JI. Cerebral interstitial tissue oxygen tension, pH, HCO3, CO2. Surg Neurol 1997; 48: 414–417.

22. Zauner A, Doppenberg EM, Woodward JJ, Choi SC, Young HF, Bullock R. Continuous monitoring of cerebral substrate delivery and clearance: initial experience in 24 patients with severe acute brain injuries. Neurosurgery 1997; 41: 1082–1091.

23. Gupta AK, Hutchinson PJA, Al-Rawi PG et al. Measurement of brain tissue oxygenation compared with jugular venous oxygen saturation for monitoring cerebral oxygenation after traumatic brain injury. Anesth Analg 1999; 88: 549–553.

24. Delgado JMR, De Feudis FV, Roth RH, Ryugo DK, Mitruka BM. Dialytrode for long-term intracerebral perfusion in awake monkeys. Arch Int Pharmacodyn Ther 1972; 198: 9–21.

25. Benveniste H. Brain microdialysis. J Neurochem 1989; 6: 1667–1679.

26. Hamberger A, Jacobson I, Nystrom B, Sandberg M. Microdialysis sampling of the neuronal environment in basic and clinical research. J Intern Med 1991; 230: 375–380.

27. Ungerstedt U. Measurement of neurotransmitter release by intracranial dialysis. In: Marsden CA, (ed.) Measurement of neurotransmitter release in vivo. John Wiley, New York, 1984, pp 81–107.

28. Ungerstedt U. Microdialysis–principles and applications for studies in animals and man. J Intern Med 1991; 230: 365–373.

29. Ungerstedt U. Microdialysis – a new technique for monitoring local tissue events in the clinic. Acta Anaesthesiol Scand 1997; 110(suppl): 123.

30. Lonnroth P. Microdialysis – a new and promising method in clinical medicine. J Intern Med 1991; 230: 363–364.

31. Whittle IR. Intracerebral microdialysis: a new method in applied clinical neuroscience research. Br J Neurosurg 1990; 4: 459–462.

32. Editorial. Microdialysis. Lancet 1992;339: 1326–1327.

33. Nicholson C, Phillips JM. Ion diffusion modified by tortuosity and volume fraction in the extracellular microenvironment of the rat cerebellum. J Physiol Lond 1981; 321: 225–257.

34. Nicholson C, Rice ME. The migration of substances in the neuronal microenvironment. Ann NY Acad Sci 1986; 481: 55–71.

35. Benveniste H, Hansen AJ, Ottoson NS. Determination of brain interstitial concentrations by microdialysis. J Neurochem 1989; 52: 1741–1750.

36. Menacherry S. In vivo calibration of microdialysis probes for exogenous compounds. Anal Chem 1992; 64: 577–583.

37. Benveniste H, Drejer J, Schousboe A, Diemer NH. Regional cerebral glucose phosphorylation and blood flow after insertion of a microdialysis fibre through the dorsal hippocampus in the rat. J Neurochem 1987; 49: 729–734.

38. Benveniste H, Diemer NH. Early postischaemic 45Ca accumulation in rat dentate hilus. J Cereb Blood Flow Metab 1987; 8: 713–719.

39. Whittle IR, Glasby M, Lammie A, Ball H, Ungerstedt U. Neuropathological findings after intracerebral implantation of microdialysis catheters. NeuroReport 1998; 9: 2821–2825.

40. Hutchinson PJA, O'Connell MT, Al-Rawi PG et al. Neuropathological findings after microdialysis catheter implantation (letter). NeuroReport 1999 (in press).

41. Kanner A, Mendelowitsch A, Langemann H, Alessandri B, Gratzl O. A new screwing device for fixing a microdialysis probe in critical care patients. Acta Neurochir Wien 1996; 67(suppl): 63–65.

42. Hutchinson PJA, O'Connell MT, Al-Rawi PG et al. Intracerebral monitoring in severe head injury – intracranial pressure, Paratrend sensor and microdialysis using a new triple bolt. Br J Neurosurg 1998; 12: 87P.

43. Church MK, Skinner SP, Burrows LJ, Bewley AP. Microdialysis in human skin. Clin Exp Allergy 1995; 25: 1027–1029.

44. Lonnroth P. Microdialysis in adipose tissue and skeletal muscle. Horm Metab Res 1997; 29: 344–346.

45. Hutchinson PJA, O'Connell MT, Maskell LB, Pickard JD. Monitoring by subcutaneous microdialysis in neuro-intensive care. In: Bullock R et al, (eds.) Neuromonitoring in brain injury. Springer Verlag, Wien, 1999: in press.

46. Rosdahl H, Hamrin K, Ungerstedt U, Henriksson J. Metabolite levels in human skeletal muscle and adipose tissue studied with microdialysis at low perfusion flow. Am J Physiol 1998; 274: E936–E945.

47. Bolinder J, Ungerstedt U, Arner P. Long-term continuous glucose monitoring with microdialysis in ambulatory insulin-dependent diabetic patients. Lancet 1993; 342: 1080–1085.

48. Rojdmark J, Blomqvist L, Malm M, Adams RB, Ungerstedt U. Metabolism in myocutaneous flaps studied by in situ microdialysis. Scand J Plast Reconstr Surg Hand Surg 1998; 32: 27–34.

49. Meyerson BA, Linderoth B, Karlsson H, Ungerstedt U. Microdialysis in the human brain: extracellular measurements in the thalamus of Parkinsonian patients. Life Sci 1990; 46: 301–307.

50. Persson L, Hillered L. Chemical monitoring of neurosurgical intensive care patients using intracerebral microdialysis. J Neurosurg 1992; 76: 72–80.

51. Persson L, Valtysson J, Enblad P et al. Neurochemical monitoring using intracerebral microdialysis in patients with subarachnoid haemorrhage. J Neurosurg 1996; 84: 606–616.

52. Enblad P, Valtysson J, Andersson J et al. Simultaneous intracerebral microdialysis and positron emission tomography in the detection of ischaemia in patients with subarachnoid haemorrhage. J Cereb Blood Flow Metab 1996; 16: 637–644.

53. Hillered L, Valtysson J, Enblad P, Persson L. Interstitial glycerol as a marker for membrane phospholipid degradation in the acutely injured human brain. J Neurol Neurosurg Psychiatry 1998; 64: 486–491.

54. Bullock R, Zauner A, Tsuji O, Woodward JJ, Marmarou AT, Young HF. Patterns of excitatory amino acid release and ionic flux after severe human head trauma. In: Tsubokawa T et al (eds.) Neurochemical monitoring in the intensive care unit. Springer-Verlag, Tokyo1995, pp 64–71.

55. Bullock R, Zauner A, Woodward J et al. Factors affecting excitatory amino acid release following severe human head injury. J Neurosurg 1998; 89: 507–518.

56. Vespa P, Prins M, Ronne-Engstrom E et al. Increase in extracellular glutamate caused by reduced cerebral perfusion pressure and seizures after traumatic brain injury: a microdialysis study. J Neurosurg 1998; 89: 971–982.

57. Goodman JC, Robertson DP, Gopinath SP et al. Measurement of lactic acid and amino acids in the cerebral cortex of head-injured patients using microdialysis. In: Tsubokawa T et al (eds.) Neurochemical

monitoring in the intensive care unit. Springer-Verlag, Tokyo, 1995. pp 78–83.

58. Goodman JC, Gopinath SP, Valadka AB et al. Lactic acid and amino acid fluctuations measured using microdialysis reflect physiological derangements in head injury. Acta Neurochir Wien 1996; 67(suppl): 37–39.

59. Robertson CS, Gopinath SP, Uzura M, Valadka AB, Goodman JC. Metabolic changes in the brain during transient ischemia measured with microdialysis. Neurol Res 1998; 20(suppl 1): S91–S94.

60. Bachli H, Langemann H, Mendelowitsch A, Alessandri B, Landolt H, Gratzl O. Microdialytic monitoring during cerebrovascular surgery. Neurol Res 1996; 18: 370–376.

61. Mendelowitsch A, Langemann H, Alessandri B, Kanner A, Landolt H, Gratzl O. Microdialytic monitoring of the cortex during neurovascular surgery. Acta Neurochir Wien 1996; 67(suppl): 48–52.

62. Mendelowitsch A, Sekhar LN, Wright DC et al. An increase in extracellular glutamate is a sensitive method of detecting ischaemic neuronal damage during cranial base and cerebrovascular surgery. An in vivo microdialysis study. Acta Neurochir Wien 1998; 140: 349–355.

63. Nilsson OG, Saveland H, Boris MF, Brandt L, Wieloch T. Increased levels of glutamate in patients with subarachnoid haemorrhage as measured by intracerebral microdialysis. Acta Neurochir Wien 1996; 67(suppl): 45–47.

64. Saveland H, Nilsson OG, Boris-Moller F, Wieloch T, Brandt L. Intracerebral microdialysis of glutamate and aspartate in two vascular territories after aneurysmal subarachnoid haemorrhage. Neurosurgery 1996; 38: 12–20.

65. Runnerstam M, Von Essen C, Nystrom B, Rosengren L, Hamberger A. Extracellular glial fibrillary acidic protein and amino acids in brain regions of patients with subarachnoid hemorrhage–correlation with level of consciousness and site of bleeding. Neurol Res 1997; 19: 361–368.

66. Hutchinson PJA, Al-Rawi PG, O'Connell MT et al. Monitoring of brain metabolism during aneurysm surgery using microdialysis and brain multiparameter sensors. Neurol Res 1999; 21: 352–358.

67. During MJ, Spencer DD. Extracellular hippocampal glutamate and spontaneous seizure in the conscious human brain. Lancet 1993; 341: 1607–1610.

68. Hamberger A, Nystrom B, Larsson S, Silfvenius H, Nordborg C. Amino acids in the neuronal microenvironment of focal human epileptic lesions. Epilepsy Res 1991; 9: 32–43.

69. Ronne-Engstrom E, Hillered L, Flink R, Spannare B, Ungerstedt U, Carlson H. Intracerebral microdialysis of extracellular amino acids in the human epileptic focus. J Cereb Blood Flow Metab 1992; 12: 873–876.

70. Meldrum BS. Metabolic factors during prolonged seizures and their relation to nerve cell death. Adv Neurol 1983; 34: 261–275.

71. Carlson H, Ronne-Engstrom E, Ungerstedt U, Hillered L. Seizure related elevations of extracellular amino acids in human focal epilepsy. Neurosci Lett 1992; 140: 30–32.

72. During MJ, Fried I, Leone P, Katz A, Spencer DD. Direct measurement of extracellular lactate in the human hippocampus during spontaneous seizures. J Neurochem 1994; 62: 2356–2361.

73. During MJ, Spencer DD. Adenosine: a potential mediator of seizure arrest and postictal refractoriness. Ann Neurol 1992; 32: 618–624.

74. Ronquist G, Hugosson R, Sjolander U, Ungerstedt U. Treatment of malignant glioma by a new therapeutic principle. Acta Neurochir Wien 1992; 114: 8–11.

11

MULTIMODAL MONITORING IN NEUROINTENSIVE CARE

Pawanjit S. Minhas & Peter J. Kirkpatrick

INTRODUCTION

One of the key principles behind the establishment of specialist neurointensive care units is that following acute brain injury (be it from head trauma, spontaneous subarachnoid or intracerebral haemorrhage or embolic stroke), continuing cerebral ischaemia is a significant factor in determining outcome.

Up to 90% of patients who die from severe head injury have histological evidence of ischaemic brain necrosis at postmortem.[1,2] Analysis of the National Institute of Neurological Disease and Stroke Traumatic Coma Data Bank indicates that mortality after severe head injury doubles from 30% in patients who remain normotensive and adequately oxygenated to 60% in those who suffer hypoxaemia or hypotension.[3] Similarly, approximately one-third of all patients with subarachnoid haemorrhage develop clinical signs of delayed ischaemic neurologic deficit, probably as a result of cerebral arterial vasospasm.[4] Vasospasm is the most important factor that prevents a good outcome in a patient with good-grade subarachnoid haemorrhage undergoing early clipping of a ruptured cerebral aneurysm. In addition to the high risk of delayed ischaemic neurologic deficit, patients with poor-grade subarachnoid haemorrhage often suffer ischaemia from the outset due to increased intracranial pressure, reduced cerebral perfusion pressure and blood pressure abnormalities. Contrary to the widely held view that poor-grade subarachnoid haemorrhage patients are unlikely to benefit from aggressive treatment and surgical intervention, Le Roux et al were able to demonstrate that 30% of these patients will have good outcome with either no or non-debilitating neurologic deficit if treated aggressively from the outset.[5]

By examining changes in cerebral blood flow (CBF) and rate of oxygen metabolism (CMRO$_2$), positron emission tomography (PET) studies have demonstrated that following embolic stroke, there are often large regions of ischaemic but potentially viable cerebral tissue.[6,7]

In all the conditions described above, the pathophysiology producing cerebral ischaemia is complex and heterogeneous and can change rapidly. Without the ability to immediately detect subtle changes in cerebral haemodynamics and oxygenation, cerebral ischaemia cannot be prevented or treated effectively. This requires continuous monitoring modalities, with well-defined thresholds, which can be easily applied at the patient's bedside. By simultaneous monitoring of several parameters sensitive to brain ischaemia, the multimodal approach provides the 'picture' from several angles, thus increasing our understanding of the pathophysiology of brain injury and our ability to prevent secondary cerebral ischaemia.

This chapter is an overview of the multimodal monitoring system currently used within the Addenbrooke's Neurosciences Critical Care Unit in Cambridge.

GENERAL CONSIDERATIONS REGARDING MULTIMODAL MONITORING

IDENTIFYING THE DIFFERENT CAUSES OF COMMON ENDPOINTS

By using multimodal monitoring, it is possible to identify different causes for a particular change in a monitored parameter. For example, an increase in ICP may be the result of an increase in cerebral blood volume in hyperperfusion (hyperaemia) or cytotoxic oedema generated by hypoperfusion (ischaemia). Monitoring ICP in isolation cannot identify the primary event leading to this increase. However, if transcranial Doppler ultrasonography is used to monitor flow velocity (FV) in the basal arteries and a jugular bulb catheter is used for cerebral oximetry (SjO$_2$), the cause of this increase in ICP may become apparent. Hyperaemia will be accompanied by an increase in FV and SjO$_2$, while hypoperfusion will result in a decrease in FV and SjO$_2$. (Figure 11.1). The most appropriate and therapeutic intervention can then be applied; hyperventilation will reduce ICP in hyperaemic patients, but may be detrimental in patients with hypoperfusion as it will further reduce cerebral blood flow.[8]

DEFINING CRITICAL THRESHOLD FOR INDIVIDUAL PATIENTS AT PARTICULAR TIME POINTS

The maintenance of adequate cerebral perfusion pressure (CPP) in brain-injured patients seems to offer the best chance of a favourable outcome. However, the 'absolute' threshold for CPP, and indeed many other parameters, below which brain ischaemia is likely remain widely debated issues.[9,10] In reality, the preferred CPP may vary between patients and even within the same patient with time and type of treatment. Multimodal monitoring can provide 'on-line' assessment of cerebral haemodynamics, thus promoting a more informed decision on what CPP level is appropriate at that particular instant in that individual patient. For example, in a patient with a raised ICP secondary to hyperaemia, a CPP of 50 mmHg may be adequate whereas a threshold of 70

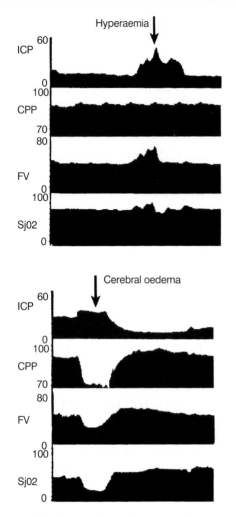

Figure 11.1   A recording of two events characterized by intracranial hypertension (ICP) in a head-injured patient receiving intensive care. By using multimodality monitoring, it is possible to identify the cause of this increase. (Top trace) The increase in ICP is secondary to an increase in cerebral blood volume (hyperaemia) as both the jugular bulb saturations ($SjO_2\%$) and blood velocity (FV cm/s) increase, with stable cerebral perfusion pressure (CPP mmHg). (Bottom trace) The rise in ICP is secondary to a fall in CPP as the FV and the SjO_2 also fall, indicating hypoperfusion. (Reproduced with permission from PJ Kirkpatrick.)

mmHg or greater would be used for the patient with a raised ICP secondary to brain ischaemic.

DISTINGUISHING ARTEFACTS FROM GENUINE CHANGES IN CEREBRAL HAEMODYNAMICS

All monitoring devices are prone to artefacts. The difficulty lies in identifying a genuine from an arte-

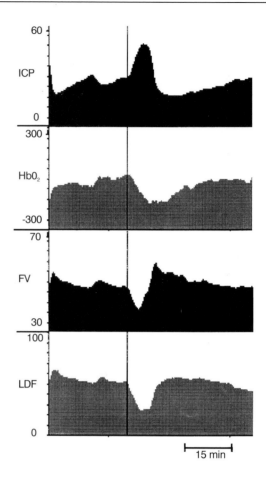

Figure 11.2   Multimodal recording of intracranial pressure (ICP), cerebral oxyhaemoglobin concentration (HbO_2) measured with near infrared spectroscopy, transcranial Doppler middle cerebral artery flow velocity (FV) and cortical laser Doppler flux during an ICP plateau wave in a patient with severe head injury. The ICP elevation is associated with features of ischaemia as FV, HbO_2 and LDF are all seen to decrease in a temporally related fashion.

factual change in a measured parameter. When several parameters are monitored, a genuine change in cerebral physiology is likely to affect more than one monitored parameter, whereas an artefact will only appear in one. Hence, multimodal monitoring will increase the sensitivity and specificity of secondary insult detection.

ABILITY TO DISTINGUISH GLOBAL FROM REGIONAL CHANGES

The injured brain is heterogeneous. Therefore, normal and injured parts of the brain may respond differently to alterations in physiology or pathophysiology. By using multimodal monitoring, it is possible to observe regional and global changes in cerebral haemodynamics. For example, the use of jugular bulb oximetry and tissue probes allows observation of changes in global (SjO_2) and regional (contused area) oxygenation with changes in $PaCO_2$, CPP and temperature.[11] Treatment can then be directed at correcting the most abnormal parameter.

TESTING CEREBRAL VASCULAR RESERVE

Cerebral vascular reactivity to carbon dioxide and an intact autoregulatory response to changes in CPP are the two hallmarks of normal cerebral vasculature. Cerebral vasoparalysis often signals that the vasculature is maximally vasodilated in response to cerebral

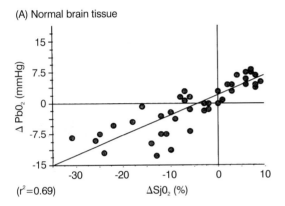

(A) Normal brain tissue

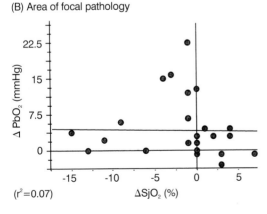

(B) Area of focal pathology

Figure 11.3   Changes in brain tissue PO_2 (PbO_2 mmHg) and jugular bulb oxygen saturation (SjO_2%) during hyperventilation in head-injured patients. (A) In areas of no focal pathology, there is a good correlation between changes in PbO_2 and SjO_2, while in areas of focal pathology this correlation is absent (B). PbO_2 = brain tissue oxygen tension; $PaCO_2$ = arterial carbon dioxide tension. (Redrawn from reference[11] with permission.)

ischaemia. It therefore represents a final common pathway for many pathological processes. The state of cerebral autoregulation after severe head injury can be as reliable in predicting outcome as the admission Glasgow Coma Score (GCS).[12] Multimodal monitoring techniques allow continuous assessment of the state of cerebral vasoreactivity to changes in CPP and $PaCO_2$. Many of these techniques are described later in this chapter.

MULTIMODAL MONITORING IS DEPENDENT ON THE AVAILABILITY OF EQUIPMENT AND STAFF

Multimodal monitoring set-ups are costly in terms of both expenditure and staff time.[13] Therefore, data of significant clinical value are only likely to be collected if the equipment is available and monitoring can be instituted easily. The availability of support staff familiar with computer hardware and software is invaluable. Best data are collected when the nursing staff caring for the patient being monitored are familiar with the set-up, regularly educated and see the benefits of multimodal monitoring in altering clinical decision making.

MONITORED MODALITIES

All patients with altered GCS admitted to our intensive care unit will have electrocardiograph, pulse oximetry, invasive blood and central venous blood pressure monitored. Pulmonary artery flotation catheters are used for continuous measurement of cardiac output when deemed necessary. Cerebral parameters that we currently monitor in patients with cerebral pathology are outlined below. The level of monitoring depends on the degree of brain injury. For greater detail on a particular modality, please consult the appropriate chapter.

INTRACRANIAL AND CEREBRAL PERFUSION PRESSURE

Although the gold standard of ICP monitoring remains the measurement of intraventricular fluid pressure either directly or via a CSF reservoir, in practice many centres, including our own, frequently use intraparenchymal microtransducers inserted via a bolt placed in the skull. These microtransducers have very low zero drift over long periods of monitoring, very good frequency response and stable linearity and are associated with a lower risk of infection than ventricular catheters.[14]

In the sedated and ventilated patient, in whom neurological state (other than pupillary response) cannot be

Table 11.1   Monitoring in the Addenbrooke's Neurosciences Critical Care Unit

Patient type	Standard of care monitors	Part of a research protocol
All patients	ECG, non-invasive blood pressure, pulse oximetry, temperature	
Patients requiring mechanical ventilation (postoperative, non-neurologic injury)	All of the above + invasive blood pressure, central venous pressure ± pulmonary artery wedge pressure and cardiac output	
Head injury (GCS <9)	All of the above + intracranial pressure monitoring (+ cerebral perfusion pressure), jugular bulb oximetry and daily transcranial Doppler ultrasonography	Near infrared spectroscopy Laser Doppler flowmetry Intracerebral microsensors Intracerebral microdialysis
Poor-grade subarachnoid haemorrhage	All of the above + intracranial pressure monitoring (+ cerebral perfusion pressure), jugular bulb oximetry and twice-daily transcranial Doppler ultrasonography	Near infrared spectroscopy Laser Doppler flowmetry Intracerebral microsensors Intracerebral microdialysis

assessed clinically, the measurement of ICP will ensure the maintenance of adequate cerebral perfusion pressure and early detection of intracranial lesions that may be surgically treatable (such as an intracranial haematoma or acute hydrocephalus). Increases in ICP >25 mmHg after severe head injury are associated with worse outcome[15] and the reduction in ICP following the early evacuation of an intracranial haematoma can significantly improve outcome.[16] Cerebral perfusion pressure-targeted therapy, shown to improve outcome after severe head injury, cannot be successfully implemented without measurement of the ICP.[9]

Impaired cerebral autoregulation after head injury has been associated with worse outcome.[11] ICP waveform analysis during spontaneous fluctuations in arterial blood pressure can provide important information about the state of cerebral autoregulation and the adequacy of cerebral perfusion in brain-injured patients.[17] Briefly, the pulsatility of an ICP waveform (expressed as the pulse amplitude in mmHg) increases with any increase in ICP. When the change in ICP pulse amplitude is linearly correlated with the change

in ICP, a regression correlation coefficient (the RAP coefficient, derived from the Regression of Amplitude and Pressure) is obtained. RAP will be positive and usually equates to +1. This relationship holds until the ICP is high enough to restrict the volume of blood flowing into the cranial compartment with each heartbeat. As less blood enters the cranium with each heartbeat, so the pressure rise with each pulsation also decreases, leading to a reduction in ICP pulse amplitude with any further increases in ICP. At this point, the RAP becomes negative (minimum of –1). Therefore a RAP of +1 indicates good cerebral perfusion while a RAP value of 0.5 to –1 is indicative of reduced intracranial compliance and compromised cerebral perfusion.

When cerebral autoregulation is intact, an increase in mean arterial pressure results in a momentary increase in CBF before reflex cerebrovascular vasoconstriction leads to an increase in cerebral vascular resistance and return of CBF to the baseline level. Cerebral vasoconstriction is accompanied by a reduction in cerebral blood volume and ICP. As the cerebral vasculature vasoconstricts, the intracranial blood volume is reduced and ICP will fall. Conversely, a fall in arterial blood pressure will result in autoregulatory cerebral vasodilatation and a concomitant increase in ICP as a result of an increase in cerebral blood volume. Therefore, when changes in ICP are correlated to changes in mean arterial pressure, a negative correlation is observed if autoregulation is intact and a positive correlation is observed when autoregulation is disrupted. The correlation coefficient of spontaneous variations in blood pressure and change in ICP can be used as a measure of cerebral autoregulation (autoregulatory index which we have termed PRx). PRx ranges from −1 for intact autoregulation to +1 (zero or positive values) when autoregulation is impaired.[11]

JUGULAR BULB OXIMETRY

Retrograde insertion of an internal jugular line to the level of the jugular bulb allows sampling of effluent blood from the brain for oximetry. Normal jugular venous blood oxygen saturation (SjO_2) ranges from 55% to 75%. SjO_2 values <50% indicate relative hypoperfusion, while those >80% indicate relative hyperaemia or 'luxury' perfusion. Episodes of jugular venous desaturation have been associated with poor outcome after head injury and this has been used for establishing therapeutic cerebral perfusion pressure thresholds (at 70 mmHg or greater).[10]

SjO_2 can be monitored using an intermittent or continuous technique (fibreoptic catheter). The use of continuous SjO_2 monitoring with a fibreoptic catheter will detect episodes of cerebral desaturation associated with intracranial hypertension, hypocapnia, hypotension and cerebral vasospasm but the readings are frequently unreliable because of artefacts, usually from the catheter lying against a vessel wall or being covered with thrombus.[13] Furthermore, SjO_2 is a measure of global hemispheric venous oxygen saturation and has obvious limitations in that it cannot detect regional ischaemia, as the blood from the remainder of the brain may dilute blood from such ischaemic regions.

The side of cannulation that provides the best indication of cerebral oxygenation remains controversial. Simultaneous SjO_2 readings from right and left jugular bulbs catheters can vary significantly.[18,19] However, as most of the blood from the superior sagittal sinus, which is responsible for the bulk of cerebral venous drainage, drains into the right internal jugular vein, the right jugular bulb is favoured in our unit.

TRANSCRANIAL DOPPLER

By using the Doppler shift principle, transcranial Doppler ultrasonography (TCD) can be used to non-invasively measure red cell velocity (FV) in the basal arteries. Although there are many ultrasonic 'windows' through which the cerebral vessels may be insonated, the middle cerebral artery (MCA) is most commonly insonated via the thin squamous temporal bone above the zygomatic arch. The MCA carries three-quarters of supratentorial blood and the probe can be easily fixed in position. Therefore, this allows continuous long-term monitoring of the instantaneous changes in FV which reflect changes in hemispheric CBF with excellent temporal resolution. Changes in FV reflect variations in CBF only when the angle of insonation and the diameter of the vessel insonated remain constant. Although by observing the basal arteries at craniotomy, Giller et al were able to show that the diameter of the main trunk of the MCA does not significantly change with changes in arterial blood pressure or carbon dioxide tension,[20] the diameter of the distal branches of the MCA may vary in size. The cerebral vessels may also behave differently after trauma or subarachnoid haemorrhage, and in the presence of intracranial pathology. For example, the presence of angiographically diagnosed vasospasm after subarachnoid haemorrhage will invalidate FV as a measure of CBF as the assumption of a constant vessel diameter is no longer tenable. A 'vasospastic' phase has been reported after head injury even in the absence of subarachnoid blood.[21] Therefore, daily variations in FV cannot be used in isolation to reflect changes in CBF.

Perhaps one of the main limitations of this technology remains the inability to reliably secure the monitoring probe in position for long periods of time. The majority of fixation devices require constant adjustment and often interfere with the intensive care of the patient. This is particularly important in patients with craniofacial trauma where even slight changes in probe position can result in the loss of FV signal. Nevertheless, TCD has many applications in patients with severe brain injury and although FV measurements may be useful in isolation, they are more valuable when used as part of multimodality.

Vasospasm or hyperaemia

TCD can be used to diagnose vasospasm in most of the basal cerebral arteries (most commonly the MCA, basilar artery, terminal internal carotid artery, anterior and posterior cerebral arteries). When the diameter of an insonated vessel is reduced, for the same volume flow, FV is increased. Vasospasm is considered present when the FV value is greater than twice the upper limit of normal.[22] However, high FV may also be a true reflection of an increased CBF: hyperaemia. In order to differentiate between the two conditions, the FV ratio between the MCA and the extracranial internal carotid artery (ICA) is used. As the MCA is supplied by the ICA, hyperaemia will result in an increase in both MCA and ICA velocities with a MCA:ICA FV ratio <2, while vasospasm will lead to a MCA:ICA FV ratio >3, indicating that the increase in MCA FV is the result of narrowing in MCA diameter and not an increase in overall CBF.[23] A change in clinical care of patients with subarachnoid haemorrhage (i.e. a move towards hypertensive, hypervolaemic therapy instead of dehydration and the routine use of calcium channel antagonists) may account for the high proportion of patients with high FV who appear to be hyperaemic rather than ischaemic or vasospastic.[24]

Multimodal monitoring can be used to differentiate hyperaemia (increased FV is usually accompanied by an increase in SjO_2) from vasospasm (FV increases may be accompanied by a normal or low SjO_2).

Detection of cerebral tamponade

Multiply injured patients with concomitant cerebral injury may require emergency abdominal or thoracic surgery prior to appropriate radiological assessment of the extent of head injury. TCD can be used to identify patients in whom brain injury is extensive and has led to intracranial circulatory arrest that is clearly not compatible with life. Although the presence of an oscillating flow pattern, where blood enters the cranium during systole and refluxes out in diastole, is not a criterion of brain death, it confirms intracranial circulatory arrest and inevitably results in death. By using TCD, the overall decision-making process may be enhanced, thus avoiding wasting time and resources.

Cerebral autoregulation

Cerebral autoregulation after brain injury can be assessed non-invasively and continuously using TCD. A detailed description of all the tests for the integrity of cerebral autoregulation can be found in Chapter 8.

By compressing the common carotid artery for a period of 5–8 s and observing the postcompression change in FV in the ipsilateral circle of Willis, it is possible to assess the integrity of cerebral autoregulation in brain-injured patients repeatedly at the bedside. When the carotid artery is compressed, FV decreases and the distal cerebrovascular bed dilates in response to the drop in perfusion pressure. When the compression is released, an increase in FV (>10% of baseline value) is observed as a result of this dilatation, which persists until the distal cerebrovascular bed constricts to its former diameter.[25] The compression

results in this 'transient hyperaemia' only when autoregulation is intact. When autoregulation is impaired, no dilatation of the distal cerebral vascular beds occurs in response to the compression and hence, no transient hyperaemia is detected.

Although this transient hyperaemic response test is reproducible and easily performed, the results depend heavily on the compression technique. The drop in FV during compression and the hyperaemia following release are also dependent on the patency of the collateral circulation at the circle of Willis.[25–29] Furthermore, in patients with carotid disease, the compression may dislodge atheroma, resulting in stroke. Therefore, the FV at the carotid bifurcation and along the ICA should first be examined by Doppler ultrasonography. The test should not be performed in those patients with high carotid FV suggestive of significant carotid stenosis, a history of carotid disease or significant risk factors for atherosclerotic disease. Nevertheless, our experience to date (over five years) has proved the test useful in the assessment of outcome after head injury without a single stroke.[25]

Cerebral autoregulation may also be assessed by observation of changes in FV in response to spontaneous small variations in CPP.[26] Briefly, in the autoregulating brain an increase in CPP will transiently increase CBF that is immediately followed by arteriolar vasoconstriction and return of CBF to baseline. Hence, increases in CPP are met by no change or a decrease in FV, with a negative correlation coefficient (termed Mx) between the FV and CPP. Conversely, in the non-autoregulating brain, increases in CPP are mirrored by increases in FV resulting in positive correlation between FV and CPP. This method has the advantage of not requiring any specific intervention (such as carotid compression) in order to 'challenge' the cerebral circulation. In addition, it can give a continuous output of autoregulatory status and may therefore be helpful in determining optimal CPP in an individual patient. For example, in patients with hypoperfusion, autoregulation is lost and Mx is positive. CPP is then increased to a level sufficient to improve perfusion and restore autoregulation (Mx positive).

The therapeutic objective is therefore to keep CPP high enough to retain a negative Mx value. The assumption is made that all patients will eventually autoregulate once CPP is high enough[9] and that loss of pressure autoregulation will always accompany ischaemia.

NON-INVASIVE ESTIMATION OF CPP

The advantages of monitoring CPP non-invasively are self-evident. We have recently published a method for non-invasively estimating CPP using mean arterial pressure, diastolic and mean FV. We were able to predict CPP value non-invasively with errors of estimation <10 mmHg in over 71% of the measurements.[30]

NEAR INFRARED SPECTROSCOPY

Near infrared spectroscopy (NIRS) uses attenuation of low levels of reflected near infrared light to measure cerebral concentrations of oxyhaemoglobin and deoxyhaemoglobin. Fibreoptic optodes transmitting and receiving near infrared light are placed approximately 6 cm apart on one side of the frontal scalp above the level of the frontal air sinuses and away from the temporalis muscle, in order to avoid undue light attenuation or extracranial tissue contamination. The technique is therefore non-invasive, simple to apply, and ideally suited to continuous monitoring and has been used extensively in neonates. In adult patients, the degree of light attenuation through a thicker skull and the relatively greater contamination of signal by extracranial tissues have led to difficulties in implementing this system to the same degree as in neonates.

We have used NIRS in the intraoperative monitoring of patients undergoing carotid surgery, in cerebrovascular reactivity testing and for monitoring brain-injured patients receiving neurointensive care. Transient falls in CPP and hypoxaemia can be readily detected by NIRS, sometimes with greater sensitivity than that given by traditional methods of cerebral oximetry (SjO_2).[31] However, as one of the major limitations of this technology lies in its inability to reliably distinguish between extracranial and intracranial changes in blood flow and oxygenation, the sensitivity and specificity of NIRS are best when used as part of multimodal system.

LASER DOPPLER FLOWMETRY

Laser Doppler flowmetry measures microcirculatory red cell flux within a small volume of brain tissue (1–2 mm^3). An invasive intraparenchymal probe can be inserted via an ICP-type supporting bolt into the superficial cortex to provide a non-quantitative measure of microcirculatory flow. The signal can be very susceptible to artefact created by movement or local tissue pressure changes but generally these problems are avoided with the technique described, which achieves a rigid fixation. Our experience with this technique has shown the ability to detect falls in microcirculatory flow in response to falls in CPP and increases in red cell flux after mannitol administration independent of changes in CPP.[32]

METABOLIC PROBES

The multimodal monitoring techniques discussed so far give information that is primarily haemodynamic in nature, although both jugular venous oxygen saturation and NIRS are actually reflecting the balance between oxygen delivery by cerebral blood flow and oxygen consumption by cerebral tissue. It is increasingly recognized that the widespread metabolic disturbances which follow acute brain injury can be detected by measuring tissue oxygen, glucose consumption and lactate levels.[33] Cerebral blood flow and metabolism are often uncoupled after brain injury. It is also likely that the glucose:oxygen ratio is altered. Excitotoxic processes involving the extracellular and synaptic release of large amounts of glutamate are also strongly implicated in the progression of brain injury after an acute insult.[34] From a research perspective, understanding these events is likely to prove critical to understanding delayed (and therefore potentially avoidable) neuronal injury. From a clinical viewpoint the ability to detect these events as part of a multimodal monitoring set-up may add further information regarding the nature and severity of injury, even though strategies such as pharmacological neuroprotection, which might deal specifically with metabolic disturbances, remain to be proven in large-scale clinical trials.

Intracerebral microdialysis techniques can provide information on extracellular concentrations of important substances such as lactate, pyruvate, glucose, glycerol and glutamate.[34,35] Although this technique is very much in its infancy, a high lactate:pyruvate ratio probably indicates an increase in anaerobic metabolism as a result of cerebral ischaemia, extracellular glucose concentration reflects the balance between blood flow and glucose metabolism, and the presence of high glycerol concentrations suggests cell membrane phospholipid breakdown and permanent structural cellular injury. As it is possible to select the pore size of semipermeable membrane used for microdialysis, it may be possible to monitor specific concentrations of proteins and drug delivery to the cerebral extracellular space.

Microprobes capable of measuring intracerebral PO_2, PCO_2 and pH can provide a range of haemodynamic and metabolic information.[36,37] Our experience suggests that these probes can be used safely in brain-injured patients to provide information about cerebral oxygenation and metabolism in agreement with published data.[37] However, these probes only provide information from a small region. The greatest yield of information will therefore be achieved by targeting probes into critical regions, such as around the ischaemic penumbra of a cerebral infarction.

INTERFACING MULTIPLE MONITORED MODALITIES

In order to provide continuous monitoring with on-line analysis of several signals in parallel, analogue signals from bedside monitors are sampled at a set frequency and the data are stored. Most bedside monitors have an analogue data bus in a range of 1 to 10 V, suitable for this kind of data acquisition. Where the range of analogue output is too low, an external amplifier can be added to take advantage of the full input range of the analogue-to-digital converter. The precision of the analogue-to-digital converter should be sufficient for the analysis of waveforms, which may contain different amplitudes (arterial blood pressure, ICP waveforms, etc.). Programming the sampling frequency provides the ability for a wide spectrum of signal processing, from simple trending to pattern recognition and modelling. The main disadvantage of analogue interfacing is the large number of cables required and the potential of electromagnetic interference. However, serial data processing (RS232) is generally unsuitable for fast on-line signal analysis and only information about 'mean' values is transmitted.

Primary analysis of data obtained will include time averaging, extreme values (minimum and maximum) and pulsatility of waveforms (TCD). Secondary analysis may include calculation of differential pressure (cerebral perfusion pressure), correlation between ICP and blood pressure changes and cerebral autoregulation indices from TCD and blood pressure signals. Both primary and secondary analysis may be possible on-line depending on the processing ability of the data acquisition system. Data may also be exported in ASCII format for more extensive examination or storage.

Finally, the large number of monitors that are likely to be in contact with the patient should conform with electrical safety standards.

FUTURE DEVELOPMENTS

In caring for patients with acute brain injury, undoubted benefits have arisen from the increased use of CT scanning and a more interventional, techno-logical approach within the neurosurgical intensive care unit. The development of multimodal monitoring has been a natural extension of this process and the need for a greater understanding of physiological as well as anatomical derangement. This information is not only of value in assessing present-day treatment but will also become increasingly important for the development of new therapies such as pharmacological

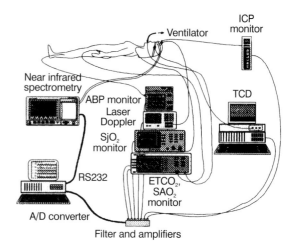

Figure 11.4 A diagramatic representation of the multimodality set-up used at the neurosciences critical care unit, Addenbrooke's Hospital, Cambridge.

neuroprotection or hypothermia. Although multi-modal systems will not replace conventional and evolving neuroimaging, the accumulation of data will undoubtedly result in the increased recognition of specific patterns of cerebral insult, a greater proportion of which will be 'filtered out' at the bedside, allowing prompt responses.

The development of computer support for multi-modal systems has to date functioned principally to amalgamate the different monitoring techniques employed and calculate indices, which provide infor-mation regarding autoregulatory status. This could be very easily extended to providing alarm warning systems when critical thresholds for important para-meters are not being satisfied. Such instances are often short-lived and frequently require a stereotypical response (e.g. increasing the rate of volume infusion or inotrope infusion to increase blood pressure) and hence the potential exists for using computer feedback control to administer treatment in the intensive care unit in a manner that is faster and more effective than human control. Important safety parameters could be programmed in to ensure that the computer's inter-vention is limited to safe levels (e.g. it may be desirable to set a maximum volume of fluid that may be infused over a given period to prevent overloading). Neural networking is a concept that allows a computer to 'learn' from its experience. In this context a statistical prediction can be derived for the success of a particular intervention in correcting an aberrant parameter and over time experience will accumulate in allowing the computer to handle more complicated therapeutic interventions.

A greater understanding of the heterogeneous nature of acute brain injury will require regional techniques able to examine the entire brain, such as positron emission tomography and functional magnetic resonance imaging (including magnetic resonance spectroscopy). These techniques can only be used intermittently, providing a 'snapshot'. However, when performed during critical time points and used in conjunction with continuous bedside monitoring, they will provide valuable additional insight.

REFERENCES

1. Graham DI, Adams JH, Doyle D. Ischaemic brain damage in fatal non-missile head injuries. J Neurol Sci 1978; 39: 213–234.

2. Graham DI, Ford I, Hume Adams J et al. Ischaemic brain damage is still common in fatal non-missile head injury. J Neurol Neurosurg Psychiatry 1989; 52: 346–350.

3. Chesnut RM. Secondary brain insults after head injury: clinical perspectives. New Horizons 1995; 3(3): 366–375.

4. Dorsch NW. Cerebral arterial spasm – a clinical review. Br J Neurosurg 1995; 9: 403–412.

5. Le Roux PD, Elliott JP, Newell DW, Grady MS, Winn HR. Predicting outcome in poor-grade patients with subarachnoid hemorrhage: a retrospective review of 159 aggressively managed cases. J Neurosurg 1996; 85: 39–49.

6. Marchal G, Beaudouin V, Rioux P et al. Prolonged persistence of substantial volumes of potentially viable brain tissue after stroke. A correlative PET-CT study with voxel based analysis. Stroke 1996; 27: 599–606.

7. Heiss WD, Huber H, Fink GR et al. Progressive derangement of periinfarct viable tissue in ischaemic stroke. J Cereb Blood Flow Metabol 1992; 12: 193–203.

8. Miller JD, Becker DP. Secondary insults to the injured brain. J Roy Coll Surg Edinburgh 1982; 27: 292–298.

9. Rosner MJ, Rosner SD, Johnson AH. Cerebral perfusion pressure: management protocol and clinical results. J Neurosurg 1995; 83: 949–962.

10. Chan KH, Miller JD, Dearden NM, Andrews PJD, Midgley S. The effect of changes in cerebral perfusion pressure upon cerebral artery blood flow velocity and jugular bulb venous oxygen saturation after severe brain injury. J Neurosurg 1992; 77: 55–61.

11. Gupta AK, Hutchinson PJ, Al-Rawi P et al. Measurement of brain tissue oxygenation compared with jugular venous oxygen saturation for monitoring cerebral oxygenation after traumatic brain injury. Anesth Analg 1999; 88: 549–553.

12. Czosnyka M, Smielewski P, Kirkpatrick PJ, Laing RJ, Menon D, Pickard JD. Continuous assessment of the cerebral vasomotor reactivity in head injury. Neurosurgery 1997; 41: 11–19.

13. Czosnyka M, Whitehouse H, Smielewski P, Kirkpatrick PJ, Guazzo EP, Pickard JD. Computer supported multimodal bedside monitoring for neuro-intensive care. Int J Clin Monit Comput 1994; 11: 223–232.

14. Czosnyka M, Czosnyka Z, Pickard JD. Laboratory testing of three intracranial pressure microtransducers: technical report. Neurosurgery 1996; 38: 219–224.

15. Miller JD, Becker DP, Ward JD, Sullivan HG, Adams WE, Rosner MJ. Significance of intracranial hypertension in severe head injury. J Neurosurg 1977; 47: 503–516.

16. Wilberger JE, Harris M, Diamond DL. Acute subdural haematoma: morbidity, mortality and operative timing. J Neurosurg 1991; 74: 212–218.

17. Czosnyka M, Guazzo EP, Whitehouse H et al. Significance of intracranial pressure waveform analysis after head injury. Acta Neurochir (Wien) 1996; 138: 531–542.

18. Stoccheti N, Paparella A, Bridelli F. Cerebral venous oxygen saturation studied with bilateral samples in the internal jugular veins. Neurosurgery 1994; 34: 38–44.

19. Metz C, Holzschuh M, Bein T et al. Monitoring of cerebral oxygen metabolism in the jugular bulb: reliability of unilateral measurements in severe head injury. J Cereb Blood Flow Metab 1998; 18: 332–343.

20. Giller CA, Bowman G, Dyer H, Mootz L, Krippner W. Cerebral arterial diameters during changes in blood pressure and carbon dioxide during craniotomy. Neurosurgery. 1993; 32: 737–742.

21. Martin NA, Patwardhan RV, Alexander MJ et al. Characterisation of cerebral hemodynamic phases following severe head trauma: hypoperfusion, hyperemia and vasospasm. J Neurosurg 1997; 87: 9–19.

22. Aaslid R, Huber P, Nornes H. Evaluation of cerebrovascular spasm with transcranial Doppler ultrasound. J Neurosurg 1984; 60: 37–41.

23. Lindegaard KF, Nornes H, Bakke SJ, Sorteberg W, Nakstad P. Cerebral vasospasm after subarachnoid haemorrhage investigated by means of transcranial Doppler ultrasound. Acta Neurochir (Wien) 1988; 42(suppl): 81–84.

24. Clyde BL, Resnick DK, Yonas H, Smith HA, Kaufmann AM. The relationship of blood velocity as measured by transcranial Doppler ultrasonography to cerebral blood flow as determined by stable xenon computed tomographic studies after aneurysmal subarachnoid hemorrhage. Neurosurgery 1996; 38: 896–905.

25. Smielewski P, Czosnyka M, Kirkpatrick PJ, Pickard JD. Evaluation of the transient hyperemic response test in head injured patients. J Neurosurg 1997; 86: 73–78.

26. Czosnyka M, Smielewski P, Kirkpatrick PJ, Menon DK, Pickard JD. Monitoring of cerebral autoregulation in head injured patients. Stroke 1996; 27: 1829–1834.

27. Giller CA. A bedside test for cerebral autoregulation using transcranial Doppler ultrasound. Acta Neurochir 1991; 108: 7.

28. Smielewski P, Czosnyka M, Kirkpatrick P et al. Assessment of cerebral autoregulation using carotid artery compression. Stroke 1996; 27: 2197.

29. Smielewski P, Czosnycka M, Kirkpatrick PJ et al. Validation of the computerised transient hyperemic response test as a method of testing autoregulation in severely head injured patients. J Neurotrauma 1995; 12: 420.

30. Czosnyka M, Matta BF, Smielewski P, Kirkpatrick PJ, Pickard JD. Cerebral perfusion pressure in head injured patients: a non-invasive assessment using transcranial Doppler ultrasonography. J Neurosurg 1998; 88: 802–808.

31. Kirkpatrick PJ, Smielewski P, Czosnyka M, Menon DK, Pickard JD. Near infrared spectroscopy use in patients with head injury. J Neurosurg 1995; 83: 963–970.

32. Kirkpatrick PJ, Smielewski P, Piechnik S, Pickard JD, Czosnyka M. Early effects of mannitol in patients with head injuries assessed using bedside multimodality monitoring. Neurosurgery 1996; 39: 714–721.

33. Bergsneider MA, Hovda DA, Shalmon E et al. Cerebral hyperglycolysis following severe traumatic brain injury in humans: a positron emission tomography study. J Neurosurg 1997; 86: 241–251.

34. Bullock R, Zauner A, Woodward JJ et al. Factors affecting excitatory amino acid release following severe head injury. J Neurosurg 1998; 89: 507–518.

35. Persson L, Valtysson J, Enblad P et al. Neurochemical monitoring using intracerebral microdialysis in patients with subarachnoid haemorrhage. J Neurosurg 1996; 84: 606–616.

36. Van Santbrink H, Maas AIR, Avezaat CJJ. Continuous monitoring of partial pressure of brain tissue oxygen in patients with severe head injury. Neurosurgery 1996; 38: 21–31.

37. Doppenberg EMR, Watson JC, Broaddus WC, Holloway KL, Young HF, Bullock R. Intraoperative monitoring of substrate delivery during aneurysm and hematoma surgery: initial experience in 16 patients. J Neurosurg 1997; 87: 809–816.

SECTION 3

INTRAOPERATIVE MANAGEMENT OF NEUROSURGICAL PATIENTS

12

SOME GENERAL CONSIDERATIONS IN NEUROANAESTHESIA

John M. Turner

INTRODUCTION

The anaesthetist in the operating theatre must endeavour to provide good intracranial operating conditions. This means ensuring that the intracranial pressure (ICP) does not rise and that, when the skull is open, brain bulk is not increased. The neurosurgeon must be able to retract the brain easily; too high a pressure on the retractors may result in neuronal damage. Understanding the mechanisms underlying the alterations in ICP in disease, the actions of drugs on ICP and the way they interrelate are important requirements for safe neuroanaesthesia. In intensive care, the manipulation and control of ICP is an important part of care of the neurosurgical patient.

Neurosurgical operations are relatively high-risk procedures. The patient with intracranial space occupation is at risk from the development of high ICP and as the space-occupying lesion (SOL) grows, the danger increases. The patient who has suffered a subarachnoid haemorrhage (SAH) is at further risk from repeated bleeds at any moment. There may also be the danger of vascular spasm and cerebral infarction. Anaesthesia and surgery in the patient with cerebral arterial insufficiency are complicated by the fact that arterial disease affects many vascular beds and the patient with cerebral arterial disease may also have significant disease in the coronary or renal circulations. A head-injured patient is not only exposed to the initial neuronal damage but also to the extension of the neuronal damage by high ICP, cerebral oedema and cerebral ischaemia. Unconsciousness may also worsen the injury by producing hypoxia and hypercarbia.

The anaesthetist must make a careful assessment of the neurosurgical patient's general condition and the extent of the neurosurgical disease. Although many clinical situations require a degree of urgency, the high-risk nature of neurosurgery means that when time allows, conditions which would affect the safety of the patient are evaluated and corrected before surgery.

ASSESSMENT

GENERAL MEDICAL CONDITION

A preoperative evaluation of pulmonary function is essential. Intraoperative hypoxia and hypercarbia will cause brain swelling, making surgery difficult or impossible, so any potential cause needs to be identified and treated preoperatively. Active pulmonary infection requires appropriate treatment before anaesthesia and surgery start. Any tendency towards asthma needs to be noted together with any treatment the patient needs. Chest X-rays only need to be ordered if there are signs or symptoms in the respiratory system but as a high proportion (at least 20%) of intracranial tumours are metastases[1] and frequently from bronchogenic carcinoma, a chest X-ray is indicated to detect a primary tumour.

The prevalence of cardiovascular disease in the population at large means that for neurosurgery, as for any major surgery, the careful assessment of cardiovascular function is essential. Pre-existing untreated arterial hypertension can predispose to cerebrovascular complications and during the perioperative period, the patient is at risk from fluctuations in blood pressure. The limits for autoregulatory control of cerebral blood flow (CBF) are reset during hypertension[2] and if inadvertent hypotension is caused, there is considerable danger of cerebral and myocardial ischaemia. In the untreated hypertensive patient, a period of high blood pressure can lead to cerebral swelling, as the autoregulatory limit is exceeded, or cause intracranial haemorrhage. If time allows, it is better to establish a previously unrecognized hypertensive patient on treatment. Treated hypertensive patients should be maintained on their treatment and the anaesthetic technique modified to take into account the drugs used. Hypertension may be a response to high ICP, especially following head injury or subarachnoid haemorrhage.

Ischaemic heart disease is also common and needs to be evaluated by a careful history of the patient's exercise tolerance and by electrocardiograph (ECG). The ECG will also show evidence of previous myocardial infarction, whether old or recent. ECG abnormalities are frequently present in patients who have had a SAH or who have raised ICP.

NEUROLOGICAL ASSESSMENT

The clinical neurological assessment needs to elucidate not only the diagnosis but also complicating factors that affect the anaesthetic. The level of consciousness, neurological deficits and occurrence of seizures need to be noted. The existence of intracranial space occupation and raised ICP (persistent headache, vomiting, papilloedema) must be evaluated.

Posterior fossa tumours may cause bulbar palsy and the lower cranial nerves should be examined for impairment of swallowing or laryngeal palsy. A history of repeated aspiration of stomach contents, perhaps with nocturnal bronchospasm, reveals laryngeal incompetence.

A skull X-ray and CT scan or MRI scan may reveal not only the presumptive diagnosis but also the extent of any secondary features such as cerebral oedema, brain shift, hydrocephalus or compression and distortion of the ventricular system. Space-occupying lesions producing more than 10 mm shift of the midline structures suggest significant compromise of the intracranial dynamics.[3]

A reduced level of response presents many problems. It may be associated with hypoxia and hypercarbia, which may in turn reduce still further the level of response by increasing ICP. Reduced ventilation will allow the development of basal pulmonary collapse and consolidation, leading to pneumonia. Dehydration will develop rapidly as the patient is unable to eat and drink and the increased blood viscosity will predispose to venous thrombosis.

Patients with epilepsy need to have their drugs continued up to the time of operation. Sudden withdrawal of antiepileptic drugs is likely to lead to a worsening of the seizure activity. Cerebral oedema complicating intracranial tumours is frequently successfully treated with steroids such as dexamethasone 8 mg tds. Such a regime often produces a significant improvement, with confused patients becoming rational and the level of response improving.

PREMEDICATION

The prospect of intracranial neurosurgery will be daunting for many patients and it is wise to limit the natural anxiety they feel by using a form of sedative or anxiolytic premedication. This is of value particularly when hypertension poses a danger for the patient, as in aneurysm surgery. Temazepam (10–30 mg) or diazepam (10–20 mg) have proved useful and safe for some years.

Spinal procedures are usefully premedicated with a non-steroidal anti-inflammatory analgesic such as diclofenac, assuming there is no contraindication to the NSAID. We have used one of the modified-release preparations of diclofenac for some years together with one of the benzodiazepines. A patient may be in quite severe pain from a prolapsed intervertebral disc and an analgesic premedication may be indicated.

INDUCTION OF ANAESTHESIA

The detailed management of anaesthesia will be discussed in the specific chapters; here the outlines only are discussed.

The anaesthetist needs to aim for a smooth induction of anaesthesia, avoiding coughing, straining or the production of undue hypo- or hypertension. In the

adult an intravenous induction of anaesthesia is normal; either thiopentone or propofol may be used and will produce a fall in ICP by lowering the cerebral metabolic rate ($CMRO_2$) and the CBF.[4,5] Propofol has been demonstrated to produce a 32% fall in cerebrospinal fluid (CSF) pressure 2 min after the induction of anaesthesia with 1.5 mg/kg. The fall in CBF and ICP may be quite short; with propofol, the CSF pressure returned to normal values within 3 min.

Nevertheless, such a fall in ICP is most valuable because many other factors are operating during the induction sequence, which tend to raise ICP. Laryngoscopy, for example, may cause a rapid rise in blood pressure and also be associated with jugular venous obstruction as the laryngoscope is pulled forward to visualize the vocal folds. This action has been implicated in kinking the jugular veins, thus causing an obstruction to cerebral venous drainage.

If non-depolarizing relaxants are used for tracheal intubation it is important to wait for complete relaxation to occur, because any attempt to intubate an incompletely relaxed patient will cause straining and a consequent elevation in blood pressure and intrathoracic pressure.[6] Adequate ventilation must be maintained as the action of the relaxant is developing so that hypoxia and hypercarbia are avoided. The delay implied means that the disturbance produced by laryngoscopy and intubation may well occur after the return to normal of the CBF and ICP following the initial dose of induction agent. Laryngoscopy and intubation provoke a transient but marked arterial hypertension and tachycardia. This is a considerable danger for many neurosurgical patients. The rapidity of the rise in blood pressure is such that it is likely to outstrip the ability of autoregulation to control CBF, so that CBF and ICP will rise with the blood pressure. If there is an area of brain in which autoregulation is impaired or absent, then any rise in blood pressure will lead to a rise in ICP. The patient with a cerebral aneurysm is in danger of aneurysmal rupture, especially if the blood pressure rise is rapid.

Control of the pressor response is important and many ways have been suggested. The administration of a second bolus of the intravenous induction agent before laryngoscopy is one and one study[7] has suggested that propofol (0.5–1.0 mg/kg) is rather more effective at preventing the development of hypertension than thiopentone. The use of opioids provides only a partial protection against the pressor response[8,9] and some authors suggest delaying the opioid until after the muscle relaxant is given to avoid the danger of increased chest wall stiffness.[10] Lignocaine (1.5 mg/kg)[11] given 90 s before intubation has been recommended to blunt the blood pressure and ICP response to laryngoscopy. β-Blockers have also been used.

AIRWAY

Neurosurgical operations may take several hours and the head may be inaccessible under the sterile drapes. It is important to make sure that the airway and pulmonary ventilation are secure for the duration of the operation. The use of an armoured tracheal tube – that is, a tube with a metal or nylon spiral reinforcing the wall – is necessary. The neurosurgeon will put the head and neck into the best position for the planned operation and this may on occasion mean that the head and neck are flexed, so that the end of the tracheal tube is advanced farther into the bronchial tree. The tracheal tube therefore must be placed with care, especially ensuring that the end of the tube is clear of the carina so that flexion of the neck does not advance the tube into the right main bronchus.

Fixation of the tracheal tube must also be done with care. Tapes should never be tied around the neck to fasten the tube in place, because there is a considerable danger of causing cerebral venous obstruction. The tube may be effectively fixed to the face by adhesive strapping, using hypoallergenic materials if required. Any method of fixation needs to take into account the length of the surgical procedure, the fact that secretions or surgical skin preparation fluids may loosen the strapping and the position required for the operation.

Neurosurgical patients may be positioned supine, in a lateral position, prone or sitting. In the prone or sitting position, there is a great danger that the tracheal tube may be dragged out. These are the positions in which it would be most difficult to reintubate the trachea, especially if the head is fixed in pins. It is clearly important, then, to fix the tube especially securely in these patients and to ensure that the weight of the anaesthetic tubing does not drag on the tracheal tube. A practice that was once commonplace is to support the tracheal tube with an oropharyngeal pack. The pack should not be placed rigidly, because it may obstruct the internal jugular veins, but firmly enough to support the tracheal tube and to keep it stationary. Even the reinforced tubes may kink in an extreme position; placing a pack supports their kink-resisting properties. Once a pack is placed, all members of the anaesthetic team must be informed that there is a pack to be removed before extubation at the end of the procedure.

CONDUCT OF A CRANIOTOMY

During intracranial surgery the head is often fixed using a frame with pins, which are applied to the skull. The fixation produces painful stimuli and a hypertensive response may occur, which obviously has the same dangers as the hypertensive response to tracheal intubation. The eyes must be carefully protected.

The start of a craniotomy is also painful, particularly the skin incision and reflecting the galea. The process of cutting the bone flap may also be painful and the physical pressure on the skull involved in drilling a burr hole may cause an increase in ICP.[6] Surgery inside the skull is not markedly painful, unless the surgeon stretches the dura, which is most likely to happen near points of dural attachment. Once the bone flap is cut, the surgeon needs to retract the brain to obtain access to deeper structures.

During this period it is important that anaesthesia is arranged to produce good operating conditions, reducing ICP and brain bulk wherever possible. When the skull is open and the ICP is low, the dura can be seen to be slack but moves in response to the cardiac impulse and the pressure changes produced by the lung ventilator. A high ICP will be seen to be distending the dura and dural pulsation in response to the cardiac cycle and the ventilator will not be visible. In such a circumstance, the ICP must be reduced before the dura is incised because a high ICP will extrude the brain through the dural incision, physically damaging the neurones, and the edge of the dura will cut off the blood supply, causing infarction.

MAINTENANCE OF ANAESTHESIA

The choice of a volatile anaesthetic agent or propofol infusion is controversial. All the volatile agents (including nitrous oxide) have the potential to increase CBF and therefore make the brain difficult to retract. The use of hyperventilation may mask the effects of some of the volatile agents on CBF but this mechanism cannot be relied on, especially when extensive space occupation means that the mechanisms compensating for space occupation are near exhaustion.[12]

The discussion was developed by Todd et al,[13] who prospectively studied three anaesthetic techniques for patients undergoing craniotomy for supratentorial tumour. The patients were assessed carefully, ICP was measured and the extent of the brain swelling noted. Patients were assigned to one of three groups. Group 1 received propofol induction and maintenance of anaesthesia with fentanyl 10 μg/kg loading dose followed by

2–3 μg/kg/h. The propofol infusion was set between 50 and 300 μg/kg/min. In group 2, anaesthesia was induced with thiopentone and maintained with nitrous oxide, oxygen and isoflurane; fentanyl up to 2 μg/kg was given after bone flap replacement. Group 3 also received thiopentone induction of anaesthesia but with fentanyl, as in group 1, and a lower dose of isoflurane. The ICP before craniotomy in group 1 was 12 ± 7 mmHg, in group 2 15 ± 12 mmHg and in group 3 11 ± 8 mmHg. Two patients in groups 1 and 3 but nine patients in group 2 had ICP greater than 24 mmHg. The authors suggest that all three anaesthetic regimes were acceptable. The group also noted speed of emergence and total stay in hospital and hospital costs.

Propofol infusion avoids the need for vasodilating anaesthetic agents and not only Todd et al but also Ravussin et al[14] reported on the successful use of propofol infusion. Ravussin et al considered that propofol gave better control of responses to painful stimuli and faster recovery than thiopentone-isoflurane. Fox et al[15] used 2.0–2.5 mg/kg of propofol for induction of anaesthesia and 12 mg/kg/h for 10 min followed by 9 mg/kg/h for another 10 min and then 3–6 mg/kg/h for the rest of the study. They showed that the responsiveness of the cerebral circulation was well maintained.

HYPERVENTILATION

Hyperventilation has been a part of neurosurgical anaesthesia for many years, notwithstanding the concern that metabolism and flow were being uncoupled. CBF changes 4% for each mmHg change in $PaCO_2$; thus at high values (10.6 kPa, 80 mmHg) the cerebral vasculature is maximally dilated and CBF is approximately doubled. Maximum vasoconstriction occurs below 2.6 kPa (20 mmHg), at which level CBF is reduced by 40%.[16] Harp and Wollman[17] studied safety of hyperventilation and found no evidence of brain hypoxia, even during marked hypocapnia. The vasoconstriction and the reduction in cerebral blood volume (CBV) reduce the ICP and although in the normal brain when hyperventilation is instituted, CBF returns to normal values in about 3 h, the ICP returns to the starting value more slowly. The difference is due to the reduction in brain extracellular fluid volume. Cerebral vasoconstriction reduces the intravascular hydrostatic pressure in the capillary, so extracellular water returns to the circulation under the influence of the plasma oncotic pressure. The result is that brain extracellular fluid volume is reduced, at least in the short term.

The introduction of jugular venous oxygen content measurement[18] has allowed the study of hyperventilation and its effects. The study quoted comments that the use of hyperventilation during neurosurgical procedures can result in cerebral venous oxygen desaturation, which the authors define as jugular venous bulb oxygen saturations less than 50%, in up to 40% of patients. The slowing of the cerebral circulation allows increased oxygen extraction by the brain and the authors comment that the desaturation is suggestive of a decreased margin of safety and possibly indicative of a limited oxygen supply with impending tissue hypoxia. In a subsequent study, they investigated the effect of high oxygen tensions (PaO_2 = 100–200, 201–300, 301–400 and >400 mmHg) on jugular venous oxygen content at two levels of hyperventilation ($PaCO_2$ = 3.3 kPa and $PaCO_2$ = 4 kPa). They suggested that hyperoxia during acute hyperventilation should be considered for those patients in whom hyperventilation is contemplated and cerebral ischaemia considered a risk. Hyperventilation should also be considered if volatile anaesthetic agents are to be used.[19]

MUSCLE RELAXANTS

A profound degree of muscle relaxation is important in the production of good operating conditions. Incomplete muscle relaxation is associated with an increased mean intrathoracic pressure and therefore central venous pressure (CVP); the increased CVP is transmitted to the cerebral veins. Good muscle relaxation is also advisable because of the obvious danger of an incompletely paralysed patient coughing during an intracranial operation.

MANAGEMENT OF HIGH ICP DURING ANAESTHESIA

An intraoperative rise in ICP will impede surgery because if the brain is bulky, it is more difficult to retract. Increased force will be needed on the brain retractors, producing local damage. If, during neurosurgery, the ICP is noted to be high, the likely cause must be identified and corrected. There are also specific methods for lowering ICP.

Checklist for causes of high ICP during surgery

- Position   Head up
                              Clear cerebral venous
                              drainage
                              No abdominal compression
- No hypoxia
- Adequate ventilation $PaCO_2$ low
                              Long expiratory pause
                              No PEEP
- CVP low
- Good muscle relaxation
- Avoid cerebral vasodilating drugs

Treatment of high ICP

Hyperosmolar diuretics

Mannitol, which is perhaps the agent most frequently used, has many systemic and cerebral effects. Given in doses of 0.5–1.0 g/kg, it raises serum osmotic pressure so that water is drawn into the vascular system from the tissues. The increased oncotic pressure draws water from the brain and reduces brain bulk. As the action develops, the circulating blood volume rises and the haematocrit falls.[20] The blood volume remains elevated for 15–30 min and during this time, the blood pressure and CVP may also be elevated. The diuresis limits the rise in blood volume. The decreased haematocrit allows a greater CBF and in patients with intact autoregulation, cerebral vasoconstriction occurs, keeping oxygen supply in balance with demand. The result is that the CBV is reduced and therefore so is the ICP. If autoregulation is impaired then the increased CBF persists, though ICP still falls, though to a small extent.[21]

Loop diuretics

Frusemide has been studied the most, though many diuretics have useful intracranial effects. Frusemide[22] 1.0 mg/kg produces a fall in ICP similar to that produced by 1 g/kg mannitol. It acts by inhibition of sodium and chloride reabsorption in the ascending limb of the loop of Henle and has a separate action in reducing CSF production by suppressing sodium transport. It lowers ICP by mobilizing normal brain extracellular fluid and cerebral oedema. The diuresis reduces blood volume and therefore the low cerebral venous pressure allows resorption of CSF. Frusemide appears not to affect the volume/pressure response, as does mannitol.

Steroids

The effect of steroids in reducing the oedema related to tumours preoperatively has been mentioned earlier. They are particularly effective in patients with focal lesions and are ineffective when there is widespread brain injury. They have little place in the control of intraoperative high ICP but may be given intraoperatively to reduce postoperative swelling. They reduce the extrachoroidal production of CSF.[23]

Hyperventilation

If high ICP occurs, then it is important to check the $PaCO_2$ with an arterial sample to avoid any inadvertent hypercapnia.

Metabolic suppression

Shapiro[24] described the use of barbiturates intravenously during periods of intraoperative high ICP.

The aim is to reduce cerebral metabolic activity, while reducing brain bulk by producing a cerebral vasoconstriction. Propofol and etomidate have also been used to lower ICP and have the advantage over the barbiturates that they are metabolized quickly.

Lignocaine (1.5 mg/kg) may also be used to lower ICP, especially in the patient with cardiovascular instability. 1.5 mg/kg lignocaine is said to be as effective as 3 mg/kg thiopentone in lowering ICP.[25]

THE END OF THE ANAESTHETIC

The end of the neurosurgical anaesthetic has been studied less than the start. Leech et al[26] measured ICP at the end of surgery, before and after the reversal of the muscle relaxants and after removal of the tracheal tube. After surgery but before reversal of the relaxants, the mean ICP was 11 mmHg but after reversal, with the patient breathing spontaneously, the mean ICP had risen to 21 mmHg. Just before return to the ward, the ICP was still high at 19 mmHg. These are surprisingly high values considering that craniotomy had been performed and CSF drainage had taken place.

The possible role of nitrous oxide in causing an increase in ICP by diffusing into the air space left in the skull after craniotomy was studied by Domino et al.[29] They found that all patients in their series had intracranial air but that nitrous oxide was not associated with an increase in ICP as the dura and skull were closed. Indeed, the patients who were maintained on nitrous oxide demonstrated a significant fall in ICP postoperatively. The air disappears only slowly; in one series[27] all patients were shown to have intracranial air immediately after craniotomy or craniectomy. In the second postoperative week, 11.8% still had an intracranial air collection large enough, in the opinion of the authors, to put them at risk if nitrous oxide was used for another anaesthetic.

Extubation

The disturbance of pharyngeal suction and extubation may cause a rise in MAP and an increase in intrathoracic pressure. Hypertension may provoke bleeding from arteries that have been cut during the surgical procedure and the increase in intrathoracic pressure may provoke bleeding from venous channels opened during surgery. The anaesthetic should be continued so that there is no tendency for the patient to cough and strain during the application of head bandages, which often results in head movement. Muscle relaxants should not be reversed until after the bandages have been applied.

The removal of the tracheal tube should be carefully performed when it is certain that the patient is able to breathe effectively. The use of IV lignocaine (1.5 mg/kg) at least 90 s before extubation[28] blunts the cardiovascular responses effectively.

POSTOPERATIVE CARE

The neurosurgical patient requires close observation postoperatively, because many of the preoperative disease processes will still be active, such as cerebral oedema. Haematomas may form and oedema may spread, raising ICP and reducing conscious level. Vascular spasm may worsen, producing local cerebral ischaemia, shown as a neurological deficit. The patient may develop seizures. Monitoring must therefore be close and include neurological observations, observation of the conscious level, such as the Glasgow Coma Scale, observation of the pupil size and reactivity and frequent measurements of pulse rate, blood pressure and respiration.

It is crucial therefore that the patient should be awake and responding at the end of the anaesthetic and choosing the anaesthetic drugs and techniques to achieve not only good operating conditions but also an awake patient without neurological deficit is part of the challenge of neuroanaesthesia.

REFERENCES

1. Kendall BE. The detection of intracranial tumours. Br J Hosp Med 1980; 23: 116.

2. Strandgaard S, Olesen J, Skinh"y E, Lassen NA. Autoregulation of brain circulation in severe arterial hypertension. BMJ 1973; 1: 507.

3. Bedford RF, Morris L, Jane JA. Intracranial hypertension during surgery for supratentorial tumor: correlation with pre-operative computed tomography scans. Anesth Analg 1982; 61: 430–433.

4. Michenfelder JD. The interdependency of cerebral function and metabolic effects following maximum doses of thiopental in the dog. Anesthesiology 1974; 41: 231.

5. Ravussin P, Guinard JP, Ralley F, Thorin D. Effect of propofol on cerebrospinal fluid pressure and cerebral perfusion pressure in patients undergoing craniotomy. Anaesthesia 1988; 43(suppl): 37–41.

6. Shapiro HM, Wyte SR, Harris AB, Galindo A. Acute intraoperative intracranial hypertension in neurosurgical patients: mechanical and pharmacological factors. Anesthesiology 1972; 37: 399–405.

7. Harris CE, Murray AM, Anderson JM, Grounds RM, Morgan M, Effects of thiopentone, etomidate and propofol on the haemodynamic response to tracheal intubation. Anaesthesia 1988; 43(suppl): 32.

8. Martin DE, Rosenberg H, Aukburg SJ et al. Low dose fentanyl blunts circulatory responses to tracheal intubation. Anesth Analg 1982; 61: 680–684.

9. Kautto UM. Attenuation of the circulatory response to laryngoscopy and intubation by fentanyl. Acta Anaesth Scand 1982; 26: 217–221.

10. Spiekermann BF, Stone DJ, Bogdonoff DL, Yemen TA. Airway management in neuroanaesthesia. Can J Anaesth 1996; 43: 820–834.

11. Bedford RF, Persing JA, Pobereskin L, Butler A. Lidocaine or thiopental for rapid control of intracranial hypertension? Anesth Analg 1980; 59: 435.

12. Grosslight K, Foster R, Colohan AR, Bedford RF. Isoflurane for neuroanesthesia: risk factors for increases in intracranial pressure. Anesthesiology 1985; 63: 533.

13. Todd MM, Warner DS, Sokoll MD et al. A prospective comparative trial of three anesthetics for elective supratentorial craniotomy. Propofol/fentanyl, isoflurane/nitrous oxide and fentanyl/nitrous oxide. Anethesiology 1993; 78: 1005–1020.

14. Ravussin P, Tempelhoff R, Modica PA, Bayer-Merger MM. Propofol vs thiopental-isoflurane for neurosurgical anaesthesia: comparison of hemodynamics, CSF pressure and recovery. J Neurosurg Anesthesiol 1991; 3: 85.

15. Fox J, Gelb AW, Enns J, Murkin JM, Farrar JK, Manninen PH. The responsiveness of cerebral blood flow to changes in arterial carbon dioxide tension is maintained during propofol-nitrous oxide anesthesia in humans. Anesthesiology 1992; 77: 453.

16. Harper AM, Glass HI. Effect of alterations in arterial carbon dioxide tension on the blood flow through the cerebral cortex at low and normal arterial blood pressures. J Neurol Neurosurg Psychiat 1965; 28: 449.

17. Harp JR, Wollman H. Cerebral metabolic effects of hyperventilation and deliberate hypotension. Br J Anaesth 1973; 45: 256.

18. Matta BF, Lam AM, Mayberg TS, Shapiro Y, Winn HR. A critique of the intraoperative use of jugular venous bulb catheters during neurosurgical procedures. Anesth Analg 1994; 79: 745–750.

19. Jung R, Reisel R, Marx W, Galicich J, Bedford RF Isoflurane and nitrous oxide: comparative impact on cerebrospinal fluid pressure in patients with brain tumours. Anesth Analg 1992; 75: 724–728.

20. Muizelaar JP, Wei EP, Kontos HA, Becker DP. Mannitol causes compensatory cerebral vasoconstriction and vasodilatation in response to blood viscosity changes. J Neurosurg 1983; 59: 822.

21. Muizelaar JP, Lutz HA, Becker DP. Effect of mannitol on ICP and CBF and correlation with pressure autoregulation in severely head injured patients. J Neurosurg 1984; 61: 700.

22. Cottrell JE, Robustelli A, Post K, Turndorf H. Furosemide and mannitol induced changes in ICP and serum osmolality and electrolytes. Anesthesiology 1977; 47: 28.

23. Martins AM, Ramirez A, Soloman LS, Weise GM. The effect of dexamethasone on the rate of formation of cerebrospinal fluid in the monkey. J Neurosurg 1974; 41: 550.

24. Shapiro HM. Intracranial hypertension: therapeutic and anesthetic considerations. Anesthesiology 1975; 43: 445.

25. Bedford RF, Persing JA, Poberskin L, Butler A. Lidocaine or thiopental for rapid control of intracranial hypertension? Anesth Analg 1980; 59: 435–437.

26. Leech PJ, Barker J, Fitch W. Changes in intracranial pressure during the termination of anaesthesia. Br J Anaesth 1974; 46: 315.

27. Reasoner DK, Todd MM, Scamman FL, Warner DS. The incidence of pneumocephalus after supratentorial craniotomy. Observations on the disappearance of intracranial air. Anesthesiology 1994; 80: 1008–1012.

28. Bidwai AV, Bidwai VA, Rogers CR, Stanley TH. Blood-pressure and pulse-rate responses to endotracheal extubation with and without prior injection of lidocaine. Anesthesiology 1979; 51: 171–173.

29. Domino KB, Hemstad JR, Lam AM. Effect of nitrous oxide on intracranial pressure after cranial dural closure in patients undergoing craniotomy. Anesthesiology 1992; 77: 421–425.

13

ANAESTHESIA FOR SURGERY OF SUPRATENTORIAL SPACE-OCCUPYING LESIONS

John M. Turner

INTRODUCTION

The challenge of any anaesthetic for neurosurgery is to provide good intracranial operating conditions, with a slack brain and low intracranial pressure (ICP). When a patient has an intracranial space-occupying lesion (SOL), the achievement of a low ICP during surgery demands a careful choice of the most appropriate anaesthetic and an attention to detail.

Patients present for craniotomy for a supratentorial SOL most often because of a tumour but space occupation may also be caused by subdural, extradural or intracerebral haematomas or an intracranial abscess. Even when a tumour is histologically benign, the processes set in train by intracranial space occupation can be fatal if the tumour is not treated. A badly administered or inappropriate anaesthetic may add to the intracranial problems generated by the space occupation, increasing ICP.

INTRACRANIAL TUMOURS

MENINGIOMAS

These arise from the arachnoid cap cell which is synthetically active but has a slow rate of cell division. They account for 15% of all intracranial neoplasms and 90% are supratentorial. Tentorial meningiomas account for 2–3% but, because of the high rate of brainstem compression, tend to present earlier, whereas frontal lobe meningiomas arising in a 'silent' area of the brain present much later and may become very large before diagnosis (see Fig. 4.3). In general, meningiomas tend to present in the fifth and sixth decades of life. Agents implicated in causation are trauma, hormonal influence and viral infection and there is a definite link with radiotherapy, when lesions arise in younger patients. They are classically benign, causing compression rather than invasion, but have a high rate of local recurrence, particularly associated with radiotherapy, and can be frankly malignant. They are generally highly vascular, deriving large 'feeding' vessels from local blood vessels, both intracranial and extracranial. They are classified using the Helsinki system which grades increasing malignancy from grade I (benign) to grade IV (sarcomatous). Seizures are common and occur in up to 60% of patients presenting for surgery. Mental deterioration is usually slow in onset but eventually focal deficit will occur with a rise in ICP. At surgery, extension outwards along the vault or skull floor may make complete removal impossible.

GLIOMAS

These are the commonest types of intracranial neoplasms, arising from brain cellular components and ranging from relatively slow-growing astrocytomas to malignant glioblastomas. The variable natural history and unpredictability of malignant transformation require a histological diagnosis. Positron emission tomography (PET) scanning may show up 'hot spots' for metabolism which are highly suggestive of malignant transformation[1]. Total excision may not be possible and surgery may need to be followed by radiotherapy.

Astrocytomas tend to present with a long history of epilepsy, with late-onset focal deficit. Glioblastomas comprise 25% of primary intracranial tumours and are always supratentorial. They have a 10% 2-year survival rate. They present with a short clinical history, rapid onset and progression of focal deficit and signs of raised intracranial pressure. Epilepsy is less common. Surgery may be required to improve the neurological deficit prior to radiotherapy. Oligodendrogliomas are uncommon and slow growing. They commonly cause epilepsy and may even calcify. Eventually localizing signs will develop.

TUMOURS OF THE VENTRICULAR SYSTEM

Whatever the histology, these tumours tend to present with obstructive hydrocephalus due to obstruction of the third ventricle outflow and aqueduct of Sylvius. Papillomas can occur in the choroid plexus. Colloid cysts arise in the third ventricle and are related to ependymomas, which usually arise in the fourth ventricle from cells lining the ventricular system. Pinealomas do not all arise directly from the pineal gland but from the area around it. They cause similar symptoms and can produce midbrain compression. With all these tumours, the presentation is usually related to the onset of hydrocephalus, the patient complaining of severe intermittent headache. Intermittent blockage of the CSF circulation may produce high ICP and occasionally this can precipitate sudden loss of consciousness. Surgical removal may be difficult because of potential damage to the ventricular system or hypothalamus. An endoscopic approach may be possible to intraventricular tumours such as colloid cysts.

OTHER PRIMARY TUMOURS

Dermoid and epidermoid neoplasms can arise although these are rare outside the posterior fossa.

METASTATIC DISEASE

Secondary lesions from primary cancers elsewhere are the commonest intracranial neoplasms; 20–40% of all cancer patients develop brain metastases.[2] Despite their frequency, care should be taken to ensure that the patient does have a metastasis and not another primary tumour.

Removal of a solitary cerebral metastasis is usually worthwhile because most patients do not die of their brain disease and improvement in neurological function after surgery may greatly improve their quality of life. Clearly, these patients may present with a range of systemic problems which may need attention preoperatively.

EXTRADURAL AND SUBDURAL HAEMATOMA

The space occupation produced by acute extradural and subdural haematomas develops rapidly and allows less time for the brain to accommodate to the SOL. Figure 4.2 shows the classic appearance of an extradural haematoma, with its biconvex shape. Chronic subdural haematomas, usually affecting the elderly, may present weeks after the initial injury. The patient may become confused and drowsy and the state of consciousness may fluctuate, with a mild hemiparesis. A history of trauma may be difficult to elicit and ICP may be normal or only slightly raised. Burr hole aspiration may be all that is required but occasionally open operation may be necessary if the haematoma recollects. Occasionally the insertion of a conduit from the haematoma cavity to the peritoneum may be required to provide for continuous decompression of the haematoma.

INTRACEREBRAL ABSCESS

The first successful removal of an intracranial abscess was in 1752, when most abscesses were secondary to gunshot wounds or other trauma. Now supratentorial abscesses usually result from local spread of a source of infection from the frontal sinus or middle ear; occasionally they arise as a result of blood borne infection.

Surgery is the mainstay of treatment despite the huge improvement in mortality which occurred following the introduction of antibiotics to neurosurgery in 1943. The key to further improvement in treatment has come with the greater ability to localize cerebral lesions. Introduction of CT scanning led to much earlier diagnosis and early, accurate drainage. The patient presents with a picture of meningitis and raised ICP occurring over a few days or weeks. Aspiration should be carried out via a burr hole and antibiotics instilled into the cavity. This may need to be repeated until the abscess cavity contracts and becomes sterile. The residual cyst may need to be removed. Some surgeons prefer craniotomy and primary excision. The mortality rate remains related to the neurological status of the patient at initial presentation.

ASSESSMENT

The diagnosis of a space-occupying lesion implies a degree of urgency for surgery because as the SOL develops, the intracranial compensating mechanisms for space occupation are being exhausted. A general history should be taken, with particular reference to cardiac and respiratory disease and to neurological deficit. An examination should be carried out in the usual way, again with special attention paid to neurological deficit which may compromise the airway, hinder safe emergence from anaesthesia or be due to raised intracranial pressure. It is particularly important to identify raised ICP and to assess the degree of intracranial space occupation preoperatively as extra care must be taken to ensure the patient's condition is not worsened by manoeuvres preoperatively or at induction. A history of headache together with papilloedema suggests that high ICP is present.

The patient's full blood count, urea and electrolytes and clotting should be checked and blood cross-matched as appropriate. The amount of blood loss depends on the type of tumour and its vascularity; a large meningioma can be associated with heavy blood loss but for most craniotomies 2–4 units of blood are sufficient. Chest X-ray and ECG should be ordered if indicated. It should be remembered that neurological disease can cause a variety of ECG changes including ischaemic changes and arrhythmias. Some patients will have been prescribed dexamethasone for several days preoperatively to reduce reactive oedema.

Normal medication, especially anticonvulsants and antihypertensive drugs, should be continued until just before surgery. Sedative premedication may be desirable in order to allay anxiety. Respiratory depression with subsequent hypercarbia should be avoided, especially in the presence of raised ICP. For this reason we avoid opiates and usually prescribe 10–20 mg of temazepam or 10–15 mg diazepam, with 10 mg metoclopramide orally 90 min preoperatively.

General anaesthesia for surgery in patients with an acute mass effect includes head elevation, osmotherapy with mannitol, artificial ventilation to prevent hypoxia and hypercarbia, with controllable hypocarbia, administration of cerebral protective agents such as barbiturates and maintenance of cerebral perfusion pressure with fluids and inotropes if necessary. Emergency craniotomy for decompression may be necessary.

The assessment of supratentorial lesions is made considerably easier by the improvement in imaging techniques, CT scanning and MRI. These allow early, precise location of lesions and give some idea of the probable histological diagnosis. The scans should be examined to give information on:

- size of mass;
- ventricular distortion or CSF obstruction;
- midline shift;
- amount of oedema;
- degree of contrast enhancement;
- proximity to venous sinus.

The size of the mass depends partly on whether the tumour is developing in a silent or an eloquent area of the brain. Tumours in a silent area may grow so large before they present that they cause a very considerable compromise of intracranial dynamics. Assessment of the degree of intracranial space occupation is important; if there is more than 10 mm shift of the midline structures, for example, volatile agents should be used with care.[3,4,5] The amount of oedema may turn a relatively small lesion into a more serious problem. The degree of enhancement with intravenous radiographic contrast shows the degree of abnormal or damaged blood–brain barrier (BBB) in the lesion and it is through this damaged BBB that the contrast penetrated to the stroma of the tumour. A vascular tumour may have a low vascular resistance and frequently in angiography cerebral veins draining the tumour fill early, during the arterial or capillary phases of the angiogram, reflecting the fast flow. Such a tumour, especially if it is near one of the venous sinuses, has the potential for causing major blood loss as resection is undertaken.

The increasing availability of metabolic imaging such as PET, MR spectroscopy and single photon emission tomography (using thallium-201 which is specifically taken up by tumour cells but not by necrotic areas) will offer more precise information on the size and location of the tumour.

Patients suspected of having an astrocytoma should undergo stereotactic biopsy prior to craniotomy to confirm the histological diagnosis.

GENERAL ANAESTHESIA FOR CRANIOTOMY

The dangers of intraoperative high ICP in the presence of a SOL mean that the anaesthetist must be especially careful to choose anaesthetic agents and techniques which lower ICP. In particular, it is important to avoid a rise in cerebral venous pressure, cerebral vaso-

dilation, hypercapnia and hypertension. All these circumstances can be provoked during the induction and maintenance of anaesthesia.

EFFECTS OF ANAESTHETIC AGENTS

The effects of anaesthetic agents and techniques on cerebral blood flow (CBF) and ICP have been discussed in earlier chapters. All volatile agents have the ability to raise CBF and ICP, though their action can be modified by hyperventilation and by the use of opioids which reduce the MAC of the agents. Adams[6] demonstrated that isoflurane combined with hypocapnia ($PaCO_2$ about 25 mmHg) was not associated with a rise in ICP and Jung[7] makes a similar point.

Muzzi has shown that 1 MAC desflurane causes a gradual but significant rise in ICP in patients with a supratentorial SOL, whereas isoflurane does not.[8] Enflurane has the potential to produce high-amplitude spike and wave EEG complexes and whilst in one study,[9] the postoperative seizure rate was no higher in the patients receiving enflurane than in those receiving isoflurane, it is probably best avoided. Sevoflurane seems to have similar effects to isoflurane.[10,11]

The potential problems of the volatile agents can be avoided by using intravenous maintenance of anaesthesia with propofol. Barbiturates and propofol reduce $CMRO_2$ and therefore CBF. The reduction in CBF and cerebral blood volume (CBV) is helpful in maintaining as low an ICP as possible. The cerebral effects of propofol, together with its rapid recovery, make possible the use of an infusion technique for maintenance of anaesthesia throughout a craniotomy. Infusion rates have been published[12] and one group[13] has used a maintenance infusion rate of 100 μg/kg/min for elective neurosurgery after a bolus dose for induction of 1.5 mg/kg. The infusion should be started at the same time as the bolus dose, to achieve an effective plasma concentration rapidly.

The opioids are a valuable adjunct to neuroanaesthesia, not least because of the cardiovascular stability they produce. They also reduce the MAC of volatile agents and therefore allow agents such as isoflurane to be used safely in lower concentrations so that the effect on CBF is lessened. Many opioids can be used as long as they do not induce a fall in MAP.[14,15,16]

INDUCTION AND INTUBATION

Induction of anaesthesia can be with either thiopentone or propofol. Neuromuscular blockade can be achieved with atracurium or vecuronium, although newer agents such as mivacurium or rocuronium[17] may also be used. Intubation should not be performed until enough time has elapsed for the muscle relaxation to be complete. The pressor response to laryngoscopy and intubation will cause an increase in the size of vascular tumours in particular, because the tumour blood supply will not be under autoregulatory control. At the same time, laryngoscopy tends to kink the jugular veins, so that cerebral venous outflow is impaired. The result is a great tendency for a dangerous rise in ICP. The pressor response should, therefore, be controlled. A second dose of the induction agent or the use of IV lignocaine 1.5 mg/kg 90 s before intubation is well established, as is the use of agents such as esmolol.

The airway should be secured with an armoured endotracheal tube, taped on the contralateral side to operation. It may be desirable to secure the tube further using a throat pack. Careful taping is required to prevent both extubation and venous congestion. Pressure ventilation of the lungs is arranged so that there is a slow rate, with a long expiratory pause; PEEP is normally not applied. A nasogastric tube should be considered for long operations.

POSITION

Operations may last several hours so the patient should be carefully positioned with bony points padded, eyes protected with tape or gel and care taken to ensure tubing is not pressed against the patient's skin. Patients may be positioned supine or slightly rotated, with one shoulder raised, or they may be placed in a lateral position. A head-up tilt of the table of about 15° is essential to aid cerebral venous drainage. Pinealomas may be approached with the patient either prone or sitting.

A urinary catheter is necessary to assess fluid status. The patient's head position on the operating table is fixed either on a horseshoe-type head rest or by the insertion of skull pins. The application of the pins represents another stimulus causing an increase in blood pressure response[18] and great care should be taken to ensure that the patient is adequately anaesthetized before the pins are applied.

MAINTENANCE OF ANAESTHESIA

The choice of volatile or intravenous agents for maintenance of anaesthesia has already been described. Todd et al,[19] in a complex and thoughtful study, effectively demonstrated that propofol/fentanyl, nitrous oxide/high-dose isoflurane or fentanyl/low-dose isoflurane techniques of anaesthesia can be used. It is interesting to note that although there were no signif-

icant intergroup differences in mean ICP, a relatively high number of patients in the nitrous oxide/high-dose isoflurane group (9/40) showed ICP greater than 23 mmHg. In the propofol/fentanyl group, there were only two patients out of 40 and in the fentanyl/low-dose isoflurane only two out of 41 patients with high ICP (greater than 23 mmHg).

Whichever technique is chosen, therefore, there remains a danger of high ICP and it is important for the anaesthetist to check on the state of the brain once the skull has been opened. A tense, bulging dura is dangerous and may prevent surgery proceeding, because if the dura is opened the brain is squeezed through the dural defect and infarcts. Reduction of ICP is necessary, first of all eliminating any faults of technique that have given rise to the high ICP and then using specific methods to lower ICP. A checklist for this has been given in Chapter 12, p. 176.

REDUCING INTRACRANIAL HYPERTENSION

The use of mannitol at the start of the craniotomy is valuable, because mannitol not only lowers ICP but also appears to reduce the volume/pressure response (VPR).[20] This reduces the pressure required on the surgical retractors and therefore reduces the extent of neuronal damage. The dose of mannitol is controversial; suggested doses have ranged from 0.5 to 2.0 g/kg body weight, given as a 20% solution. Smaller doses (0.5–1.0 g/kg) can be given over 15–20 min at the start of an operation, but the larger doses should be infused over 1–1.5h. Mannitol exerts its action in a number of ways. The administration of mannitol raises serum oncotic pressure, so that water is drawn into the vascular system. The withdrawal of brain extracellular fluid reduces brain bulk and therefore ICP. The increased vascular volume is demonstrated by a temporary increase in blood pressure and CVP before the onset of the diuresis. It also produces a reduction in the haematocrit.

Muizelaar et al[21,22] suggested that the reduction in haematocrit is associated with an increase in cerebral blood flow so that oxygen supply is greater than metabolic demand. When cerebral autoregulation is intact, the balance of oxygen supply and demand is restored by cerebral vasoconstriction which, by producing a fall in CBV, also reduces ICP. In patients with intact autoregulation, there was a 27% fall in ICP but in a group of head-injured patients with impaired autoregulation, mannitol produced a rise in CBF of 17.9%, but a fall in ICP of 4%. Ravussin et al[23] infused mannitol rapidly and found that there was a 25% increase in CBV and ICP. The rise in ICP lasted for a short time

(5 min), but the rise in CBV lasted for 15 min. They suggested that the ICP begins to fall after mannitol only when the dehydrating effect has begun to counteract the initial increase in CBV.

Mannitol may theoretically worsen oedema by crossing a damaged BBB.

Frusemide may be used either on its own or in combination with mannitol to reduce intracranial hypertension. Frusemide (1 mg/kg) reduces ICP to the same extent as mannitol (1 g/kg).[24] It has the advantage of mobilizing oedema fluid more effectively than mannitol and lowering CVP, so that cerebral venous pressure is low and therefore reabsorption of CSF optimal.

Metabolic suppression with thiopentone,[25] propofol and lignocaine[26] may also be used to reduce intracranial hypertension.

MONITORING

Careful monitoring is essential and must include oxygen saturation, ECG and end-tidal CO_2 analysis. Two large-bore venous cannulae must be placed when a vascular tumour is being excised. Continuous direct measurement of arterial pressure and central venous pressure is essential. A central venous line is also valuable for administration of hypotensive agents when the tumour is vascular. A temperature probe is placed in the oesophagus. Arterial blood gases should be taken early in the procedure to check the validity of the end-tidal reading.

Blood loss

Vascular tumours (notably meningiomas) can be associated with very fast blood loss and if the tumour is on the convexity of a cerebral hemisphere, the blood loss may occur during the cutting of the bone flap, when the surgeon may not be in a position to stop the bleeding.

The anaesthetist thus needs to have everything needed for rapid transfusion ready at the start of a craniotomy for a vascular tumour. Crossmatched blood needs to be in the theatre suite and there must be a large-bore venous cannula in place, together with arterial and CVP measurement. A blood warmer needs to be set up and acid–base estimations available quickly.

Further significant and persistent blood loss may occur during the subsequent resection of a meningioma, so it is important that the initial blood loss is replaced. The cerebral vasoconstriction that occurs with haemorrhage reduces CBF significantly,[27] especially in the junctional areas between the major cerebral vessels.

INDUCED HYPOTENSION

The need for induced hypotension has lessened in neuroanaesthesia following the improvements in surgical techniques. The use of propofol infusion with opioid analgesics and moderate hyperventilation provides a satisfactory surgical field for most neurosurgical operations but occasionally the resection of a large vascular tumour may still require hypotension.

Before hypotension is used, the patient's physical state should be carefully assessed, particularly looking for signs of ischaemia in the cerebral or coronary circulations or a history of hypertension. Hypotension should not normally be applied until the dura is open and the length of hypotension should be kept as short as possible. Hypovolaemia should not be allowed to coexist with induced hypotension; blood replacement must parallel blood loss. CBF is maintained constant as long as the MAP is between 60 and 160 mmHg, so hypotension to a MAP of 60–70 mmHg, which will provide a surgical field with reduced oozing, may be of value.

Monitoring must be extensive and reliable; as well as the monitoring mentioned, jugular venous oxygen content measurements are valuable, as are transcranial Doppler measurements of flow velocity.

Hypotension is most easily induced by the combination of labetalol (10–20 mg) followed by sodium nitroprusside infusion (0.01%). The infusion is best given along the central venous line, so that the time lag between changing the infusion rate and observing the effect on blood pressure is kept to a minimum.

Sodium nitroprusside causes cerebral vasodilatation[28] but the effect can be overcome by ensuring that the arterial pressure is lowered to at least 70% of the control value. If the anaesthetic has been so arranged that the patient's cardiovascular system is stable and not responding to painful stimuli, hypotension should be easily achieved with such small doses of propofol that toxicity[29] is not invoked. If the patient develops a tachycardia or is resistant to sodium nitroprusside, it is better to supplement the action of sodium nitroprusside by another drug, such as labetalol or propranolol to control heart rate, or to increase the infusion of propofol or the inhaled concentration of isoflurane, rather than using excessive infusion rates of sodium nitroprusside.

Other hypotensive agents are available, such as trimetaphan[28] and trinitroglycerine[30,31] (GTN). GTN, like sodium nitroprusside, causes an increase in ICP and also a marked tachycardia. Trimetaphan is a less effective drug than either but does not cause a rise in

ICP, unless the patient is suffering from extreme degrees of intracranial space occupation, in which case the ganglionic blockade may produce an increase in CBF by blocking the sympathetic supply to the cerebral vessels.[28]

When induced hypotension is being used, it is important that the surgeon knows this and that, after the tumour is resected, blood pressure is returned to normal before the dura is closed. This is essential so that the bleeding points can be visualized and sealed.

INTRAVENOUS FLUIDS

Intravenous fluids should be chosen with care; over-transfusion will lead to a high CVP and therefore predispose to high ICP and use of solutions of glucose in water worsen cerebral oedema. Patients with severe intracranial hypertension may have been drowsy or vomiting preoperatively and therefore may be hypovolaemic. If mannitol has been used, fluids should be given to replace the deficit produced by diuresis. Mannitol may also produce hyponatraemia and hypokalaemia.

Normal saline or Hartmann's solution is indicated for fluid therapy during the procedure and should be given to replace fluid losses and controlled by the CVP to avoid overtransfusion. Colloid solutions, such as modified gelation (Gelofusine), may be given and blood loss over 1 litre should be replaced as appropriate.

EMERGENCE FROM ANAESTHESIA

The closure of a craniotomy may take a little time. Following surgery for a space-occupying lesion, some postoperative brain swelling is likely and great care should be taken to ensure that the end of the anaesthetic is smooth, without undue hypertension, coughing or straining. During the closure period, the propofol and relaxant infusions can be reduced, the aim being to ensure that the patient is awake at the end of the procedure, but reversal of the muscle relaxant must be left until after any dressings or head bandages have been applied. Much movement of the head may take place then and the patient should not cough or strain.

In order to avoid hypertension on extubation, removal of the endotracheal tube and suctioning of the pharynx may be covered with IV lignocaine 1.5 mg/kg 90 s before extubation. Labetalol can also be given to obtund these responses.[32]

Patients in whom a tight brain was present during surgery or where there was excessive blood loss or in whom oedema spread is marked should be considered

for postoperative pressure ventilation in an intensive care unit. Normally, however, anaesthetic technique should be so judged as to produce an awake, responding patient in the recovery area, so that neurological monitoring to detect the postoperative complications of haematoma formation may be started.

REFERENCES

1. De Witte O, Levivier M, Vioon P et al. Prognostic value positron emission tomography with [1 8F] fluoro-2-deoxy-D-glucose in the low-grade glioma. Neurosurgery 1996; 39: 470-476.

2. Kendall BE The detection of intracranial tumours. Br J Hosp Med 1980; 23: 116.

3. Bedford RF, Morris L, Jane JA. Intracranial hypertension during surgery for supratentorial tumor: correlation with pre-operative computed tomography scans. Anesth Analg 1982; 61: 430–433.

4. Campkin TV, Flynn RM. Isoflurane and cerebrospinal fluid pressure – a study in neurosurgical patients undergoing intracranial shunt procedures. Anaesthesia 1989; 44: 50.

5. Grosslight K, Foster R, Colohan AR, Bedford RF. Isoflurane for neuroanesthesia: risk factors for increase in intracranial pressure. Anesthesiology 1985; 63: 533.

6. Adams RW, Cucchiara RF, Gronert GA, Messick JM, Michenfelder JD. Isoflurane and cerebrospinal fluid pressure in neurosurgical patients. Anesthesiology 1981; 54: 97–99.

7. Jung R, Reisel R, Marx W, Galicich J, Bedford RF Isoflurane and nitrous oxide: comparative impact on cerebrospinal fluid pressure in patients with brain tumours. Anesth Analg 1992; 75: 724–728.

8. Muzzi DA, Losasso TJ, Dietz NM, Faust RJ, Cucchiara RF, Milde LN. The effect of desflurane and isoflurane on cerebrospinal fluid pressure in humans with mass lesions. Anesthesiology 1992; 76: 720–724.

9. Christys AR, Moss E, Powell D. Retrospective study of early postoperative convulsions after intracranial surgery with isoflurane of enflurane anaesthesia. Br J Anaesth 1989; 62: 624–627.

10. Scheller MS, Teteishi A, Drummond JC, Zornow MH. The effects of sevoflurane on cerebral blood flow, cerebral metabolic rate for oxygen, intracranial pressure, and the electroencephalogram are similar to those of isoflurane in the rabbit. Anesthesiology 1988; 68: 548–551.

11. Takahashi H, Murata K, Ikeda K. Sevoflurane does not increase intracranial pressure in hyperventilated dogs. Br J Anaesth 1993; 71: 551–555.

12. Roberts FL, Dixon J, Lewis GTR, Tackley RM, Prys-Roberts C. Induction and maintenance of propofol anaesthesia. A manual infusion scheme. Anaesthesia 1988; 43(suppl): 14–17.

13. Ravussin P, Guinard JP, Ralley F, Thorin D. Effect of propofol on cerebrospinal fluid pressure and cerebral perfusion pressure in patients undergoing craniotomy. Anaesthesia 1988; 43(suppl): 37–41.

14. Fitch W, Barker J, Jennett WB, McDowall DG. The influence of neuroleptanalgesic drugs on cerebrospinal fluid pressure. Br J Anaesth 1969; 41: 800.

15. Werner C, Kochs E, Bause H, Hoffman WE, Schulte am Esch J. Effects of sufentanil on cerebral hemodynamics and intracranial pressure in patients with brain injury. Anesthesiology 1995; 83: 721–726.

16. Warner DS, Hindman BJ, Todd MM et al. Intracranial pressure and hemodynamic effects of remifentanil versus alfentanil in patients undergoing supratentorial craniotomy. Anesth Analg 1996; 83: 348–353.

17. Schramm WM, Strasser K, Bartunek A, Spiss CK. Effects of rocuronium and vecuronium on intracranial pressure, mean arterial pressure and heart rate in neurosurgical patients. Br J Anaesth 1996; 77: 607–611.

18. Shapiro HM, Wyte SR, Harris AB, Galindo A. Acute intraoperative intracranial hypertension in neurosurgical patients: mechanical and pharmacological factors. Anesthesiology 1972; 37: 399–405.

19. Todd MM, Warner DS, Sokoll MD et al. A prospective comparative trial of three anesthetics for elective supratentorial craniotomy. Propofol/fentanyl, isoflurane/nitrous oxide and fentanyl/nitrous oxide. Anesthesiology, 1993; 78: 1005–1020.

20. Leech P, Miller JD. Intracranial volume/pressure relationships during experimental brain compression in primates. 3. The effect of mannitol and hypocapnia. J Neurol Neurosurg Psychiat 1974; 37: 1105.

21. Muizelaar JP, Wei EP, Kontos HA, Becker DP. Mannitol causes compensatory cerebral vasoconstriction and vasodilatation in response to blood viscosity changes. J Neurosurg 1983; 59: 822.

22. Muizelaar JP, Lutz HA, Becker DP. Effect of mannitol on ICP and CBF and correlation with pressure autoregulation in severely head injured patients. J Neurosurg 1984; 61: 700.

23. Ravussin P, Archer DP, Meyer E, Abou-Madi M, Yamamotu L, Trop D. The effect of rapid infusions of saline and mannitol on cerebral blood volume and intracranial pressure in dogs. Can Anaesth Soc J 1985; 32: 506.

24. Cottrell JE, Robustelli A, Post K, Turndorf H. Furosemide and mannitol induced changes in ICP and serum osmolality and electrolytes. Anesthesiology 1977; 47: 28.

25. Shapiro HM. Intracranial hypertension: therapeutic and anesthetic considerations. Anesthesiology 1975; 43: 445.

26. Bedford RF, Persing JA, Poberskin L, Butler A. Lidocaine or thiopental for rapid control of intracranial hypertension? Anesth Analg 1980; 59: 435–437.

27. Brierley JB, Brown AW, Excell BJ, Meldrum BS. Brain damage in the rhesus monkey resulting from profound arterial hypotension. 1. Its nature, distribution and general physiological correlates. Brain Res, 1969; 13: 68.

28. Turner JM, Powell D, Gibson RM, McDowall DG. Intracranial pressure changes in neurosurgical patients during hypotension induced with sodium nitroprusside or trimetaphan. Br J Anaesth 1977; 49: 419.

29. McDowall DG, Keaney NP, Turner JM, Lane JR, Okuda Y. Toxicity of sodium nitroprusside. Br J Anaesth 1974; 46: 327.

30. Morris PJ, Todd M, Philbin D. Changes in canine intracranial pressure in response to infusion of sodium nitroprusside and trinitroglycerin. Br J Anaesth 1982; 54: 991.

31. Burt DER, Verniquet AJW, Homi J. The response of canine intracranial pressure to hypotension induced with nitroglycerin. Br J Anaesth 1982; 54: 665.

32. Muzzi DA, Black S, Losasso TJ, Cucchiara RF. Labetalol and esmolol in the control of hypertension after intracranial surgery. Anesth Analg 1990; 70: 68–71.

14

ANAESTHESIA FOR INTRACRANIAL VASCULAR SURGERY

Leisha S. Godsiff & Basil F. Matta

INTRODUCTION

Recent improvements in neurosurgical and neuroanaesthetic techniques have reduced the morbidity and mortality traditionally associated with intracranial haemorrhage. Even patients presenting with significant neurologic deficit may achieve good outcome provided appropriate therapy is instituted early in their illness. The success of the combined aggressive anaesthetic and surgical management is most notable in those patients with subarachnoid haemorrhage or traumatic intracranial haematomas. Neuronaesthetists play an important role in the preoperative resuscitation and optimization, the intraoperative management and the postoperative neurointensive care of patients with intracranial vascular lesions.

This chapter discusses the anaesthetic management of intracranial vascular lesions with particular emphasis on subarachnoid haemorrhage (SAH) and arteriovenous malformations (AVM).

AETIOLOGY

The pathological classification of intracranial haematomas is provided in Box 14.1.

TRAUMATIC HAEMATOMAS

Traumatic intracranial haematomas secondary to head injury usually occur in young males early in their working lives, with significant social and economic implications. Extradural, subdural and intracerebral haematomas often occur in association with other significant injuries such as cervical spine or intraabdominal trauma which may take priority in treatment. However, as 40% of comatose head-injured patients

---

Traumatic
Non-traumatic
   Hypertensive
   Amyloid angiopathy
   Drug induced
   Coagulopathy
   Neoplasia
   Vascular:
      aneurysm
      arteriovenous malformations
      cavernous malformations

Box 14.1   Classification of intracranial haematomas

---

have an intracranial mass, an early CT scan once the patient is stabilized will differentiate operative from non-operative lesions.

Extradural haematoma (EDH)

The majority of extradural haematomas are traumatic. EDHs are often found in the temporal region in association with a skull fracture involving the middle meningeal artery. Less frequently, they originate from the venous sinuses following disruption of the dural membranes. Whereas most EDHs are acute, they can present up to 48 h after the initial trauma and are an important cause of late clinical deterioration.[1]

The clinical presentation depends on the size, position and rate at which the haematoma forms. Only one-third of patients with EDH present with the classic initial loss of consciousness followed by a lucid interval and then a rapid decline in consciousness. Not all patients develop ipsilateral pupillary dilatation and focal neurological deficits. Although poor outcome is associated with coma on admission, bilateral dilated pupils, a subdural component and delays in surgical intervention,[2,3] the overall mortality following an extradural haematoma is less than 5%.[2]

Subdural haematoma (SDH)

A SDH is often associated with an underlying cerebral injury and is therefore associated with poorer prognosis. Bleeding occurs from torn cerebral tissues and bridging cortical veins. Over 50% of patients will be unconscious from the start, with a mortality of 40–80%.[4] Poor outcomes are associated with a low Glasgow Coma Scale score (GCS 3–5) on presentation, age >60 years, unreactive dilated pupils, high intracranial pressure, hypotension and hypoxaemia.[5]

Intracerebral haematoma (ICH)

Traumatic ICHs can follow all types of blunt cranial trauma. Penetrating skull injuries (stab or gunshot wound) and depressed skull fractures are also commonly associated with intracerebral bleeds. In the elderly and in alcoholics with cerebral atrophy, the associated trauma may be modest and the haematoma may only produce symptoms 48 h after the initial trauma.

Posterior fossa haematoma (PFH)

Although uncommon, PFHs can lead to rapid deterioration as a result of brainstem compression. Occipital abrasions, an occipital fracture, respiratory irregularities and/or hypertension should alert the clinician to the possibility of a posterior fossa haematoma. Without rapid decompression mortality is very high.[6]

NON-TRAUMATIC HAEMATOMAS

The causes of non-traumatic intracerebral haemorrhage vary with age. Hypertension and tumours predominate in the elderly, whilst vascular abnormalities predominate in younger patients.[7]

Hypertensive haematomas

Hypertension is probably the most significant risk factor for intracerebral haemorrhage in the elderly.[7] Evidence of preexisting high blood pressure, such as left ventricular hypertrophy, is common. The mechanisms believed to be responsible for hypertensive bleeds include the formation and rupture of microaneurysms affecting the lenticulostriate vessels and the degeneration of the media affecting small penetrating arteries (hyalinosis).

Amyloid angiopathy

This is associated with the deposition of amyloid in the media and adventitia of cerebral vessels causing calcific degeneration and rupture of the vessel wall in the elderly.[8] The arteries and arterioles of the leptomeninges and the superficial layers of the cortex are involved, causing lobar haemorrhages (most commonly the parietal and occipital lobes). Subarachnoid and subdural haemorrhages can also occur.

Drug and alcohol abuse

Cocaine[9, 10] and amphetamines[11] cause intense sympathetic activity which can lead to extreme rises in blood pressure. In such circumstances, especially with amphetamine abuse, an intracerebral haemorrhage can occur without an underlying vascular lesion. Intravenous drug abusers are at an increased risk of bacterial endocarditis with the subsequent development and rupture of cerebral mycotic aneurysms. Alcoholics can develop systemic hypertension and liver abnormalities, which predispose them to spontaneous intracerebral haemorrhages.

Coagulopathies

All types of coagulopathies predispose to spontaneous intracerebral bleeds.[12] These can be intrinsic (idiopathic thrombocytopenia, disseminated intravascular coagulation, haemophilia) or drug related (aspirin, anticoagulants, fibrinolytics). Intracranial haematomas secondary to anticoagulant therapy are common.

Neoplasia

Patients with primary or secondary cerebral tumours may deteriorate suddenly because of haemorrhage into the lesion.[13] This is more likely to occur in the more vascular tumours, which include malignant gliomas, malignant melanomas, bronchogenic carcinomas, choriocarcinomas and renal cell carcinomas.

Vascular anomalies

These include cerebral aneurysms, arteriovenous malformations (AVM) and cavernous malformations. The majority of patients present with either an intracerebral haematoma or a subarachnoid haemorrhage. Rarely, they may present with cerebral irritation, seizures or neurological deficits from an intracranial mass effect.

PATHOPHYSIOLOGY

Autoregulation, arterial carbon dioxide and oxygen tension and cerebral metabolism influence cerebral blood flow (CBF). In normal individuals, CBF remains constant over a wide range of cerebral perfusion pressures (CPP), CPP being the difference between mean arterial pressure (MAP) and intracranial pressure (ICP). In the awake resting normotensive individual, changes in cerebrovascular resistance (CVR) maintain CBF at an average of 50ml/100g/min despite changes in CPP between 60 and 160 mmHg. This process is termed autoregulation and occurs in seconds. Hypocapnia can increase or restore impaired autoregulation[14] whereas hypercapnia impairs autoregulation. At CPP outside this range CBF becomes pressure dependent.

In normal individuals, changes in cerebral blood volume (CBV) mirror changes in CBF. Therefore, following intracranial haemorrhage when autoregulation is often impaired either focally or globally, rapid changes in blood pressure have profound effects on CBF. While hypotension will lead to cerebral ischaemia, hypertension will result in increased CBV, raised ICP and secondary brain ischaemia.

Carbon dioxide is one of the major determinants of CBF.[14,15] CBF changes almost linearly with changes in arterial carbon dioxide tension ($PaCO_2$) between 3 and 10 kPa. While hyperventilation reduces CBF, CBV and ICP, hypoventilation has opposite effects. In subarachnoid haemorrhage, cerebral vasoreactivity to carbon dioxide may be reduced. Therefore, hyperventilation may be ineffectual in reducing ICP. Furthermore, as the relationship between CBF, CBV and ICP may no longer exist, hyperventilation may reduce CBF without changing CBV or ICP, thus exacerbating brain ischaemia.

Arterial oxygen tension (PaO_2) has little effect on CBF within the physiologic range. However, if PaO_2 decreases below 6kPa, tissue oxygen delivery is maintained by cerebral vasodilatation, which overrides any vasoconstriction induced by hyperventilation. At a PaO_2 >100kPa cerebral vasoconstriction occurs.[16] However, a combination of moderate hyperventilation and hyperoxia may be used to reduce brain bulk while maintaining cerebral oxygen delivery.[17]

Cerebral blood flow and cerebral metabolism are tightly coupled. Any increase in regional or global cerebral activity will lead to an increase in cerebral metabolism and therefore CBF. This relationship may be uncoupled by an intracerebral bleed or head injury, a finding which is central to the management of intracranial haemorrhage.

PRINCIPLES OF MANAGEMENT

Regardless of the causes of intracranial haemorrhage, the above pathophysiological mechanisms may precipitate cerebral ischaemia. Therefore, the management of all patients with intracerebral haematomas irrespective of cause is aimed at maintaining adequate CBF and preventing and treating secondary cerebral ischaemia. The anaesthetic management of traumatic intracranial haematomas is described in detail in Chapter 20.

SUBARACHNOID HAEMORRHAGE

EPIDEMIOLOGY

Cerebral aneurysms account for 75–80% of spontaneous subarachnoid haemorrhage (SAH),[18] cerebral arteriovenous malformations for 4–5%,[19] and in 15–20% of patients no source of haemorrhage can be found. Other causes of SAH include trauma, dural and spinal arteriovenous malformations, mycotic aneurysms, sickle cell disease, cocaine abuse and coagulation disorders.

Cerebral aneurysms mainly occur at vascular bifurcations within the circle of Willis or proximal cerebral artery. Most are supratentorial and approximately 20% of patients will have multiple aneurysms.[20] The incidence of aneurysmal SAH is 12–15 per 100,000 population per year with a peak incidence between 55 and 60 years of age. Females are affected more than males and genetic factors may contribute.[21, 22]

Despite improvements in anaesthetic and surgical care, SAH is associated with high morbidity and mortality.[23]

One-third of patients will die before reaching hospital[24] and the remaining patients will have a 30–50% mortality.[25] The major risks facing patients who reach hospital are recurrent haemorrhage,[26] the development of delayed ischaemic neurological deficits (vasospasm) and hydrocephalus. Conservative non-surgical management of SAH is associated with much higher mortality than surgical management (40% vs <10% respectively within six months of the bleed). However, conservative medical management has been recently advocated in elderly patients (>64 years) with unruptured aneurysms less than 1 cm diameter as in the risks of surgery outweigh the benefits.[27, 28]

CLINICAL PRESENTATION

SAH classically presents with sudden-onset severe headache radiating to the occipital or cervical region with or without loss of consciousness. Photophobia, nausea, vomiting, lethargy and signs of meningism are all common. Hypertension, hyperpyrexia, seizures, motor or sensory deficits, cranial nerve palsies (third and sixth) and visual field defects may also occur. Elevated intracranial pressure and meningeal irritation cause loss of consciousness, headaches and neurological deficits. A sudden rise in intracranial pressure, in conjunction with normal coagulation, is thought to prevent continuing bleeding from the aneurysm site.

EARLY MANAGEMENT

The immediate management of patients with SAH follows the principles of airway, breathing and circulation. Patients unable to protect their airway or, obey commands and those with a GCS <9 should have their airway secured by intubation and ventilation. Hypoxaemia and hypercarbia may result in a rapid increase in ICP that could precipitate a rebleed and aggravate cerebral ischaemia from the initial insult. Heart rate, blood pressure and tissue perfusion are assessed and treated when abnormal. Neurological examination includes level of consciousness, spontaneous movement, orientation, ability to follow commands, pupillary size, shape, reactivity, ocular movement, muscle tone and reflexes.

Information regarding previous trauma, intracerebral haemorrhages, hypertension and hypertensive treatments, known vascular malformations or tumours, anticoagulant use, coagulopathies, prosthetic heart valves, ischaemic cerebrovascular disease and drug abuse should be obtained at the same time.

The clinical condition of the patient is graded using the World Federation of Neurological Surgeons[29] (WFNS) system as shown in Table 14.1. Although the morbidity and mortality vary widely between centres, it is commonly accepted that a higher WFNS grade generally results in worse outcome. This may be due to a combination of initial damage and the increased risk of developing intracranial hypertension, vasospasm, reduced CBF and impaired autoregulation.

A CT scan will identify the site and extent of the haemorrhage and assess ventricular size. It may also indicate the most likely site of the aneurysm.[30] Once an intracranial bleed is identified, immediate referral to a neurosurgical centre is advisable. Although we will consider patients with SAH of all grades at our centre including those with unreactive pupils, in reality those greater than 70 years of age with a poor quality of life, extensive SAH on CT scan and with bilateral fixed dilated pupils are not usually suitable for neurosurgical intervention. Decisions on further management should not be based on pupillary size in isolation, as dilated pupils can accompany subclinical seizures[31] and hydrocephalus and therefore are not an absolute contraindication for transfer.

When no SAH is detected on CT scan but the history is strongly suggestive of it, a lumbar puncture is performed. If xanthochromia is present the patient should be transferred to a neurosurgical centre for cerebral angiography. Lumbar puncture should only be performed after a negative CT scan and in the absence of signs of raised ICP, as the procedure may cause a rebleed or brain herniation with disastrous consequences.

Once a diagnosis of SAH has been made, the WFNS grade and the premorbid state of the patient influence further treatment. Patients with grades I–II are monitored on the neurosurgical high-dependency unit. Neurological assessments, vital signs and fluid balance are recorded hourly. A daily fluid intake of at least 3 l is recommended. Intravenous fluids can supplement oral intake but 5% dextrose solutions are best avoided because of hypotonicity and the possible risk of hyperglycaemia with its associated adverse effects in brain injury. Oral nimodipine (60mg four-hourly) is started in an attempt to prevent delayed cerebral ischaemia. However, nimodipine can cause hypotension and the dose may need to be reduced or divided in more frequent doses (30 mg 2 hourly). Ideally the systolic blood pressure should be maintained at 140–150mmHg (slightly higher in previously hypertensive individuals). Paracetamol or codeine phosphate is prescribed for pain. Any electrolyte abnormalities are corrected and a haematocrit of 30% is aimed for. A central venous line or a pulmonary artery flotation catheter may be required to guide therapy in those with cardiac disease and the elderly, aiming for a filling pressure of 10–14 mmHg. Cerebral angiography should be performed within 24 h.

Patients with WFNS grades iii–iv are cared for on the neurocritical care unit. The CT scan is studied for factors contributing to the poor grade of the patient. If hydrocephalus is present, an extraventricular drain is inserted. If a large intracerebral haematoma is present and the patient's condition is stable, urgent angiography is performed before clot evacuation and aneurysm clipping. However, in the event of deterioration with mass effect (such as a fixed pupil) surgical decompression is performed immediately.

Patients with evidence of raised intracranial pressure on CT scan should have their ICP monitored to help guide management (see Ch. 7). After resuscitation these patients are assessed neurologically. Neuromuscular relaxants and sedation are withdrawn and at an appropriate time, the response to a painful stimulus observed. If the patient exhibits purposeful movement they are resedated and cerebral angiography performed with a view to definite aneurysm clipping. In the case of multiple aneurysms only the culprit aneurysm is treated. Residual aneurysms may

Table 14.1   World Federation of Neurological Surgeons (WFNS) grading of subarachnoid haemorrhage

Grade	Glasgow Coma Score	Motor deficit aphasia and/or hemiparesis or hemiplegia)
0	15	Absent
I	15	Absent
II	13–14	Absent
III	13–14	Present
IV	7–12	Present or absent
V	3–6	Present or absent

be treated electively a minimum of three months later depending on the outcome of the current episode.

If the patient displays no purposeful movement to painful stimuli, CBF studies are performed and cerebral perfusion supported with ICP management and blood pressure control. Patients are assessed periodically for improvements in their neurological status. If no improvement occurs, outcome is likely to be poor and a decision regarding further treatment should be discussed with the relatives at an early stage.

Although CT scanning and magnetic resonance angiography can diagnose vascular lesions, cerebral angiography remains the gold standard.[32] An acceptable angiogram must show all the intracranial vessels in at least two planes to identify the neck of the aneurysm and its surrounding vessels. Any radiographic evidence of vasospasm is noted. If multiple aneurysms are detected, the patient's symptoms, the location, appearance and the presence of regional vasospasm help identify the culprit aneurysm. For angiogram-negative patients in whom other causes have been excluded (such as dural fistulae, cerebral vasculitis and venous thrombosis), repeat angiography is performed 14 days later.

THE TIMING OF SURGERY

Definitive surgery can be early (1–3 days after SAH) or late (10–14 days after SAH). Historically, 'late' surgery was preferred as surgical exposure and aneurysm clipping were considered easier when less cerebral oedema and inflammation are present. However, although technically more difficult, 'early' surgery decreases the probability of rebleeding with its associated high morbidity and mortality.[33–36] Furthermore, by removing the blood clot early the risk of developing a delayed ischaemic deficit may be reduced.[37,38] If a deficit should develop as a result of vasospasm, then induced hypertension can be used safely if the aneurysm is secured.[39] Recent experience shows that early surgery does not increase the risk of intraoperative complications compared to later surgery.[40]

Our policy is to perform definitive surgery within four days of the primary event, especially in patients with good-grade SAH. This is based on published evidence suggesting that rebleeding is commonest in the first day post-SAH and 70% of patients who rebleed will die.[41] This has been recently confirmed in a prospective audit at our hospital, which identified a 2% risk of rebleeding within the first four days rising to 18% in the first two weeks, with 85% mortality as a result of the second bleed. Surgery is performed during the day on elective lists except when a space-occupying mass needs urgent evacuation.

PREOPERATIVE EVALUATION

A routine general anaesthetic assessment will include the patient's past medical history, medications, allergies and previous general anaesthetics. The extent of the neurologic and myocardial injury are of particular interest.[42] In addition, blood results, ECG and echocardiography when indicated, chest X-ray, CT scans, angiography and transcranial Doppler findings should be available. Proper communication between the anaesthetist and the operating surgeon is likely to lead to the best perioperative care.

Cardiovascular assessment

Although seen in the majority (50–100%) of patients with a SAH, ECG changes are more frequent in those with severe neurologic impairment.[43, 44] They include T-wave abnormalities, ST segment depression, prominent U-waves, prolonged QT intervals and both atrial and ventricular dysrhythmias.[45] The ECG abnormalities occur within 48 h of the SAH and may last up to six weeks. Whilst the degree of myocardial dysfunction does not correlate with the SAH-induced ECG changes, the greatest degree of myocardial dysfunction occurs in those patients with worse WFNS grades.[46] Postmortem and CPK isoenzyme studies have shown that the majority of SAH-induced ECG changes are related to subendocardial ischaemia or localized areas of myocardial necrosis. It is postulated that these changes are caused by posterior hypothalamic stimulation leading to an acute increase in sympathetic activity.[43] The resulting increase in myocardial and systemic noradrenaline levels may (by a direct toxic effect or by increasing myocardial afterload) cause this subendocardial ischaemia. The coronary arteries are usually normal. Some patients will develop pathological Q-waves following a SAH.[47] This is often misinterpreted as evidence of a recent myocardial infarction. However, the differentiation between SAH-associated and myocardial ischaemia-related ECG changes is difficult especially in patients with coexisting cardiac disease. An echocardiogram and/or a pulmonary artery catheter may be valuable in these patients.

Although non-specific ECG changes not accompanied by symptoms or signs of myocardial dysfunction are probably insignificant and should not delay surgery, it is probably prudent to wait as long as possible before proceeding with the surgery in those patients with changes suggestive of myocardial infarction as the risk of malignant dysrhythmias is high. The benefits of early surgery have to be weighed against possible perioperative myocardial ischaemia. Our policy is to wait at least 72 h unless there are mass effects or the patient's condition allows a 10–14 day wait.

Blood pressure abnormalities are frequent after SAH. When hypertension is a compensatory response to maintain CPP in the presence of an elevated ICP, it should not be treated unless it is severe. Systolic blood pressure >160 mmHg increases the risk of rupture and rebleeding in an unsecured aneurysm and therefore a compromise needs to be achieved. Patients with systolic blood pressures >160mmHg may be treated judiciously with labetalol, which appears to have little if any effect on cerebral blood flow or intracranial pressure. Sodium nitroprusside and hydralazine are vasodilators which may increase CBF and therefore should not be used whilst the dura is closed especially in the presence of raised intracranial pressure. In patients with symptomatic vasospasm higher blood pressures may be tolerated.

Hypotension should be avoided at all costs and the blood pressure below which neurological deterioration occurs recorded. This can be used to guide blood pressure management intraoperatively.

Respiratory assessment

Respiratory dysfunction, common after SAH, can be the result of poor ventilatory drive, decreased level of consciousness and aspiration of stomach contents, or neurogenic pulmonary oedema. Therefore, a thorough evaluation of the respiratory system must include examination for evidence of pulmonary oedema, basal atelectasis and aspiration pneumonia. The oxygen and ventilatory requirements, arterial blood gases and chest X-ray are assessed. Patients requiring high levels of inspired oxygen and positive end-expiratory pressure to maintain borderline arterial blood gases should have their operation postponed until their respiratory function improves. Avoiding secondary hypoxaemic insults is paramount.

Volume status and blood chemistry

Autonomic hyperactivity is thought to be responsible for the reduction in plasma and red blood cell volume. Other factors include bedrest, negative nitrogen balance and diuretics. A haematocrit of 30% is considered optimum. A central venous pressure line or a pulmonary artery flotation catheter may be required to guide fluid management.

Hyponatraemia is common (10–34%)[48,49] and can be associated with an impaired level of consciousness, cerebral oedema, seizures and vasospasm. Hyponatraemia may be iatrogenic because of the administration of hypnotic maintenance fluids instead of 0.9% sodium chloride. It may also result from either the cerebral salt wasting syndrome or the inappropriate secretion of antidiuretic hormone (SIADH).[50] In both groups the plasma sodium concentration is low (<134 mmol/l). Patients with the salt wasting syndrome are hypovolaemic and require fluid to prevent intravascular volume contraction. Atrial natriuretic factor may also be involved.[51] In contrast, patients with SIADH secretion require fluid restriction. Central venous pressure monitoring is required in these circumstances.

Normoglycaemia should be maintained as hyperglycaemia is associated with worse neurologic outcome after brain injury.[52, 53] Dextrose-containing solutions are best avoided and an insulin infusion may be required to control stress-induced hyperglycaemia when present.

Neurologic assessment

A detailed examination to assess the level of consciousness and the presence of focal neurological deficits should be performed. Evidence of raised intracranial pressure, cerebral vasospasm, hydrocephalus and an intracranial mass effect should be sought.

Blood in the subarachnoid space may occlude the arachnoid villie and lead to the development of hydrocephalus. Mortality is higher in patients who develop hydrocephalus. Symptoms include headache, drowsiness, confusion and agitation. If hydrocephalus develops before the aneurysm has been secured, a ventricular drain may improve the neurological state of the patient. The CSF should be drained to 15–20 cmH$_2$O to avoid excess ventricular decompression, which may cause the aneurysm to re-rupture.[54]

Seizures can occur following a SAH and lead to acute increases in blood pressure and rebleeding. When present, seizures should be controlled with anticonvulsants but there is currently no evidence to support the prophylactic use of anticonvulsants in patients following SAH and hence, they are not routinely administered at our institution.

Medications

Preoperative drugs are usually continued unless contraindicated; for example, diuretics are discontinued if the patient is dehydrated. Patients presenting for aneurysm surgery after SAH are usually receiving calcium channel blockers (nimodipine) to reduce the risk of developing delayed ischaemic deficits. Therefore, relative hypotension secondary to systemic vasodilatation, with an increased cardiac output is not an uncommon finding in these patients.[55] Patients must be well hydrated before general anaesthesia to prevent hypotension on induction of anaesthesia.[56]

PREMEDICATION

The use of sedative premedications is controversial as pre- and postoperative neurologic assessment may be difficult. Premedicants may also cause respiratory depression leading to hypercarbia, hypertension and increased CBF, CBV and ICP. Generally, grade III–V patients rarely require sedative premedication. Grade I–II patients may require an anxiolytic to prevent the haemodynamic fluctuations associated with anxiety. Midazolam IV can be administered in the anaesthetic room. Midazolam reduces the cerebral metabolic rate and hence CBF and CBV without significantly affecting cerebral CO_2 reactivity or autoregulation. However, the agent should be titrated carefully as hypotension must be avoided. Patients at risk of aspiration will need standard antacid prophylaxis.

MONITORING

Routine monitoring will include ECG, pulse oximetry end-tidal capnography, urinary output and temperature. Direct blood pressure measurement is established before induction of anaesthesia as this will allow accurate, beat-to-beat observation of blood pressure. It will also be useful for intraoperative blood gas and haemoglobin measurements. Central venous pressure is measured in all patients presenting for aneurysm surgery to guide fluid management as these patients often receive repeated doses of diuretics and/or mannitol. A pulmonary artery catheter is used in elderly patients, those with cardiac disease and in poor grade subarachnoid haemorrhage patients, especially if hypertensive, hypervolaemic and haemodilutional therapy is contemplated.

A jugular bulb catheter measures jugular venous oxygen saturation and lactate and is used to monitor alterations in ventilation and blood pressure.[57, 58] A cerebral function analysing monitor is used when burst suppression is planned (e.g. prolonged temporary clipping). An intraparenchymal probe, which measures cerebral oxygenation, carbon dioxide, pH and temperature, can be sited in the territory of the operative site by the surgeon.

INDUCTION OF ANAESTHESIA

The aims are to titrate the depth of anaesthesia and the blood pressure to match surgical need, control ICP, minimize cerebral metabolic demands, prevent cerebral ischaemia, ensure good operating conditions and allow rapid awakening. As transmural pressure determines the likelihood of aneurysmal rupture, abrupt increases in arterial blood pressure or sudden decreases in ICP may cause a rebleed. Although rebleeding is rare during induction of anaesthesia and tracheal intubation (<0.5% at this institution), it is associated with high mortality and postoperative morbidity. Aneurysmal rupture is suspected when a sustained rise in blood pressure with or without a bradycardia is observed on or shortly after induction or tracheal intubation. The surgery is best deferred for 24–48 h during which detailed assessment of the patient is made.

With the exception of ketamine, any intravenous induction agent can be used. Thiopentone, etomidate and propofol are the main agents used for induction of anaesthesia, with muscle relaxation usually achieved with vecuronium, atracurium or pancuronium. When rapid control of the airway is required, suxamethonium can be used but it may result in a transient increase in ICP.[59] This potential increase in ICP and its possible effect on aneurysmal rupture is balanced against the risk of aspiration, hypoxaemia and hypercapnia.

If a rapid sequence is not required, the patient's lungs are denitrogenated and anaesthesia is induced with the intravenous agent of choice in combination with a short-acting opioid (e.g. fentanyl 1 μg/kg). The agent is titrated to blood pressure and heart rate. There is no place for high-dose opioid anaesthesia as this will result in catastrophic hypotension, cerebral vasodilatation, reduced CPP and cerebral ischaemia. Once the patient is judged ready for tracheal intubation (by the use of peripheral nerve stimulator), further aliquots of induction agent, fentanyl, labetolol, esmolol or lignocaine can be used to attenuate the response to laryngoscopy and intubation. The lungs are then ventilated to mild hypocapnia at $PaCO_2$ ~4 kPa. Marked hyperventilation reduces ICP and may increase transmural pressure leading to aneurysmal rupture. The endotracheal tube is then secured, wide-bore intravenous access established and the eyes protected. Local anaesthesia or further doses of induction agent or opioid can be used to attenuate the response to head pin insertion.[60] Lumbar drains, although not routinely used, may be employed for posterior circulation and giant aneurysms where a greater degree of brain retraction is anticipated. Rapid decompression should be prevented when a lumbar drain is inserted as this will lead to a sudden reduction in ICP and rebleeding. Patients are then transferred into theatre and positioned 15–30° head up to aid venous drainage.

MAINTENANCE

There is currently no evidence from prospective randomized trials to suggest a particular anaesthetic technique is superior in patients undergoing aneurysm surgery. However, the 'best' anaesthetic technique produces a 'slack' brain so that retraction pressure is low while ensuring maximal cerebral protection by keeping cerebral metabolic requirements to a minimum. Those agents that maintain cerebral vasoreactivity to CO_2 and autoregulation may reduce fluctuations in CBF, ICP and CPP when blood pressure changes with varying surgical stimuli.

A combination of a propofol infusion and an opioid is increasingly used to maintain anaesthesia during aneurysm surgery. Propofol allows rapid adjustment of anaesthetic depth with more rapid recovery than either thiopentone or isoflurane.[61] Propofol has no intrinsic vasodilatory effect and therefore does not result in increases in CBF, CBV or ICP. Furthermore, propofol has been shown not to affect cerebral autoregulation or carbon dioxide reactivity even at doses high enough to produce EEG isoelectricity.[62] It also reduces the cerebral metabolic rate, with cortical structures being depressed to a greater extent than subcortical structures, and may be neuroprotective.

Inhalational anaesthetic agents have a dual effect on CBF: a reduction consequent on to the decrease in cerebral metabolism and an increase secondary to their direct cerebral vasodilatory effect. The 'net' effect of an inhalational agent on CBF is therefore dependent on the level of cerebral metabolism at the time the agent is introduced.[63] When cerebral metabolism is low, as in patients with SAH grades III or IV, the net effect may be vasodilatory with increases in CBF and ICP accompanying the introduction of the agent. However, in patients with good-grade SAH I or II in whom cerebral metabolism is high, inhalational agents primarily reduce CBF secondary to the reduction in cerebral metabolism. Therefore, inhalational agents can be safely used in patients with good-grade SAH. When there is uncertainty about the level of cerebral metabolism or when signs of significant cerebral oedema are present, total intravenous anaesthesia is the preferred option.

Inhalational agents with the exception of sevoflurane impair autoregulation in a dose-dependent manner.[64] Therefore, isoflurane in concentrations less than 1.0% can be used to supplement intravenous anaesthesia. The epileptic activity of enflurane prevents its use in neurosurgery. Desflurane increases ICP and this may be related to its sympathoadrenal effects.[65] Sevoflurane has been shown not to alter cerebral autoregulation in concentrations up to 1.5 MAC.[66-68] However, at 1.5 MAC sevoflurane, brain oxygen consumption was shown to be reduced by 25% and therefore a degree of luxury perfusion may occur.[69]

Nitrous oxide has a number of advantages. It has a rapid onset and offset, is easy to use and is relatively inexpensive. However, its routine use in neuroanaesthesia is discouraged at our institution as there is evidence to suggest that N_2O increases ICP and CBF by stimulating cerebral metabolism.[70] Although nitrous oxide increased CBF velocity when used in combination with isoflurane,[71] this effect can be attenuated by hyperventilation[72] and propofol.[73]

Opioids generally have negligible effects on CBF and metabolism. However, the newer synthetic opioids fentanyl, sufentanil and alfentanil can increase ICP in patients with tumours and head trauma.[74] This increase, originally assumed to be secondary to an increase in CBF, is more likely to be the result of changes in $PaCO_2$ and systemic hypotension.[75-77] Irrespective of the actual mechanism causing the increase in ICP, these observations underscore the importance of administering these agents judiciously and carefully to avoid systemic hypotension. Fentanyl, with its medium duration of action and its negligible cerebral vascular effects, is the agent of choice in many neurosurgical intensive care units. Remifentanil, a new opioid with a rapid onset and short half-life, is being investigated for neurosurgery. Remifentanil appears to compare favourably to fentanyl in patients undergoing elective supratentorial surgery.[78] We have shown that remifentanil when combined with 0.5 MAC sevoflurane does not alter cerebral autoregulation in individuals undergoing non-intracranial neurosurgical procedures.[79]

Brain relaxation

The aim is to produce a 'slack' brain so that retraction pressure can be kept to a minimum. There are several methods employed to reduce the brain bulk, CSF volume and CBV. These include a 15–30° head-up position, mild hypocarbia (~4 kPa), mannitol and frusemide.

Mannitol is an osmotic diuretic used to reduce cerebral tissue water.[80,81] It is usually administered (0.5–1.0 g/kg) as a 20% solution and probably acts on all three intracranial compartments via different mechanisms. It may reduce brain bulk by osmotic dehydration, CBV by improving rheology of red blood cells thus decreasing blood viscosity,[82] and CSF production.[83,84] Mannitol is also a free radical scavenger. Mannitol's high osmolarity causes an immediate but transient increase in intravascular volume, CBF, CBV and ICP. This is followed by a reduction in ICP and CBV, which is maximum at 45–60 min. Therefore, care must be taken when administering mannitol to patients with poor cardiac function as they may develop congestive cardiac failure and pulmonary oedema. Frusemide can be used in conjunction with mannitol or it can be used alone in those patients with poor myocardial function who may be sent into cardiac failure with mannitol.[81] Hypertonic saline has been advocated as an alternative to mannitol, although its action is transient and its overall effects remain untested in SAH.[85]

The potential ischaemic effects of marked hyperventilation must be balanced against the benefits of reducing CBV. When used properly, hyperventilation is a quick and effective tool for reducing CBV, provided a measure of cerebral oxygenation is employed. Although it cannot detect regional ischaemia, jugular bulb oximetry (SjO_2) will reflect the balance between cerebral oxygen supply and demand. It is probably unwise to induce hypocapnia if the SJO_2 <50%.

Cerebral blood volume can also be reduced pharmacologically by reducing cerebral metabolism and hence CBF. This is achieved by bolus intravenous administration of thiopentone (3–5 mg/kg), propofol (1–2 mg/kg) or lignocaine (1.5 mg/kg). If brain condition improves after the bolus, a continuous infusion is started.

The amount of fluid given intraoperatively depends on the maintenance requirements, blood loss and filling pressures. Urine output is a poor marker of circulatory volume in the presence of mannitol and frusemide. We maintain hypervolaemia prior to clipping to optimize CBF and reduce the effects of perioperative vasospasm.

Hyponatraemia is associated with an increased incidence of delayed ischaemic neurological deficits and glucose solutions are avoided as they may worsen cerebral acidaemia and ischaemia.

With difficult aneurysms, measures are taken to reduce the transmural pressure across the wall of the aneurysm before a permanent clip is placed. This reduces the risk of rupture and the rate of bleeding should the aneurysm rupture during dissection. There are two methods by which this can be achieved: deliberate hypotension and temporary clipping.

Deliberate hypotension

Although the use of induced hypotension during surgical clipping of cerebral aneurysms is in decline, many North American neurosurgical centres continue to use it regularly. Hypotension increases 'slack' in the structures around the aneurysm and aneurysmal sac and decreases the risk of rupture during surgical dissection and clipping of the aneurysm. Hypotension also decreases bleeding from surrounding small vessels which allows better visualization of the anatomy of the aneurysm and the perforating vessels. Some of the drugs used include isoflurane, thiopentone (3–5 mg/kg), propofol (1–4 mg/kg), labetalol in 5–10 mg increments, esmolol and sodium nitroprusside. The MAP is not usually reduced below 50 mmHg in normotensive individuals and chronically hypertensive patients may require a higher mean pressure (systolic is best kept > than the preoperative diastolic value). However, there are numerous problems associated with deliberate hypotension. Many SAH patients will have impaired autoregulation or cerebral vasospasm and hypotension may therefore lead to focal or global cerebral ischaemia.[86] Futhermore, the ischaemic threshold cannot be predicted accurately. Hypotension is rarely employed at our institution.

Temporary clipping

This is the preferred technique in our unit. When exposure of the aneurysm is difficult and temporary clip placement is anticipated, maximal cerebral protection is aimed for: moderate hypothermia (33° C), induced hypertension (20% above baseline) and propofol or thiopentone-induced burst suppression. A temporary clip occludes the vessels feeding the aneurysm and reduces transmural pressure, thus decreasing the risk of rupture. Although the safe length of time for which temporary clipping can be used before cerebral infarction occurs is unknown, the risk of infarction increases with the duration of clip application and varies from 15 to 120 min.[87,88] Factors thought to contribute to new neurological deficit include age >61 years and poor preoperative neurological condition.

Cerebral protection

Various cerebroprotective methods have been used including hypothermia, additional doses of intravenous or inhalational anaesthetics, deliberate hypertension and drugs such as mannitol, phenytoin and calcium channel blockers.[89] These methods may be used routinely or their use may be guided by changes to the EEG or evoked potentials. Although the exact mechanism for neuroprotective action of anaesthetic agents is not fully understood, barbiturates and propofol may produce their effect by reducing the cerebral metabolic rate. However, doses of intravenous anaesthetic high enough to suppress EEG activity cause marked cardiovascular depression.[90] The cerebral protective effects of barbiturates may be secondary to their ability to reduce calcium influx, inhibit free radical formation, potentiate GABA-ergic activity, reduce cerebral oedema and inhibit glucose transfer across the blood–brain barrier.

In contrast to pharmacological agents which only reduce the active component of cerebral metabolism, hypothermia reduces both the active and basal components thereby increasing the period of ischaemia tolerated.[91,92] Cerebral metabolism is approximately 15% of normal at 20°C. It is now commonly accepted that hypothermia may be neuroprotective because it affects factors other than cerebral metabolism: cytokines, free radicals and glutamate.[93–95]

Problems associated with hypothermia include reliability of temperature measurement, the optimal temperature needed to offer the best benefit:risk ratio and the best method of rewarming the patient safely[96] so that normothermic temperatures are reached before emergence. Other problems include delayed awakening, postoperative shivering, coagulation disorders and aggravation of myocardial disease.

Ketamine, an NMDA receptor antagonist,[97] has been traditionally avoided in neurosurgery because it increases CBF and ICP. However, NMDA receptor antagonists can prevent neuronal injury by decreasing cellular influx of calcium. There is renewed interest in the use of ketamine for neuroanaesthesia as it has been shown to be neuroprotective in an experimental head-injured rat model.[98] Furthermore, when ketamine is administered (1 mg/kg) during isoflurane and N_2O anaesthesia in mechanically ventilated patients it reduced ICP, CBF velocity and total EEG power.[99] The role of ketamine in neuroprotection requires further evaluation. For a full account of cerebral protection please see Ch. 3.

Induced hypertension

This is often employed to improve collateral blood flow during temporary clipping and in patients with areas of critical perfusion. Adequate volume loading and inotropes such as dopamine are often sufficient for producing the desired hypertension. However, in patients with abnormal autoregulation, CBF is pressure dependent and increases in MAP will increase CBF and may result in blood–brain barrier damage and vasogenic oedema. Patients with myocardial disease or unsecured aneurysms are at risk for myocardial ischaemia and aneurysm rupture respectively.

Intraoperative rupture

If the aneurysm ruptures intraoperatively, intravenous fluids are increased to maintain the cerebral perfusion pressure. Cerebral protection is provided by propofol or thiopentone-induced EEG burst suppression.

Normovolaemia must be maintained.[100] The afferent and efferent blood vessels supplying the aneurysm may be temporarily occluded by the surgeon. However, if bleeding persists, a short period of induced hypotension may be used to facilitate control.

GIANT ANEURYSMS AND CIRCULATORY ARREST

Approximately 2% of cerebral aneurysms are greater than 2.5 cm in diameter.[23] These giant aneurysms are a challenge because of their size, the lack of an anatomic neck and the perforating vessels that often originate from their walls. They often present with symptoms of mass lesion such as headaches and nerve palsies. Although improvements in microsurgical techniques and neuroanaesthesia have improved outcome considerably after giant aneurysm surgery, the morbidity and mortality remain higher than after surgery for smaller aneurysms.[101]

Three main techniques are used: temporary clipping, hypothermic circulatory arrest and arterial bypass surgery (e.g. EC-IC bypass).[102,103] Temporary clipping and EC-IC bypass have been discussed elsewhere (Ch. 15).

Circulatory arrest ensures haemorrhage during dissection and exposure of the aneurysm is minimized. After induction of anaesthesia and with all routine monitors in place, surface cooling is started. Barbiturates are administered to induce and maintain burst suppression (5 mg/kg bolus followed by 5–10 mg/kg/h infusion). Haemodilution to a haematocrit of 30% is achieved by collecting blood and administering cold intravenous saline containing potassium. After the aneurysm is dissected, femoral artery to vein bypass is established following the administration of heparin 300 IU/kg aiming for an ACT between 450 and 500 s. The patient is cooled to 18°C. Cardiac fibrillation, which commonly begins at temperatures <28°C, is stopped by potassium chloride.

Once the desired temperature is reached and the EEG is isoelectric, circulatory arrest is performed. This should only be for the duration of clip application and should not exceed 60 min. Once the aneurysm is secured, bypass is reestablished and warming at a rate not exceeding 0.5°C/min proceeds with the help of a vasodilator (sodium nitroprusside). Normal sinus rhythm is established by cardioversion when the heart fibrillates and by the administration of antiarrhythmic drugs. Bypass is discontinued when the patient's temperature reaches 36°C. Heparin is reversed with protamine and coagulation factors and blood are administered as necessary. The bypass is best coordinated with a cardiac anaesthetist.

ARTERIOVENOUS MALFORMATIONS

Arteriovenous malformations (AVM) are congenital abnormalities which shunt blood from the arterial to the venous side with flow rates out of proportion to the low metabolism within this abnormal vascular network. The majority of AVMs are supratentorial and superficial. In approximately 5% of cases, they are found in association with cerebral aneurysms. While the risk of bleeding averages 2% per year, the risk of rebleeding is closer to 5% per year.

Patients with AVMs commonly present with intracranial haemorrhage and less frequently with seizures, headaches and/or sign of intracranial hypertension. In our institution, the majority of AVMs are embolized and only small superficial ones are resected surgically. The embolization is carried out as staged procedures over a period of several weeks. AVM 'feeder' vessels are characterized by high blood flow, low resistance, low perfusion pressure and decreased CO_2-reactivity.[104] Embolization or resection of the AVM results in normalization of flow velocity and CO_2 reactivity.[105]

The principles of intraoperative management are similar to those already described for aneurysm surgery. A notable exception is the meticulous control of blood pressure control both intra- and postoperatively.[106] It is well recognized that some patients are at risk of brain swelling and haemorrhage after AVM resection. Risk factors include the volume of the AVM (>20 cm³), the presence of deep feeders, the location of the AVM (rolandic, inferior limbic and insular region) and the preexcision mean feeder transcranial Doppler, velocity (>120 cm/s).[107] According to the normal perfusion pressure breakthrough theory initially proposed by Spetzler et al,[108] the hyperaemia occurred as a result of the loss of autoregulatory capacity in normal brain tissue adjacent to the AVM. However, Young et al were unable to demonstrate this loss of autoregulation with xenon wash-out studies.[109, 110] Occlusive hyperemia was recently proposed as the cause of this hyperperfusion.[111]

Regardless of the underlying mechanism, there is little doubt that brain swelling/haemorrhage that occurs after AVM resection is related to an increase in hemispheric perfusion,[109] and the only effective treatment is adequate control of blood pressure and optimal cerebral vasoconstriction. High-dose propofol infusion and labetalol are effective in controlling blood pressure.

RECOVERY

In patients with initial good-grade SAH, a rapid return of consciousness is aimed for to allow early neurologic assessment. Provided no untoward events occurred intraoperatively, grade I–II patients are extubated. In patients with WFNS grade III, recovery depends on their preoperative conscious level and ventilatory state. Grade IV–V patients are usually transferred to the neurocritical care unit for a 24–48 h period of elective postoperative ventilation.

When surgery is complete, the anaesthetic agents are discontinued and 100% oxygen is given. Residual neuromuscular blockade is reversed, the airway suctioned and the patient extubated on regaining consciousness. Boluses of short-acting opioids, propofol or lignocaine can be used to facilitate extubation and control the blood pressure. Uncontrolled hypertension in the immediate postoperative phase can precipitate intracerebral haemorrhage. In patients with unsecured aneurysms, the blood pressure is kept to within 20% of normal. If the patient remains hypertensive (systolic pressure greater than 200 mmHg) in recovery despite adequate pain relief, esmolol, labetalol or nifedipine is used.

If the patient fails to regain their preoperative neurological state, the following need to be excluded:

- anaesthetic causes (partial neuromuscular blockade);
- residual narcotic and sedative drugs;
- hypoxia and hypercarbia;
- metabolic factors (hyponatraemia);
- Postictal state.

It is important that the airway is not compromised postoperatively and hypercapnia and hypoxaemia are avoided. Reintubation will be required in those patients unable to protect their airway or maintain adequate gas exchange. Once the above possible causes have been excluded, a CT scan is performed to exclude hydrocephalus, cerebral oedema, intracranial haemorrhage, haematoma or a rebleed (multiple aneurysms). If the scan is negative, a cerebral angiogram is required to exclude vascular occlusion (e.g. misplaced clip). Vasospasm can be detected using transcranial Doppler.

All patients are transferred to the neurocritical care unit or high-dependency unit for their postoperative management. Cerebral vasospasm and delayed ischaemic neurological deficits remain the major postoperative complications once the aneurysm has been clipped. The management of this condition is described in Ch. 23.

CONCLUSION

The maintenance of adequate cerebral perfusion, the avoidance of hypotension and the prevention and treatment of raised intracranial pressure are essential for good recovery in patients with intracranial haemorrhage, cerebral trauma or encephalopathies. Therefore, clinicians caring for these patients must have a thorough understanding of cerebral physiology and the factors that affect cerebral haemodynamics. The principles of anaesthetic management of patients with SAH described above are applicable to any patient with an intracranial vascular lesion.

REFERENCES

1. Poon WS, Rehman SU, Poon CYF et al. Traumatic extradural haematoma of delayed onset is not a rarity. Neurosurgery 1992; 30: 681.

2. Rivas JJ, Lobato RD, Sarabia R et al. Extradural haematoma: analysis of factors influencing the courses of 161 patients. Neurosurgery 1988; 23: 44.

3. Bricolo AP, Paust LM. Extradural haematoma: toward zero mortality. A prospective study. Neurosurgery 1985; 63: 30

4. Wilberger JE, Harris M, Diamond DL. Acute subdural hematoma. J Trauma 1990; 30: 733.

5. Newfield P, Pitts LH, Kaktis J et al. Influence of shock on survival after head injury. Neurosurgery 1980; 6: 596.

6. Garza-Mercado R. Extradural haematoma of the posterior cranial fossa. Report of seven cases with survival. J Neurosurg 1983; 59: 664.

7. Brott TG, Hayley EC, Levy DE et al. Hypertension as a risk factor for spontaneous intracerebral hemorrhage. Stroke 1986; 17: 1078.

8. Vinters HV. Cerebral amyloid angiopathy: a critical review. Stroke 1987; 18: 311–324.

9. Levine SR, Brust JC, Futrell N et al. A comparative study of the cerebrovascular complications of cocaine: alkaloid versus hydrochloride – a review. Neurology 1991; 41: 1173–1177.

10. Green RM, Kelly KM, Gabrielson T et al. Multiple intracerebral hemorrhages after smoking 'crack' cocaine. Stroke 1990; 21: 957.

11. Harrington H, Heller HA, Dawson D et al. Intracerebral hemorrhage and oral amphetamine. Arch Neurol 1983; 4: 503–507.

12. Franke CL, De Jonge J, Van Swieten JC et al. Intracerebral hematomas during anticoagulant treatment. Stroke 1990; 21: 72–730.

13. Little JR, Dial B, Belanger G, Carpenter S. Brain hemorrhage from intracranial tumor. Stroke 1979; 10: 283–288.

14. Paulson OB, Olesen J, Christensen MS. Restoration of autoregulation of cerebral blood flow by hypocapnia. Neurology 1972; 22: 286–293.

15. Aaslid R, Lindegaard K-F, Sorteberg W et al. Cerebral autoregulation dynamics in humans. Stroke 1989; 20: 45–52.

16. Plum F, Posner JB, Smith WW. Effects of hyperbaric hyperoxic hyperventilation on blood, brain and CSF lactate. Am J Physiol 1968; 215: 1240–1244.

17. Matta BF, Lam AM, Mayberg TS. The influence of arterial hyperoxygenation on cerebral venous oxygen content during hyperventilation. Can J Anaesth 1994; 41: 1041–1046.

18. Inagawa T, Hirano A. Autopsy study of unruptured incidental intracranial aneurysms. Surg Neurol 1982; 20: 13–17.

19. Phillips LH, Whisnant JP, O'Fallon WM, Sundt TM. The unchanging pattern of subarachnoid haemorrhage in a community. Neurology 1980; 30: 1034–1040.

20. Sacco RL, Wolf PA, Bharucha NE et al. Subarachnoid and intracerebral hemorrhage: natural history prognosis, and precursive factors in the Framingham study. Neurology 1984; 34: 847–854.

21. Norrgaard O, Angqvist KA, Fodstad H et al. Intracranial aneurysms and heredity. Neurosurgery 1987; 20: 236–239.

22. Bromberg JEC, Rinkel GJE, Algra A et al. Subarachnoid haemorrhage in first and second degree relatives of patients with subarachnoid haemorrhage. BMJ 1995; 311: 288–289.

23. Kassell NF, Torner JC, Haley EC et al. The International Cooperative Study on the timing of aneurysm surgery. Part 1: overall management results. J Neurosurg 1990; 73: 18–32.

24. Schievink WI, Wijdicks EFM, Parisi JE et al. Sudden death from aneurysmal subarachnoid hemorrhage. Neurology 1995; 45: 871–874.

25. Hijdra A, Braakman R, Van Gijn J et al. Aneurysmal subarachnoid hemorrhage. Complications and outcome in a hospital population. Stroke 1987; 18: 1061–1067

26. Rosenorn J, Eskesen V, Schmidt K, Ronde F. The risk of rebleeding from ruptured intracranial aneurysms. J Neurosurg 1987; 67: 329–332.

27. International Study of Unruptured Intracranial Aneurysms Investigators. Unruptured intracranial aneurysms – risk of rupture and risks of surgical intervention. N Engl J Med 1998; 339(24): 1725–1733.

28. Caplan LR. Should intracranial aneurysms be treated before they rupture? (editorial). N Engl J Med 1998; 339(24): 1774–1775.

29. Drake CG, Hunt WE, Sano K et al. Report of World Federation of Neurological Surgeons Committee on a Universal Subarachnoid Hemorrhage Grading Scale. J Neurosurg 1988; 68: 985–986.

30. Lim ST, Sage DJ. Detection of subarachnoid blood clot and other thin flat structures by computed tomography. Radiology 1977; 123: 79–84.

31. Hart RG, Byer JA, Slaughter JR et al. Occurrence and implications of seizures in subarachnoid hemorrhage due to ruptured intracranial aneurysms. Neurosurgery 1981; 8: 417–421.

32. Schwartz RB, Tice HM, Hooten SM et al. Evaluation on cerebral aneurysms with helical CT: correlation with conventional angiography and MR angiography. Radiology 1994; 192: 717–722.

33. Kelly DF. Timing of surgery for ruptured aneurysms and initial critical care. J Stroke Neurovasc Dis 1997; 6(4): 235–236.

34. Ohman J, Heiskanen O. Timing of operation for ruptured supratentorial aneurysms: a prospective randomised study. J Neurosurg 1989; 70: 55–60.

35. Kassell NF, Torner JC, Haley C et al. The International Study on the Timing of Aneurysm Surgery. Part I: Overall management results. J Neurosurg 1990; 73: 18–36.

36. Broderick JP, Brott TG, Duldner JE et al. Initial and recurrent bleeding are major causes of death following subarachnoid haemorrhage. Stroke 1994; 25: 1342–1347.

37. Romner B, Ljunggren B, Brandt L, Saveland H. Correlation of transcranial Doppler sonography findings with timing of aneurysm surgery. J Neurosurg 1990; 73: 72–76.

38. Mizukami K, Kawase T, Usami T, Tazawa T. Prevention of vasospasm by early operation with removal of subarachnoid blood. Neurosurgery 1982; 10: 301–307.

39. Kassell NF, Torner JC, Jane JA et al. The International Cooperative Study on the timing of aneurysm surgery. Part II: Surgical results. J Neurosurg 1990; 73: 37–47.

40. Kassell NF, Peerless SJ, Durward QJ et al. Treatment of ischaemic deficits from vasospasm with intravascular volume expansion and induced arterial hypertension. Neurosurgery 1982; 11: 337–343.

41. Broderick JP, Brott TG, Duldner JE et al. Initial and recurrent bleeding are major causes of death following subarachnoid haemorrhage. Stroke 1994; 25: 1342–1347.

42. Solenski NJ, Haley EC, Kassell NF et al. Medical complications of aneurysmal subarachnoid hemorrhage: a report of the multicenter, cooperative aneurysm study. Crit Care Med 1995; 23: 1007–1017.

43. Marion SW, Segal R, Thompson ME. Subarachnoid hemorrhage and the heart. Neurosurgery 1986; 18: 101–106.

44. Mayer SA, Swarup R. Neurogenic cardiac injury after subarachnoid hemorrhage. Curr Opin Anaesthesiol 1996; 9: 356–361.

45. Goldman MR, Rogers EL, Rogers MC. Subarachnoid hemorrhage–association with unusual electrocardiographic changes. JAMA 1975; 234: 957–958.

46. Manninen PH, Ayra B, Gelb AW, Pelz D. Association between electrocardiographic abnormalities and intracranial blood in patients following acute subarachnoid hemorrhage. J Neurosurg Anesthesiol 1995; 7: 12–16.

47. White JC, Parker SD, Rogers MC. Preanesthetic evaluation of a patient with pathologic Q waves following subarachnoid hemorrhage. Anesthesiology 1985; 62: 351.

48. Doczi T, Bende J, Huszka E, Kiss J. Syndrome of inappropriate secretion of antidiuretic hormone after subarachnoid hemorrhage. Neurosurgery 1981; 9: 394–397.

49. Hasan D, Vermeulen M, Wijdicks EFM et al. Management problems in acute hydrocephalus after subarachnoid hemorrhage. Stroke 1989; 20: 747–753.

50. Nelson PB, Seif SM, Maroon JC, Robinson JC. Hyponatremia in intracranial disease: perhaps not the syndrome of inappropriate secretion of antidiuretic hormone (SIADH). J Neurosurg 1981; 55: 938–941.

51. Diringer M, Ladenson PW, Stern BJ et al. Plasma atrial natriuretic facor and subarachnoid hemorrhage. Stroke 1988; 19: 1119–1124.

52. Young B, Ott L, Dempsey R et al. Relationship between admission hyperglycaemia and neurologic outcome of severely brain-injured patients. Ann Surg 1989; 210: 466–473.

53. Lam AM, Winn HR, Cullen BF et al. Hyperglycemia and neurological outcome in patients with head injury. J Neurosurg 1991; 75: 545–551.

54. Pare L, Delfino R, LeBlanc R. The relationship of ventricular drainage to aneurysmal rupture during angiography. J Neurosurg 1992; 76: 422–427.

55. Warner DS, Sokoll MD, Maktabi M et al. Nicardipine HCl: clinical experience in patients undergoing anaesthesia for intracranial aneurysm clipping. Can J Anaesth 1985; 36: 219–223

56. Stullken EH, Balestrieri FJ, Prough DS, McWhorter JM. The hemodynamic effects of nimodipine in patients anesthetised for cerebral aneurysm clipping. Anesthesiology 1985; 62: 346–348.

57. Sheinberg M, Kanter MJ, Robertson CS et al. Continuous monitoring of jugular venous oxygen saturation in head injured patients. J Neurosurg 1992; 76: 212–217.

58. Matta BF, Lam AM, Mayberg TS et al. A critique of the intraoperative use of jugular venous bulb catheters during neurosurgical procedures. Anesth Analg 1994; 79: 745–750.

59. Cottrell JE, Hartung J, Griffi JP et al. Intracranial and hemodynamic changes after succinylcholine administration in cats. Anesth Analg 1983; 62: 1006–1009.

60. Colley PS, Dunn R. Prevention of the blood pressure response to skull-pin head-holder by local anaesthesia. Anesth Analg 1979; 4: 223–226.

61. Ravussin P, De Tribolet N. Total intravenous anesthesia with propofol for burst suppression in cerebral aneurysm surgery: preliminary report of 42 patients. Neurosurgery 1993; 32: 236–240.

62. Matta BF, Lam AM, Strebel S, Mayberg TS. Cerebral pressure autoregulation and CO_2-reactivity during propofol-induced EEG suppression. Br J Anaesth 1995; 4: 159–163.

63. Matta BF, Mayberg TS, Lam AM. Direct cerebrovasodilatory effects of halothane, isoflurane, and desflurane during propofol induced isoelectric electroencephalogram in humans. Anesthesiology 1995; 83: 980–985.

64. Strebel S, Lam AM, Matta BF et al. Dynamic and static cerebral autoregulation during isoflurane, desflurane and propofol anesthesia. Anesthesiology 1995; 83: 66–76.

65. Ebert TJ, Muzi M. Sympathetic hyperactivity during desflurane anesthesia in healthy volunteers. A comparison with isoflurane. Anesthesiology 1993; 79: 444–453.

66. Gupta S, Heath K, Matta BF. Effect of incremental doses of sevoflurane on cerebral pressure autoregulation in humans. Br J Anaesth 1997; 79: 469–472.

67. Cho S, Fujigaki T, Uchiyama Y et al. Effects of sevoflurane with and without nitrous oxide on human cerebral circulation. Anesthesiology 1996; 85: 755–760.

68. Katsuyasu K, Hisatoshi O, Masakazu K et al. Effects of sevoflurane on cerebral circulation and metabolism in patients with ischemic cerebrovascular disease. Anesthesiology 1993; 79: 704–709.

69. Heath KJ, Gupta S, Matta BF. The effects of sevoflurane on cerebral hemodynamics during propofol anesthesia. Anesth Analg 1997; 85: 1284–1287.

70. Matta BF, Lam AM. Nitrous oxide increases cerebral blood flow velocity during pharmacologically induced EEG silence in humans. J Neurosurg Anesthesiol 1995; 7: 89–93.

71. Strebel S, Kaufmann M, Anselmi L, Schaefer HG. Nitrous oxide is a potent cerebrovasodilator when added to isoflurane. A transcranial doppler study. Acta Anaesthesiol Scand 1995; 39: 653–658.

72. Hormann CH, Schmidauer CH, Haring HP et al. Hyperventilation reverses the nitrous oxide-induced increases in cerebral blood flow velocity in humans. Br J Anaesth 1995; 74: 616–618.

73. Eng C, Lam AM, Mayberg TS et al. The influence of propofol with and without nitrous oxide on cerebral blood flow velocity and CO_2 reactivity in humans. Anesthesiology 1992; 77: 872–879.

74. Albanese J, Durbec O, Viviand X et al. Sufentanil increases intracranial pressure in patients with head trauma. Anesthesiology 1993; 79: 493–497.

75. Trindle MR, Dodson BA, Rampil IJ. Effects of fentanyl versus sufentanil in equianesthetic doses on middle cerebral artery blood flow velocity. Anesthesiology 1993; 78: 454–460.

76. Mayer N, Weinstabl C, Podreka I et al. Sufentanil does not increase cerebral blood flow in healthy human volunteeers. Anesthesiology 1990; 73: 240–243.

77. Werner C, Kochs E, Bause H et al. Effects of sufentanil on cerebral hemodynamics and intracranial pressure in patients with brain injury. Anesthesiology 1995; 83: 721–726.

78. Guy J, Hindman BJ, Baker KZ et al. Comparison of remifentanil and fentanyl in patients undergoing craniotomy for supratentorial space-occupying lesions. Anesthesiology 1997; 86: 514–524.

79. Godsiff LS, Matta BF, Gupta AK, Summers A. The effect of sevoflurane and remifentanil anesthesia on dynamic cerebral pressure autoregulation. J Neurosurg Ansthesiol 1998; 10: A267.

80. Archer D. Mannitol, osmotherapy, and fluid management in neuroanaesthesia. Curr Opin in Anesthesiol 1996; 9: 362–364.

81. Pollay M, Fullenwider C, Roberts PA, Griffin G. Effect of mannitol and furosemide on blood-brain osmotic gradient and intracranial pressure. J Neurosurg 1983; 59: 445–452.

82. Muizelaar JP, Wei EP, Kontos HA et al. Mannitol causes compensatory cerebral vasoconstriction and vasodilatation in response to blood viscosity changes. J Neurosurg 1983; 59: 822–828.

83. Sahar A, Tsipstein E. Effects of mannitol and furosemide on the rate of formation of cerebrospinal fluid. Exp Neurol 1978; 60: 584–591.

84. Donato T, Shapira Y, Artru A et al. Effect of mannitol on cerebrospinal fluid dynamics and brain tissue edema. Anesth Analg 1994; 78: 58–66.

85. Gemma M, Cozzi S, Tommasino C et al. 7.5% hypertonic saline versus 20% mannitol during elective neurosurgical supratentorial procedures. J Neurosurg Anesthesiol 1997; 9(4): 329–334.

86. Ruta TS, Mutch WAC. Controlled hypotension for cerebral aneurysm surgery: are the risks worth the benefits? J Neurosurg Anesthesiol 1991; 3: 153–156.

87. Samson D, Hunt B, Bowman G et al. A clinical study of the parameters and effects of temporary arterial occlusion in the management of intracranial aneurysms. Neurosurgery 1994; 34: 22–27.

88. Ljunggren B, Saneland H, Brandt L et al. Temporary clipping during early operation for ruptured aneurysm: preliminary report. Neurosurgery 1983; 12: 525–530.

89. Warner DS. Perioperative neuroprotection. Curr Opin Anaesthesiol 1994; 7: 416–420.

90. Todd MM, Drummond JC, Hoi SU. Hemodynamic effects of high dose pentobarbital: studies in elective neurosurgical patients. Neurosurgery 1987; 20: 559–563.

91. Steen PA, Newberg L, Milde JH et al. Hypothermia and barbiturates: individual and combined effects on canine cerebral oxygen consumption. Anesthesiology 1983; 58: 527.

92. Doppenberg EMR, Bullock R. Clinical neuroprotection trials in severe head traumatic brain injury: lessons from previuos studies. J Neurotrauma 1997; 14: 71–80.

93. Bart RD, Takaoda S, Pearlstein RD, Dexter F, Warner DS. Interactions between hypothermia and the latency to ischemic depolarisation – implications for neuroprotection. Anesthesiology 1998; 88: 1266–1273.

94. Marion DW, Penrod LE, Kelsey SF et al. Treatment of traumatic brain injury with moderate hypothermia. N Engl J Med 1997; 336: 540–546.

95. Lei B, Adachi N, Arai T. The effect of hypothermia on H_2O_2 production during ischemia and reperfusion: a microdialysis study in gerbil hippocampus. Neurosci Lett 1997; 222: 91–94.

96. Cheney F, Posner K, Caplan R, Gild W. Burns from warming devices in anesthesia: a closed claims analysis. Anesthesiology 1994; 80: 806–810.

97. Hirota K, Lambert DG. Ketamine: its mechanism(s) of action and unusual clinical uses. Br J Anaesth 1996; 77: 441–444.

98. Church J, Zerman S, Lodge D. The neuroprotective action of ketamine and MK-801 after transient cerebral ischemia in rats. Anesthesiology 1988; 69: 702–709.

99. Mayberg TS, Lam AM, Matta BF et al. Ketamine does not increase cerebral blood flow velocity or intracranial pressure during isoflurane/nitrous oxide anesthesia in patients undergoing craniotomy. Anesth Analg 1995; 81: 84–89.

100. Giannotta SL, Oppenheimer JH, Levy ML, Zelman V. Management of intraoperative rupture of aneurysms without hypotension. Neurosurgery 1991; 28: 531–535.

101. Lawton MT, Raudzens PA, Zabramski JM, Spetzler RF. Hypothermic circulatory arrest in neurovascular surgery: evolving indications and predictors of patient outcome. Neurosurgery 1998; 43: 10–21.

102. Weill A, Cognard C, Levy D, Robert G, Moret J. Giant aneurysms of the middle cerebral artery trifurcation treated with extracranial-intracranial arterial bypass and endovascular occlusion. Report of two cases. J Neurosurg 1998; 89: 474–478.

103. Lawton MT, Spetzler RF. Surgical management of giant intracranial aneurysms: experience with 171 patients. Clin Neurosurg 1995; 42: 245–266.

104. De Salles AA, Manchola I. CO2 reactivity in arteriovenous malformations of the brain: a transcranial Doppler ultrasound study. J Neurosurg 1994; 80: 624.

105. Kader A, Young WL, Massaro AR et al. Transcranial Doppler changes during staged surgical resection of cerebral arteriovenous malformations: a report of three cases. Surg Neurol 1993; 39: 392.

106. Young Wl, Prohovnick I, Ornstein E et al. Monitoring of intraoperative cerebral haemodynamics before and after arteriovenous malformations. Stroke 1994; 25: 611.

107. Pasqualin A, Barone G, Cioffi F, Rosta L, Scienza R, Da Pian R. The relevance of anatomic and hemodynamic factors to a classification of cerebral arteriovenous malformations. Neurosurgery 1991; 28: 370–379.

108. Spetzler RF, Wilson CB, Weinstein P et al. Normal perfusion pressure breakthrough theory. Clin Neurosurg 1978; 25: 651–672.

109. Young WL, Kader A, Prohovnik I et al. Pressure autoregulation is intact after arteriovenous malformation resection. J Neurosurg 1993; 32: 491–496.

110. Young WL, Pile-Spellman J, Prohovnik I, Kader A, Stein BM. Evidence for adaptive autoregulatory displacement in hypotensive cortical territories adjacent to arteriovenous malformations. Neurosurgery 1994; 34: 601–610.

111. Al-Rodhan NRF, Sundt TM, Piepgras DG et al. Occlusive hyperemia: a theory of the hemodynamic complications following resection of intracerebral arteriovenous malformations. J Neurosurg 1993; 78: 167–175.

15

ANAESTHESIA FOR CAROTID SURGERY

Sanjeeva Gupta & Basil F. Matta

INTRODUCTION

Carotid endarterectomy (CEA) prevents stroke in patients with symptomatic severe carotid stenosis (>70%). However, its superiority over medical therapy alone is yet to be proven in those patients with mild (0–29%) or moderate (30–69%) symptomatic carotid stenosis.[1–3] Furthermore, despite recently published evidence claiming some benefit for CEA in carefully selected asymptomatic patients,[4,5] its role in preventing stroke in asymptomatic patients remains controversial.

The aim of CEA is to prevent stroke. The major indications for CEA are recurrent strokes, transient ischaemic attacks (TIA) and reversible ischaemic neurological deficit (RIND). The prevalence of moderate internal carotid artery stenosis (>50% reduction in lumen diameter) rises from about 0.5% in people in their 50s to around 10% in those over the age of 80 years.[6] As the incidence of coronary artery disease also increases with age, it is not surprising that the major cause of mortality and morbidity from carotid endarterectomy is myocardial infarction (MI). Irrespective of the surgical and anaesthetic technique used, the procedure-related risk of stroke of death should be less than 3% in asymptomatic patients and less than 6% in symptomatic patients.[7] A complication rate exceeding these figures should prompt a review of the surgical and/or anaesthetic technique. Over the two-year period 1996–7, of the 210 CEA performed at our centre, the mortality rate stands at just over 1% with a 2.9% stroke rate. However, the incidence of perioperative MI approximates 4%.

Although the major indication of CEA is stroke, its major complication is stroke. Therefore, a thorough understanding of the pathophysiology of carotid artery disease and the anaesthetic implications is essential for maximizing the benefit of this procedure.

PREOPERATIVE ASSESSMENT

By retrospectively reviewing their series at the Mayo Clinic, Sundt et al identified neurological, medical and angiographical factors that can be used to assess the risk of postoperative complications (Tables 15.1 and 15.2).[8,9] Although the risk factors in individuals vary, patients with the greatest risk are also those most likely to suffer a severe stroke and therefore have the most to gain from prophylactic surgery.

Patients presenting for carotid surgery are elderly and often have co-existing medical problems common to patients with vascular disease. These include coronary

---

Table 15.1 Perioperative risk factors

Medical risk factors
Angina
Myocardial infarction within six months of surgery
Congestive cardiac failure
Uncontrolled hypertension
Advanced peripheral vascular disease
Chronic obstructive pulmonary disease
Obesity

Neurologic risk factors
Progressive neurologic deficit
Recent deficit (within 24 h)
Active transient ischaemic attacks (TIA)
Recent cerebral infarction (<7 days)
Generalized cerebral ischaemia

Angiographic risk factors
Contralateral occlusion of ICA
Coexisting ipsilateral carotid siphon disease
Extensive plaque extension >3 cm distally or >5 cm proximally
Thrombus extending from an ulcerative lesion
Carotid bifurcation at cervical vertebral level C2 with short thick ICA

---

artery disease, chronic obstructive airway disease and diabetes mellitus. As part of the routine preoperative assessment, special emphasis should be laid on a thorough evaluation of:

1. the cardiovascular system;
2. the neurological system;
3. the respiratory system;
4. the endocrine system.

CARDIOVASCULAR SYSTEM

Stroke and TIA are markers of general atherosclerosis. Many patients presenting for carotid endarterectomy will have concomitant coronary artery disease and up to 20% have a history of myocardial infarction.[10] The annual long-term mortality rate from cardiac disease in these patients is 5%, similar to the 6% rate among patients with symptomatic triple vessel coronary artery disease and far exceeding the mortality rate from stroke.[10] The cardiac risk is further increased by other associated medical conditions such as hypertension and obesity. The high prevalence of coronary artery disease, as determined by history, electrocardiography or cardiac catheterization present in over 55% of these patients, is responsible for the increased risk of postoperative

Table 15.2	Grading of patients undergoing carotid endarterectomy			
Grade	Neurological findings	Medical findings	Angiographical risk	Risk of MI/RND
1	Stable	No defined risk	No major risk	1%
2	Stable	No defined risk	No major risk	2%
3	Stable	Major risk	With or without risk	7%
4	Unstable	With or without risk	With or without risk	10%

MI = myocardial infarction; RND = residual neurological deficit
Patients are at increased risk if they have suffered an acute ICA occlusion or recurrent carotid stenosis having previously undergone carotid endarterectomy.

myocardial infarction (5%) when compared to those patients without coronary artery disease (0.5%).[11,12] Evidence of cardiac disease should be sought by careful history and thorough examination, noting the presence of angina and its severity, previous myocardial infarction and symptoms and signs of cardiac failure. The ECG should be examined for abnormalities of rhythm and evidence of previous infarction and ischaemia. When indicated, chest radiograph is examined for evidence of cardiac failure. Further cardiac work-up, including an exercise ECG, radionuclide studies or coronary angiography, may be necessary and is best co-ordinated with a cardiologist.

Hypertension, present in up to 70% of patients presenting for CEA, must be well controlled. Postoperative hypertension and transient neurological deficits are more frequent in patients with poor preoperative blood pressure control (BP > 170/95 mmHg).[12,13] Sudden normalization of blood pressure should be avoided in order to reduce the risk of hypoperfusion and stroke.

Elective surgery should be postponed in those patients with uncontrolled blood pressure, unstable angina, congestive cardiac failure or myocardial infarction in the previous six months, as the perioperative cardiac risk is greatly increased. In some unstable patients, combined coronary artery bypass and CEA may be necessary and is discussed later in this chapter.

NEUROLOGICAL SYSTEM

Evaluation of the cerebrovascular system should carefully document the presence of transient or permanent neurological deficit. This is essential for assessing postoperative progress as well as quantifying perioperative risk of stroke. Frequent daily TIAs, multiple neurologic deficits secondary to cerebral infarctions or a progressive neurological deficit increases the risk of new postoperative neurological deficit.[8] Results of tests assessing the cerebral vascular system, such as

duplex ultrasound scan, cerebral angiography and CO_2 reactivity, should be available.

RESPIRATORY SYSTEM

Chronic obstructive pulmonary disease is often present in these patients and needs optimal medical treatment preoperatively, which may include bronchodilators, corticosteroids, physiotherapy and incentive spirometry. Cigarette smoking should be stopped 6–8 weeks preoperatively. If necessary, preoperative pulmonary function tests like PEFR, $FVC:FEV_1$ ratio and a baseline arterial blood gas analysis with the patient breathing air should be carried out to guide perioperative care of the patient.

ENDOCRINE SYSTEM

Diabetes mellitus has been shown to exist in about 20% of patients presenting with CEA and most of these patients are insulin dependent.[14] Adequate blood glucose control with absence of ketoacidosis preoperatively must be established. In experimental studies, even modest elevations in blood glucose have been shown to augment postischaemic cerebral injury.[15] Manifestations of diabetes mellitus such as renal failure, silent myocardial infarction, autonomic and sensory neuropathy and ophthalmic complications must be looked for.

It is very important that the patient's preoperative medication should be reviewed. These patients are often receiving cardiac and antihypertensive drugs, antiplatelet agents, antacids, steroids, insulin and anticoagulants. Most of the drugs should be continued except for the antiplatelet agents and anticoagulants.

ANAESTHETIC MANAGEMENT

The aim of perioperative anaesthetic management is to minimize the risk of occurrence of the two major complications, stroke and myocardial infarction. Strokes are either haemodynamic or embolic in origin. No randomized clinical trial has identified a superior anaesthetic technique. Therefore, many of the anaesthetic techniques advocated, including the one provided here, are the result of indirect evidence based on animal data or surrogate endpoints and are biased by personal experience.

PREMEDICATION

Good rapport should be established with the patient in the preoperative period. This will help to reduce anxiety which may exacerbate the perioperative blood pressure abnormalities with increased risk of myocardial ischaemia and cardiac arrhythmias. An anxiolytic premedicant is especially important in those patients undergoing the procedure under regional or local blockade. Regional anaesthesia allows neurological assessment during and immediately following the procedure, but necessitates judicious use of preoperative sedation. A balance must be struck between adequate sedation and 'over' sedation as the latter depresses neurologic function. Oversedation often leads to hypoventilation with CO_2 retention and blood pressure abnormalities, often with detrimental effects on the cerebral circulation.[16] Benzodiazepines are routinely used in our institution for premedication.

REGIONAL OR LOCAL VERSUS GENERAL ANAESTHESIA

The type of anaesthetic used seems to depend on individual practice rather than hard evidence. Local anaesthesia or cervical plexus block allows evaluation of neurological status during carotid cross-clamping to assess the need for shunting and therefore prevention of stroke from hypoperfusion. However, perioperative strokes are more likely to be embolic than low flow in origin.[17,18] Other potential advantages include a lower incidence of postoperative hypertension and a lesser need for vasoactive drugs with shorter stay in the intensive care unit.[19]

Unfortunately, this technique has numerous disadvantages. It requires patient cooperation and the ability to remain supine for the duration of the procedure. Many patients presenting for carotid endarterectomy are unable to lie flat and suppress cough for the duration of surgery. The procedure may be uncomfortable for the patient, many of whom would prefer to be unaware during surgery. Anxiety, especially with the proximity of the surgical drapes, may lead to hyperventilation with a concomitant reduction in cerebral blood flow and increased risk of cerebral ischaemia. Autonomic responses to surgical manipulation of the carotid bulb may be excessive, resulting in hypotension, hypertension or bradycardia. There is also an ever-present risk of airway obstruction, as well as the occurrence of nausea and vomiting. Uncontrolled haemorrhage or sudden neurological deterioration may require general anaesthesia with rapid tracheal intubation.

Nevertheless, when used properly in carefully selected patients by experienced surgeons, regional anaesthesia has a good safety record and is not associated with any increase in the rate of perioperative myocardial infarction.[20] A recent publication, in which 215 CEA were performed under cervical block anaesthesia, reported a substantial decrease in complications, length of hospital stay and cost.[21]

REGIONAL OR LOCAL ANAESTHESIA

The patient is attached to all the standard monitors as for general anaesthesia. An appropriate dose of sedation is given. Regional anaesthesia is achieved with a deep cervical plexus block. This may be performed by a single injection or a multiple injection technique (performed by the surgeon). For the single injection technique,[22] the patient is placed supine with the head turned to the opposite side. The area is prepped and draped. The lateral margin of the clavicular head of the sternocleidomastoid muscle is identified at the level of C4 (level with the superior margin of the thyroid cartilage). The middle and index fingers are rolled laterally over the anterior scalene muscle until the interscalene groove, between the anterior and middle scalene muscle, is palpated. Asking the patient to lift the head off the table slowly may further enhance the groove. After raising a skin wheal with 1% lignocaine, a short bevel needle is then inserted between the palpating fingers, perpendicular to all levels and slightly caudad in direction until paraesthesia is elicited. After careful aspiration, 5–6 ml of local anaesthetic suitable for the duration of surgery is injected (1% lignocaine or 0.5% bupivacaine with 1:200 000 adrenaline). The local anaesthetic should spread in the fascial sheath extending from the cervical transverse processes to beyond the axilla, investing the cervical plexus in between the middle and anterior scalene muscles. The slight caudad direction is important as, should the nerve not be encountered, advancing the needle in this direction is less likely to result in epidural or subarachnoid puncture, as this complication is prevented by the transverse process of the cervical vertebra.

There is no need to perform a superficial cervical plexus block with this technique, as the nerve roots are already anaesthetized. It may be more comfortable for the patient, who is going to have their head turned laterally intraoperatively, if 5 ml of local anaesthetic is deposited below the attachment of the sternocleidomastoid muscle, thus anaesthetizing the accessory nerve. Local infiltration by the surgeon may be required if the upper end of the incision is in the trigeminal nerve area or if the midline is crossed. Judicious administration of intravenous midazolam or propofol can provide sedation without compromising the ability to evaluate the patient's neurologic function.

Possible complications of interscalene cervical plexus block include epidural, subarachnoid and intervertebral artery injection, which can be minimized by the caudad direction of the needle and by repeated aspiration before injecting the local anaesthetic. Hoarseness may occur if the recurrent laryngeal nerve is blocked and Horner's syndrome if the cervical sympathetic chain is blocked. The lower roots of the brachial lexus may also be blocked by spread of local anaesthetic. Local infiltration with or without superficial cervical plexus block has been used. A large volume of local anaesthetic is required and the results are not as satisfactory as deep cervical plexus block.

GENERAL ANAESTHESIA

These patients in general have a tendency for extreme blood pressure liability under general anaesthesia. However, general anaesthesia reduces cerebral metabolic demand and may offer some degree of cerebral protection.[23] It also allows for the precise control and manipulation of systemic blood pressure and arterial carbon dioxide tension to optimize cerebral blood flow. Several techniques are available and the precise one used depends on the experience and preference of the anaesthetist. A balanced general anaesthesia that maintains the blood pressure at the preoperative level is preferred to 'deep' general anaesthesia that may necessitate the use of vasopressors to maintain blood pressure, as the risk of myocardial ischaemia may be increased in the latter.[12,24]

Induction

The aim is to maintain cerebral and myocardial perfusion as close to baseline values as possible. A preinduction intra-arterial line is useful to monitor blood pressure during and after induction. Anaesthesia can be induced in several ways. After preoxygenation, fentanyl and etomidate or thiopentone or propofol are given in incremental doses, titrated against the patient's haemodynamic responses. Muscle relaxation is achieved using a cardiostable non-depolarizing agent such as vecuronium and a peripheral nerve stimulator is used to monitor the neuromuscular junction. To obtund the intubation response, lignocaine 1–1.5 mg/kg may be given 2–3 min before laryngoscopy and intubation. When muscle relaxation is complete, laryngoscopy and intubation are performed. After confirmation of tracheal tube placement by breath sounds and end-tidal capnometry, the tube is secured away from the operative side. Some surgeons may prefer nasotracheal placement of the tube to allow maximum extension of the neck and therefore better exposure. The lungs are ventilated to maintain adequate arterial oxygen saturation and normocarbia.

Maintenance

As during induction of anaesthesia, the aim is to provide stable cerebral perfusion while minimizing stress to the myocardium. We prefer to use a balanced general anaesthesia with fentanyl, isoflurane, nitrous oxide and muscle relaxants. Although theoretically, nitrous oxide is thought to enlarge an air embolus that can occur during the course of the operation, it is often used for its sympathomimetic effect in maintaining blood pressure. The use of isoflurane is associated with a lower critical cerebral blood flow needed to maintain a normal EEG,[25] as well as a lower incidence of ischaemic EEG changes compared to halothane and enflurane, and therefore should be the agent of choice if general anaesthesia with inhalational agent is used.[26] In spite of its controversial coronary steal phenomenon, isoflurane has been shown to be associated with a lower incidence of fatal MI (0.25%) than either enflurane (0.5%) or halothane (1.0%).[27] Total intravenous anaesthesia with propofol and fentanyl or alfentanil infusion may also be used, but systemic hypotension is more likely with these combinations and may be problematic, especially if remifentanil, the newly introduced ultra short-acting opioid, is used. Regardless of the anaesthetic agents used, the regimen should be one that allows early awakening so that neurological function can be assessed.

Sevoflurane, a recently introduced inhalational agent, has properties which favour its use in carotid surgery. In addition to its low blood gas solubility coefficient allowing early awakening, sevoflurane maintains cerebral autoregulation[28] and has minimal direct cerebral vascular effect.[29] Although remifentanil, an ultra short-acting opioid which is metabolized rapidly after its infusion is stopped, allows rapid awakening and neurological assessment, it may have profound effects on blood pressure and heart rate, especially in combination with propofol and vecuronium. Nevertheless, we have used remifentanil as part of a balanced anaesthetic with encouraging results. Adequate analgesia must be provided before remifentanil infusion is discontinued to avoid excessive post-operative hypertension.[30]

Before carotid cross-clamping, heparin (75–100 units/kg) is administered intravenously. Application of the carotid cross-clamp is often associated with an increase in blood pressure. Mild increases in blood pressure up to about 20% above preoperative levels are acceptable, but excessive increases should be controlled. Heparin is generally not reversed after closure of the artery but if the surgeon is not satisfied with haemostasis at the time of wound closure, a small dose of protamine (0.5 mg/kg) may be given.

Blood pressure and arterial CO_2 management

Arterial blood gases are checked after tracheal intubation and when necessary during the surgical procedure to ensure adequate oxygenation and normocapnia. Hypercapnia should be avoided as it will only vasodilate blood vessels supplying the normal brain without affecting those supplying the ischaemic regions which are presumably already maximally dilated. This diverts blood from the ischaemic areas to the normal areas (intracranial steal), thus further aggravating cerebral ischaemia. Hypocapnia, on the other hand, may increase flow to the ischaemic area by constricting the blood vessels in the normal areas (Robin Hood effect) and could be beneficial. However, hypocapnia causes a global reduction in cerebral blood flow and it is generally accepted that the changes in cerebral blood flow associated with changes in CO_2 in these individuals are unpredictable. Normocapnia is therefore preferred.

The preoperative blood pressure of individual patients should give guidance to a 'target' mean arterial blood pressure in the perioperative period. Cerebral autoreguation in these patients may be impaired and the autoregulation curve is shifted to the right in uncontrolled or poorly controlled hypertensive patients. As autoregulation may be completely lost in ischaemic areas, maintaining an adequate blood pressure is a critical factor in the maintenance of cerebral blood flow. If the blood pressure decreases below the individual patient's normal level, 'lightening' anaesthesia by reducing isoflurane concentration or decreasing propofol infusion rate within acceptable limits should be done before using a vasopressor. Use of vasopressor to elevate the blood pressure during cross-clamp may be necessary, but it has been shown to induce ventricular dysfunction[24] and in one early series was associated with a four-fold increase in the incidence of myocardial infarction,[31] although a recent study has disputed these findings.[32] If necessary, phenylephrine (0.1–0.5 μg/kg/min)

infusion can be administered judiciously. On the other hand, patients who remain hypertensive during anaesthesia may require intravenous hypotensive agents (nitroglycerine infusion 1–5 μg/kg/min) for control. Surgical manipulation of the carotid sinus may cause marked alteration in heart rate and blood pressure. These reflexes can be minimized by prior local infiltration with lignocaine. Should EEG changes occur shortly after infiltration, one must be aware that the injection may have been into the carotid artery, resulting in transient CNS lignocaine toxicity.[33]

Monitoring

Cardiovascular and respiratory monitoring

In addition to routine monitoring, an intra-arterial cannula is placed under local anaesthesia before induction, to continuously monitor blood pressure throughout the perioperative period and facilitate the sampling of arterial blood gas analysis. Alternatively, in low-risk patients, a rapidly cycling non-invasive blood pressure device can be used during induction and the arterial cannula place before surgery starts. Central venous pressure, pulmonary capillary wedge pressure, cardiac output and/or urine output are indicated in patients with high cardiac risks, such as those who have had a recent myocardial infarction or those with significantly compromised left ventricular function. End-tidal CO_2, checked against an arterial blood gas sample obtained after induction, facilitates the continuous maintenance of $PaCO_2$ within the patient's normal range.

CNS monitoring

No special monitoring is required in awake patients operated on under regional anaesthesia. When general anaesthesia is employed, although no difference in stroke rate has been convincingly demonstrated between patients treated with routine carotid shunting or selective shunting and without shunting,[34–37] physiological considerations dictate that it is still prudent to monitor brain function during crossclamping of the carotid artery. A summary of available modalities can be found in Table 15.3.

Electrophysiological monitoring

Electroencephalogram: the 16-channel conventional EEG remains the gold standard as a sensitive indicator of inadequate cerebral perfusion.[38] The unprocessed EEG displays voltage as a function of time. Proper use of this technique is tedious and time consuming and interpretation of the raw EEG is not easy – certainly in the setting of an operating theatre! Furthermore, at the

Table 15.3   Summary of available CNS Monitoring during CEA

Monitor	Advantages	Disadvantages
Awake patient	Continuous neurological assessment Avoids the risks of general anaesthesia Lower incidence of postoperative hypertension Shorter ICU stay	Requires patient cooperation, ability to lie flat, anxiety, hyperventilation with potential risk of cerebral ischaemia, risk of autonomic disturbances, nausea, vomiting and airway obstruction
EEG (16-channel)	Gold standard	Cumbersome, difficult to interpret Not suitable for theatre environment
EEG (computer processed) CFM, DSA, etc.	Easier to use than 16 channel Less cumbersome set-up	More than one channel needed for reasonable detection of ischaemia Embolic events not easily detectable
Somatosensory evoked potentials	Can detect subcortical ischaemia	Cumbersome Intermittent monitor with 'time lag' Affected by anaesthetic agents
Stump pressure	Measures retrograde perfusion pressure Easy to perform Cheap	Unreliable, does not reflect regional blood flow
rCBF	Measures cerebral blood flow	Expensive Invasive Requires steady state Intermittent
TCD	Continuous Non-invasive Relatively easy to use Can be used pre-, intra- and postoperatively Detects emboli Detects shunt malfunction	Not as sensitive as EEG Measures flow velocity and not CBF 5–10% failure rate due to lack of ultrasonic window
NIRS	Continuous Non-invasive Easy to use	Extracranial contamination a problem No defined ischaemic thresholds yet

usual rate of 25 mm/s, a 270 m strip of paper is produced for a three-hour case. Nevertheless, intraoperative neurological complications have been shown to correlate well with EEG changes indicative of ischaemia.[38,39] Ipsilateral or bilateral attenuation of high-frequency amplitude or development of low-frequency activity seen during carotid crossclamping is indicative of cerebral hypoperfusion. The computer-processed EEG[40–42] and somatosensory evoked potential[43–47] have also been found to be useful.

The processed EEG generally simplifies the raw data and displays them as either average power or voltage. This allows less experienced observers to concentrate on how the parameters are changing with respect to time instead of trying to mentally analyse them. Although computer-processed EEG are easier to interpret, they have been shown to be less accurate than the 16-channel EEG.[48] Despite extensive studies on the use of EEG to detect haemodynamic insufficiency during carotid cross-clamping and reported success in individual series, review of the literature fails to establish a definite and conclusive role for EEG monitoring in reducing the incidence of perioperative stroke (Table 15.3).

Somatosensory evoked potentials

SSEPs (medial nerve stimulation) have been shown to be useful during carotid endarterectomy.[43–47] Early studies indicate that intraoperative loss of late cortical components has been associated with a worsening of neuropsychological abilities and in some instances with subsequent stroke.[49] With the exception of one study,[50] recent studies suggest that SSEP monitoring is useful for cerebral perfusion during carotid cross-clamping and has similar sensitivity and specificity to conventional EEG. Because of the need for computer averaging, it does not provide continuous real-time monitoring. Stable anaesthesia must also be maintained to minimize the influence of anaesthetic agents on the amplitude. In general, >50% reduction or complete loss of amplitude of the cortical component is considered to be a significant indicator of inadequate cerebral perfusion. In contrast to conventional EEG, SSEP monitors the cortex as well as the subcortical pathways in the internal capsule, an area not reflected in the cortical EEG.[51]

Measurement of stump pressure (internal carotid artery back pressure)

Since one important determinant of cerebral blood flow is perfusion pressure, it seems reasonable to assume that the distal arterial pressure in the ipsilateral hemisphere during carotid occlusion would provide some indication of collateral CBF.[52] Stump pressure represents the mean arterial pressure measured in the carotid stump (the internal carotid artery cephalad to the common carotid cross-clamp) after cross-clamping of the common and external carotid arteries. Stump pressure measurement represents the pressure transmitted retrograde along the ipsilateral carotid artery from the vertebral and contralateral carotid arteries and has been postulated to provide a useful indicator of the adequacy of collateral circulation.[53,54] Early reports of stump pressure measurements concluded that stump pressure <50 mmHg required the placement of a shunt to avoid postoperative neurological complications.[53,55] Unfortunately, several studies have demonstrated the unreliability of stump pressures, with ischaemic EEG changes reported despite stump pressures in excess of 50 mmHg and a normal CBF (>24 ml/min/100g) with stump pressures <50 mmHg.[56,57] On balance, extreme values (<25 mmHg or >50 mmHg) are probably useful indicators of the state of the cerebral circulation, but not the intermediate values.[58,59]

Intraoperative measurement of CBF

Intraoperative CBF measurement has also been used to determine the need for placement of shunts,[40] but the associated cost makes it prohibitive for general use. This involves the intra-arterial injection of 20 mCi of the inert radioactive gas xenon 133 and measuring the wash-out of β emissions by extracranial collimated sodium iodide scintillation counter focused on the parietal cortex. The initial slope or fast component of the wash-out curve relates directly to regional blood flow. Newer measurement techniques involve single-photon emission computed tomography of inhaled xenon. Both techniques are useful as research tools, but very few centres have the equipment and expertise required to produce accurate results.

Transcranial Doppler Ultrasonography

TCD is an attractive technique for the detection of cerebral ischaemia during cross-clamping of the carotid artery because it is continuous and non-invasive and the transducer probes can be used successfully without impinging on the surgical field. It is also an important tool in the preoperative assessment and postoperative care of patients with carotid disease.[60–66]

Cerebral ischaemia is considered severe if mean velocity in the middle cerebral artery (FV) after clamping is 0–15% of preclamping value, mild if 16–40% and absent if >40%. This criterion correlates well with subsequent ischaemic EEG changes and hence can be used as an indication for shunt placement. TCD has been successfully used to detect intraoperative cerebral ischaemia,[61] malfunctioning of shunts due to kinking,[64] high-velocity states associated with hyperperfusion syndromes,[65] as well as intra- and postoperative emboli.[67,68] TCD appears to be a useful adjunct to other monitoring modalities such as EEG.[69]

Emboli, high-intensity 'chirps', are easily detectable using TCD and, interestingly, surgeons will tend to adapt their operative technique to minimize embolus generation.[67] Emboli can occur throughout the operation but are more frequent during dissection of the carotid arteries, upon release of ICA cross-clamp and during wound closure.[68,70–72] Although the clinical significance of TCD-detected emboli is not yet fully understood, they probably represent adverse embolic events during surgery.[68,72] The rate of microembolus generation can indicate incipient carotid artery thrombosis, has been related to intraoperative infarcts and can predict postoperative neuropsychological morbidity.[70,73] Following the introduction of intraoperative TCD monitoring, some centres have reported a reduction in operative stroke rates.[74]

Following closure of the arteriotomy and release of carotid clamps, FV will typically increase immediately to levels above baseline and gradually correct back to the preclamping baseline over the course of a few minutes.[73] This hyperaemic response is to be expected as the dilated vascular bed vasoconstricts in autoregulatory response to an increased perfusion pressure. However, approximately 10% of patients are at increased risk of cerebral oedema or haemorrhage because of gross hyperaemia with velocities 230% of baseline value lasting from several hours to days.[75,76]

This persistent postoperative hyperaemia, likely to occur in patients with high-grade stenosis, is probably the result of defective autoregulation in the ipsilateral hemisphere as a reduction in blood pressure is effective in normalizing FV and alleviating the symptoms.[77] TCD provides the means of early detection and effective treatment of this potentially fatal complication.

Finally, a progressive fall in velocity postoperatively to below preclamping baseline levels can be indicative of postoperative occlusion of the ipsilateral carotid artery and can be an indication for reexploration of the endarterectomy. The development of sudden symptoms postoperatively should prompt an immediate TCD examination and early reexploration.

Near infrared spectroscopy

NIRS, first described by Jobsis, continues to receive considerable attention as a monitor of cerebral oxygenation.[78] By using near infrared light, cerebral oximetry can theoretically be used to monitor haemoglobin oxygen saturation (HbO_2) in the total tissue bed including capillaries, arterioles and venules. One of the limitations of this technology is its inability to reliably differentiate between intra- and extracranial blood. However, during CEA, as the external carotid artery is clamped, most of the contamination due to extracranial blood flow is removed. There is now some evidence to suggest that it is possible to obtain useful intraoperative information about cerebral oxygenation in those undergoing CEA using NIRS. In patients undergoing CEA under general anaesthesia, changes in jugular venous oxyhaemoglobin saturation and middle cerebral artery blood velocity correlate well with changes in cerebrovascular haemoglobin oxygen saturation (Sco_2).[79] Similarly, Samara et al demonstrated that NIRS can be used to track changes in carotid blood flow in the majority of patients undergoing CEA under regional anaes-

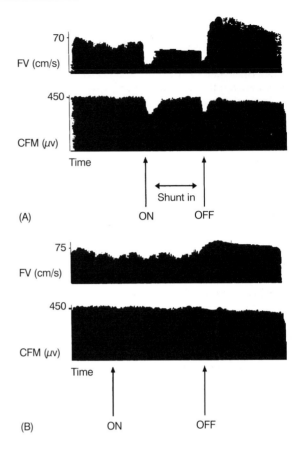

Figure 15.1 Graphic display of right middle cerebral artery flow velocity (FV) and cerebral function analyzing monitor (CFM) in two patients undergoing carotid endarterectomy. (A) On cross-clamping the carotid artery (IN), FV and CM decrease, indicating cerebral ischaemia. Insertion of a shunt restores the signals to the preclamping value. Hyperaemia is observed upon release of carotid artery cross-clamp at the end of the procedure (OFF). (B) Cross-clamping of the carotid artery results in no significant change in either FV or CFM, hence no shunt was used. Hyperaemia is also observed upon release of clamp but to a lesser degree than in (A).

Table 15.4   Intraoperative shunting and cerebral blood flow velocity (FV) in 1495 CEAs (compiled from reference[68])

Change in cerebral blood flow velocity on cross-clamping	Shunt used	% of patients with postoperative stroke
<15%	Yes	0
<15%	No	46
16–40%	Yes	3.9
16–40%	No	0.6
>40%	Yes	4.4
>40%	No	0.7

thesia.[80] Kirkpatrick et al observed that NIRS-based measurements can provide a warning of severe cerebral ischaemia (SCI) with high specificity and sensitivity provided the extracranial vascular contamination is accounted for.[81] There was a good correlation between the % reduction in FV on cross-clamp application and the internal carotid artery associated change in $HB_{diff}(ICA-\Delta Hb_{diff})$. An $ICA-\Delta Hb_{diff}>6.8$ μmol/l was 100% specific for SCI and $ICA-\Delta HB_{diff}<0.5$ μmol/1 was 100% sensitive for excluding ischaemia.

Despite numerous publications on the use of NIRS in carotid endarterectomy, its use as a monitoring tool for detecting cerebral ischaemia remains undefined.

Intraoperative cerebral protection

Although a detailed account of this appears in Chapter 3, a rational approach to cerebral protection from an anaesthetist's viewpoint is discussed briefly here. The approach is dependent on the surgeon's decision regarding the placement of shunts. Where the carotid shunt is never used, it is reasonable to administer a bolus of thiopentone 5 mg/kg prior to cross-clamping of the carotid artery. With selective shunting according to EEG, thiopentone should not be given as it will interfere with monitoring (although it can be used if SSEP monitoring is used). Shunting would be a more effective cerebral protective manoeuvre under these circumstances. If routine carotid shunting is used, thiopentone is not necessary if the shunt is functioning adequately, but may be given if additional pharmacological protection is desired. Administration of thiopentone is always associated with systemic cardiovascular depression and therefore should always be used with caution.

The decision on whether to shunt or not is generally made by the surgeon. There are those who shunt routinely, some who never use shunts and others that shunt selectively according to signs of cerebral ischaemia detected by monitoring of the CNS during carotid artery cross-clamping. Gummerlock and Neuwelt reviewed the literature and found no difference in stroke or mortality rates, although they favour the use of shunts routinely.[82] We have combined the results from these studies to compile Table 15.5.

Propofol, etomidate and benzodiazepines have also been shown to produce dose-related decreases in cerebral metabolic rate and cerebral blood flow. Although each of these drugs has properties that may make it useful during CEA,[83,84] available data based on animal models have yet to establish a definitive cerebroprotective effect associated with the administration of these agents.[85–87] Similarly, conflicting evidence surrounds the issue of a potential cerebroprotective effect associated with isoflurane during CEA.[25,26,88]

In addition to the above anaesthetic drugs, several other drugs are being evaluated for use as cerebroprotective agents. Nimodipine, a calcium channel blocker, has been shown to be efficacious in this regard. It has been of proven benefit in the treatment of vascular spasm after subarachnoid haemorrhage.[89] Interestingly, it is not clear whether this drug acts by an effect on the vascular smooth muscle or if its primary mechanism of action is directly on the neurone. Free radical scavenging may provide a means of defence against ischaemic brain damage. If given within 8 h of injury, methylprednisolone has been shown to improve outcome in patients with spinal cord injury,[90] but whether it has a place in cerebral protection is yet to be demonstrated. Other drugs like dizocilipine maleate,[91] an excitatory neurotramsmitter antagonist, and U74006F,[91] a free radical scavenger, are being investigated for cerebroprotective effect.

Non-pharmacological methods of cerebral protection include mild hypothermia (temperature about 35°C) which may be achieved easily and may decrease cerebral metabolism sufficiently with no obvious disadvantages.

Table 15.5 Combined results of carotid endarterectomy series from the literature

Procedure	Patients	Neurological deficit Number of patients (%, range)	Mortality Number of patients (%, range)
Without shunt*	4253	165 (3.8, 1.1–80)	59 (1.4, 0–2.0)
With shunt	4303	163 (3.8, 21–71)	71 (1.7, 05–3.5)
Selective use of shunt	4287	197 (4.6, 14–62)	46 (1.1, 0.5–1.5)

*Data compiled from the literature based on reference[72].

Combined or staged CEA and coronary artery bypass grafts

As mentioned earlier, more than 50% of patients undergoing CEA have overt coronary artery disease: previous infarct, angina or ischaemic electrocardiographic abnormalities.[92] Similarly, up to a fifth of patients undergoing coronary artery bypass grafting have duplex ultrasound-detected moderate carotid stenosis (>50%); of those, 5.9–12% have stenosis >80%.[93–95] Therefore, it is not surprising that stroke complicates 1–4% of all coronary bypass operations.[96,97] There are many potential causes for coronary bypass-related stroke, namely embolization from the carotid arch, endocardium or pump oxygenator, hypoperfusion related to occlusive arterial lesion or intracerebral haemorrhage.[98] Coronary angiography, advocated by some as a routine investigation for all patients undergoing CEA,[99] has been used to select high-risk patients for staged CEA or combined with coronary artery bypass graft (CABG).[99,100]

However, when the procedures are combined, the risk of both stroke and mortality is increased up to 21% and 11.7% respectively.[103–108] Although this may in part be due to a selection bias towards high-risk patients, the unacceptably high rate of complications has prompted us to abandon this procedure at our instiution.[100–103] When staged procedures are planned, it is preferable to operate on the presenting lesion first.[104,105]

Extracranial/intracranial bypass grafting

Anastomosing the extracranial to the intracranial arterial circulation (EC/IC bypass) should in theory increase cerebral blood flow to ischaemic areas thus reducing the risk of stroke.[104–106] Unfortunately, controversial as they are, the results of the only large prospective randomized study on EC/IC failed to demonstrate a superior outcome in those patients who had EC/IC bypass performed and medical therapy alone.[112] As a result, the popularity of this procedure for preventing strokes in patients with carotid stenosis has declined markedly. However, prophylactic EC/IC bypass procedures are increasingly performed for patients in whom therapeutic occlusions are required for controlling aneurysmal or vascular legions not amenable to surgical clipping, such as giant internal carotid artery aneurysms with wide necks. Nevertheless, the procedures carry a significantly higher mortality than carotid endarterectomy, which in part may be due to patient selection.

Although the perioperative management of patients presenting for EC/IC bypass surgery is similar to those presenting for CEA, particular attention is focused on preventing coughing and control of blood pressure to ensure patency of the graft.

POSTOPERATIVE CARE

In order not to negate the benefits of a carefully conducted anaesthetic, recovery should be smooth and prompt to allow immediate postoperative neurological assessment. We find that careful reduction in anaesthetic concentration with discontinuation upon wound closure results in satisfactory haemodynamics. Lignocaine 1–1.5 mg/kg may be given intravenously to minimize coughing during emergence. When the patient is responsive and awake, the trachea is extubated. It is advisable to leave the intra-arterial cannula in the immediate postoperative period to permit continuous blood pressure monitoring and blood gas analyses. All our patients receive supplemental oxygen and are monitored in recovery for two hours postoperatively. This allows rapid intervention should wound haematoma or intimal flap thrombosis develop.

Although the need for intensive care depends on the premorbid state and the intraoperative course, development of a 'neurovascular unit', allows most patients to be closely monitored for cardiac, respiratory and neurologic complications without the need for intensive care.

CAROTID CHEMORECEPTOR AND BARORECEPTOR DYSFUNCTION

Postoperative haemodynamic instability is common (incidence >40%) after CEA and is thought to be due to carotid baroreceptor dysfunction.[11,113] It is postulated that the atheromatous plaques dampen the pressure wave reaching the carotid sinus baroreceptors and with the removal of these plaques, increased stimulation of baroreceptors may result in bradycardia and hypotension.[114] The hypotension can be prevented or treated by blocking the carotid sinus nerve with a local anaesthetic,[115,116] intravenous fluid administration or, if necessary, the administration of vasopressor drugs, such as phenylephrine.[114,117]

Hypertension after CEA is less well understood and has been reported to be more common in patients with preoperative hypertension, particularly if poorly controlled,[11,113,118] and in patients who undergo CEA in which the carotid sinus is denervated. Hypertension after CEA in which the sinus nerve is preserved has been postulated to be due to temporary dysfunction of the baroreceptors or nerve, caused by intraoperative trauma.[113] Mild increases in blood pressure are acceptable (up to about 20% above preoperative levels), but marked increases are treated with an infusion of antihypertensive drugs such as nitroglycerine or esmolol[119] or repeated bolus doses of labetalol, depending on the patient's condition in the immediate postoperative period.

Other causes of haemodynamic instability after CEA include myocardial ischaemia/infarction, dysarrhythmias, hypoxia, hypercarbia, pneumothorax, pain, confusion and bladder distension, which should be treated appropriately.

Hypotension may lead to hypoperfusion and ischaemic infarction of the brain. Hypertension may increase the incidence of wound haematoma formation with possible airway obstruction. Similarly, myocardial ischaemia/infarction may occur as a result of either complication. Therefore, the blood pressure must be closely monitored and controlled in the immediate postoperative period. Regional anaesthesia appears to be associated with a higher incidence of postoperative hypotension while general anaesthesia is more often associated with postoperative hypertension.

CEA may result in loss of carotid body function with reduced ventilatory response to hypoxemia and hypercarbia.[120] This effect is further exaggerated in patients with coexisting pulmonary disease, especially in the presence of respiratory depressant drugs. Provision of supplemental oxygen and close monitoring of ventilatory status is particularly important in these patients and if necessary, they should be admitted to the high-dependency/intensive care unit for observation.

HYPERPERFUSION SYNDROME

Patients who become hypertensive in the postoperative period (defined as systolic BP >200 mmHg) are at a much greater risk of developing neurological deficit (10.2%) than patients who remain normotensive (3.4%).[118] Hypertension may cause excessive cerebral perfusion in a circulation unable to autoregulate, resulting in the hyperperfusion syndrome and intracerebral haemorrhage.[76] Patients at greatest risk include those with reduced preoperative hemispheric CBF caused by bilateral high-grade stenosis, unilateral high-grade carotid stenosis with poor collateral crossflow or unilateral carotid occlusion with contralateral high-grade stenosis.[121] The syndrome is thought to develop after restoration of perfusion to an area of the brain that has lost its ability to autoregulate because of chronic maximal vasodilatation. Restoration of blood flow after carotid endarterectomy thus leads to a state of hyperperfusion until autoregulation is reestablished, which occurs over a period of days.[76,122] Clinical features of this syndrome include headache (usually unilateral), face and eye pain, cerebral oedema, seizures and intracerebral haemorrhage.[76,121] Patients at risk for this syndrome should be closely monitored in the perioperative period and blood pressure should be meticulously controlled.

MYCOCARDIAL ISCHAEMIA AND INFARCTION

Perioperative myocardial infarction is the most frequent cause of mortality following CEA.[12] In general, the reported incidence of fatal postoperative myocardial infarction is 0.5–4% and the proportion of total perioperative mortality (within 30 days of operation) attributed to cardiac causes is at least 40%.[20,92,94,95,123] All causes of increased cardiac work must be minimized in order to avoid myocardial ischaemia. The patient should be warm, pain free, well oxygenated and normotensive with no tachycardia. Any signs of myocardial ischaemia should be treated immediately.

HAEMORRHAGE AND AIRWAY OBSTRUCTION

Persistent oozing from deep tissues, insecure ligation of vessels and the disruption of suture lines may all lead to bleeding into the wound site. This can be further aggravated by compromised coagulation due to the use of anticoagulants or antiplatelet agents. An expanding haematoma in the neck may cause airway obstruction and may necessitate reexploration of the wound site. Difficult intubation may result from this complication and the unwary may mismanage these patients with catastrophic results. Clinical assessment of the airway can underestimate the potential hazard of a rapid-sequence induction technique. Opening the sutures and letting the haemotoma out or surgical evacuation of the haematoma under local anaesthesia are possible options. If general anaesthesia is necessary, an inhalational induction with halothane or sevoflurane or a fibreoptic awake intubation are the methods of choice.

NEUROLOGICAL COMPLICATIONS

Postoperative neurological deficit occurs in 1–7% of patients after CEA, regardless of the anaesthetic technique.[11] Neurological deficits following CEA are multifactorial in origin: they may result from embolization at the site of surgery, cerebral ischaemia due to hypoperfusion or thrombosis at the endarterectomy site and intimal flap, or intracerebral haemorrhage. The manifestations include transient deficits and ischaemic strokes. All potentially treatable causes including thrombosis must be sought and re-exploration may be necessary. Re-exploration for evacuation of haematoma requires meticulous airway management as discussed above. Cranial nerve injuries have also been reported, the most commonly injured nerves being the hypoglossal and recurrent laryngeal nerves, leading to possible problems with upper airway control.[124] Damage to the recurrent laryngeal nerves may reduce the upper airway protective reflexes and place the patient at risk of aspiration, as well as cause airway obstruction (if the abductor fibres are the only ones affected).

CONCLUSION

CEA reduces the incidence of stroke in patients with symptomatic high-grade carotid artery stenosis. This benefit is only seen if the perioperative complications, mainly stroke and myocardial infarction, are kept to a minimum. Therefore, to realize the potential surgical benefits of this increasingly popular procedure, it is essential to provide the optimal physiological environment during surgery and this requires a thorough understanding of the pathophysiology of carotid artery disease and careful anaesthetic management. Research directed at areas of controversy, such as the application of neurological monitors, methods for the prevention and/or treatment of cerebral ischaemia and the development and evaluation of effective interventions to reduce the high cardiac morbidity and mortality associated with CEA are needed urgently.

REFERENCES

1. North American Symptomatic Carotid Endarterectomy Trial Collaborators. Beneficial effect of carotid endarterectomy in symptomatic patients with high-grade carotid stenosis. N Engl J Med 1991; 325: 445.

2. European Carotid Surgery Trialists Collaborative Group. MRC European Carotid Surgery Trial: interim results for symptomatic patients with severe (70–90%) stenosis or with mild (0–29%) stenosis. Lancet 1991; 337: 1235.

3. Mayberg MR, Wilson SE, Yatsu F et al. Carotid endarterectomy and prevention of cerebral ischemia in symptomatic carotid stenosis. Veterans Affairs Cooperative Studies Program 309 Trialist Group. JAMA 1991; 266: 3289.

4. Hobson RW, Weiss DG, Fields WS et al and the Veterans Affairs Co-operative Study Group. Efficacy of carotid endarterectomy for asymptomatic carotid stenosis. N Engl J Med 1993; 328(4): 221.

5. Executive Committee for the Asymptomatic Carotid Atherosclerosis Study. Endarterectomy for asymptomatic carotid artery stenosis. JAMA 1995; 273: 1421.

6. Parry A, McCollum C. Cerebrovascular disease. Surgery 1997; 16: 25–30.

7. Zarins CK. Carotid endarterectomy: the gold standard. J Endovasc Surg 1996; 3: 10–15.

8. Sundt TM Jr, Sandok BA, Whisnant JP. Carotid endarterectomy: complications and preoperative assessment of risk. Mayo Clin Proc 1975; 50: 301.

9. Sieber FE, Toung TJ, Diringer MN, Long DM. Preoperative risks predict neurological outcome of carotid endarterectomy related stroke. Neurosurgery 1992; 30: 847.

10. Adam HP Jr, Kassell NF, Mazuz H. The patient with transient ischemic attacks. Is this the time for a new therapeutic approach? Stroke 1984; 15: 371.

11. Asiddao CB, Donegan JH, Whitesell RC, Kalbfleisch JH. Factors associated with perioperative complications during carotid endarterectomy. Anesth Analg 1982; 61: 631.

12. Riles TJ, Kopelman I, Imparato AM. Myocardial infarction following carotid endarterectomy: a review of 683 operations. Surgery 1979; 85: 249.

13. Dyker ML, Wolf PA, Barner HJM et al. Risk factors in stroke. Stroke 1984; 1105–1111.

14. Frost EAM. Some inquiries in neuroanesthesia and neurological supportive care. J Neurosurg 1984; 60: 673.

15. Lanier WL, Stangland KJ, Scheithauer BW, Milde JH, Michenfelder JD. The effects of dextrose infusion and head position on neurological outcome after complete ischemia in primates: examination of a model. Anaesthesiology 1987; 66: 39.

16. Fieschi C, Agnoli A, Battistini N, Bozzao L, Prencipe M. Derangement of regional cerebral blood flow and of its regulatory mechanisms in acute cerebrovascular lesions. Neurology 1968; 18: 1166–1179.

17. Toronto Cerebrovascular Study Group. Risks of carotid endarterectomy. Stroke 1986; 17: 848.

18. Krul JMJ, Van Gijn J, Ackerstaff RGA, Theodoeides T, Vermevlen FE. Site and pathogenesis of infarcts associated with carotid endarterectomy. Stroke 1989; 20: 324.

19. Corson JD, Chang BB, Shah DM, Leather RP, Leo BM, Karmody AM. The influence of anesthetic choice on carotid endarterectomy outcome. Arch Surg 1987; 122: 807.

20. Prough DS, Scuderi PE, Stullken E, Davis CH Jr. Myocardial infraction following regional anaesthesia for carotid endarterectomy Can Anaesth Soc J 1984; 31: 192.

21. Harbaugh RE. Carotid surgery using regional anesthesia. Tech Neurosurg 1997; 3(1); 25–33.

22. Winnie AP, Ramamurthy S, Durrani Z, Radonjic R. Interscalene cervical plexus block: a single injection technique. Anesth Analg 1975; 54: 370.

23. Wells BA, Keats AS, Cooley DA. Increased tolerance to cerebral ischaemia produced by general anesthesia during temporary carotid occlusion. Surgery 1963; 54: 216.

24. Smith JL, Roizen MF, Cahalan MK et al. Does anesthetic technique make a difference? Augmentation of systolic blood pressure during carotid endarterectomy: effects of phenylephrine versus light general anesthesia and of isoflurane versus halothane on the incidence of myocardial ischemia. Anesthesiology 1988; 69: 846.

25. Messick JM Jr, Casement B, Sharborough F, Milde LN, Michenfelder JD, Shundt TM Jr. Correlation of regional cerebral blood flow (rCBF) with EEG changes during isoflurane anesthesia for carotid endarterectomy: critical rCBF. Anesthesiology 1987; 66: 344.

26. Michenfelder JD, Sundt TM, Fode N, Sharbrough FW. Isoflurane when compared to enflurane and halothane decreases the frequency of cerebral ischemia during carotid endarterectomy. Anesthesiology 1987; 67: 336.

27. Cucchiara RF, Sundt TM, Michenfelder JD. Myocardial infraction in carotid endarterectomy patients anesthetized with halothane, enflurane or isoflurane. Anethesiology 1988; 69: 783.

28. Gupta S, Heath K, Matta BF. The effect of incremental doses of sevoflurane on cerebral pressure autoregulation in humans: a transcranial Doppler study. Br J Anaesth 1997; 79: 469–472.

29. Heath K, Gupta S, Matta BF. The effect of sevoflurane on cerebral haemodynamics during propofol anesthesia. Anesth Analg 1997; 85: 1284–1287.

30. Guy J, Hindman BJ, Baker KZ et al. Comparison of remifentanil and fentanyl inpatients undergoing craniotomy for supratentorial space-occupying lesions. Anesthesiology 1997; 86: 514–524.

31. Riles TS, Kopelman I, Unoarati AM. Myocardial infarction following carotid endarterectomy: a review of 683 operations. Surgery 1979; 85: 249.

32. Mutch WA, White IW, Donen N et al. Haemodynamic instability and myocardial ischaemia during carotid endarterectomy: a comparison of propofol and isoflurane. Can J Anasth 1995; 42: 577–587.

33. Perkins WJ, Lanier WL, Sharbrough FW. Cerebral and haemodynamic effects of lidocaine accidentally injected into the arteries of patients having carotid endarterectomy. Anesthesiology 1988; 69: 787.

34. Ferguson GG. Intra-operative monitoring and internal shunts: are they necessary in carotid endarterectomy? Stroke 1982; 13–287.

35. Green RM, Messick WJ, Ricotta JJ et al. Benefits, shortcomings, and costs of EEG monitoring. Ann Surg 1985; 201: 785.

36. Van Alphen HAM, Polman CH. The value of continuous intra-operative EEG monitoring during carotid endarterectomy. Acta Neurochir (Wien) 1988; 91: 95.

37. Reddy K, West M, Anderson B. Carotid endarterectomy without indwelling shunts and intraoperative electrophysiologic monitoring. Can J Neurol Sci 1987; 14: 131.

38. Sundt TM, Sharbrough FW, Piepgras DG. Correlation of cerebral blood flow and electroencephalograhic changes during carotid endarterectomy with results of surgery and hemodynamics of cerebral ischemia. Mayo Clin Proc 1981; 56: 533.

39. McFarland HR, Pinkerton JA, Flyre D. Continuos electroencephalographic monitoring during carotid endarterectomy. J Cardiovasc Surg 1988; 29: 12.

40. Rampil IJ, Holzer JA, Quest DO, Rosenbaum SH, Correl JW. Prognostic value of computerized EEG analysis during carotid endarterectomy. Anesth Analg 1983; 62: 186.

41. Spackman TN, Faust RJ, Cucchiara RF, Sharbrough FW. A comparison of aperiodic analysis of the EEG with standard EEG and cerebral blood flow for detection of ischemia. Anesthesiology 1987; 66: 229.

42. Tempelhoff R, Modica PA, Grubb RL Jr, Rich KM, Holtmann B. Selective shunting during carotid endarterectomy based on two channel computerized electroencephalographic compressed spectral array analysis. Neurosurgery 1989; 24: 339.

43. Lam AM, Manninen PH, Ferguson GG, Nantau W. Monitoring electrophysiologic function during carotid endarterectomy: a comparison of somatosensory evoked potential and conventional electroencephalogram. Aneshesiology 1991; 75: 15.

44. Dinkel M, Schweiger H, Goerlitz P. Monitoring during carotid surgery: somatosensory evoked potentials vs. carotid stump pressure. J Neurosurg Anesth 1992; 4: 167.

45. Fava E, Bortolani E, Ducati A, Schieppati M. Role of SEP in identifying patients requiring temporary shunt during carotid endarterectomy. Electroenceph Clin Neurophysiol 1992; 84: 426.

46. Tiberio G, Floriane M, Giulini SM et al. Monitoring of somatosensory evoked potentials during endarterectomy: relationship with different haemodynamic parameters and clinical outcome. Eur J Vasc Surg 1991; 5: 647.

47. Haupt WF, Horsch S. Evoked potential monitoring in carotid surgery: a review of 994 cases. Neurology 1992; 42: 835.

48. Young WL, Moberg RS, Omstein E et al. Electroencephalographic monitoring for ischemia during carotid endarterectomy: visual versus computer analysis. J Clin Monit 1988; 4: 78.

49. Brinkman SD, Braun P, Gangi S, Morrell RM, Jacobs LA. Neuropsychological performance one week after carotid endarterectomy reflects intraoperative ischemia. Stroke 1984; 15: 497.

50. Kearse LA Jr, Brown EW, McPeck K. Somatosensory evoked potentials sensitivity relative to electroencephalography for cerebral ischemia during carotid endarterectomy. Stroke 1992; 23: 498.

51. Gerwetz BL, McCaffrey M. Intraoperative monitoring during carotid endarterectomy. Curr Probl Surg 1987; 24: 478.

52. Michal VV, Heighal L, First P. Zeitweilige shunts in der vaskularen chirurgie. Thoraxchirurgie 1966; 14: 35.

53. Hayes RJ, Levinson SA, Wylie EJ. Intraoperative measurement of carotid back pressure as a guide to operative management for carotid endarterectomy. Surgery 1972; 72: 953–960.

54. Moore WS, Hall AD. Carotid artery backpressure: a test of cerebral tolerance to temporary carotid occlusion. Arch Surg 1969; 99: 702–710.

55. Ricotta JJ, Charlton MH, Deweese JA. Determining Criteria for shunt placement during carotid endarterectomy: EEG versus backpressure. Ann Surg 1983; 198: 642.

56. Kelly JJ. Callow AD, O'Donnel TF et al. Failure of carotid stump pressures: its incidence as a predictor for a temporary shunt during carotid endarterectomy. Arch Surg 1979; 114: 1361.

57. McKay RD, Sundt TM, Michenfelder JD et al. Internal carotid artery stump pressure and cerebral blood flow during carotid endarterectomy. Anesthesiology 1976; 45: 390.

58. Modica PA, Tempelhoff R. A comparison of computerized EEG with internal carotid artery stump pressure for detection of ischemia during carotid endarterectomy. J Neurosurg Anesth 1989; 1: 211.

59. Cherry KJ Jr, Roland CF, Hallett JW Jr et al. Stump pressure, the contralateral carotid artery, and electroencephalographic changes. Am J Surg 1991; 162: 185.

60. Halsey JH, McDowell HA, Gelman S, Morawetz RE. Blood velocity in the middle cerebral artery and regional cerebral blood flow during carotid endarterectomy. Stroke 1989; 20: 53.

61. Jorgensen LG, Schroeder TV. Transcranial Doppler for detection of cerebral ischemia during carotid endarterectomy. Eur J Casc Surg 1992; 6: 142.

62. Padayachee TS, Bishop CCR, Gosling RG, Browse NL. Monitoring cerebral perfusion during carotid endarterectomy. Case report. J Cardiobasc Surg 1990; 31: 112.

63. Powers AD, Smith RR, Graeber MC. Transcranial Doppler monitoring of cerebral flow velocities during surgical occlusion of the carotid artery. Neurosurgery 1989; 25: 383.

64. Spencer MP, Thomas GI, Moehring MA. Relationship between middle cerebral artery blood flow velocity and stump pressure during carotid endarterectomy. Stroke 1992; 23: 1439.

65. Steiger HJ, Schaffler L, Boil J, Leichti S. Results of microsurgical carotid endarterectomy: a prospective study with transcranial doppler sonography and EEG monitoring and elective shunting. Acta Neurochir (Wien) 1989; 100: 31.

66. Aaslid R, Markwalder TM, Nornes H. Noninvasive transcranial doppler ultrasound recording of flow velocity in basal cerebral arteries. J Neurosurg 1982; 57: 769.

67. Spencer PM, Thomas GI, Nicholls SC, Savage LR. Detection of middle cerebral artery emboli during carotid endarterectomy using transcranial doppler ultrasonography. Stroke 1990; 21: 415.

68. Halsey JH. Risks and benefits of shunting in carotid endarterectomy. Stroke 1992; 23: 1583.

69. Bornstein NM, Rossi GB, Treves TA, Shifrin EG. Is transcranial Doppler effective in avoiding the hazards of carotid surgery? Cardiovasc Surg 1996; 4(3): 335–337.

70. Jansen C, Ramos LM, Van Heesewijk JP et al. Impact of microembolism and hemodynamic changes in the brain during carotid endarterectomy. Stroke 1994; 25: 992.

71. Gravilescu T, Babikian VL, Cantelmo NL et al. Cerebral microembolism during carotid endarterectomy. Am J Surg 1995; 170: 159.

72. Gaunt ME, Martin PJ, Smith JJ et al. Clinical relevance of intraoperative embolisation detected by transcranial Doppler ultrasonography during carotid endarterectomy: a prospective study of 100 patients. Br J Surg 1994; 81: 1435.

73. Naylor AR, Whyman M, Wildsmith JAW et al. Immediate effects of carotid clamp release on middle cerebral artery blood flow velocity during carotid endarterectomy. Eur J Vasc Surg 1993; 7: 308.

74. Jansen C, Vriens EM, Eikelboom BC et al. Carotid endarterectomy with transcranial Doppler and electroencephalographic monitoring. A prospective study in 130 operations. Stroke 1993; 24: 665.

75. Sbarigia E, Speziable F, Gianoni MF et al. Post-carotid endarterectomy hyperperfusion syndrome: preliminary observations for identifying at risk patients by transcranial Doppler sonography and the acetzolamide test. Eur J Vasc Surg 1993; 7: 252.

76. Schroeder T, Sillesen H, Sorensen O et al. Cerebral hyperperfusion syndrome following carotid endarterectomy. J Neurosurg 1987; 28: 824.

77. Jorgensen LG, Schroeder TV. Defective cerebrovascular autoregulation after carotid endarterectomy. Eur J Vasc Surg 1993; 7: 370.

78. Jobsis FF. Noninvasive, infrared monitoring of cerebral and myocardial oxygen sufficiency and circulatory parameters. Science 1977; 198: 1264–1267.

79. Williams IM, Picton A, Farrell A, Mead DE, Mortimer AJ, McCollum CN. Light-reflective cerebral oximetry and jugular bulb venous oxygen saturation during carotid endarterectomy. Br J Surg 1994; 81: 1291–1295.

80. Samra SK, Dorje P, Zelenock GB, Stanley JC. Cerebral Oximetry in patients undergoing carotid endarterectomy under regional anesthesia. Stroke 1996; 27: 49–55.

81. Kirkpatrick PJ, Lam J, Al-Rawi P, Smielewski P, Czosnyka M. Defining thresholds for critical ischaemia using near infrared spectroscopy (NIRS) in the adult brain. J Neurosurg 1998; 89: 389–394.

82. Gummerlock MK, Neuwelt EA. Carotid endarterectomy: to shunt or not to shunt? Stroke 1988; 19: 1485.

83. Farling PA. Intravenous anaesthetics. Curr Opin Anaesthesiol 1990; 3: 689–693.

84. Renou AM, Vernhiet J, Macrez P et al. Cerebral blood flow and metabolism during etomidate anaesthesia in man. Br J Anaesth 1979; 50: 1047–1050.

85. Hoffman WE, Prekezws C. Benzodiazepines and antagonists: effects on ischemia. J Neurosurg Anesth 1989; 1: 272–277.

86. Milde LN, Milde JH. Preservation of cerebral metabolites by etomidate during incomplete ischemia in dogs. Anesthesiology 1986; 65: 272–277.

87. Weir DL, Goodchild CS, Graham DI. Propofol: effects on indices of cerebral ischemia. J Neurosurg Anesth 1989; 1: 284–289.

88. Young WL, Prohovnik I, Correll JW et al. Cerebral blood flow and metabolism in patients undergoing anesthesia for carotid endarterectomy. A comparison of isoflurane, halothane and fentanyl. Anesth Analg 1989; 68: 712–717.

89. Allan GS, Ahn HS, Preziose TJ et al. Cerebral arterial spasm – a controlled trail of nimodipine in patients with subarachnoid hemorrhage. N Engl J Med 1983; 308: 619–624.

90. Bracken MB, Shephard MJ, Collins WF et al. A randomized, controlled trial of methylprednisolone or naloxone in the treatment of acute spinal-cord injury. Results of the second National Acute Spinal Cord Injury Study. N Engl J Med 1986; 314: 397–403.

91. Michenfelder JD. Cerebral Protection and control of elevated intracranial pressure. Annual Refresher Course Lectures. J Assoc Anesthsiol 1990; 115: 1–4.

92. Masckey WC, O'Donnell TF, Callow AD. Cardiac risks inpatients undergoing carotid endarterectomy: impact on perioperative and long term mortality. J Vasc Surg 1990; 11: 226–234.

93. Brener BJ, Brief DK, Alpert J, Goldenkranz RJ, Parsonnet V. The risk of stroke in patients with asymptomatic carotid stenosis undergoing cardiac surgery: a follow-up study. J Vasc Surg 1987; 5: 269–279.

94. Schwartz LB, Bridgeman AH, Kieffer RW et al. Asymptomatic carotid artery stenosis and stroke in patients undergoing cardiopulmonary bypass. J Vasc Surg 1995; 21: 146–153.

95. Bernes ES, Kouchoukos NT, Murphy SF, Waring TH. Preoperative carotid artery screening in elderly patients undergoing cardiac surgery. J Vasc Surg 1992; 15: 313–323.

96. Ricotta JJ, Faggioli GL, Castilone A, Hassett JM. Risk factors for stroke after cardiac surgery: Buffalo Cardiac Cerebral Study Group. J Vasc Surg 1995; 21: 359–364.

97. Kuroda Y, Uchimoto R, Keieda R et al. Central nervous system complications after cardiac surgery: a comparison between coronary artery bypass and valve surgery. Anesth Analg 1993; 76: 222–227.

98. Mackey WC, Khabbaz K, Boyar R, O'Donnell TF Jr. Simultaneous carotid endarterectomy and coronary bypass: perioperative risk and long term survival. J Vasc Surg 1996; 24: 58–64.

99. Hertzer NR, Lees CD. Fatal Myocardial infraction following carotid endarterectomy. Ann Surg 1981; 194: 212–218.

100. Dunn EJ. Concomitant cerebral and myocardial revascularization. Surg Clin North Am 1986; 66: 385–395.

101. Fode NC, Sundt TM Jr, Robertson JT et al. Multicenter retrospective review and complication of carotid endarterectomy in 1981. Stroke 1986; 17: 370–376.

102. O'Donnell TF, Callow AD, Willet C et al. The impact of coronary artery disease on carotid endarterectomy. Ann Surg 1983; 198: 705–712.

103. Hertzer NR, Loop FD, Beven EG, O'Hara PJ, Krawjewski LP. Surgical staging for simultaneous coronary and carotid disease: a study including prospective randomization. J Vasc Surg 1989; 9: 455–463.

104. Rizzo RJ, Whittemore AD, Couper GS et al. Combined carotid and coronary revascularization: the preferred approach to the severe vasculopath. Ann Thorac Surg 1992; 54: 1099–1109.

105. Cambria RP, Ivarsson BL, Akins CW, Moncure AC, Brewster DC, Abbott WM. Simultaneous carotid and coronary disease: safety of the combined approach. J Vasc Surg 1989; 9: 56–64.

106. Chang BB, Darling C, Shah DM, Paty PSK, Leather RP. Carotid endarterectomy can be safely performed with acceptable mortality and morbidity in patients requiring coronary artery bypass grafts. Am J Surg 1994; 168: 94–97.

107. Curl GR, Lakshmikumar P, Raza ST, Lenely GA, Castilone AS, Ricotta JJ. Staged vs combined carotid endarterectomy in coronary bypass patients. Presented at the Ninth Eastern Vascular Society Meeting, Buffalo, May 5–7, 1995.

108. Coyle KA, Gray BC, Smith RB et al. Morbidity and mortality associated with carotid endarterectomy: effect of adjunctive coronary revascularization. Ann Vasc Surg 1995; 9: 21–27.

109. Takagi Y, Hashimoto N, Iwama T, Hayashida K. Improvement of oxygen metabolic reserve a after extracranial-intracranial bypass surgery in patients with server haemodynamic insufficiency. Acta Neurochir (Wien) 1997; 139: 52–56.

110. Schick U, Zimmermann M, Stolke D. Long-term evaluation of EC-IC bypass patency. Acta Neurochir (Wein) 1996; 138: 938–942.

111. Ishikawa T, Houkin K, Abe H, Isobe M, Kamiyama H. Cerebral haemodynamics and long-term prognosis after extracranial-intracranial bypass surgery. J Neurol Neurosurg Psychiatry 1995; 59: 625–628.

112. The EC/IC Bypass Study Group. Failure of extreacranial-intracranial arterial bypass to reduce the risk of ischemic stroke: results of an international randomized trail. N Engl Med 1985; 313: 1191–1200.

113. Bove EL, Fry WJ, Gross WS et al. Hypotension and hypertension as consequences of baroreceptor dysfunction following carotid endarterectomy. Surgery 1979; 85: 633–637.

114. Taylor E, Schmidex H, Scott RM, Wepsic JG, Ojemann RG. Reflex hypotension following carotid endarterectomy: mechanisms and management. J Neurosurg 1973; 39: 323.

115. Cafferata HT, Merchant RF, DePalma RG. Avoidance of postcarotid endarterectomy hypertension. Ann Surg 1982; 196: 465–472.

116. Pine R, Avellone JC, Hoffman M et al. Control of post-carotid endarterectomy hypotension with baroreceptor blockade. Am J Surg 1984; 147: 763–765.

117. Prough DS, Scuderi PE, McWhorter JM et al. Hemodynamic status following regional and general anesthesia for carotid endarterectomy. J Neurosurg Anesth 1989; 1: 35–40.

118. Towne JB, Bernhard VM. The relationship of postoperative hypertension to complications following carotid endarterectomy. Surgery 1980; 88: 575–580.

119. Cucchiara RF, Benefiel CJ, Matteo RS, DeWood M, Arbin MS. Evaluation of esmolol incontrolling increases in heart rate and blood pressure during endotracheal intubation in patients undergoing carotid endarterectomy. Anesthesiology 1986; 65: 528–531.

120. Wade JG, Larson CP, Hickey RF, Ehrenfield WK, Severinghaus JW. Effect of carotid endarterectomy on carotid chemoreceptors and baroreceptors in man. N Engl J Med 1970; 282: 823.

121. MarFarlane R, Moskowitz MA, Saskas DE et al. The role of neuroeffector mechanisms in cerebral hyperperfusion syndrome. J Neurosurg 1991; 75: 845–855.

122. Bernstein M, Fleming JFR, Deck JHN. Cerebral hyperperfusion after carotid endarterectomy: a cause of cerebral hemorrhage. Neurosurgery 1984; 15: 50–56.

123. Rubin JR, Pitluk HC, King TA et al. Carotid endarterectomy in a metropolitan community: the early results after 8535 operations. J Vasc Surg 1988; 7: 256–260.

124. Spiekermann BF, Stone DJ, Bogdonoff DL, Yemen TA. Airway management in neuroanaesthesia. Can J Anaesth 1996; 43: 820–834.

16

PRINCIPLES OF PAEDIATRIC NEUROANAESTHESIA

Fay Gilder & John M. Turner

INTRODUCTION

The spectrum of paediatric neurosurgical disease differs from that of adult disease and, additionally, varies according to the age group to which the child belongs. Clinical presentation is also very much dependent on age. A good working knowledge of normal neonatal, infant and child physiology and pharmacology and paediatric neurophysiology and neuropharmacology is required for the practice of paediatric neurosurgical anaesthesia. Furthermore, an understanding of the particular requirements for safe paediatric anaesthetic practice is mandatory.

THE NEONATE

It is beyond the scope of this book to give a detailed account of normal neonatal physiology and pharmacology and therefore the following discussion will be brief, highlighting the particular problems that need attention.

THE PRETERM INFANT

Preterm infants can be grouped as those born between 31 and 36 weeks gestation (moderate preterm) and those born between 24 and 30 weeks gestation. Both groups have several problems in common which are usually more severe in the more premature. Deaths in the older group are uncommon (5% mortality at 31/40, <1% by 36/40) while deaths in the younger age group account for 70% of neonatal mortality. The commonest causes are respiratory distress syndrome, sepsis and intraventricular haemorrhage. Medical management of the latter disorder may involve neurosurgical intervention.

Normal neonatal physiology is markedly different from that of any other age group due to immature organ systems, particularly the lungs (surfactant deficient), liver and kidneys. The circulation is transitional between foetal and adult and the ductus arteriosus may remain patent or be reopened by hypoxia or fluid overload. Blood volume is 90–100 ml/kg and the preterm infant is more susceptible to hypoglycaemia due to limited glycogen stores.

Neonatal neuroanatomy and physiology varies with age. At term the brain weighs approximately 335g (10–15% total body weight). It doubles in weight by six months, triples by one year and reaches adult weight by 12 years of age. The skull at birth consists of ossified plates (calvaria) separated by fibrous sutures and two fontanelles, anterior and posterior. The posterior fontanelle closes by the second or third month while the anterior fontanelle may remain open until 16 months of age. Complete ossification occurs by 12–16 years.

Table 16.1 summarizes the differences in paediatric neurophysiology with age. Intracranial pressure is positive on the first day of life but may become subatmospheric for the next few days.[6,7] It is at this time that preterm infants in particular are at risk of intracranial haemorrhage. Acute rises in intracranial pressure are poorly tolerated despite the presence of open fontanelles because of the rigidity of the dura mater. The neurological status of the child deteriorates rapidly under these conditions. However, a slow increase in intracranial pressure is accommodated more easily due to expansion of the fontanelles and separation of the sutures. The intracranial pressure may be estimated by palpation of, or by the use of a transducer placed on, the anterior fontanelle.

Normally the neonatal cerebral vessels are able to autoregulate throughout a range of systolic blood pressure (45–160 mmHg).[8] Trauma, infection or other intracranial pathology and anaesthesia may impair or abolish autoregulation and under these circumstances cerebral perfusion is determined by intracranial pressure and mean arterial pressure (CPP = MAP – ICP). Cerebral blood flow varies directly with changes in arterial carbon dioxide tension between 20 and 80 mmHg.[9]

Intracerebral steal and inverse intracerebral steal occur in children. The former is when vasodilatation of normal cerebral vessels reduces blood flow through vessels that have lost the ability to autoregulate (for example, arteriovenous malformations, vascular tumours). Inverse steal occurs when normal vessels vasoconstrict, resulting in diversion of blood flow to the abnormal vessels.

The overall metabolic rate for brain tissue in children is higher than that of adults although is lower in premature infants (see Table 16.1).

Preoperative assessment of the preterm neonate must therefore include an assessment of the intracranial pressure, an appreciation of the risk of intraventricular haemorrhage and the likelihood of apnoea postoperatively. Table 16.2 summarizes the information required from the preoperative assessment of the preterm neonate.

Conditions presenting in the premature infant

The commonest conditions presenting in this age group are those related to the presence of hydrocephalus requiring neurosurgical intervention.

Table 16.1	Paediatric neurophysiology					
	Adult	Child (mean age 6)	3–12 y	6–40 months	Neonate	Preterm
Brain metabolic rate for O_2 (ml O_2/min/100g)	3.5	5.8	5.2[1]	2.3*[2]		
CBF (ml/100g/min)			100[1,2]	90[3]	40–42[4,5]	40–42[4,5]
ICP (mmHg)	8–18	2–4			Positive ICP day 1 subatmospheric for next few days[6]	

*anaesthetized

TERM INFANTS (37/40–44/40 GESTATIONAL AGE)

Term infants are at much lower risk of the hazards associated with prematurity. The organ systems, however, are still immature, in particular the liver. The airway and ventilation are more difficult to manage, not only because of the difficulties expected in the neonate (large head and tongue, anterior and cephalad larynx, large floppy epiglottis, narrowest point in the airway the cricoid ring) but also because of the increased size of the skull due to hydrocephalus. Ventilatory difficulties may also exist since the pulmonary reserve may be poor due to a small volume functional residual capacity and because the higher metabolic rate results in an increased oxygen consumption. Cardiac output is age dependent and therefore bradycardia is poorly tolerated. Blood volume is 80 ml/kg. Intravenous access may be awkward. Neurophysiology is as described in the previous section.

Assessment of the term infant must take into account much of what was written for the preterm infant but particular attention must be paid to the following:

- history of birth and presentation of neurological condition;
- current neurological status and risk of deterioration;
- evidence and assessment of other congenital abnormalities;
- maternal history;
- whether vitamin K has been administered.

Conditions presenting in this age group

Hydrocephalus, intracranial haemorrhage, craniosynostosis, arteriovenous malformations, meningomyelocoele and encephalocoele.

THE INFANT FROM FOUR WEEKS TO TWO YEARS OF AGE

By this time most of the organ systems have matured and the major problem is likely to be that of the underlying neurological condition and any associated congenital abnormalities. Conditions seen in this age group are similar to those in the previous age groups but the incidence of intracranial tumours is increased. The Arnold–Chiari malformation may present at this age.

CHILDREN OVER TWO YEARS OF AGE

The spectrum of disease presenting to neurosurgeons is different in this age group. The peak incidence of paediatric intracranial tumours is between the ages of five and eight years.[9] There is also a higher incidence of head injury.

NEUROPHARMACOLOGY

The sensitivity of children to anaesthetic drugs varies with age. All inhalational agents increase cerebral blood flow and therefore have a tendency to raise ICP. Nitrous oxide also increases intracranial pressure and cerebral metabolic rate for oxygen ($CMRO_2$). Halothane raises intracranial pressure, may reduce the vascular reactivity to carbon dioxide (CO_2) and reduces $CMRO_2$. Isoflurane increases cerebral blood flow but less so than halothane and at less than 1 MAC autoregulation is thought to be preserved. It has very

Table 16.2	Preoperative assessment of the preterm neonate
History	Cause and extent of neurosurgical disorder, incidence of apnoeas, neonatal course so far, birth trauma, maternal drug history, medication
Examination	*Cardiovascular system* Evidence of congenital heart defects (in particular patent ductus arteriosus, ventricular septal defect and patent foramen ovale), congestive cardiac failure *Respiratory system* Respiratory distress syndrome, bronchopulmonary dysplasia, pulmonary barotrauma, ventilatory requirements, apnoeas *Central nervous system* Lack of primitive reflexes (suck, swallow, gag), intraventricular haemorrhage, hydrocephalus, fits *Gastrointestinal* Necrotizing enterocolitis, source of nutrition (parenteral/enteral), herniae *Metabolic* Electrolyte derangements, hypo- or hyperglycaemia *Haematological* Coagulopathies (N.B. hepatic function is immature), anaemia, thrombocytopaenia, DIC *Miscellaneous* Evidence of sepsis, evaluation of state of hydration and evidence of hypovolaemia
Investigations	Full blood count, urea and electrolytes, coagulation studies, serum glucose, echocardiography, ultrasound examinations, appropriate radiographs

little effect on CO_2 reactivity but does raise intracranial pressure. There are no published data on the cerebral effects of enflurane, sevoflurane and desflurane in children.

All intravenous induction agents either have no effect on cerebral blood flow (CBF) or reduce it, with the exception of ketamine. Thiopentone reduces ICP and $CMRO_2$ although it does not attenuate the hypertensive response to intubation as well as propofol. Propofol, in addition to the effects for thiopentone, preserves autoregulation. Ketamine increases CBF, $CMRO_2$ and CSF pressure and therefore is not used in neuroanaesthetic practice.

Opioids have little effect on CBF and $CMRO_2$ providing ventilation is maintained; benzodiazepines (midazolam, diazepam) decrease CBF and $CMRO_2$, while non-depolarizing muscle relaxants have minimal effects. Suxamethonium slightly increases CBF and ICP.

BRIEF PRINCIPLES OF PAEDIATRIC NEUROANAESTHESIA

This section includes both the general principles of paediatric anaesthesia and issues specific to neuroanaesthesia.

PREOPERATIVE PREPARATION

The theatre should be warmed to a temperature of 24°C and efficient warming equipment provided. Table 16.3 includes a list of equipment that must be available. Consideration must be given to the position of the child required for the procedure and all necessary bolsters, supports and padding must be to hand.

PREMEDICATION

Children with intracranial pathology should not be given sedative premedication. This is because heavy premedication may depress respiration, while the associated risks of hypoxia and hypercapnia, delay recovery from anaesthesia and complicate neurological assessment in the recovery period. An exception is made in children with vascular lesions at risk of or with a previous history of subarachnoid haemorrhage. Atropine (0.02 mg/kg) may be given to minimize vagal effects on the heart (in children under six months of age). β-Blockers are sometimes used to reduce systemic hypertension.

INDUCTION OF ANAESTHESIA

An ideal induction will avoid increases in ICP, include rapid control of the airway and achieve haemodynamic stability, resulting in prevention of hypoxia,

Table 16.3 Equipment for paediatric anaesthesia

Intravenous access	An assortment of peripheral, central venous and arterial cannulae
Airway management	Laryngoscopes, blades, airways, facemasks, t-piece, introducers, armoured endotracheal tubes
Temperature measurement	Core and peripheral devices
Temperature maintenance	Warming mattress, forced air blanket, wrapping
Infusions	Pumps, infusion/blood warmers, giving sets with burettes
Monitoring	Oesophageal stethoscopes of different diameters, urometer, ECG, SpO_2, NIBP, invasive pressure monitoring, neuromuscular monitoring
Miscellaneous	Urinary catheters, nasogastric tubes

hypoventilation and systemic hypertension. Induction of anaesthesia can be inhalational or intravenous with assisted bag and mask ventilation. A sleep dose of thiopentone (5–7 mg/kg) or propofol (2–4 mg/kg) is administered; sevoflurane provides a useful alternative for inhalational induction. Muscle relaxation is achieved by the use of a non-depolarizing muscle relaxant or suxamethonium if rapid airway control is necessary. Fentanyl, sufentanil or lignocaine can be given to attenuate the hypertensive response to intubation. After intubation with an armoured oral endotracheal tube (or nasotracheal tube), an oesophageal or precordial stethoscope, an oesophageal or nasopharyngeal temperature probe and throat pack should be placed. There is considerable risk of endotracheal tube displacement on positioning, particularly in the small child. From full flexion to full extension of the head in the neonate, the tip of the endotracheal tube (ETT) moves an average of 14.3 mm(7–28 mm).[10] It must be obsessively checked once in position and secured appropriately (without obstructing central venous return). Considerable attention must be paid to maintaining body temperature. The surface area of the head is large in comparison to that of the child's body and considerable heat loss will occur here. Continuous monitoring of core temperature is essential. The eyes must be protected.

MAINTENANCE OF ANAESTHESIA

A balanced anaesthetic technique of oxygen, nitrous oxide, a short-acting opioid, a muscle relaxant and a low-dose inhalational agent (isoflurane or sevoflurane) is probably the technique of choice for most neuroanaesthetics. Air may be substituted for nitrous oxide, particularly where intracranial air is likely, but this requires the use of an increased concentration of the volatile agent. A continuous infusion of propofol may also be used as an alternative to a volatile agent.

Fluid balance is important. A combination of crystalloid (to replace normal fluid requirements), colloid and blood may be needed. Dextrose-containing solutions are avoided except in infants or where there is documented hypoglycaemia because hyperglycaemia is thought to worsen tissue damage caused by local cerebral ischaemia. Volume status can be estimated by peripheral perfusion (normal capillary refill time less than 3 s), heart rate, blood pressure and central venous pressure and also by the degree of respiratory swing on the arterial or oximetric trace.

Agents used to control intracerebral volume include mannitol and frusemide. Both are given after induction with the aim of reducing brain bulk and therefore intracranial pressure and the pressures required for surgical retraction. The dose of mannitol is 0.5–1.0 g/kg and of frusemide is 0.5 mg/kg.

HYPOTENSIVE TECHNIQUES

Hypotensive techniques, though required infrequently, may be used when considerable blood loss is anticipated, for example in spinal surgery and craniofacial operations. Systolic blood pressures of 50 mmHg and above are well tolerated by children under the age of 10 and of 70 mmHg and above in children over 10.

Techniques advocated include the use of isoflurane, sodium nitroprusside, tubocurarine and trimetaphan. Invasive pressure monitoring is mandatory and the length of hypotension should be kept to a minimum.

EMERGENCE AND RECOVERY

Emergence should be smooth with no coughing on the ETT (this can be facilitated by lignocaine 1–1.5 mg/kg). A speedy recovery aids neurological assessment. This can be achieved by withholding opioid supplement for the last 30 min of the operation, reducing inhalational agent concentration and giving boluses of short-acting sedatives (propofol) to maintain the required anaesthetic depth. Full neuro-muscular function must have returned (child – eyes open, hip flexion; older child – neck flexion). Planned admission to ICU for postoperative ventilation may be appropriate for certain major cases.

POSTOPERATIVE CARE

This includes regular frequent neurological assessment as well as routine physiological assessment (heart rate, respiratory rate, blood pressure, urine output).

ANAESTHESIA FOR SPECIFIC NEUROSURGICAL PROCEDURES

HYDROCEPHALUS

Hydrocephalus occurs because an imbalance exists between CSF production and absorption. The cerebral ventricles become dilated and there may be a dispro-portionate increase in head size. Hydrocephalus is classified as follows.

- *Non-obstructive*: this is very rare. It is due to either an overproduction of CSF by a choroid plexus papilloma or a lack of brain matter with subsequent ventricular dilatation.
- *Obstructive, communicating*: CSF is not reabsorbed by the arachnoid granulations. This may be caused by an arachnoiditis following meningitis or intraven-tricular haemorrhage.
- *Obstructive, non-communicating*: there are three common sites of obstruction:
  1. the aqueduct of Sylvius (due to stenosis or atresia);
  2. occlusion of the foramina of Luschka and Magendie due to basal adhesions (this is the commonest site of obstruction and is usually due to IVH);
  3. the Arnold–Chiari malformation.

Clinical Features

Congenital hydrocephalus may be diagnosed antena-tally as part of a routine ultrasound examination or after birth when accelerated head growth will predate symptoms and signs of raised intracranial pressure. Posthaemorrhagic hydrocephalus is usually detected by ultrasound examination in the neonatal period. Hydrocephalus in the older child usually presents with signs or symptoms of raised intracranial pressure or of the underlying condition (tumour, inflammation). The sunset sign and abducens nerve palsy are very late signs and indicate advanced hydrocephalus.

Investigations

Investigations include serial ultrasound scans, occip-itofrontal circumference measurements, skull radiog-raphy to detect suture separation and computed tomography.

Management

Management depends on the underlying cause and the degree of ventricular dilatation. Medical management includes the use of acetazolamide or isosorbide but these are only temporizing measures. Surgical procedures performed depend on the nature of the hydrocephalus.

Non-communicating hydrocephalus

Ventriculoperitoneal shunt (lateral ventricle to peri-toneum) is the commonest surgical shunt procedure and has the advantage of reducing the need for shunt revision as a result of growth of the child. The most common complications are infection and obstruction of the shunt, necessitating shunt revision.

Ventriculoatrial shunt (lateral ventricle to right atrium) is much less common. Disadvantages of this procedure include the higher incidence of complica-tions (infection, obstruction, pulmonary thromboem-bolism leading to cor pulmonale) and the need for more frequent revisions with growth of the child.

Ventriculopleural shunt (lateral ventricle to pleural cavity) is rarely performed unless placement of a ventriculoperitoneal or ventriculoatrial shunt is not possible.

Anterior third and fourth ventriculostomy are opera-tions which re-establish CSF drainage routes from the third or fourth ventricle into the basal cisterns. Third ventriculostomy is commonly performed as an endo-scopic procedure using a rigid ventriculoscope, which is inserted into one of the lateral ventricles and guided into the third ventricle. Diathermy and a balloon dilatational technique are used to establish an opening in the floor of the third ventricle.

Communicating hydrocephalus

Lumboperitoneal shunt (lumbar subarachnoid space to peritoneum) is used when the ventricles are small or for managing communicating hydrocephalus.

Anaesthetic Considerations

Preoperative management should include a general assessment of the child and a neurological exami-nation for evidence of raised intracranial pressure.

Any associated conditions should be optimized. While sedative premedication should not be prescribed, atropine may be useful. Preoperative preparation includes planning for positioning of the child, particularly if the head is large. Intubation under these circumstances can be difficult. Attention must also be paid to maintaining body temperature.

Induction may be intravenous or inhalational with the aim of maintaining oxygenation and haemodynamic stability and preventing an acute rise in intracranial pressure. Spontaneous ventilation is contraindicated when the cranium is open and during the positioning of ventriculoatrial (risk of air embolus) or ventriculopleural (risk of pneumothorax) shunts. During the course of the procedure the following should be anticipated: hypotension at the time of cerebrospinal fluid tap and bradycardia or other arrhythmias at the time of ventricular catheter placement. If a ventriculoatrial shunt is being placed using the atrial tip as an endocardial ECG lead, monitoring the change in QRS complex allows correct placement of the atrial tip.

Recovery should be rapid and postoperatively routine craniotomy observations are usually all that are required. Codeine phosphate (1 mg/kg IM or orally) can be used for analgesia.

SKULL ABNORMALITIES

Craniosynostosis and craniofacial dysmorphism are the commonest skull abnormalities seen in the paediatric population.

Craniosynostosis occurs as a result of premature fusion of the cranial vault sutures. It is classified according to the shape of the skull reflecting the underlying prematurely closed suture. The sutures that are involved include the left or right coronal (anterior plagiocephaly), the metopic (trigonocephaly), the sagittal (scaphycephaly), the left or right lambdoidal (posterior plagiocephaly), the bilateral coronal (anterior brachycephaly) or the bilateral lambdoidal (posterior brachycephaly).

In the craniofacial dysostosis syndromes (Crouzon's, Apert's) additional cranial base and facial sutures are involved. Particular anaesthetic considerations are as for craniosynostosis with the additional problem of the management of a potentially difficult airway. These children may also have severe nasal obstruction.

Elevated intracranial pressure secondary to rapid brain growth within the rigid skull may occur depending on how many sutures are fused and how quickly the problem is recognized. Hydrocephalus affects 5–10% of the patients with craniofacial anomalies. The aetiology is not always clear but may be secondary to cranial base stenosis.

Anaesthetic Considerations

Preoperative assessment will include particular attention to examination of the airway, for evidence of raised intracranial pressure and other associated congenital anomalies. Preoperative preparation must take into consideration the position of the patient, the potential requirement for massive blood transfusion and maintenance of body temperature. Surgery involves division of the skull along the suture lines (craniectomy). Deformities of the eyebrow and forehead may require the use of bone from the skull, rib or pelvis. There is the potential for considerable blood loss and a high risk of air embolus.

Induction may be inhalational or intravenous with the aim of rapid control of the airway. A nasotracheal tube may be used if there is no associated choanal atresia. A wide-bore intravenous cannula should be placed and an intraarterial cannula may be useful in all but the simplest of craniectomies. Hyperventilation and a forced diuresis may be required to reduce the volume of the intracranial contents. A precordial Doppler probe may be used to detect air embolism.

While some cases may require postoperative care in an intensive care unit, most can be woken up immediately. Codeine phosphate is used for postoperative analgesia and routine postcraniotomy observations are all that is necessary.

CRANIAL AND SPINAL DYSRAPHISM

These are disorders of an embryonic stage called dorsal induction. Dorsal induction occurs in the third and fourth weeks of gestation and is the formation and migration of the neural tube with subsequent development of the anterior tube into the primitive brain structures. Defects include anencephaly, encephalocoele, myelomeningocoele and meningocoele.

Encephalocoele occurs as a result of failure of midline closure of the skull. The defect is usually occipital but frontal encephalocoeles do occur and carry a better prognosis in the long term. Diagnosis is usually made antenatally on ultrasound. Prognosis depends on the degree of accompanying brain herniation. Treatment is neurosurgical closure.

Spina bifida results from failure of fusion of the vertebral column. It can be accompanied by herniation of the meninges and spinal cord. The abnormalities that occur are classified according to their severity.

Spina bifida occulta has an incidence within the general population of 10%. It is usually of no clinical significance. The vertebrae are bifid with no associated herniation of meninges or spinal cord. In a small population there may be tethering of the spinal cord which, if not corrected, may result in irreversible neurological abnormalities of the bladder and lower limbs as the child grows. There is often an associated cutaneous abnormality (sinus, naevus, tuft of hair) in the lumbar region. All children with such cutaneous markers need to be investigated by ultrasound and referred if necessary to a neurosurgeon.

Spina bifida cystica has an incidence of one in 1000 live births in the United Kingdom. Twenty per cent of the lesions are meningocoeles while 80% are meningomyelocoeles; 70% occur in the lumbosacral area. The sac is usually covered by the meninges but may have ruptured with a resulting CSF leak. Nerve lesions may be sensory (asymmetrical) or motor, involving the bladder and/or anus (causing a neurogenic bladder and a patulous anus with faecal incontinence). The neurological examination is usually consistent with the level of the meningomyelocoele. As many as 80% of affected infants will have accompanying hydrocephalus and a proportion of meningomyelocoeles are associated with the Arnold–Chiari malformation (see below). Children with spina bifida may also have orthopaedic (talipes, congenital dislocation of the hip, kyphosis, scoliosis), renal, cardiac, visceral and chromosomal defects. Most cases are diagnosed antenatally. MRI scanning is used to accurately map the region. Early surgical closure is attempted in order to prevent infection of the defect. A ventricular shunt may also be needed if hydrocephalus is present.

Anaesthetic Considerations

Preoperative assessment should include a thorough work-up to exclude any associated congenital anomalies and an awareness of the preexisting neurological deficits. In the case of a cervical encephalocoele the neck is often short and rigid, making endotracheal intubation potentially difficult. Infants with meningomyelocoeles may be volume depleted secondary to evaporative and third space losses from the exposed area so rehydration may be necessary preoperatively.

Surgery takes place with the patient in the prone position so padding and appropriate head support must be planned in advance. Fluid losses (both blood and evaporative) may be considerable so equipment for administering and warming replacement fluids will be needed. Hypothermia should be anticipated and measures taken to prevent it.

Induction may be performed with the child in the lateral or supine position (with the infant's body supported on a ring bolster protecting the defect) and may be inhalational or intravenous (although some centres advocate awake intubation). Care should be taken when fixing the endotracheal tube both because displacement may occur on repositioning the child and because oral secretions may loosen the tapes. Placement of a throat pack may help to absorb some of the secretions. A large-bore intravenous cannula should be placed and for encephalocoeles requiring craniotomy, an arterial line may be useful. Additional monitoring includes core temperature and urine output. The need to use a nerve stimulator to identify the nerves intraoperatively necessitates the use of short-acting neuromuscular blockers and peripheral neuromuscular monitoring.

Once prone, bolsters should be placed under the shoulders and hips to allow the abdomen to move freely with respiration. The child should be mechanically ventilated and anaesthesia maintained with an appropriate gaseous mixture. Intraoperative pitfalls include large fluid and heat losses.

Most patients can be extubated immediately postoperatively when fully awake. Codeine phosphate and paracetamol are usually all that is required for analgesia.

THE ARNOLD–CHIARI MALFORMATION

The Arnold–Chiari malformation is an abnormality of the brain and skull base, a prolapse of the medulla, cerebellum and fourth ventricle through an abnormal foramen magnum into the cervical canal. Syringomyelia may also be present. Signs and symptoms include difficulty swallowing, recurrent aspiration, apnoeic episodes, stridor and an absent gag reflex. Ultrasound scanning will reveal ventricular dilatation, usually with hydrocephalus. Surgery is complex and fraught with risk and includes posterior fossa decompression, enlargement of the foramen magnum and cervical laminectomy.

Anaesthetic Considerations

Ventilatory control may be abnormal in these patients, necessitating pre- and postoperative ventilation. Pulmonary disease secondary to aspiration may be present. Stridor may occur which does not resolve immediately postoperatively and may ultimately require placement of a tracheostomy. In patients with Arnold–Chiari malformation care must be taken to avoid excessive rotation of the neck when turning the patient prone. Anaesthesia management is as for posterior fossa exploration (see later).

NEUROLOGICAL TUMOURS (ANTERIOR, MIDDLE AND POSTERIOR FOSSA)

Intracranial tumours are the second most common childhood neoplasms. There are significant differences in the presentation, site and incidence according to age. The peak incidence of childhood tumours is between five and eight years of age, and, unlike adults, up to 70% are found in the posterior fossa. Table 16.4 summarizes briefly a few of the more common neoplasms and some of the ways in which they may present. Childhood tumours may present with signs of obstructive hydrocephalus, raised intracranial pressure and focal neurological deficits. The diagnosis and investigation of intracranial neoplasms include MRI and CT scanning and, in older children, stereotactic biopsy.

Anaesthetic Considerations

Preoperative assessment must focus on the identification of raised intracranial pressure and elucidation of focal neurological deficits. If cranial nerve palsies are likely, the presence of a gag reflex should be sought. Brainstem vital centres may be involved and potential respiratory problems could therefore also exist. If the tumour is likely to be neuroendocrine in origin or is situated close to the hypothalamic-pituitary axis the child may exhibit symptoms and signs of hormonal deficit or excess. The surgery may include the placement of an extraventricular drain or ventricular shunt or the child may already have had one placed previously. If so, it is important to ascertain if the shunt is working adequately. It is likely that corticosteroids (dexamethasone) will have been administered and prophylactic anticonvulsants may have been prescribed. These should continue intraoperatively and through into the postoperative period.

Preoperative preparation must anticipate requirements for positioning, reduction of brain mass, large blood and fluid losses, avoidance of hypothermia and electrolyte disturbances. Tumours in the anterior and middle fossae usually require the patient to be positioned supine with a 15–20° head-up tilt. Positioning for posterior fossa surgery depends on the neurosurgical preference. The operation can be performed in either the prone, semiprone or sitting position. It is very difficult to position children under the age of 3–4 years in the sitting position so they are placed prone or semiprone. However, older children may be operated on in the sitting position. If the sitting position is to be used the legs should be bandaged to promote venous return and all pressure points padded aggressively.

Table 16.4	Presentation of common childhood neoplasms	
Tumour	Age of presentation	Clinical presentation
Supratentorial astrocytoma	Variable	Focal neurological signs. Signs of ↑ICP
Cystic cerebellar astrocytoma	2–10	Midline cerebellar signs
Ependymoma	1st decade of life (somewhat later with spinal tumours)	Space-occupying lesions with focal signs. Obstructive hydrocephalus common at presentation
Optic nerve glioma	Peak incidence 0–5	Impaired vision
Brainstem glioma	5–15	Obstructive hydrocephalus, progressive brainstem signs
Medulloblastoma a/PNET	Bimodal, 3–4y, 8–9y	Raised ICP arising from obstructive hydrocephalus caused by IV ventricular compression. Cerebellar signs not a common presentation
Cranial germ cell tumours	Teenage children	Commonly pineal tumours with obstructive hydrocephalus secondary to obstruction of aqueduct
Craniopharyngioma	Occur throughout childhood	Hydrocephalus, ↑ICP, hypothalamic-pituitary dysfunction

PNET = primitive neuroectodermal tumour

The conduct of anaesthesia is as described for hydrocephalus surgery with some important additions.

- Nasotracheal tubes are often used both for ease of fixation and the potential for less movement as the head is manipulated. Alternatively, armoured orotracheal tubes may be used.
- Monitoring for posterior fossa surgery involves positioning of either a precordial (or oesophageal) stethoscope or precordial Doppler probe to detect venous air emboli. Continuous capnography is also valuable in this regard.
- Central venous pressure monitoring aids assessment of fluid losses and if the catheter tip is positioned near the right atrium, it may be possible to aspirate air emboli should they occur. Once again, this is an essential requirement if the patient is positioned sitting.
- If surgery occurs close to the brainstem or other eloquent areas, evoked potential monitoring may be required. Brainstem function can also be monitored by observing for arrhythmias or changes in blood pressure.
- Urinary catheterization may well be required although in very small children efforts are made to avoid doing so. This is because of the potential for meatal damage and introduction of infection. In these instances the bladder can usually be expressed intraoperatively.
- Diabetes insipidus is a complication of pituitary surgery and may occur intraoperatively. All cases require continuous monitoring of urine output and fluid balance as well as regular serum and urine electrolyte estimations. If it occurs, it should be treated early on with 1-deamino-8d-arginine vasopressin (DDAVP).

Postoperatively the patient should have recovered fully from the effects of the anaesthesia. All brainstem and cranial nerve reflexes must be intact. Frequent temperature monitoring is necessary after surgery near the hypothalamus as body temperature may rise. Diabetes insipidus may occur, as may the syndrome of inappropriate antidiuretic hormone secretion. Seizures are common postoperatively, hence the need for prophylactic anticonvulsants. Elective admission to a paediatric intensive care unit may be required.

ARTERIOVENOUS MALFORMATIONS

Arteriovenous malformations (AVM) are congenital or acquired and arise from abnormal development of the arteriolar-capillary bed. Clinically AVMs present most commonly during adolescence. Symptoms and signs may include those of an intracranial bleed, raised intracranial pressure and seizures and sometimes the presenting complaint is headache. Congestive heart failure may be the clinical presentation in infants and small children if the AVM is particularly large. Some AVMs may require embolization before surgery. Indeed, as interventional radiological techniques become more sophisticated, embolization may be the only treatment required.

Anaesthetic considerations

The anaesthetic management is similar to that of a craniotomy for tumour surgery. Blood losses are difficult to manage and may be great. Intraoperative hypertension should be avoided and as mentioned earlier, a sedative premedication may be administered to smooth induction in a distressed child. In experienced hands the surgical mortality is less than 5%.

ANEURYSM OF THE VEIN OF GALEN

This arteriovenous malformation is rare. However, it a significant challenge to both the neuroanaesthetist and neurosurgeon. The surgical mortality is 75%. There are two clinical pictures.

1. The neonate with congestive heart failure, macrocrania and a bruit heard over the anterior fontanelle. The operative risk is highest at this age. Embolization of the aberrant vessels may be attempted before surgery.
2. Older children often present with migraine-like headache. Mortality is much lower in this group.

Surgical mortality is high due to uncontrollable blood loss. The use of techniques such as profound hypothermia and extracorporeal circulation have been attempted but with poor results.

Anaesthetic considerations

Management of anaesthesia involves aggressive cardiovascular monitoring and avoidance of hypotension, hypovolaemia and low diastolic blood pressure (which will jeopardize myocardial perfusion). Clipping of the aneurysm results in an acute rise in ventricular afterload and cardiac failure which may necessitate the use of inotropes and vasodilators. Nitrous oxide is avoided because of its negative inotropy and ability to increase pulmonary vascular resistance.

SPINAL CORD SURGERY

Conditions necessitating surgery on the spine or spinal cord include spinal cord tumours, haematomata, abscesses, spondyloses, syringomyelia and tethered cord. Clinical presentation may include signs of motor and sensory deficits, pain and bladder and bowel symptoms.

Anaesthetic Considerations

Potential problems include positioning, blood loss and spinal cord monitoring. The patients are prone and care must be taken to prevent abdominal compression as an increase in intraabdominal pressure may divert blood from the abdominal veins to the vertebral plexi, increasing blood loss and worsening conditions at the surgical site. Several methods are used to monitor the spinal cord intraoperatively.

The wake-up test

Here anaesthesia is lightened, allowing the patient to wake up in a controlled fashion. The advantage of this test is the ability to assess anterior spinal cord (motor) function. Its disadvantages are the potential for the patient to cough and buck on the endotracheal tube, the risk of extubation in a prone patient and the fact that it assesses cord function at one point in time only.

Somatosensory evoked potentials (SSEPs)

Cortical SSEPs measure cortical response to peripheral nerve (posterior tibial nerve at the ankle or median nerve at the wrist) stimulation from the scalp adjacent to the somatosensory area. While these responses are modified variably by anaesthesia (more so by halothane than enflurane), perhaps the greatest difficulty in interpreting SSEPs is due to varying anaesthetic concentrations which make interpretation of changes impossible. Spinal SSEPs are also used and record responses from the epidural space by an electrode placed by the surgeon. The peripheral nerve is then stimulated and interference with spinal cord function during surgery can be detected by a marked drop in amplitude from control values. The major disadvantage of the technique is that it only assesses the sensory component.

Motor evoked potentials (MEPs)

This test involves stimulation of the motor cortex with a transcranial electric current or pulsed magnetic field.

EPILEPSY AND CORTICAL MAPPING

Surgery for epilepsy involves identification of the epileptogenic focus by cortical mapping followed by excision of the area. The technique for younger children (less than 4–6 years of age) involves general anaesthesia. In older more cooperative children, the technique of neuroleptanaesthesia is used (a combination of fentanyl and droperidol).

Anaesthetic Considerations

Drugs that modify the EEG must be avoided. As mentioned above, the patient must be awake and compliant so the technique of neuroleptanaesthesia is used. This will require explanation to the patient before they get to theatre. There is the potential for considerable blood loss which may be difficult to measure so a central line and arterial line should be placed under local anaesthesia before the start of the procedure. Equipment and drugs for emergency intubation may be required. Mannitol and frusemide are used to reduce intracranial volume and so optimize conditions for the neurosurgeon.

REFERENCES

1. Ogawa A, Sakurai Y, Kayama Y. Regional cerebral blood flow with age: changes in cerebral blood flow in childhood. Neurol Res 1989; 11: 173.

2. Settergen G, Lindblad B, Andpersson B. Cerebral blood flow and exchange of oxygen, glucose, ketone bodies, lactate, pyruvate and amino acids in anaesthetised children. Acta Paediat Scand 1980; 69: 457.

3. Mehta S, Kalsi H, Nai C, Menkes J. Energy metabolism of brain in human protein calorie malnutrition. Paediat Res 1977; 11: 290.

4. Younkin D, Reivich M, Jaggi J et al. Noninvasive method of estimating newborn regional cerebral blood flow. J Cereb Blood Flow Metab 1982; 2: 415.

5. Cross K, Dear P, Hathorn M et al. An estimation of intracranial blood flow in the newborn infant. J Physiol 1985; 289: 329.

6. Welch K. Intracranial pressure in infants. J Neurosurg 1980; 52: 693.

7. Raju T, Vidyasagar D, Papazafiratou C: Intracranial pressure monitoring in the neonatal ICU. Crit Care Med 1980; 8: 575.

8. Steward DJ. Neurosurgery. In: Steward DJ (ed) Manual of pediatric anesthesia, 4th edn. Churchill Livingstone, New York, 1995, p. 190.

9. Harwood-Nash DC. Primary neoplasms of the central nervous system in children. Cancer 1991; 67: 1223–1228.

10. Todres ID, De Bros F, Kramer SS et al. Endotracheal tube displacement in the newborn infant. J Paediat 1976; 89: 126.

17

THE ANAESTHETIC MANAGEMENT OF SPINAL INJURIES AND SURGERY TO THE CERVICAL SPINE

Karen J. Heath & Richard E. Erskine

INTRODUCTION

The management of the spine, especially the cervical spine during surgery and also during the resuscitation of patients with spinal injuries, has many important considerations for the anaesthetist, not least the potential to cause severe irreversible injury during tracheal intubation.

Trauma is the most common cause of spinal cord injury with an incidence of 3–4 per 100 000 population per year in the United States,[1] while estimates for the UK are 8.1 traumatic cases per 1 000 000 population.[2] These injuries can be devastating and often affect young adults with a long life expectancy.[3,4]

The cost of spinal injuries is immense, not only because the cost of caring for patients with spinal injuries is very high and may be spread over many years, but also because the victims of these injuries are usually young, healthy, tax-paying individuals.

Operations on the cervical spine are common neurosurgical procedures for congenital or acquired conditions which may result in compression of closely related neural structures.

Anaesthetists will be closely involved with the immediate resuscitation of patients with spinal injuries, the elective and emergency operative procedures to the spine and patients with chronic paraplegia presenting for emergency or elective surgery.

The aims of this chapter are to:

- outline the anatomy and biomechanics of the cervical spine;
- describe the emergency management of patients with cervical spine injuries;
- discuss anaesthesia for elective spinal surgery;
- discuss anaesthetic considerations for patients with acquired and congenital spinal pathology presenting for surgery;
- discuss the anaesthetic management of patients with paraplegia.

CLINICAL ANATOMY AND BIOMECHANICS

A basic understanding of the anatomy and biomechanics of the cervical spine is essential to the anaesthetist managing patients with neck injuries or for definitive surgery to the cervical spine.

The upper two and the lower five cervical vertebrae differ both anatomically and functionally and need to be discussed separately.[5,6]

UPPER CERVICAL SPINE

The occipitoatlantoaxial unit is the most complex osseous-articular structure within the human body. Its function is to support the head and to protect the spinal cord within its immediate surrounding structures while enabling flexion, extension and rotation of the upper neck to take place.

The first cervical vertebra, the *atlas*, has thick anterior and posterior arches that blend laterally into large masses. The upper convex surface articulates with the occipital condyles. The flatter inferior aspects of the masses articulate with the superior facet joints of the second cervical vertebra, the *axis*.

The transverse ligament of the atlas arises from two tubercles situated on the inner anterolateral aspect to enclose the odontoid peg (*dens*) of the axis on its posterior aspect. The dens arises as a central upward extension of the body of the axis. Alar and apical ligaments fan up from the dens to insert into the anterior margins of the foramen magnum.

LOWER CERVICAL SPINE

The five lower vertebrae of the neck conform to the typical shape of cervical vertebrae. They provide a protective bony canal for the spinal cord and at the same time allow flexion, extension and rotation of the neck. The laterally projecting transverse processes are well developed and contain a fenestration to permit the passage of the vertebral artery.

The facet joints between the cervical vertebral arches face downwards and forwards. The cervical intervertebral discs extending from the inferior surface of the body of C2 are attached above and below to hyaline articular cartilage on the surfaces of the adjacent vertebral bodies.

Anterior and posterior longitudinal ligaments extend the length of the spine.

The anterior longitudinal ligament passes upwards attached to the anterior aspects of the vertebral bodies, intervertebral discs and the anterior aspect of the arch of the atlas; it inserts into the base of the skull as the anterior atlantooccipital ligament. The posterior longitudinal ligament attaches to the dorsal surfaces of the vertebral bodies and the cartilages and fans out over the posterior aspects of the body of the axis, the odontoid peg and transverse ligament; it inserts into the basiocciput as the tectorial membrane.

The ligamentum flavum, less substantial in the neck than lower in the vertebral column, connects adjacent laminae and is complemented posteriorly by the interspinous and supraspinous ligaments. The supraspinous ligament termed the ligamentum nuchae in the neck terminates by inserting into the nuchal line on the base of the skull.

BLOOD SUPPLY TO THE SPINAL CORD[7]

The substance of the spinal cord is supplied by two posterior spinal arteries and the anterior spinal artery which runs along the anterior median fissure spinal. The anterior spinal artery is formed by the confluence of the two vertebral arteries and it is supplemented by anterior radicular arteries entering the subarachnoid space with each anterior spinal root. A few posterior radicular arteries enter with the posterior nerve roots but only make a small contribution to the blood supply of the spinal cord. The largest radicular arteries (the arteries of Adamkiewicz) enter with the T1 and T11 nerve roots; the T11 artery supplies the cord upwards and downwards, but the T1 artery only supplies the cord downwards.

The lower cervical part of the cord is thus a region of relative ischaemia and is vulnerable should the anterior spinal artery be compromised between the foramen magnum and C8, the 'cervical watershed'.[8] Spinal veins form loose-knit plexuses and drain into the segmental veins along the nerve roots.

Hickey has demonstrated a close rheological similarity between the perfusion of the spinal cord and the brain.[9]

MOVEMENT

The neck moves through 90° from full flexion to full extension. A third of this takes place in the upper segment and the rest in the lower cervical region, mostly around the C5–7 segments. Extension within the occipitoatlantoaxial complex is limited by contact of the posterior arch of the atlas with the occiput above and the axial arch below. The distance from the posterior arch of the atlas to the occiput is the *atlantoocipital gap* (AOG). A short AOG has been described as a common cause of difficult intubation.[10] Attempts to extend the head in a patient with a narrow AOG result in anterior bowing of the lower cervical vertebra and anterior displacement of the larynx.

Flexion and extension of the neck are reduced by 20% by the seventh decade. Most of this reduction occurs within the lower cervical segments and does not have a significant effect on the ease of direct laryngoscopy.[11]

The correct position to facilitate laryngoscopy for oral tracheal intubation is with the neck flexed and the head

extended at the atlantooccipital joint. This optimum position is often unachievable in patients with cervical spine pathology.[12]

STABILITY

Stability is defined as the ability of the spine, under conditions of physiological loading, to maintain relationships between vertebrae, so as not to damage the neural structures contained within the spinal column.[13] The stability of the spine is almost entirely the result of ligamentous attachments to bone and cartilage rather than muscle tone.

The transverse ligament normally permits a separation of 3 mm between the dens and the posterior aspect of the anterior arch of the atlas – the *atlas–dens interval* (ADI).

The area of the vertebral canal at the C1 level may be considered to be one-third odontoid peg, one-third cord and one-third space (Steel's rule of thirds).[14] Any posterior displacement of the odontoid peg from the arch of the atlas reduces the space available for the spinal cord (SAC). The SAC is measured on a lateral radiography as the luminal distance from the posterior aspect of the odontoid peg to the posterior border of the vertebral canal at the level of C1; this is normally 20 mm.

In the lower cervical spine the posterior longitudinal ligament and the structures anterior to it are considered to be the *anterior column*. Behind the posterior longitudinal ligaments are the structures which comprise the *posterior column*. If all the components of either column are disrupted, the stability of the cervical spine is lost. If one element of either column remains intact and the other column is disrupted, the spine will be stable.[15]

AETIOLOGY AND INCIDENCE OF SPINAL INJURIES

The main causes of spinal cord injuries are motor vehicle accidents, falls, assaults and sporting accidents particularly related to diving and horse riding.[16,17]

Spinal cord injury may be immediate, occurring at the time of injury; alternatively, an injury may result in an unstable vertebral column with the potential for spinal cord damage if uncontrolled movements occur during resuscitation and treatment. The recognition of the great potential for damage to the spinal cord in patients with unstable vertebral injuries is of vital importance.

The cervical spine is particularly vulnerable to injury; 50% of spinal injuries affect the cervical spine and of these 32–45% will be tetraplegic at the time of the injury. Below the cervical spine, 54% of injuries result in complete paraplegia.[4,6,18]

Injuries to the thoracic spine are associated with complete spinal injuries in 62–80% of cases, due to the significant force required to cause injury in this relatively protected area of the body and also due to the narrower thoracic spinal canal. Thoracolumbar and lumbar spine fractures account for 20–30% of all spine fractures; neurological injury here will affect the cauda equina.[4,18]

Injuries to the cervical spine may be considered in terms of upper injuries to the C1–2 complex and lower injuries to C3 through C7.[19] There is a lower incidence of serious neurological injury associated with injuries to the C1–2 complex than with injuries to the lower cervical spine. This may reflect a high incidence of fatality in patients suffering injuries at this level but the increased space available for the spinal cord at this level may also be an important factor. Subsequent neurological deterioration has been reported resulting from injuries to the atlantoaxial complex not identified at the time of early radiological assessment.[20]

Injuries to the upper spine result from forces transmitted from the head downwards and the disrupted forces transmitted depend on the position of the head in relation to the occipitoatlantoaxial complex at the time of impact. The history and clinical examination may help to identify the forces involved. Type III anterior displaced fractures of the dens which carry with it its base from the anterior arch of the axis are associated with a high incidence of neurological damage.

The main cause of immediate death following spinal cord injury is respiratory failure. The spinal cord respiratory centre, mainly the C4 motor nucleus with small contributions from C3 and C5, emerge as the phrenic nerve to innervate the diaphragm. If C4 remains intact under cervical voluntary control, voluntary breathing is maintained with a vital capacity of 20–25% of normal.[21]

EMERGENCY MANAGEMENT OF PATIENTS WITH CERVICAL SPINE INJURIES

The incidence of cervical spine fracture following major trauma is variously quoted as between 1.7% and 4.3%.[22–24] Patients are often victims of high-impact blunt trauma and have often sustained head or craniofacial injuries.

Radiological evaluation of these patients is essential although 20% of patients with cervical spine injuries will have a normal crosstable lateral cervical spine radiograph.[6,20] The sensitivity of radiographic evaluation is increased to 93% by adding an odontoid peg view.[25] It is essential, however, to assume an unstable cervical spine in any patient with a head injury or injury above the level of the clavicle until complete radiological, neurological and clinical examinations have been undertaken.[6,26]

There are many reports of injured patients suffering neurological damage during attempts to secure the airway.[27–29] The incidence of neurological damage in patients with unrecognized cervical spine injuries is approximately 10%[30–32] but when injuries are recognized and the neck is immobilized during airway manipulation, the incidence is reduced to 1–2%.[30,33,34] Cervical spine immobilization is therefore vital in all patients at risk of cervical spine injuries.[24,26,34]

Most upper cervical spine injuries may be treated conservatively, at least in the first instance. Early operative fixation, with the disadvantage of reduced neck movements later on, may be required for patients with head injuries and a depressed level of consciousness. This will facilitate early management, especially when turning patients on an intensive care ward. Pharyngeal haematoma may cause swelling, and airway compromise may be an early life-threatening complication of high cervical spine injuries, requiring early intubation to secure the airway.

METHODS FOR STABILIZING THE CERVICAL SPINE FOR AIRWAY MANAGEMENT

Basic manoeuvres to open the airway, such as the chin lift and jaw thrust manoeuvres, insertion of an oesophageal obturator airway and oral endotracheal intubation with a Macintosh laryngoscope blade, have all been shown to produce extension of the head on the neck.[32,35,36] Ventilation using a facemask, inflating bag and one-way valve will also result in cervical spine displacement.[37] These movements can cause spinal cord injury in a patient with an unstable cervical spine.

The Advanced Trauma Life Support protocol recommends the use of a rigid collar combined with tape across the forehead securing the patient to a long spinal board and sandbags at the side of the head to restrict neck movements.[26] The use of a rigid collar alone may still allow between 19% and 35% of unrestricted cervical spine movements, depending on the type of collar used.[38,39] When combined with taping the patient's head to a spinal board, these movements may be reduced to 14–20%.[38–40]

A rigid collar significantly impedes the view obtained at laryngoscopy[41] and manual in-line stabilization

(MIS) of the cervical spine without traction is the preferred method to prevent neck movements when oral tracheal intubation is required in an emergency or elective situation.[26,41–44]

EMERGENCY ANAESTHETIC MANAGEMENT OF CERVICAL SPINE INJURIES

Several reviews outline the optimum anaesthetic management of patients with potential cervical spine fractures who require immediate tracheal intubation and ventilation in the emergency situation.[6,45–47] Table 17.1 outlines a protocol for managing patients with potential cervical spine injuries who require immediate tracheal intubation.

ALTERNATIVE METHODS FOR SECURING THE AIRWAY IN PATIENTS WITH POTENTIAL CERVICAL SPINE INJURIES

It is important to assess whether the need to secure the airway is immediate or whether time exists to allow a more elective procedure. In the emergency situation where there is an immediate need for oxygenation, it may be necessary to proceed directly to a surgical technique such as cricothyroidotomy. This technique is advocated by the Advanced Trauma Life Support program[26] and involves a surgical incision through the cricothyroid membrane with the insertion of a size 6 tracheostomy.[53] The need for surgical cricothyroidotomy in emergency situations is rare at 1.4–2.8%[54–56] and the complication rate from emergency cricothyroidotomy is variously reported at 0–39%.[54,56,57]

The alternative technique in a patient *in extremis* is to puncture the cricothyroid membrane with a 14G cannula attached to a high-pressure oxygen source and insufflate oxygen.[26] This technique does not protect the airway from soiling with blood or vomit present in the pharynx and is also limited to a period of 30 min by the accumulation of carbon dioxide; it is, however, a useful immediate life-saving procedure.

Other techniques may be used for securing the airway in a patient who is difficult to intubate and who

---

Table 17.1   **Protocol for managing patients with potential cervical spine injuries who require immediate tracheal intubation**

Protocol	Notes and references
1 Immediate assessment of the airway and MIS of cervical spine Administration of high-flow oxygen	26
2 Rigid collars should be removed prior to intubation	41
3 A rapid-sequence anaesthetic induction technique is safe in most patients with cervical spine injuries requiring emergency airway control	48,49 Avoid multiple attempts at laryngoscopy in unanaesthetized patients with head injuries as this will cause catastrophic rises in intracranial pressure
4 Preoxygenation is vital prior to tracheal intubation and may be effectively carried out with cricoid pressure in place	50,51
5 Cricoid pressure as part of a rapid-sequence intubation technique does not aggravate cervical spine injuries	47,49,50,52
6 Anaesthetic induction agents facilitate tracheal intubation and attenuate the rise in intracranial pressure	Drug doses should be reduced appropriately in hypovolaemic patients
7 Suxamethonium (1.5–2.0 mg/kg) is the drug of choice to produce satisfactory intubating conditions within 30 s	The advantage of rapidly securing the airway and facilitating ventilation outweighs any potential side effects of suxamethonium
8 Suxamethonium should be used with caution in patients with maxillofacial trauma or other injuries likely to make tracheal intubation impossible	The consequences of paralysing a breathing patient with a partially patent airway and then being unable to intubate or ventilate him are dire
9 Patients who are unsuitable for rapid-sequence tracheal intubation require alternative methods for securing the airway	

requires cervical spine immobilization;[58] these are described in Table 17.2.

ANAESTHESIA FOR ESTABLISHED SPINAL OR VERTEBRAL INJURIES AND ELECTIVE CERVICAL SPINE SURGERY

The anaesthetic management of patients presenting for elective surgery for spinal fractures or other pathology differs from the emergency situation as there is more time to assess the patient and to plan the anaesthetic, especially the method of securing the airway. The most important consideration is to secure the airway without excessive cervical spine movements that may lead to neurological deterioration.

A variety of methods have been described for assessing the difficulty of tracheal intubation.[72–74] These methods

are not always specific or sensitive for predicting difficulty in intubation,[75–77] but they are useful for assessing the patient and planning the best method of securing the airway. Alternative techniques for securing the airway have been described in Table 17.2.

A variety of laryngoscopes and blades have been designed to aid intubation when head movements are limited, as in the instance of an unstable cervical spine (Table 17.3).

PATIENT POSITIONING

Once the patient is anaesthetized and the airway secured, care must be taken when positioning the patient on the operating table. Excessive and awkward movements must be avoided and the surgeon responsible for the patient's care should supervise the transfer of the patient on to the operating table as this can be particularly hazardous, especially if the patient is to be placed in a prone position. All pressure areas must be carefully padded for these operations, which may be very lengthy.

Table 17.2   Techniques and adjuncts to aid tracheal intubation in patients with unstable cervical spines

Adjunct or technique	Notes
Blind nasal intubation	Can be achieved in a spontaneously breathing patient and has the advantage that cervical spine movements are minimal.[32] Advocated as a method for securing the airway in patients with potential cervical spine injuries,[26] but the technique is not widely practised in the UK and is a difficult skill to maintain.[59]
Gum elastic bougie	Aids intubation when the laryngoscopy view is limited by the need for cervical spine immobilization.[44]
Laryngeal mask airway (LMA)	May be used as a temporizing measure to maintain an airway in a patient with an unstable cervical spine. Tracheal intubation may be performed through the laryngeal mask. The LMA does not protect the patient from aspiration of vomit.[60,61]
Fibreoptic intubation	Becoming more widely used and is accepted as the method of choice when difficult laryngoscopy is anticipated.[62,63] It is generally safer and easier to perform fibreoptic intubation in awake or lightly sedated patients with adequate topical anaesthesia to the upper airway and trachea. A variety of techniques have been suggested for providing adequate anaesthesia to the upper airway.[64,65] Of limited use in the acute emergency situation as it is time consuming and requires patient cooperation and the presence of blood, vomit or secretions in the airway may obscure the view of the larynx.[66–68]
Retrograde catheter techniques	A guidewire followed by a catheter is passed through the cricothyroid membrane and into the mouth. An endotracheal tube may then be passed over the catheter and into the trachea.[69,70]
Light wand	A flexible stilette with a distal light bulb which may be passed blindly into the glottis and tracheal intubation achieved over it.[71]
Awake intubation	With topical anaesthesia to the airway, conventional tracheal intubation techniques have been successfully used in awake patients with cervical spine injuries.[34]

Table 17.3 Types of laryngoscope that may aid tracheal intubation	
Blade type	**Notes**
Macintosh blade	The most commonly used laryngoscope blade; a larger size blade may help to improve the view at laryngoscopy.
McGill blade	A straight blade, designed to lift up the epiglottis, and may improve intubating conditions.[12] Excessive vagal stimulation may occur, causing cardiac arrhythmias.
Polio blade	A Macintosh blade which articulates with the handle of the laryngoscope at an angle of 150° rather than 90°. It may be useful when cricoid pressure is being applied as it moves the hand of the laryngoscopist away from the hand of the assistant providing cricoid pressure.
McCoy blade	A modified Macintosh blade, the tip of which is designed to lever when placed in the vallecula; this acts on the hyoepiglottic ligament to lift up the epiglottis, exposing more of the glottis. It has been shown to significantly improve the laryngoscopy view in patients with simulated cervical spine injuries and MIS undergoing oral tracheal intubation.[78]
Bullard laryngoscope	A rigid fibreoptic laryngoscope that causes less head and cervical spine extension than conventional laryngoscopes and produces a more favourable view at laryngoscopy in patients in whom cervical spine movement is limited or undesirable.[79]

TRANSORAL ODONTOID PEG PROCEDURES

The anaesthetic management of these patients has been reviewed by Marks et al.[80] Both tracheostomy and nasotracheal intubation have been used to secure the airway.

Patients undergoing odontoid peg surgery by the transoral route may develop considerable postoperative swelling of the pharynx with the risk of airway obstruction. It is useful to keep these patients intubated and ventilated in the immediate postoperative period and to extubate them after the swelling has subsided in a high-dependency nursing care area or intensive care unit.

A nasogastric tube should be positioned preoperatively as it will be very difficult to place postoperatively; it prevents soiling of the pharyngeal wound with gastric contents and aids feeding in the immediate postoperative period when swallowing may be difficult. Dexamethasone 4–8 mg may also be useful in the perioperative period to reduce pharyngeal swelling.

RHEUMATOID CERVICAL JOINT DISEASE (RCJD)

Rheumatoid arthritis is a multisystem disease which presents challenges to the anaesthetist responsive for perioperative care. The incidence of neck involvement in rheumatoid disease have been estimated at between 15–80%[81] and patients with RCJD

may be at risk of developing life-threatening neurological sequelae following general anaesthesia either for procedures to stabilize the neck or for other operations.

The problems in patients with severe RCJD are often compounded by concomitant rheumatoid disease resulting in ankylosis of the temporomandibular joint which impedes mouth opening.

The abnormalities occurring in RCJD have been classified by Macarthur et al, who suggest a 'lesion-specific' approach to anaesthesia.[82]

Early pathological changes result from erosion of bone and laxity of the ligaments leading to subluxation and this may progress to ankylosis of the neck.

The disease is considered in two sections:

- **atlantoaxial subluxation**: occurs in 15–35% of rheumatoid patients;[83]
- **subaxial subluxation**: involving the lower neck, present in 10–20% of patients with long-standing disease.

Atlantoaxial subluxation (AAS)

This is described by the directions in which the axis and atlas change their relationship to each other and the base of the skull as a result of rheumatoid destruction of the ligaments, facet joints and vertebral bodies.

Anterior AAS

This is the commonest form of RCJD and often occurs in addition to vertical AAS. It is defined by a distance of greater than 3 mm between the odontoid peg and the atlas. The transverse ligament is destroyed, allowing C1 to move forward on C2 and the odontoid peg to encroach onto the anterior aspect of the cervical cord. The condition is exaggerated, and may be diagnosed, by lateral radiographs of the neck in flexion. Magnetic resonance imaging helps to identify the extent to which neural compression has taken place.[84]

Posterior AAS

C1 moves backwards on C2 as a result of destruction of the odontoid peg. This abnormality is worse in extension radiographs of the cervical spine but it is less common than anterior AAS.

Vertical AAS

The lateral masses of C1 are destroyed by erosion of the atlantooccipital and atlantoaxial joints. The odontoid peg subluxes upwards through the foramen magnum above Macgregor's line (the line drawn from the superior surface of the posterior aspect of the hard palate to the most caudal aspect of the occipital curve) where it may compress the cervical medullary junction. When neurological damage occurs or when the condition is progressive, the surgical treatment is odontoidectomy via a transoral approach. This may be combined with posterior fixation of the cervical spine.[85]

Lateral/rotatory AAS

Changes in the C1, C2 facets, usually more on one side than the other, result in C1 moving rotationally with respect to C2. Non-reducible rotational head tilt, spinal nerve compression or vertebral artery insufficiency may result. This condition is rare.

Subaxial subluxation

Facet joint destruction below C2 in the neck results in a steplike movement of upper vertebral bodies on those beneath, the so-called 'staircase spine'. These changes are most common around C5–6 levels. Neurological changes are an early feature because of the smaller diameter of the vertebral canal and larger diameter of the cord at this level. When indicated for subaxial subluxation, surgery is usually via a posterior approach. In time, the bony components may fuse, resulting in a shortened stiff neck referred to as 'settling'.

Anaesthetic complications in RCJD

Difficult intubation is more prevalent in patients with cervical spine disease;[86] 20% have grade 3 or 4 laryngoscopy views.[87] Fifty percent of patients with no atlantooccipital gap and 80% of patients with no atlantoaxial gap are difficult to intubate. The best predictor of difficult laryngoscopy is reduced separation of the posterior elements of C1 and C2 on lateral cervical spine radiographs.[86]

A useful clinical test has been described to assess flexion/extension movements at the craniocervical junction.[75] The patient is asked to maximally flex the cervical spine and the examiner's hand is placed on the back of the neck to immobilize further movements. The patient is then asked to nod the head and the range of movement is assessed as normal or reduced depending on the examiner's experience.

The anaesthetic problems encountered in RCJD are related to difficult laryngoscopy in patients with stiff necks and the potential for damaging the neural structures in the cervical cord when the neck is unstable. In addition, the general systemic manifestations of rheumatoid arthritis need to be assessed in terms of the cardiovascular, respiratory, haematological and dermatological systems (for a recent review, see Skues and Welchew).[88] All patients are safe with the neck maintained in a neutral position so if it is possible to intubate them in this position, they may be anaesthetized in the normal way (maintaining manual inline stabilization of the cervical spine). Patients with AAS have stable necks in extension and may be intubated via direct laryngoscopy, avoiding flexion of the neck. Patients with posterior AAS, temporomandibular joint fixation and 'settling' or vertical AAS should be intubated awake using local anaesthesia to the airway and a fibreoptic bronchoscope.

CONGENITAL DISEASE

A variety of congenital abnormalities present for surgical stabilization of the neck (Table 17.4). All these patients have actual or potential reduction in the lumen of the spinal cord and reduction in the space available for the cord may be made worse or may occur during movements of the cervical spine, especially extension of the neck prior to intubation.

Down's syndrome is commonly associated with atlantoaxial instability.[89,90] A lax transverse ligament permits an increase in the ADI and excessive laxity of other joints correlates well with this defect. Older patients with Down's syndrome often suffer from cervical spondylitis which may require surgical relief.

Table 17.4   Congenital conditions causing neck instability[6]

Lesion	Syndrome
Odontoid hypoplasia	Morquio syndrome
	Klippel–Feil syndrome
	Down's syndrome
	Spondyloepiphyseal dysplasia
	Disproportionate dwarfism
	Congenital scoliosis
	Osteogenesis imperfecta
Atlantoaxial subluxation	Down's syndrome
	Odontoid anomalies
	Mucopolysaccharidoses

Hypoplasia of the odontoid peg and non-union of the dens with the body of the axis is commonly associated with a variety of congenital abnormalities (Table 17.4). Extension of the head results in anterior displacement of the atlas on the axis, reduction in the SAC and possible pressure on the neural elements.

ANAESTHETIC CONSIDERATIONS FOR PARAPLEGIC PATIENTS AND SPINAL SHOCK

Patients with spinal cord transaction present a variety of problems to the anaesthetist.[16] Spinal cord injuries have been subdivided on a temporal basis into:[91]

- acute injuries (spinal shock) (less than three days);
- intermediate injuries (three days to three months);
- chronic injuries (more than three months).

ACUTE INJURIES TO THE SPINAL CORD

Acute injury to the spinal cord occurs as a result of several phenomena:

- direct mechanical disruption to axons and other neural elements of the spinal cord;
- spinal cord oedema;
- secondary ischaemic damage as a result of damage to local blood vessels or to the vertebral arteries.

Injury to the spinal cord is defined by the completeness of the injury and the spinal level.[92] A *complete* injury is a total loss of neurological function below the level of cord injury; the prognosis for recovery is very poor. An *incomplete* injury implies preservation of some neurological function below the injury site and has greater potential for recovery.

Various syndromes have been described associated with incomplete spinal cord injuries:[92] central cord syndrome, anterior spinal cord syndrome, Brown–Sequard syndrome, conus medullaris lesions and injuries to the cauda equina. The spinal level of the lesion is designated as the most distal uninvolved segment of the spinal cord.

Management of acute spinal cord injury

The main goal of treatment in acute spinal injury is to prevent further damage to the spinal cord that could increase the level of the injury. Careful handling of patients and the prevention of hypoxaemia and hypo-volaemia are very important.

Large doses of methylprednisolone (30 mg/kg within 8 h of injury followed by 5.4 mg/kg/h for 23 h) have been shown to cause slight but significant improvement in motor function and sensation at six months in patients with both complete and incomplete lesions.[93] The efficacy of this regime has, however, been questioned, particularly in patients with penetrating trauma to the spinal cord.[94]

Spinal shock is the term for the acute phase following spinal cord disruption due to interruption of descending autonomic pathways with loss of all somatic and reflex activity, which lasts from a few days to several weeks. Spinal injuries at a high level result in significant respiratory and cardiovascular instability.

Respiratory effects

Very high cervical lesions interrupt diaphragmatic function (C3, 4, 5) and may present as a respiratory arrest. Lower cervical and thoracic lesions result in a degree of respiratory impairment due to failure of the intercostal muscles.

Neurogenic pulmonary oedema may be associated with acute spinal cord trauma. The mechanism is thought to be due to intense autonomic discharge following acute spinal cord injury resulting in hyper-tension, bradycardia and intense vasoconstriction.[95] The rapid increase in cardiac afterload can precipitate left ventricular failure and high systolic blood pressures may disrupt the pulmonary capillary endothelium, leading to alveolar haemorrhage or pulmonary oedema.

Cardiac effects

Loss of the cardiac nerves (T1–4) results in an unopposed vagal bradycardia and loss of sympathetic vasoconstrictor tone leads to peripheral vasodilatation and hypotension.

The condition of hypotension and bradycardia associated with a high spinal injury is termed *neurogenic shock*, which should not be confused with spinal shock. The initial management of neurogenic shock involves careful fluid replacement guided by central venous pressure monitoring, the use of vagolytic agents such as atropine 0.3–0.6 mg and vasopressors such as methoxamine, phenylephrine or noradrenaline.

The potential for cardiovascular instability is increased during anaesthesia and patients require careful invasive cardiovascular monitoring and intermittent positive pressure ventilation.

Abdomen

Loss of sensation below the waist can mask signs of intraabdominal pathology such as an acute ileus, a perforated viscus or haemorrhage.

Gastric stasis may develop in patients with acute spinal cord injury, making aspiration of gastric contents a risk. Rapid-sequence induction of anaesthesia is required and a nasogastric tube should be passed to empty the stomach and reduce the risk of aspiration.

Patients with acute spinal injuries are at risk of acute gastric ulceration and H_2 antagonists should be administered.

Temperature control is lost below the level of the spinal cord injury and patients become poikilothermic, so attention to temperature monitoring and the use of warmed intravenous fluids and warming devices is essential.

Urinary retention commonly occurs so patients should be catheterized to prevent overdistension of the bladder. The hourly measurement of urine output is also useful as a monitor of intravascular fluid volume and to guide fluid replacement therapy.

Deep vein thrombosis and pulmonary embolism are also increased in paraplegic patients and may occur at any time following injury. Prophylactic measures are essential.

INTERMEDIATE PHASE

The initial posttraumatic spinal shock phase declines after 2–3 weeks.[16] The intermediate phase (three days to three months) is important to the anaesthetist as it is the time when elevated serum potassium may occur in response to depolarizing neuromuscular blocking drugs.[96] This response may persist for up to one year. Levels of serum potassium as high as 11 mEq/l have been reported following administration of suxamethonium during this phase of spinal injury and can result in ventricular fibrillation.[97,98]

CHRONIC PHASE

Problems that the anaesthetist may face in patients with chronic spinal cord injuries and paraplegia include:

- postural hypotension;
- autonomic hyperreflexia;
- respiratory control;
- renal failure and electrolyte imbalance;
- loss of normal temperature control;
- decubitus ulcers;
- thromboembolism.

Postural hypotension

This occurs in patients with high thoracic lesions above the level of T4 due to failure of cardiovascular responses. A degree of adaptation occurs but care should be taken when positioning these patients.

Autonomic hyperreflexia

This develops after a period of three months or longer following spinal cord transection associated with spinal cord lesions above the level of T7. It is characterized by hyperreflexia, spasticity and involuntary muscle spasm.[16] Hyperreflexia is due to the coordinating sympathetic centres in the hypothalamus losing control over the spinal sympathetic nervous system between T1 and L2.[99] Stimulation of the bladder, genital region, bowel and cutaneous perineal area triggers afferent impulses travelling in the sacral roots and results in excessive sympathetic outflow up to the level of the spinal lesion. This causes sweating and vasoconstriction in the dependant part of the body; if the spinal cord lesion is above T1–4 (cardiac nerves) tachycardia will occur. Hypertension stimulates a baroreceptor-mediated reflex parasympathetic response causing flushing and swelling of the nasal mucosa and vagal activity resulting in bradycardia or even asystole.[100] Severe autonomic dysfunction is rare in injuries below the mid-thoracic region.

Careful anaesthetic management is required in patients with the potential for autonomic hyperreflexia. A deep general anaesthetic is generally recommended to reduce the risk of stimulation.[16,91] Spinal anaesthesia is an alternative to deep general anaesthesia although there are risks from hypotension and bradycardia and the need to use vasopressor drugs. Epidural anaesthesia may not adequately block the sacral routes and is not recommended.[16,91]

Respiratory control

Chronic respiratory impairment may exist as a result of reduced vital capacity[21] and expiratory reserve volume;

the development of kyphoscoliosis may also impair ventilation. Intermittent positive pressure ventilation is recommended for general anaesthesia and postoperative ventilatory support may be required.

Renal failure

Patients may develop chronic renal failure with resultant electrolyte imbalances[91] and may require long-term haemodialysis. Postoperative bladder spasms and subsequent attacks of autonomic hyperreflexia have also been reported.[99]

Decubitus ulcers

Patients very easily develop decubitus ulcers as a result of poor skin perfusion. Every care should be taken to avoid them during surgery as they may take many weeks or months to heal.

REFERENCES

1. Woolsey RM. Modern concepts of therapy and management of spinal cord injuries. Crit Rev Neurobiol 1988; 4: 137.

2. McNeilly RH. Oxford Regional Health Authority. The National Spinal Injuries Centre, Stoke Mandeville Hospital, 1979.

3. Young JS. Spinal cord injury statistics: experience of the regional spinal cord injury systems. Good Samaritan Medical Center, Phoenix, 1988.

4. Kennedy EJ. Spinal cord injury: the facts and figures. University of Alabama, Birmingham, 1986, p1.

5. Moore KL. Clinically orientated anatomy. Williams and Wilkins, Baltimore, 1980, pp 610–638.

6. Crosby ET, Lui A. The adult cervical spine: implications for airway management. Can J Anaesth 1990; 37: 77–93.

7. Last RJ. Anatomy: regional and applied, 6th edn. Churchill Livingstone, Edinburgh, 1979, p 536.

8. Jellinger K. Spinal cord atherosclerosis and progressive vascular myopathy. J Neurol Neurosurg Psychiatry 1967; 30: 195–206.

9. Hickey R, Albin MS, Bunegin L, Gelineau J. Autoregulation of the spinal cord blood flow: is the cord a microcosm of the brain? Stroke 1986; 17: 1183–1189.

10. Nichol HC, Zuck D. Difficult larnygoscopy, the 'anterior' larynx and the atlanto-occipital gap. Br J Anaesth 1983; 55: 141–144.

11. Hayashi H, Okada K, Hamada M, Tada K, Ueno R. Etiological factors of myelopathy. A radiological evaluation of the ageing changes in the cervical spine. Clin Orthop 1987; 214: 200–209.

12. Fell D. The conduct of anaesthesia and tracheal intubation. In: Nimmo WS, Smith G (eds). Anaesthesia, vol 1. Blackwell Scientific Publications, Oxford, 1989, pp 451–452.

13. White AA, Southwick WO, Panjabi MM. Clinical instability in the lower cervical spine. Spine 1976; 1: 15–27.

14. Steel HH. Anatomical and mechanical considerations of the atlanto-axial articulations. J Bone Joint Surg 1968; 50: 1481–1490.

15. White AA, Johnson RM, Panjabi MM, Southwick WO. Biomechanical analysis of clinical stability in the cervical spine. Clin Orthop 1975; 109: 85–95.

16. Fraser A, Edmonds-Seal J. Spinal cord injuries. A review of the problems facing the anaesthetist. Anaesthesia 1982; 37: 1084–1098.

17. Suderman VS, Crosby ET, Lui A. Elective oral tracheal intubation in cervical spine-injured adults. Canadian J Anaesth 1991; 38: 785–789.

18. Roye WP Jr, Dunn EL, Moody JA. Cervical spinal cord injury – a public catastrophe. J Trauma 1988; 28: 1260.

19. Levine AM, Edwards CC. Treatment of injuries in the C1 and C2 complex. Orthop Clin North Am 1986; 17: 31–44.

20. Davis JW, Phreaner DL, Hoyt DB, Mackersie RC. The etiology of missed cervical spine injuries. J Trauma 1993; 34: 342–346.

21. Stauffer ES, Bell GD. Traumatic respiratory quadriplegia and pentaplegia. Orthop Clin North Am 1978; 9: 1081–1089.

22. Roberge RJ, Wears RC, Kelly M et al. Selective application of cervical spine radiology in alert victims of blunt trauma: a prospective study. J Trauma 1988; 28: 784–787.

23. Kreipke DL, Gillespie KR, McCarthy MC, Mail JT, Lappas JC, Broadie TA. Reliability of indications for cervical spine films in trauma patients. J Trauma 1989; 29: 1438–1439.

24. Criswell J, Parr MJA, Nolan JP. Emergency airway management in patients with cervical spine injuries. Anaesthesia 1994; 49: 900–903.

25. Ringenberg BJ, Fisher AK, Urdaneta LF, Midthun MA. Rational ordering of cervical spine radiographs following trauma. Ann Emerg Med 1988; 17: 792–796.

26. American College of Surgeons Committee on Trauma. Advanced trauma life support program for physicians: instructor manual. American College of Surgeons, Chicago, 1993.

27. Hastings RH, Kelley SD. Neurologic deterioration associated with airway management in a cervical spine-injured patient. Anesthesiology 1993; 78: 580–583.

28. Mace SE. The unstable occult cervical spine fracture: a review. Am J Emerg Med 1992; 10: 136–142.

29. Cloward RB. Acute cervical spine injuries. Clin Symposia 1980; 32: 3–32.

30. Reid DC, Henderson R, Saboe L, Miller JDR. Etiology and clinical course of missed spine fractures. J Trauma 1987; 27: 980–986.

31. Bohlman HH. Acute fractures and dislocations of the cervical spine: an analysis of three hundred hospitalised patients and review of the literature. J Bone Joint Surg 1979; 61: 1119–1142.

32. Aprahamian C, Thompson DM, Finger WA, Darin JC. Experimental cervical spine injury model: evaluation of airway management techniques. Ann Emerg Med 1984; 13: 584–587.

33. Graham JJ. Complications of cervical spine surgery: a five year report on a survey of the membership of the Cervical Spine Research Society by the Morbidity and Mortality Committee. Spine 1989; 14: 1046–1050.

34. Meschino A, Devitt JH, Koch JP, Szalai JP, Schwartz ML. The safety of awake intubation in cervical spine injury. Can J Anaesth 1992; 39: 114–117.

35. Sawin PD, Todd MM, Traynelis VC et al. Cervical spine motion with direct laryngoscopy and orotracheal intubation: an in vivo cinefluoroscopic study of subjects without cervical abnormality. Anesthesiology 1996; 85: 26–36.

36. Horton WA, Fahy L, Charters P. Disposition of the cervical vertebrae, atlanto-axial joint, hyoid and mandible during X-ray laryngoscopy. Br J Anaesth 1989; 63: 435–438.

37. Hauswald M, Sklar DP, Tandberg D, Garcia JF. Cervical spine movement during airway management: cinefluoroscopic appraisal in human cadavers. Am J Emerg Med 1991; 9: 535–538.

38. Johnson RM, Hart, DL, Simmons EF. Cervical orthoses. J Bone Joint Surg 1977; 59A: 332–339.

39. Chandler DR, Nemejc C, Adkins RH, Waters RL. Emergency cervical spine immobilisation. Ann Emerg Med 1992; 21: 1185–1188.

40. Podolsky S, Baraff LJ, Simon RR, Hoffman JR, Larmon B, Ablon W. Efficacy of cervical spine immobilisation methods. J Trauma 1983; 23: 461–465.

41. Heath KJ. The effect on laryngosocoy of different cervical spine immobilisation techniques. Anaesthesia 1994; 49: 843–845.

42. Hastings RH, Wood PR. Head extension and laryngeal view during laryngoscopy with cervical spine stabilisation manoeuvres. Anesthesiology 1994; 81: 1081–1082.

43. Majernick TG, Bieniek R, Houston JB, Hughes HG. Cervical spine movements during orotracheal intubation. Ann Emerg Med 1986; 15: 417–420.

44. Nolan JP, Wilson ME. Orotracheal intubation in patients with potential cervical spine injuries. An indication for the gum elastic bougie. Anaesthesia 1993; 48: 630–633.

45. Bogdonoff DL, Stone DJ. Emergency management of the airway outside the operating room. Can J Anaesth 1992; 39: 1069–1089.

46. Hastings RH, Marks JD. Airway management for trauma patients with potential cervical spine injuries Anesth Analg 1991; 73: 471–482.

47. Nolan JP. Resuscitation of the trauma patient. Care of the Critically Ill 1995; 11: 222–226.

48. Redan JA, Livingston DH, Tortella BJ, Rush BF. The value of intubating and paralysing patients with suspected head injury in the emergency department. J Trauma 1991; 31: 371–375.

49. Talucci RC, Shaikh KA, Schwab CW. Rapid sequence induction with oral endotracheal intubation in the multiple injured patient. Am Surg 1988; 54: 185–187.

50. Grande CM, Barton CR, Stene JK. Appropriate techniques for airway management of emergency patients with suspected spinal cord injury. Anesth Analg 1988; 67: 714–715.

51. Lawes EG, Campbell I, Mercer D. Inflation pressure, gastric insufflation and rapid sequence induction. Br J Anaesth 1987; 59: 315–318.

52. Doolan LA, O'Brien JF. Safe intubation in cervical spine injury. Anaesth Intens Care 1985; 13: 319–324.

53. Narrod JA, Moore EE, Rosen P. Emergency cricothyrostomy – technique and anatomical considerations. J Emerg Med 1985; 2: 443–446.

54. DeLaurier GA, Hawkins ML, Treat RC, Mansberger AR Jr. Acute airway management: the role of cricothyroidotomy. Am Surg 1990; 56: 12–15.

55. Salvino CK, Dries D, Gamelli R, Murphy-Macabobby M, Marshall W. Emergency cricothyroidotomy in trauma victims. J Trauma 1993; 34: 503–505.

56. McGill J, Clinton JE, Ruiz E. Cricothyrotomy in the emergency department. Ann Emerg Med 1982; 11: 361–364.

57. Esses B, Jafek BW. Cricothyroidotomy: a decade of experience in Denver. Ann Otol Rhinol Laryngol 1987; 96: 519–524.

58. Wood PR, Lawler PGP. Managing the airway in cervical spine injury: a review of the Advanced Trauma Life Support protocol. Anaesthesia 1992; 47: 792–797.

59. McHale SP, Brydon CW, Wood MLB, Liban JB. A survey of nasotracheal intubating skills among Advanced Trauma Life Support course graduates. Br J Anaesth 1994; 72: 195–197.

60. Logan AStC. Use of the laryngeal mask in a patient with an unstable fracture of the cervical spine. Anaesthesia 1991; 46: 987.

61. Calder I, Ordman AJ, Jackowski A, Crockard HA. The Brain laryngeal mask. An alternative to emergency tracheal intubation. Anaesthesia 1990; 45: 137–139.

62. Benumof JL. Management of the difficult adult airway. Anesthesiology 1991; 75: 1087–1110.

63. Ovassapian A. Fiberoptic tracheal intubation. In: Ovassapian A (ed) Fiberoptic airway endoscopy in anesthesia and critical care. Raven Press, New York, 1990.

64. Sidhu VS, Whitehead EM, Ainsworth QP, Smith M, Calder I. A technique of awake fiberoptic intubation. Anaesthesia 1993; 48: 910–913.

65. Ovassapian A, Krejcie TC, Yelich SJ, Dykes MHM. Awake fiberoptic intubation in the patient at high risk of aspiration. Br J Anaesth 1989; 62: 13–16.

66. Ovassapian A, Yelich SJ, Dykes MHM, Brunner EE. Fiberoptic nasotracheal intubation – incidence and causes of failure. Anesth Analg 1983; 62: 692–695.

67. Delaney KA, Hessler R. Emergency flexible fiberoptic nasotracheal intubation: a report of 60 cases. Ann Emerg Med 1988; 17: 919–926.

68. Mlineck EJ, Clinton JE, Plummer D, Ruiz E. Fiberoptic intubation in the emergency department. Ann Emerg Med 1990; 19: 359–362.

69. McNamara RM. Retrograde intubation of the trachea. Ann Emerg Med 1987; 16: 680–682.

70. Barriot P, Riou B. Retrograde technique for tracheal intubation in trauma patients. Crit Care Med 1988; 16: 712–713.

71. Fox DJ, Castro T, Rastrelli AJ. Comparison of intubation techniques in the awake patient: the Flexi-lum surgical light (lightwand) versus blind nasal approach. Anesthesiology 1987; 66: 69–71.

72. Mallampati SR, Gatt SP, Gugino LD et al. A clinical sign to predict difficult tracheal intubation: a prospective study. Can Anaesth Soc J 1985; 32: 429–434.

73. Wilson ME, Spiegelhalter D, Robertson JA, Lesser P. Predicting intubation. Br J Anaesth 1988; 61: 211–216.

74. Frerk CM. Predicting difficult intubation. Anaesthesia 1991; 46: 1005–1008.

75. Calder I. Predicting difficult intubation. Anaesthesia 1992; 47: 528–529.

76. Wilson ME, John R. Problems with the Mallampati sign. Anaesthesia 1990; 45: 486–487.

77. Oates JDL, Macleod AD, Oates PD, Pearsall FJ, Howie JC, Murray GD. Comparison of two methods for predicting difficult intubation. Br J Anaesth 1991; 66: 305–310.

78. Laurent SC, De Melo AE, Alexander-Williams JM. The use of the McCoy laryngoscope in patients with simulated cervical spine injuries. Anaesthesia 1996; 51: 74–75.

79. Hastings RH, Vigil AC, Hanna R, Yang BY, Sartoris DJ. Cervical spine movement during laryngoscopy with the Bullard, Macintosh and Miller laryngoscopes. Anesthesiology 1995; 82: 859–869.

80. Marks RJ, Forrester PC, Calder I, Crockard HA. Anaesthesia for transoral craniocervical surgery. Anaesthesia 1986; 41: 1049–1052.

81. Bland JH. Rheumatoid arthritis subluxation of the cervical spine (editorial). J Rheumatol 1990; 17: 134–137.

82. Macather A, Kleinman S. Rheumatoid cervical joint disease: a challenge to the anaesthetist. Can J Anaesth 1993; 40: 154–159.

83. Sherk H. Atlanto/axial instability and acquired basilar invagination in rheumatoid arthritis. Orthop Clin North Am 1978; 9: 1053–1063.

84. Foley-Nolan D, Stack JP, Ryan M. Magnetic resonance imaging in the evaluation of patients with rheumatoid arthritis: a comparison with plain film radiographs. Br J Rheumatol 1991; 30: 101–106.

85. Crockard HA, Calder I, Ransford AO. One-stage transoral decompression and posterior fixation in rheumatoid atlanto-axial subluxation. J Bone Joint Surg (Br) 1990; 72: 682–685.

86. Calder I, Calder J, Crockard HA. Difficult direct laryngoscopy in patients with cervical spine disease. Anaesthesia 1995; 50: 756–763.

87. Cormack RS, Lehane J. Difficult tracheal intubation in obstetrics. Anaesthesia 1984; 39: 1105–1111.

88. Skues MA, Welchew EA. Anaesthesia and rheumatoid arthritis. Anaesthesia 1993; 48: 989–997.

89. Morton RE, Khan MA, Murray-Leslie C, Elliott S. Atlanto-axial instability in Down's syndrome: a five year follow up study. Arch Dis Child 1995; 72: 115–119.

90. Powell JF, Woodcock T, Luscombe FE. Atlanto-axial subluxation in Down's syndrome. Anaesthesia 1990; 45: 1049–1051.

91. Kadis LB. Neurological disorders. In: Katz J, Berumof J, Kadis LB (eds). Anaesthesia and uncommon diseases: pathophysiologic and clinical correlations, 2nd edn. WB Saunders, Philadelphia, 1981, pp 485–508.

92. Highland T, Salciccioli G, Wilson RF. Spinal cord injuries. In: Wilson RF, Walt AJ (eds) Management of trauma: pitfalls and practice, 2nd edn. Williams and Wilkins, Baltimore, 1996, pp 212–213.

93. Braken MB, Shepard MJ, Collins WF et al. A randomised, controlled trial of methylprednisolone or naloxone in the treatment of acute spinal cord injury. Results of the second National Acute Spinal Cord Injury Study. N Engl J Med 1990; 322: 1405–1411.

94. Prendergast MR, Saxe JM, Ledgerwood AM, Lucas CE, Lucas WF. Massive steroids do not reduce the zone of injury after penetrating spinal cord injury. J Trauma 1994; 37: 576–580.

95. Theodore J, Robin ED. Speculations on neurogenic pulmonary edema. Am Rev Respir Dis 1976; 113: 405–411.

96. John DA, Tobey RE, Homer L, Rice CL. Onset of succinylcholine-induced hyperkalaemia. Anesthesiology 1976; 45: 294–299.

97. Tobey RE. Paraplegia, succinylcholine and cardiac arrest. Anesthesiology 1970; 32: 359.

98. Stone WA, Beach TP, Hamilberg W. Succinylcholine – danger in the spinal-cord injured patient. Anesthesiology 1970; 32: 168.

99. Raeder JC, Gisvold SE. Perioperative autonomic hyperreflexia in high spinal cord lesion: a case report. Acta Anaesthesiol Scand 1986; 30: 672–673.

100. Erickson RP. Autonomic hyperreflexia; pathophysiology and medical management. Acta Physiol Med Rehab 1980; 61: 431–440.

18

ANAESTHESIA FOR NEUROSURGERY WITHOUT CRANIOTOMY

Andrew C. Summors & Richard E. Erskine

TRANSSPHENOIDAL HYPOPHYSECTOMY

INTRODUCTION

The transsphenoidal surgical route has become the preferred approach for most operations on the pituitary gland. The common indication for operation is tumour. This may secrete an active hormone in an uncontrolled non-feedback loop fashion. The anaesthetist needs to understand the endocrine status of the patient to enable assessment for surgery and management of the endocrine sequelae within the perioperative period.

CLINICAL IMPLICATIONS

Pituitary tumours originate from five types of adenohypophyseal cells. They are quite common, being responsible for 8–15% of all symptomatic intracranial tumours and are twice as common in women than men. They were previously classified according to their staining characteristics by haemotoxylin and eosin histological stains into eosinophilic, basophilic and chromophobic types. Adenomas are now identified using immunocytochemical techniques to distinguish the cell types within tumours and the hormones they produce. Trouillas and Girod[48] have reviewed 709 pituitary tumours; Table 18.1 summarizes their findings. The description of microadenomas less than 10 mm in diameter and confined within the pituitary fossa and macroadenomas larger in size and often extending either above the sella turcica or into a laterally situated cavernous sinus, is of neurosurgical assistance and does not carry with it any pathological or prognostic significance. The adenomas tend to be locally invasive but do not metastasize.

PITUITARY PHYSIOLOGY AND ANATOMY

The anterior pituitary (*adenohypophysis*) is a source of at least six hormones: growth hormone (GH), adrenocorticotrophic hormone (ACTH), prolactin (PRL), thyroid-stimulating hormone (TSH), luteinizing hormone (LH) and follicle-stimulating hormone (FSH), released in pulsatile fashion that regulate growth and development, thyroid function, the adrenal cortex, breast and gonad. The anterior lobe comprises 80% of the gland.

The posterior pituitary (*neurohypophysis*) has terminal neurones from the supraoptic and paraventricular nuclei of the hypothalamus. These synthesize oxytocin and antidiuretic hormone (ADH) which are secreted directly into the circulation.[1]

The pituitary gland is located in the sella turcica enveloped by the dura mater lining the sella. Superiorly, the sella diaphragma forms the roof of the sella with a ~5 mm wide central opening through which runs the hypophyseal stalk. A wider opening may lead to transmission of CSF pressure, giving rise

Table 18.1	Immunochemical classification of the pituitary adenomas and frequency in the series (from reference[48])		
Types of adenoma	Subtype and hormonal secretion	Frequency	(%)
Somatotrophic adenoma	Monohormonal – GH only	59	26
	Pleurihormonal (GH-PRL; GHαSU)	125	
Prolactinoma	Monohormonal	137	20
	Pleurihormonal	4	
Corticotrophic adenoma	Monohormonal	9	13
	Pleurihormonal	2	
Gonadotrophic adenoma	Monohormonal (FSH-LH; FSHαSU)	140	21
	Pleurihormonal	9	
Thyrotrophic adenoma	Monohormonal	4	2
	Pleurihormonal	10	
Hormonal non-immuno reactive adenoma	No hormone detected	127	18

It is important to differentiate hyperplasia from adenoma.

eventually to the empty sella syndrome. The sphenoid bone surrounds it bilaterally and inferiorly.

The pituitary is close to several structures affected by its enlargement.

- The lateral walls of the sella are close to the cavernous sinus containing the internal carotid artery, oculomotor nerve, trochlear and abducens nerve and the first two divisions of the trigeminal nerve.
- Tumour can spread into the sphenoid sinus lying anteriorly and inferiorly below the thin inferior sella.
- The optic chiasm lies directly above the sella diaphragma in front of the hypophyseal stalk and is easily compressed by suprasellar extension.
- The hypothalamus and third ventricle of the brain lie above the roof of the sella. Compression by space-occupying lesions may give rise to hypo-thalamic abnormalities.

The circulation of the pituitary gland is complex. Arterial supply arises from two paired arteries, the superior and inferior hypophyseal arteries arising from the internal carotid arteries. A portal circulation provides 80–90% of the blood supply to the anterior lobe from the infundibulum of the posterior lobe and pituitary stalk. This contains high concentrations of hypothalamic neuroregulatory hormones controlling anterior hormone synthesis and release. The posterior pituitary receives blood from the inferior hypophyseal artery and some branches of the superior hypophyseal artery and has a rich nerve supply of unmyelinated fibres from the supraoptic and paraventricular nuclei and other areas of the hypothalamus. ADH and oxytocin are synthesized in the hypothalamus and transported via neurones to the posterior pituitary. From here, they are released into the peripheral circulation.[1,2]

ACROMEGALY

Acromegaly occurs as a result of an increase in growth hormone produced by a pituitary adenoma. Growth hormone (GH), a 191 amino acid polypeptide, is produced by the anterior pituitary in a pulsatile fashion. The temporal pattern of these pulses is deter-mined by a hypothalamic pulse-generating mech-anism, influenced in turn by other areas of the brain such as the limbic system, the amygdaloid nucleus and the brainstem. The pulsatile release of hormone into the blood results from the influence of GH-releasing factor, which stimulates, and somatostatin, which inhibits release of the hormone from the anterior pitu-itary. The most important of these influences is the sleep-stage cycle. Slow-wave sleep stimulates and REM sleep inhibits release.

Like ACTH and prolactin, GH is produced as part of the stress response. In addition, GH secretion is influ-enced by metabolism. Hypoglycaemia and fasting stimulate its release while hyperglycaemia and food inhibit its release. This is the basis of the oral glucose tolerance test (OGTT) utilized to test GH secretion. Blood is taken half-hourly for 2 hours after adminis-tration of 100 g glucose. GH should remain below its nadir of 1 µg/l. In the liver and at the growth plate of longitudinal bones, activation of GH receptors results in the production of insulin-like growth factor 1 (IGF-1). It is produced in the liver under the influence of GH but also other influences and thus has to be considered a hormone in its own right. IGF-1 is trans-ported in the blood bound to a protein, insulin-like growth factor binding protein 3 (IGFBP-3). The concentration of this binding protein is regulated by GH. Unlike GH, IGFBP-3 levels in the blood are fairly constant and can be used as an index of GH activity.

Physical findings

The head is elongated due to growth of the mandible with resultant malocclusion of the teeth. The tongue is enlarged, making intubation difficult. In addition, there is an increase of the lymphoid tissue mass in the upper airway. These patients are prone to develop a nocturnal oxygen deficit which may be compounded by a central sleep apnoea.[3] Kyphoscoliosis may be present, leading to restrictive lung disease.

Hypertension is a feature and may be the result of the direct antinaturetic effect of GH, leading to the acti-vation of the renin-angiotensin system and an increase in blood volume.[4,5] Patients with long-standing acromegaly develop cardiomegaly. Thickening of the left ventricle is the most consistent finding.[6] This hypertrophy is reversible when the GH returns to normal.[7]

An excess of GH prior to closure of the epiphyseal plates leads to gigantism. After the plates have fused, the bony growth is by apposition, i.e. thickening of the cortices. The muscles are paradoxically weak as a result of both a specific acromegalic myopathy and a peripheral neuropathy resulting from endo- and perineural connective tissue thickening.

GH plays a pivotal role in intermediate metabolism. It acts with insulin to encourage protein production and, in insulin-depleted states, as a fat-mobilizing agent. It increases amino acid uptake into muscle. In excess, it causes glucose intolerance and a third of acromegalics present with diabetes mellitus which reverts to normal after the acromegaly is successfully treated. Lean body mass is increased as protein is laid down at the expense of fat. This is accompanied by an increase in total body water, possibly resulting from the antinaturetic effect of GH. Acromegaly is diagnosed by the demonstration of autonomous GH production which is not inhibited by oral glucose. However, some response to oral glucose load may persist. Because IGF-1 has a longer half-life it does not exhibit the same pulsatility in the blood and hence its blood level is used as a diagnostic test. It is also used to measure the response of acromegalic patients to treatment. PRL is raised in a third of acromegalic patients. In some cases this is because both hormones are produced in the same cell (mammosomatotroph cell) or because a GH-producing macroadenoma has expanded to compress the pituitary stalk and reduce the hypothalamic dopaminergic inhibition of PRL production. As with other pituitary adenomas, the expanding GH-secreting tumour may compress the normal areas of the gland and inhibit the production of, in ascending order of occurrence: gonadotrophins, prolactin, ACTH and, rarely, TSH. This results in secondary inhibition of the peripheral glands. After treatment, either medical or by surgery or irradiation, the response is measured by oral glucose tolerance or by estimation of IGF-1 in the blood.

Anaesthetic considerations

The patient with acromegaly, or gigantism if excess growth hormone is secreted prior to pubertal closure of bony epiphyses, presents a variety of challenges to the anaesthetist. Acromegalic symptoms are present before surgery on average for 6–7 years. This means most patients have anatomical and physiological changes when they present for anaesthesia. Anatomical distortions of the face, tongue, vocal cords and pharyngeal and glottic structures, cardiovascular disease including hypertension and idiopathic cardiomyopathy, pulmonary disease and endocrine dysfunction such as diabetes mellitus are not uncommon.[8] The airway probably presents the most significant problem. Difficulty may be experienced with intubation due to both the long jaw and the connective tissue disturbances of the vocal cords. A fibreoptic bronchoscope may be needed to facilitate intubation. Problems with the upper airway may be suspected with exertional dyspnoea, hoarseness, stridor, macroglossia and decreased mobility of the neck and temporomandibular joints. Hypertrophy of pharyngeal and laryngeal soft tissue obscures the glottis. Thyroid enlargement may distort the airway and cause glottic stenosis. Elective tracheostomy has been suggested for the severe grades of airway involvement but fibreoptic-guided intubation has also been used.[9] Indirect laryngoscopy, soft tissue X-ray assessment of the neck and inspiratory or expiratory flow volume studies may also be helpful.[10]

The heart needs to be carefully assessed for involvement as described above. The commonly present diabetic state needs to be recognized and treated. This usually reverts back to normal when GH levels return to more physiological levels in the postoperative period.

Muscle relaxants should be used with caution and each increment monitored with a peripheral nerve stimulator. As for any transsphenoidal pituitary operation, the patient needs to be observed carefully for any signs of generalized hypopituitarism and specifically for the development of diabetes insipidus (DI).

Close attention to the use of narcotic analgesics during anaesthesia and supervision in the postoperative period is required. Postoperatively, these patients are prone to airway obstruction due to both their preoperative anatomy and nasal packing and a sleep apnoea caused by the central disturbance of ventilation that occurs with elevated growth hormone. Nasal airway catheters through the nasal packing have been used to overcome this and provide a means of positive pressure ventilation if required.[8] Their use has been well described and advantages include: suctioning and airway toilet; bypassing the tongue with a high FiO_2; avoiding unnecessary and complex tracheostomies; and avoiding the problems of mechanical ventilation.[11,12]

Large respiratory volumes may be necessary to maintain $PaCO_2$, especially in the patient with gigantism. These patients pose special problems with moving and positioning.[10] Raised intracranial pressure may be a problem if extrasellar extension is present but it is likely a transcranial route would be used for large extrasellar extensions.

Surgical treatment of acromegaly

Acromegaly almost always results from an adenoma of the pituitary. The treatment is surgical in the first instance. Surgery is additionally indicated for those patients in whom upward pressure on the optic chiasm above has resulted in visual field defects. Fifty percent of patients will be cured by surgery alone, as tested by a GH level persistently below 2 μg/l on OGTT. A further half of the remainder will respond satisfactorily to additional measures. These include medical treatment with the dopaminergic agent bromocriptine or the somatostatin analogue octreotide, or radiotherapy applied to the gland. Factors which predispose to a less favourable surgical result include tumour involvement of the dura lining the pituitary cavity, extention out of the sella and younger patients in whom gigantism may be a factor.

CUSHING'S DISEASE

Cushing's disease, first described by Harvey Cushing in 1912, is an adenoma of corticotrophic cells of the anterior pituitary.

Physiologically, corticotrophin-releasing hormone (CRH) from the hypothalamus stimulates the synthesis and release of ACTH and other pro-opiomelanocortin (POMC)-derived peptides in the pituitary. ACTH in turn induces secretion of cortisol and adrenal androgens by the adrenal gland with complex feedback mechanisms regulating plasma cortisol. Normal levels of urine free cortisol are under 250 nmol/day[13] and this can be used as a basis for screening. Total plasma cortisol levels vary widely as most is protein bound to cortisol-binding globulin (80%) or albumin (10%) and protein levels change with various disease states.

Most ACTH-secreting tumours are microadenomas, less than 1 cm diameter, lying centrally in the anterior pituitary;[14] 10% are large enough to produce changes in the sella turcica. Most tumours are basophilic. Immunochemical stains detect ACTH and POMC-related peptides. A minority are chromophobic or mixed basophilic/chromophobic with minimal ACTH. These are often larger, faster growing and less hormonally active.[15] Diagnosis of adenoma can be confirmed with a low-dose overnight dexamethasone suppression test causing feedback decrease in ACTH secretion and subsequent cortisol release. A plasma cortisol level <140 nmol/l is normal after 0.5 mg dexamethasone every 6 h for two days or 1mg dexamethasone the night before and blood sampled at 8.00 am the following morning. High-dose dexamethasone can still partly suppress ACTH from adenomas and is used to distinguish pituitary adenomas from ectopic ACTH sources.[15,16]

Physical findings

Symptoms and signs depend on the degree and duration of disease and are caused by:

- endocrine effects of ACTH on cortisol, adrenal androgens and aldosterone, to a lesser degree;
- mass effects.

Patient appearance is one of generalized obesity of face, neck, trunk and abdomen with atrophic limb muscles. The neck appears short and thick from the dorsocervical fat pad that may cause difficulty with intubation. Changes in cellular glucose transport may result in steroid-induced diabetes mellitus.[17] Mild hypertension is common and hypertension is severe in 10% with diastolic BP >130 mmHg due to both low renin and an elevated response to vasoactive substances.[18]

Congestive cardiac failure is common. The skin is atrophic, thin and very fragile with loss of connective tissue. Osteoporosis and bone fractures are common and care is needed when gaining vascular access and positioning the patient. Wound healing is slow and the immune response is suppressed by glucocorticoids. Psychiatric symptoms occur in over half of patients.

Hypokalaemia is rare in contrast to other causes of hypercortisolism. Peptic ulcers usually occur if NSAIDS have been given. Mass effects usually produce headaches and visual field defects.[15]

Treatment and outcomes

The preferred treatment is surgical in most instances. Remission rates of 85–95% can be expected following surgery in experienced hands. Determination of ACTH levels in the inferior petrosal veins has helped to identify the position of the microadenoma in the pituitary gland.

PROLACTINOMA

Prolactinoma is the most common pituitary disorder. Symptoms relate to central decrease in gonadotrophin secretion, giving menstrual disturbances in females and loss of libido in men, and to stimulation of the mammary gland, giving galactorrhoea (Table 18.2). Over half are microadenomas, sometimes occurring as part of the multiple endocrine neoplasia syndrome type 1. Their small size means adequate functioning pituitary gland often remains after surgery.[19]

Table 18.2   Symptoms and signs of prolactinoma (reproduced in part from reference[21])

Space occupation
  Visual field defects
  Hydrocephalus (blockage of foramen of Monro)
  Anterior pituitary insufficiency
  Ophthalmoplegia

Endocrine disturbance

Males	Females
Decreased libido	Amenorrhoea
Hypogonadism (decreased androgen-dependent hair growth, testicular atrophy)	Oligomenorrhoea
	Anovulatory cycles
	Galactorrhoea
	Virilization
Galactorrhoea	
Gynaecomastia	

PRL is the only anterior pituitary hormone under the dominant tonic inhibitory control of dopamine from the hypothalamus. Stress or suckling has a stimulatory effect on PRL secretion via hypothalamic TSH release. Prolactin levels correlate well with adenoma size, in contrast to other pituitary adenomas. Normal levels in males are ≤15 μg/l and in non-pregnant females 5–20 μg/l.[20,21]

Treatment and outcomes

Prolactinomas tend to be very slow growing and remain stable in size and the amount they secrete over many years. Most prolactinomas are treated with the dopamine agonist bromocriptine which is successful in reducing PRL levels to normal in 60–90% of patients. Treatment needs to be continued for a very long time, often for life. Surgery is successful mainly when the tumour is small and is thus considered when patients do not tolerate medical treatment or for a small tumour that does not respond adequately to bromocriptine.

ENDOCRINE INACTIVE ADENOMAS

Up to 30% of patients with pituitary adenomas have endocrinologically silent tumours and present with symptoms secondary to mass effects (headache, visual field disturbance) or pituitary hypofunction secondary to destruction of normal gland. Compression of the optic chiasm often results in visual field defects and extension into the cavernous sinus may cause cranial nerve palsies. Headache is the most frequent presenting symptom of mass effect (Table 18.2).

The absence of specific hormone markers makes it difficult to distinguish these tumours from other intrasellar and suprasellar lesions such as meningiomas, craniopharyngiomas or metastases.[22]

PITUITARY APOPLEXY

Pituitary apoplexy is a clinical syndrome characterized by a sudden onset of headache, accompanied by a loss of vision and impairment of ocular mobility due to the rapid enlargement of a pituitary adenoma subsequent to a vascular event. The rise in pressure within the pituitary fossa constitutes a neurosurgical emergency to reduce this pressure, usually by operation via the transnasal route. Enlargement upwards compresses the optic pathways and may produce effects on the function of the midbrain and hypothalamus. This may result in altered levels of autonomic function and a deterioration in conscious level. The hypothalamic-pituitary axis (HPA) is nearly always compromised and systemic steroid replacement should be immediately commenced in the diagnosis of pituitary apoplexy.[23]

OTHER SELLA MASSES

Craniopharyngiomas

These histologically benign tumours are formed of epithelial remnants in the region of the pituitary stalk and may represent a persistent form of Rathke's pouch. They are mostly suprasellar but present for surgery via the transseptal route if intrasellar and require biopsy or cyst decompression. The anaesthetist should be aware that they are usually adherent to critical vascular, endocrine and cerebral structures, making surgery difficult. Stereotactic irradiation under local anaesthesia may be an option for some.[19,24]

Empty sella syndrome

This is a dynamic process due to prolapse of arachnoid through an incomplete diaphragmatic sella or from previous pituitary surgery or irradiation. The sella is enlarged by CSF and pituitary tissue is compressed against the posterior floor of the sella.[19]

SURGERY

Transseptal pituitary surgery is a safe and effective method of management of pituitary adenomas and related parasellar anomalies. The extracranial approach to the hypophysis was first described by Schloffer in 1906, who reported the removal of a pituitary tumour through the nose.[19]

Four transseptal approaches to the pituitary fossa are described (direct transnasal transsphenoidal, transethmoidal, sublabial transseptal and transantral), the most common approach today being the direct transnasal transsphenoidal route.[25] Since the 1970s the transsphenoidal has been the preferred route for removal of pituitary tumours, even those with suprasellar extensions.[26] In comparison with a transcranial approach, a transsphenoidal approach is faster and less traumatic. There is a better cosmetic outcome afterward and less frequent panhypopituitarism. The posterior pituitary often remains intact, decreasing the incidence of DI. There is a faster recovery and shorter hospitalization and no external scarring. Transfusion requirements are also less. A more selective resection of tumour avoids injury to the frontal lobes, olfactory tracts, pituitary stalk and optic chiasm.[1,26] However, all the transsphenoidal operations are liable to have complications relating to damage within and adjacent to the pituitary fossa, e.g. CSF leak, meningitis, diabetes insipidis, carotid and cavernous sinus injury and optic chiasm injury. It is not the best route to use if spread is extensive. There are also complications due to the route of access to the fossa, e.g. hypertensive responses and dental or septal complications.[1,25,27]

ANAESTHETIC CONSIDERATIONS

Position

The patient is intubated via the the mouth and the throat is packed loosely with moistened gauze. The eyes are closed and covered to prevent corneal abrasions. The patient is placed with the head on a headrest. The anaesthesia machine is placed on the patient's left and the breathing circuit is secured to prevent drag on the endotracheal tube. The surgeon may operate from the patient's right side or from above the head, so the patient will be semirecumbent or supine. The image intensifier is placed for lateral views of the fossa with the C-arm below the head. Surgical access is via the nose to approach the pituitary fossa, using the image intensifier to check position. The patient's thigh is exposed for autografts to help seal the sella at the conclusion of surgery.

Anaesthetic management

Anaesthetic management of patients for transsphenoidal surgery is similar to that for transcranial surgery. The patient should undergo appropriate preoperative investigation and preparation, including baseline endocrine function tests and investigation of anatomical manifestations (e.g. changes in airway). The patient should receive appropriate premedication and explanation, a smooth induction, stable maintenance and recovery with appropriate monitoring and fluid management with control of intracranial pressure.

Preoperative assessment

Patients routinely have a clinical examination for neurological deficit including ophthalmoscopy, examination of visual fields and visual acuity, an ENT examination, full blood count, nose swabs for microbial growth and antibiotic sensitivity, a detailed neuroradiological investigation for size and location of pathology including high-resolution unenhanced and intravenous contrast- enhanced CT scan of the pituitary fossa and surrounding structures. Patients may also undergo MRI scan or, less frequently, sellar tomograms for bone thickness and sinus symmetry and carotid angiography.[19]

A number of investigations may be required to assess endocrine dysfunction, including:

- baseline glucose, cortisol, ACTH, GH, FSH, LH, TSH, PRL and testosterone in males, with repeat levels after stimulation;
- thyroid function tests;

- water deprivation tests for DI (measurement of serum electrolytes and plasma and urine osmolalities).

Coagulopathy is a rare problem with primary brain tumours but has been reported with chronic activation of the coagulation system during episodes of chronic DIC. The risk of DIC often worsens with surgery with the risk extending to several days postoperatively.[28] An explanation of the operative risk should be given. A 1% mortality has been reported.[19] The patient should also be given an explanation of packing of the nose and nasopharyngeal space that will require mouth breathing postoperatively. Admission to the intensive care unit may also be required after surgery.

Evidence suggests that the current amount of peroperative glucocorticoid coverage is excessive and based on anecdotal information. New recommendations based on preoperative glucocorticoid dose, preoperative glucocorticoid duration and the nature and duration of surgery have been proposed. Transsphenoidal hypophysectomy may equate to minor or moderate surgical stress with targets of 25–50 mg hydrocortisone equivalents per day for 1–2 days based on daily cortisol secretion rates and static plasma cortisol measurements. There is no information suggesting that these new recommended equivalent doses need to be exceeded, so a patient receiving maintenance glucocorticoid therapy exceeding the estimated stress requirement will not need more steroid cover during the stress period. After uncomplicated surgery, circulating cortisol concentration returns to normal by 24–48 h in most patients.[29]

Premedication

Our practice is to administer a small dose of benzodiazepine orally to reduce anxiety. Assessment of the HPA axis will establish the requirement for glucocorticoid replacement. Thyroid function should be controlled and diabetes stabilized. Antibiotic prophylaxis is commonly given.

Explanations are given for mouth breathing postoperatively, intensive care admission or awake fibreoptic intubation if required.

Maintenance of anaesthesia

Vascular access is established with a 16G peripheral intravenous cannula. Invasive arterial monitoring can be achieved with cannulation of a radial artery or dorsalis pedis if collateral flow is inadequate.[30]

Capnography is used to ensure adequate ventilation and a moderate reduction in $PaCO_2$ to 4–4.5 kPa.

Hypocapnoea is induced before adding a volatile anaesthetic agent but it is rare to have raised intracranial pressure without suprasellar extension. Surgical access may be aided by normalization of $PaCO_2$ to induce descent of the gland as CO_2 rises to normal. The surgeon may request a Valsalva manoeuvre at the end of surgery to check for CSF leaks.

Anaesthesia and choice of drugs

Techniques and agents are chosen based on their effects on CMR, CBF and intracranial blood volume. Thus, thiopentone, propofol and fentanyl are used frequently. Volatile agents can be used after modest hyperventilation, with isoflurane being safer than enflurane or halothane, but care should still be exercised with midline shift on CT scan. Sevoflurane also has advantages in maintaining cerebral autoregulation.[31–33] A TIVA technique with propofol is favoured by some neuroanaesthetists.

Generally, CPP is controlled and cerebral vasodilatation avoided with hypocapnia. One study with a large number of patients showed no major untoward effect of nitrous oxide in transsphenoidal hypophysectomy but isoflurane requirements decreased. Nitrous oxide increases cerebral blood flow and intracranial pressure and, unlike other inhaled agents, gives no brain protection by decreasing cerebral metabolic rate. A trend toward a higher incidence of early postoperative nausea and vomiting may be seen with nitrous oxide after transsphenoidal hypophysectomy.[34] The same authors found an association with an increased incidence of atrioventricular dissociation and a trend toward more premature ventricular contractions in these same patients receiving infiltrations of lignocaine with adrenaline for haemostasis.[35]

Blood pressure control is important for haemostasis, enabling the surgeon to perform an optimal resection. Blood pressure should be maintained at least at preoperative levels. Bleeding is more likely in Cushing's disease and acromegaly, with hypertension and fragile blood vessels, and in metastatic cancer, with thrombocytopaenia due to bone marrow invasion. These problems can be exacerbated with the severe cardiovascular reactions that have been reported with transsphenoidal surgery. Hypertension can be severe and uncontrollable, obscuring the operative field. Use of at least 1% lignocaine with the adrenaline has been shown to minimize hypertensive responses.[27]

Cocaine and adrenaline combinations may sometimes be used to help achieve haemostasis. Cocaine provides topical anaesthesia and vasoconstriction and adrenaline increases vasoconstriction further and decreases cocaine absorption. However, life-threatening complications with arrhythmias and hypertension have occurred when maximum recommended doses are exceeded, especially with the high-concentration solutions and pastes used to shorten the onset time and improve duration. The value of adding cocaine to adrenaline has recently been called into question.[36]

Moderate hypotension has been used to improve the surgical view by reducing bleeding. However, hypotension may be best avoided, as one study of intrasellar pressures suggests that the blood supply to the pituitary is mixed arterial and venous with the arterial supply pressure lower than normal arterial pressure. Hence a small decrease in mean blood pressure or an increase in intrasellar pressure may give rise to pituitary apoplexy.[37]

Small amounts of vasopressors may be required to support the circulation but hypertension is frequently seen initially.

A mean blood pressure between 60 and 80 mmHg at the highest point of the skull maintains cerebral perfusion pressure and minimizes blood in the surgical field. At the conclusion of the operation, a piece of muscle or fascia taken from the the the thigh may be used to seal the operation site and reduce the risk of CSF leak. The muscle relaxant is reversed, the pack removed and the oropharynx suctioned under direct vision. The patient is extubated when responsive to command with adequate ventilation, given humidified oxygen and reminded to mouth breathe.[38] The patient is positioned 30° head up to minimize CSF leakage and a mini neuroexam may be performed.

Intravenous fluids and blood loss

Blood loss is usually less than 100 ml and a normal perioperative fluid regimen includes 1 l of Hartmann's solution intraoperatively and for the first 8 h thereafter followed by a further 1 l over the next 16 h. Most patients have resumed normal oral intake by then. Blood transfusion is rare and occurs in 1–2%.[38]

POSTOPERATIVE COURSE AND COMPLICATIONS

As the transcranial route is avoided, neurological complications are rare and the postoperative course is generally smooth. The patient is closely monitored in the recovery area for 1–2 h for assessment of vital signs, neurologic examination and fluid monitoring. Most patients are ambulatory and resuming normal oral intake in 48 h. Hypertension lasting more than 12 h is common, especially in Cushing's syndrome, and may only resolve after nasal packs are removed on the fifth or sixth postoperative day.

Particular care with ventilation may be required depending on the level of consciousness. Problems with acromegaly and gigantism have been detailed above. Ventilation may also be required postoperatively in the patient with advanced Cushing's disease who has a reduced chest wall compliance.

Antibiotic prophylaxis is continued for at-risk patients including those with nasal or sinus infections, previous pituitary surgery and Cushing's syndrome. Corticosteroid substitution is continued for 24 h (e.g. 25–50 mg hydrocortisone/day) and decreased to a maintenance dose depending on preoperative adrenal function and the amount of pituitary tissue remaining.

Complications of sellar region surgery

Cranial DI is a well-recognized cause of fluid balance disturbance after pituitary surgery and can occur in up to 20% of patients. A greater than 90% destruction of the paraventricular and supraoptic nuclei is usually associated with permanent DI. Most patients tend to retain fluids on the day of surgery followed by a slight diuresis theraffer but without the signs of DI. Transient DI from manipulation of the posterior lobe or irritation of the pituitary stalk resolves after several days and a urine output of up to 2.5 l/day may be normal. DI is suspected when dilute urine is excreted in volumes greater than the fluid intake. Most cases have polyuria (UO $\geqslant$ 30 ml/kg/h), hypernatraemia and elevated plasma osmolality. Patients with a complete DI have urine volumes in excess of 10 l/day with urine osmolality 50–200 mosmol/kg and specific gravity of 1.001–1.005. They are sensitive to exogenous ADH. Partial DI patients have smaller urine volumes and urine osmolalities between 290 and 600 mosmol/kg. The diagnosis can be confirmed with the ADH synthetic analogue desmopressin (DDAVP) which causes the urine output to fall and urine osmolality to increase. Other causes of polyuria include osmotic diuretics (e.g. mannitol, radiocontrast agents), severe hyperglycaemia and fluid overload. Comparison of plasma and urine osmolalities may help (Figure 18.1).

Treatment consists of adequate fluid resuscitation and correction of electrolytes with regular monitoring of intake and output. Severe polyuria can be treated with IV desmopressin 1–4 µg/day. The duration of DDAVP is dose dependent and ranges from 8 to 12 h. SIADH due to inappropriate release of ADH from damaged posterior pituiary cells is much more rare but has also been reported, usually in the late postoperative period after discharge.[39]

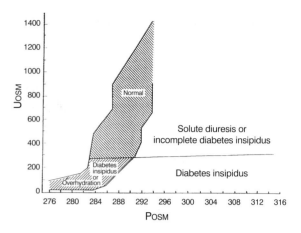

Figure 18.1 Plasma and urine osmolalities (redrawn from Moses AM, Blumenthal SA, Streeten DH. Acid-base and electrolyte disorders associated with endocrine disease: pituitary and thyroid. In: Arief AI, Defronzo RA (eds) Fluid, electrolyte and acid-base disorders. Churchill Livingstone, New York, 1985, pp 851–892).

CSF rhinorrhoea associated with diaphragmatic lesions may occur and be complicated by bacterial meningitis from nasal flora. Some centres routinely continue antibiotic prophylaxis.

Vision changes are rare and cranial nerve palsies affecting the third, fourth and sixth cranial nerves are usually transient if they occur.

Anterior pituitary function after surgery depends on the size of the tumour.[40]

Lesions to adjacent anatomical structures occur, including bleeding from the carotid artery and cavernous sinus or hypothalamic lesions leading to hyperthermia, electrolyte disturbance and cerebral coma.[41] Venous air embolism is rare with the supine patient.

Sinusitis, fractures from surgical instruments, deviated nasal septum with obstruction of nasal ventilation and dental problems have all been described.

STEREOTACTIC BIOPSY

Image-guided stereotactic surgery allows the biopsy or destruction of intracranial lesions without the need for craniotomy. It gives greater accuracy and diagnostic yield in tissue sampling and may be of great benefit in deciding the question of histology prior to a major surgical undertaking.[42] It is most commonly used for biopsy of lesions seen on CT and to locate small lesions difficult to find visually, especially lesions deep to the brain's surface. It also enables the surgeon to biopsy lesions adjacent to vital centres more safely, thereby avoiding the risks of freehand techniques.

Stereotaxis is also used for radiotherapy with radioactive wires placed through plastic cannulae or sheaths.

METHOD

A mechanical frame is attached to the patient's head and a scan obtained as usual. The scanner's computer calculates the 3D coordinates of points in the brain and relates them to the stereotactic space outlined by the frame. Simple calculations then convert these radiographic coordinates to the coordinate system used by the frame. These coordinates are set on the micrometers on the frame through which biopsy instruments can be directed with an accuracy of 1 mm.[43]

Many of these procedures can be carried out under local anaesthesia (together with supplementation by IV sedation). This has the advantage of continuous patient evaluation during biopsy. General anaesthesia is used for patient comfort in prolonged procedures and particularly in children.

A potential complication of the technique is intracerebral haemorrhage from accidental puncture of major arteries, sinuses and bridging veins. This may require urgent transfer of the patient for CT or even urgent craniotomy.[43]

ANAESTHESIA

Anaesthetic technique aimed at cardiovascular and respiratory stability throughout will maintain a stable CBF and thus ICP and CPP. Localized or general oedema is thus minimized and therefore lesion movement with respect to the skull. Bone and Bristow[44] describe results from a year's experience with total intravenous anaesthesia for stereotactic surgery. The technique consists of a combination of propofol, fentanyl, vecuronium and O_2 in air. It provides good cardiovascular stability and adequate depth of anaesthesia for all stages in stereotaxis and a reliable rapid recovery. Furthermore, it can also be useful for transferring head-injured patients from the ICU to the CT scanner. Propofol is also believed to be the ideal agent for easing the discomfort of siting the stereotactic frame if the procedure to follow requires the patient to be awake, e.g. thalamotomy.[45]

After careful preoperative assessment, a short-acting benzodiazepine premed is given and large-bore IV access is established. A level of monitoring is chosen that maintains patient care in transit, commonly NIBP, SpO_2, ECG, $EtCO_2$. All monitors, pumps, O_2 cylinder and ventilator are fixed to the trolley securely if transported and arranged for easy observation from outside the CT scanner

Bone and Bristow[44] used IV lignocaine 1 mg/kg, fentanyl 2 µg/kg, propofol 1–2 mg/kg over 30 s, vecuronium 0.1 mg/kg followed by intubation and positive pressure ventilation with a portable ventilator with fresh gas flow titrated against $EtCO_2$. Anaesthesia was then maintained by a propofol infusion according to Roberts et al,[46] i.e. 10 mg/kg/h for the first 10 min, followed by 8 mg/kg/h for the next 10 min and 6 mg/kg/h thereafter and adjusted according to depth of anaesthesia. A volatile agent is not required. This has the advantage of avoiding the need for an anaesthetic machine during transfer and avoiding the adverse effects of a volatile agent on the cerebral vasculature. The problem of pollution and scavenging requirements is also overcome. Muscle relaxant was provided with boluses or infusion of vecuronium.

After skin preparation, a minimum of four cranial fixation pins are applied to the skull. This stimulus requires careful attention to anaesthetic technique to avoid increases in ICP (a bolus of propofol or opiate is commonly used at this point to deepen anaesthesia quickly and overcome any sympathetic response). The propofol infusion is stopped just prior to reversal with neostigmine and glycopyrrolate. The patient usually remains supine throughout.

The advantages of this total intravenous technique are the haemodynamic and respiratory stability during the stereotactic procedures, patient transfer between CT and operating theatre and after use of radiocontrast in CT. It is a simple technique and the same anaesthetic technique can be continued in the operating room.

Postoperative patient care includes frequent neurological monitoring. There is a potential risk of air embolism through transgressed venous channels in bone.

Overall, there is a low incidence of nausea and vomiting and morbidity and mortality are very low.[44]

VENTRICULOPERITONEAL SHUNTS

Hydrocephalus is usually due to obstruction of CSF flow giving rise to increases in volume and thus intracranial pressure. Surgical treatment aims are to provide a shunt through which excess fluid can drain to a site to be absorbed. The most common drains are to the peritoneal cavity but the right atrium, cisterna magna and pleural cavity are also sometimes used.

VP shunts drain CSF from the fourth or lateral ventricles to the peritoneal cavity. Systems usually involve three components: a ventricular catheter, a one-way valve and a distal catheter. Other devices may also be used (on–off valves, siphon control devices and chambers for flushing the system). The ventricular catheter is inserted through a burr hole (usually on the right), connected to the one-way valve that determines the draining pressure from the ventricle and then connected to the peritoneal catheter, passed over the chest wall and inserted into the peritoneal cavity through a small incision.

POSITION

Children

For VP shunts the child is placed supine with the head turned to the opposite side for the occipital insertion of the ventricular catheter. A towel is placed under the nape of the neck so the head, neck and abdomen are in one plane for the passage of the subcutaneous tunneller for shunt placement (Fig. 18.2). Children are usually positioned with towels, rolls and pillows rather than table adjustment. The tunneller theoretically reduces chest wall compliance and may cause underventilation or dangerous increases in airway pressures.

Adults

Adults are placed supine with the head turned to the opposite side and a roll or pad under the ipsilateral shoulder and neck giving a straight path for the tunnelling device.

The shunt tubing is passed subcutaneously from the scalp incision over the occipitoparietal region to the abdominal incision made either in the midline above

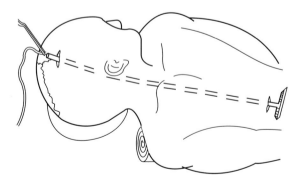

Figure 18.2 The shunt is passed subcutaneously from the cranial end to the peritoneal incisions through a shunt-passing device (redrawn from reference[47]).

the umbilicus or just lateral to and above the umbilicus. Local anaesthetic with adrenaline may be injected along the incision lines. Intravenous antibiotics are given perioperatively.[47]

ANAESTHETIC MANAGEMENT

The child presenting for insertion of VP shunt or shunt revision must be considered to have overt or potentially raised intracranial pressure. Anaesthetic technique should be tailored to minimize sympathetic responses and steps taken to reduce intracranial pressure.

Preoperative respiratory depressant drugs are avoided in the presence of a raised ICP. A smooth induction is desirable as crying will further increase the ICP. An inhalation induction is acceptable if the fontanelle and sutures are opened, otherwise an intravenous induction is preferred. EMLA cream is used over the venepuncture site. For induction, thiopentone and propofol have the advantage of decreasing cerebral metabolic rate and cerebral blood flow.

Vecuronium has the fewest cardiovascular effects during induction but the other muscle relaxants have also been used satisfactorily. Other measures may be used to limit the pressor responses to laryngoscopy and intubation, such as the use of a bolus of lignocaine or fentanyl. This, however, seems less of a problem in children with open sutures than in adults. A RAE tube or armoured tube is used either orally or nasally and fixed well to prevent movement. The chest is auscultated for breath sounds bilaterally after the patient is placed in their final position. The breathing circuit is secured firmly to prevent dragging on the endotracheal tube. The eyes and limbs are protected from injury.

Anaesthesia is maintained with a total intravenous technique using propofol or with volatile agents and IV analgesics such as fentanyl or alfentanil or with combinations of these.

TIVA with propofol decreases $CMRO_2$, may give neuroprotection, reduces relaxant needs and gives rapid wakening postoperatively. Isoflurane also decreases $CMRO_2$ and relaxant requirements and gives easy control of blood pressure if required. Opioids are adjusted to avoid postoperative respiratory depression. Their use increases the incidence of postoperative nausea and vomiting.

Moderate hypocapnia using capnography to monitor ventilation reduces brain mass by cerebral vasoconstriction.

Surgical infiltration with adrenaline reduces bleeding but the addition of at least 1% lignocaine provides scalp analgesia and helps reduces any hypertensive response.[27]

Intravenous fluids without glucose are used as elevated levels of glucose worsen outcome.

At the conclusion of surgery, the pharynx is cleared of secretions under direct vision, muscle relaxants reversed and the patient extubated, avoiding coughing if possible.

REFERENCES

1. Messick JM, Laws ER, Abboud CF. Anesthesia for transsphenoidal surgery of the hypophyseal region. Anesth Analg 1978; 57: 206–215.

2. Riskind PN, Martin JB. Functional anatomy of the hypothalamic-anterior pituitary complex. In: DeGroot LJ (ed) Endocrinology, 3rd edn. WB Saunders, Philadelphia, 1995, pp 151–159.

3. Ho KY, Sullivan CE. Sleep apnea in acromegaly. Ann Intern Med 1991; 115: 527–532.

4. Ho HI, Weissberger JA. The antinaturetic effect of biosynthetic human growth hormone in man invoves activation of the renin-angiotensin mechanism. Metabolism 1990; 39: 133–137.

5. Hirsch EZ, Sloman JG, Martin FIR. Cardiac function in acromegaly. Am J Med Sci 1969; 257: 1–8.

6. Savage DD, Henry WL, Eastman RC. Echocardiographic assessment of cardiac anatomy and function in acromegalic patients. Am J Med 1979; 67: 823–829.

7. Lim MJ, Barkan AL, Buda AJ. Rapid reduction of left ventricular hypertrophy in acromegaly after suppression of growth hormone hypersecretion. Ann Intern Med 1992; 117: 719–726.

8. Young ML, Hanson CW. An alternative to tracheostomy following transsphenoidal hypophysectomy in a patient with acromegaly and sleep apnoea. Anesth Analg 1993; 76: 446–449.

9. Southwick JP, Katz J. Unusual airway difficulty in the acromegalic patient – indications for tracheostomy. Anesthesiology 1979; 51: 72–73.

10. Chan VWS, Tindall S. Anaesthesia for transsphenoidal surgery in a patient with extreme gigantism. Br J Anaesth 1988; 60: 464–468.

11. Singelyn FJ, Scholtes JL. Airway obstruction in acromegaly: a method of prevention. Anaesth Inten Care 1988; 16: 491–492.

12. Perks WH, Horricks PM, Cooper RA et al. Sleep apnoea in acromegaly. BMJ 1980; 280: 894–897.

13. Burke CW, Beardwell CG. Cushing's syndrome: an elevation of the clinical usefulness of urinary free cortisol and other urinary steroid measurements in diagnosis. Quart J Med 1973; 42: 175–204.

14. Hardy J. Cushing's disease: 50 years later. Can J Neurol Sci 1982; 9: 375–380.

15. Schulte HM, Petersenn S. Cushing's disease – clinical findings and endocrinology. In: Landolt AM, Vance ML, Reilly PL (eds) Pituitary adenomas. Churchill Livingstone, New York, 1996, pp 101–110.

16. Liddle GW. Test of pituitary-adrenal suppressibility in the diagnosis of Cushing's syndrome. J Clin Endocrinol Metab 1960; 20: 1539–1560.

17. Murray DK, Hill ME, Nelson DH. Inhibitory action of sphigosine, sphinganine and dexamethasone on glucose uptake: studies with hydrogen peroxidase and phorbol esters. Life Sci 1990; 46: 1843–1849.

18. Ritchie CM, Sheridan B, Fraser R et al. Studies on the pathogenesis of hypertension in Cushing's disease and acromegaly. Quart J Med 1990; 76: 855–867.

19. Kern EB, Pearson BW, McDonald TJ, Laws ER. The transseptal approach to lesions of the pituitary and parasellar regions. Laryngoscope 1979; 89 (5 pt 2 suppl 15): 1–34.

20. Vance ML, Thorner OM. Prolactin and hyperprolactinaemic syndromes and management. In: DeGroot L (ed) Endocrinology. WB Saunders, Philadelphia, 1989, pp 408.

21. Von Werder K. Prolactinoma: clinical findings and endocrinology. In: Landolt AM, Vance ML, Reilly PL (eds) Pituitary adenomas. Churchill Livingstone, New York, 1996, pp 111–126.

22. Katznelson L, Klibanski A. Endocrine-inactive, FSH, LH and -subunit adenomas: clinical findings and endocrinology. In: Landolt AM, Vance ML, Reilly PL (eds) Pituitary adenomas. Churchill Livingstone, New York, 1996, pp 127–131.

23. McFadzean RM, Teasdale GM. Pituitary apoplexy. In: Landolt AM, Vance ML, Reilly PL (eds) Pituitary adenomas. Churchill Livingstone, New York, 1996, p 485.

24. Pollack IF, Lunsford LD, Slamovits TL, Gunerman LW, Levine G, Robinson AG. Stereotaxic intracavitary irradiation for cystic craniopharyngiomas. J Neurosurg 1988; 68: 227–233.

25. Cooke RS, Jones RAC. Experience with the direct transnasal transsphenoidal approach to the pituitary fossa. Br J Neurosurg 1994; 8: 193–196.

26. Peter M, DeTribolet N. Visual outcome after transsphenoidal surgery for pituitary adenomas. Br J Neurosurg 1995; 9: 151–157.

27. Abou-Madi MN, Trop D, Barnes J. Aetiology and control of cardiovascular reactions during transsphenoidal resection of pituitary microadenomas. Can Anaesth Soc J 1980; 27: 491–495.

28. Weinberg S, Phillips L, Twersky R, Cottrell JE, Braunstein KM. Hypercoagulability in a patient with a brain tumor. Anesthesiology 1984; 61: 200–202.

29. Salem M, Tainsh RE Jr, Bromberg J, Loriaux DL, Chernow B. Perioperative glucocorticoid coverage. A reassessment 42 years after emergence of a problem. Ann Surg 1994; 219: 416–425.

30. Campkin TV: Radial artery cannulation. Potential hazard in patients with acromegaly. Anaesthesia 1980; 35: 1008–1009.

31. Grosslight K, Foster R, Colohan AR, Bedford RF. Isoflurane for neuroanesthesia: risk factors for increases in intracranial pressure. Anesthesiology 1985; 63: 533–536.

32. Messick JM Jr, Newberg LA, Nugent M, Faust RJ. Principles of neuroanesthesia for the neurosurgical patient with CNS pathophysiology. Anesth Analg 1985; 64: 143–174.

33. Gupta S, Heath K, Matta BF. The effect of incremental doses of sevoflurane on cerebral pressure autoregulation in humans: a transcranial doppler study. Br J Anaesth 1997; 79: 469–472.

34. Eger EI II, Lampe GH, Wauk LZ, Whitendale P, Calahan MK, Donegan JH. Clinical pharmacology of nitrous oxide: an argument for its continued use. Anesth Analg 1990; 71: 575–585.

35. Lampe GH, Donegan JH, Rupp SM et al. Nitrous oxide and epinephrine induced arrythmias. Anesth Analg 1990; 71: 602–605.

36. Nicholson KEA, Rogers JEG. Cocaine and adrenaline paste: a fatal complication. BMJ 1995; 311: 250–251.

37. Kruse A, Astrup J, Cold GE, Hansen HH. Pressure and blood flow in pituitary adenomas measured during transsphenoidal surgery. Br J Neurosurg 1992; 6: 333–342.

38. Landolt AM, Schiller Z. Surgical technique – transsphenoidal approach. In: Landolt AM, Vance ML, Reilly PL (eds) Pituitary adenomas. Churchill Livingstone, New York, 1996, pp 315–331.

39. Tymms J, Griffith HB, Hartog M, Clark JDA, Reckless JPD. Pituitary surgery and inappropriate antidiuretic hormone secretion. J Roy Soc Med 1992; 85: 302.

40. Maclanahan CS, Christy JH, Tindall GT. Anterior pituitary function before and after transsphenoidal microsurgical resection of pituitary tumors. Neurosurgery 1978; 3: 142–144.

41. Fahlbusch R, Buchfelder M. Surgical complications. In: Landolt AM, Vance ML, Reilly PL (eds) Pituitary adenomas. Churchill Livingstone, New York, 1996, pp 394–408.

42. Apuzzo MJL, Chandrasoma PT, Cohen D, Zee CJ, Zelman V. Computed imaging stereotaxy: experience and perspective related to 500 procedures applied to brain masses. Neurosurgery 1987; 20: 930–937.

43. Salcman M. The surgical management of gliomas. In: Tindall GT, Cooper PR, Barrow PL (eds) The practice of neurosurgery. Williams & Wilkins, Baltimore, 1996, pp 649–670.

44. Bone ME, Bristow A. Total intravenous anaesthesia in stereotactic surgery – one years clinical experience. Eur J Anaesthesiol 1991; 8: 47–54.

45. Anderson BJ, Marks PV, Futter ME. Propofol – contrasting effects in movement disorders. Br J Neurosurg 1994; 8: 387–388.

46. Roberts FL, Dixon J, Lewis GTR, Tackley RM, Prys-Roberts C. Induction and maintenance of propofol anaesthesia. Anaesthesia 1988; 43(suppl): 14–17.

47. Roth PA, Cohen AR. Management of hydrocephalus in children. In: Tindall GT, Cooper PR, Barrow PL (eds) The practice of neurosurgery. Williams & Wilkins, Baltimore, 1996, pp 2707–2728.

48. Trouillas J, Girod C. Pathology of pituitary adenomas. In: Landolt AM, Vance ML, Reilly PL (eds) Pituitary adenomas. Churchill Livingstone, New York, 1996, pp 27–46.

19

ANAESTHESIA FOR POSTERIOR FOSSA SURGERY

Catherine Duffy

The posterior fossa is a small, rigid compartment which houses the cerebellum, pons, medulla oblongata and fourth ventricle. Life-threatening symptoms can result from compression of these vital structures. Because of the narrow outflow of cerebrospinal fluid (CSF), intracranial hypertension can develop suddenly. The common goal of the anaesthetist and surgeon is an operation in which the need for retraction, with consequent tissue damage, is minimized. This is achieved by optimizing the surgical approach and patient position and by minimizing congestion of cerebral vasculature.

ANATOMY

The anterior portion of the posterior fossa is the dorsum sellae and basilar portion, or clivus, of the occipital bone. Laterally are the petrous portions of the temporal bones. The roof is the tentorium cerebelli and the floor contains the foramen magnum. Cranial nerve V arises from the pons and cranial nerves VI–XII from the medulla. The posterior fossa is traversed by the transverse, superior petrosal, occipital and sigmoid sinuses.[1]

POSTERIOR FOSSA LESIONS

TUMOURS

Intraaxial lesions tend to be malignant whereas extraaxial lesions are usually benign. Posterior fossa

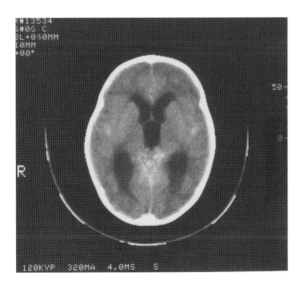

Figure 19.1   Acute hydrocephalus in a child with medulloblastoma.

tumours are more common in children than in adults, with 55% occurring in children and 45% in adults. 54–70% of childhood brain tumours originate in the posterior fossa. Primitive neuroectodermal tumours (PNET)/medulloblastomas, ependymomas and astrocytomas all occur in infants and children. Mixed gliomas are unique to childhood. In the adult population, 15–20% of brain tumours occur in the posterior fossa. Metastases, haemangioblastomas and lymphoma are all more common in adults than in children.

Signs and symptoms

Headache and vomiting are the most common symptoms in patients with posterior fossa tumours. Hemicerebellar lesions are characterized by unilateral ataxia, dysmetria, intention tremor and hypotonia. Vermian lesions tend to present with a wide-based gait, truncal ataxia and abnormal extraocular movements. Brainstem tumours present with bulbar palsies, secondary to cranial nerve dysfunction, and contralateral motor and sensory deficits. Depending on the level of the lesion, respiratory changes may occur.

When a posterior fossa lesion is complicated by obstructive hydrocephalus, headache and vomiting are exacerbated. The patient develops an unsteady gait, mental state changes, diplopia, incontinence and signs of meningism.

Intraaxial tumours

PNET/medulloblastoma

These tumours represent 25% of childhood intracranial tumours. They occur mainly in the 5–9-year-old age group with equal sex distribution. Because of their midline position, they tend to present early with intracranial hypertension due to obstructive hydrocephalus (Figure 19.1).

Cerebellar astrocytoma

These account for 12–28% of childhood brain tumours. They are relatively benign lesions with very good long-term survival following surgical resection.

Brainstem glioma

These represent 25–30% of posterior fossa tumours in childhood. Most are low-grade astrocytomas. They tend to be slow growing with insidious onset of symptoms. The exception is pontine gliomas which are malignant and present with a short and aggressive history.

Ependymoma

These lesions tend to occur in childhood and adolescence, with 50% occurring in children less than three years old. They arise from the floor of the fourth ventricle. Treatment involves surgical removal and adjuvant irradiation. Complete removal may not always be possible if there is brainstem involvement.

Choroid plexus papilloma/carcinoma

These are rare lesions arising from the fourth ventricle. They account for only 3% of paediatric intracranial tumours. They hypersecrete CSF and are associated with communicating hydrocephalus.

Dermoid tumour

These are childhood tumours involving the cerebellar midline. They often present with recurrent episodes of bacterial or aseptic meningitis due to rupture. Eventually arachnoid scarring may result in hydrocephalus. The surgical goal is total excision.

Haemangioblastoma

These are histologically benign tumours which can occur throughout the central nervous system but are most commonly seen in the posterior fossa. They account for 7–12% of adult posterior fossa tumours. They may occur as part of the Von Hippel–Lindau syndrome, an inherited disorder characterized by visceral cysts and tumours, retinal haemangiomas and polycythaemia. Due to their vascular nature, preoperative embolization is desirable. Complete surgical resection is usually curative.

Metastatic tumour

These are the most common posterior fossa tumours in adults. The usual primary tumour sites are lung, breast, skin and kidney. Surgical removal is indicated when the lesions cause a mass effect. In the case of a solitary lesion, excision may improve survival.

Extraaxial tumours

Schwannoma

An acoustic neuroma is a schwannoma arising from the vestibular portion of cranial nerve VIII. The usual presenting symptom is hearing loss. Schwannomas do not invade tissues but tend to displace them. They may cause compression of cranial nerves V and VII, manifesting as tic douloureux and hemifacial spasm respectively. If large, they may be associated with hydrocephalus. Acoustic neuromas occur in the fifth and sixth decades with equal sex distribution. Total resection is usually feasible. Acoustic neuromas may occur as part of a type II neurofibromatosis syndrome in which case they are multiple and behave more aggressively than single lesions.

Schwannomas may also affect cranial nerves V, VII, IX, X and XII.

Meningioma

Ten percent of all meningiomas are in the posterior fossa. They may arise from the petrous ridge of the temporal bone and extend into the cerebellopontine angle. Other possible sites are the clivus, tentorium cerebelli, fourth ventricle and, rarely, foramen magnum. Because they are vascular lesions, preoperative embolization is usually attempted.

Clival tumour

These are rare tumours and comprise chordomas, chondrosarcomas and carcinomas. Surgery is technically difficult and local recurrence rates are high.

Arachnoid cyst

These are common congenital lesions affecting sites throughout the central nervous system. In the posterior fossa, they are found around the foramen magnum, the cerebellopontine angle and in the pineal region. They are often asymptomatic. Should a mass effect occur, surgical treatment involves marsipualization of the cyst.

Glomus jugulare tumour

These are tumours of the extraadrenal paraganglion system. They arise in the region of the middle ear and may extend through the jugular foramen or through the petrous bone to the cerebellopontine angle.

Epidermoid cyst

These are benign tumours arising from epithelial cells. They are usually found in the cerebellopontine angle where they may enlarge to cause cranial nerve or brainstem dysfunction.

Because of the proximity of the skull base to perinasal sinuses, the mouth and upper respiratory tract, carcinomas originating in these regions can readily invade the posterior fossa. In recent years, combined surgical approaches involving neurosurgery, ear, nose and throat and plastic surgery have been utilized to treat these tumours aggressively.

VASCULAR LESIONS

Aneurysm

Fifteen percent of cerebral aneurysms occur in the posterior circulation. Of these, half occur at the basilar bifurcation and require a supratentorial or oral approach. Lesions of the vertebral and vertebrobasilar artery are treated through a suboccipital approach. For those aneurysms which are likely to be surgically technically difficult, consideration may be given to coiling in the neuroradiology suite (see Ch. 28).

Arteriovenous malformations

Arteriovenous malformations (AVMs) may occur anywhere in the posterior fossa but most frequently involve the brainstem. Rate of haemorrhage is significant at 2–3% per year.[4] Preoperative staged embolization reduces flow and may reduce intraoperative bleeding. Performing embolization in stages theoretically allows the surrounding normal brain to accommodate changes in blood flow, thereby minimizing the risk of 'normal perfusion pressure breakthrough'.[5]

Cerebellar infarction

Cerebellar infarction may be atherosclerotic, embolic or traumatic in origin. It presents as a neurosurgical emergency. Infarcted tissue swells to compress the brainstem and may cause obstructive hydrocephalus. Urgent ventriculostomy and removal of infarcted tissue may be a life-saving procedure.

Cerebellar haematoma

Cerebellar haematoma is usually associated with systemic hypertension but may be due to underlying metastatic tumours or AVMs. As with infarction, brainstem compression or obstructive hydrocephalus necessitates urgent decompression and evacuation.

CRANIAL NERVE COMPRESSION

Cranial nerves V, VII, VIII, IX and X are susceptible to compression by vascular structures at their entry zone into the pons. Microvascular decompression via a small retromastoid craniectomy has been performed for cranial nerve disorder, namely, trigeminal neuralgia (V), hemifacial spasm (VII), tinnitus or vertigo (VIII), glossopharyngeal neuralgia (IX) and hypertension (X). Surgery is reserved for those patients who are refractory to medical treatment and who have a reasonable life expectancy. It is important that underlying pathology be excluded in the work-up of candidates for microvascular decompression.

CRANIOCERVICAL ABNORMALITIES

Instability of the atlantooccipital and atlantoaxial joints may be traumatic, inflammatory, metabolic or congenital in origin. Lesions which cause brainstem compromise from the dorsal aspect require posterior fossa decompression craniectomy. When brainstem compromise is from the ventral aspect, the surgical approach is usually anterior through the transoral route.

The congenital Chiari malformations have been categorized as types I, II and III. Syringomyelia is often a feature of types I and II. Type I lesions present in early adulthood and are characterized by caudal displacement of the cerebellar tonsils below the foramen magnum (Figure 19.2). In type II malformations, there is caudal displacement of the cerebellar vermis, fourth ventricle and lower brainstem. Type II lesions present in the neonatal period with lower cranial nerve dysfunction. They tend to be associated with spina bifida. A type III lesion is herniation of the hindbrain into an occipital encephalocoele.

Hydrocephalus is usually associated with the Chiari malformations and needs to be controlled preoperatively. Definitive surgical treatment consists of suboccipital craniectomy with an upper cervical laminectomy and dural augmentation. Associated fluid-filled cavities, or syrinxes, may require shunting.[6]

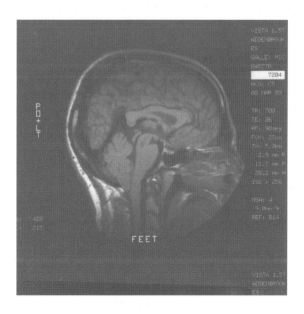

Figure 19.2   Tonsillar herniation in an adult with Chiari malformation.

PATIENT POSITIONING

During posterior fossa surgery, the optimal patient position should facilitate surgical access without jeopardizing patient safety. Important considerations are access to the patient, security of the airway and adequate protection of the eyes, skin and peripheral nerves. The potential hazards of each position can be minimized through appropriate patient selection, careful positioning and vigilance throughout the procedure.

SUPINE POSITION

The lateral posterior fossa may be accessed with the patient in the supine position and the head maximally rotated to the contralateral side. Use of the supine position overcomes many of the complications associated with other positions used in posterior fossa surgery. However, this is not a feasible position in patients with reduced lateral neck movement. There is the potential for impaired venous drainage, with consequent cerebral venous engorgement, and for macroglossia. The tongue should be checked to ensure it does not protrude beyond the teeth. A small soft bite block, rather than an oropharyngeal airway, should be used. A support should be placed under the shoulder on the side of the operation to reduce stretching of the brachial plexus.

The straight supine position is used when the posterior fossa or upper cervical spine is approached transorally. Because of the risk of infection with this surgical approach, it is rarely used.

LATERAL POSITION

The lateral position facilitates gravitational retraction of the dependent cerebellum and CSF and venous drainage from the uppermost posterior fossa. This makes it a suitable position for unilateral surgical procedures. Compared with other positions, the incidence of venous air embolism (VAE) and postural hypotension is minimized and the patient is easily accessed. The principal disadvantage is the potential for peripheral nerve damage.

Meticulous attention must be paid to positioning of patients. The upper arm may need to be taped to prevent the shoulder obscuring the surgeon's view. However, care should be taken to avoid excessive traction of the brachial plexus. Tilting the operating table head-up may allow the shoulder to fall away from the surgeon and enhance drainage of CSF and blood from the surgical site. A roll is placed under the chest just caudal to the dependent axilla. Migration of

the axillary roll can result in compression injuries to the brachial plexus. It should be checked once the patient is finally positioned. The dependent arm is usually positioned along the patient's side. The dependent leg is at risk of lateral popliteal nerve damage. It should be positioned straight with adequate padding. The upper leg should be flexed with a pillow placed between the knees. The patient's head is usually in three-point skull fixation. If it is on a headrest, care should be taken to avoid undue pressure on the dependent ear and eye.

PARK BENCH

This is a modification of the lateral position so called because the patient is positioned to resemble a drunk reclining on a park bench. The patient is positioned semiprone and the head rotated and flexed so the brow faces the floor. This allows greater access to midline structures than with the straight lateral position. The same principles apply to protection of peripheral nerves as with the lateral position. There is the same potential for venous engorgement and macroglossia as with lateral rotation of the head in the supine position.

PRONE POSITION

The prone position facilitates access to midline posterior fossa structures, the craniocervical junction and upper spinal cord. Appropriate patient selection is important. In patients with fixed neck extension, exposure of the cervical region may be inadequate. The prone position poses particular hazards for the obese patient because of restricted diaphragmatic movement and high intrathoracic pressures.[7]

The importance of secure fixation of the endotracheal tube cannot be overemphasized. There should be as little infringement on normal ventilation as possible. Whatever support is used, the abdomen and thorax should not be compressed. The head and neck should be held in alignment during transfer to the prone position. Horseshoe frames are best avoided because of the risk of pressure necrosis of the face and the potential for orbital compression due to movement of the head during surgery. For this reason, three-point skull fixation is preferred. Once the patient is finally positioned, a check is made to ensure the chin is clear of the end of the operating table. The arms should be padded and tucked by the side. The knees and ankles should be slightly flexed and padded.

Reduction in venous return due to venous pooling may be poorly tolerated, especially in elderly patients. The risk of VAE is less than with the sitting position[8] but is not eliminated since the head is usually elevated to assist drainage of fluid from the surgical site.[9]

The disadvantages of the prone position are that access to the airway and monitoring apparatus is restricted. Cardiopulmonary resuscitation, should it be required, is considerably hampered by inadequate access to the chest wall. Costly delays are incurred by having to reposition the patient.

SITTING POSITION

The sitting position provides the surgeon with excellent exposure of midline structures and the cerebellopontine angle. It promotes drainage of blood and CSF and allows the cerebellar hemispheres to fall away, thus minimizing the need for surgical retraction. The anaesthetist is able to access the patient's airway and monitoring apparatus without difficulty. Should resuscitation be required, the chest wall is accessible. Free diaphragmatic excursion makes ventilation much better than with other positions. Vital capacity and functional residual capacity are improved in the sitting position.

However, the sitting position has largely fallen into disrepute because of its potential for life-threatening complications when alternative positions can be used more safely. The sitting position is associated with significant hypotension, VAE, paradoxical air embolism (PAE), quadriplegia and pneumocephalus.[10] Macroglossia and peripheral nerve injuries can occur with other posterior fossa positions but are much more likely to occur with the sitting position. Bilateral posterior compartment syndrome has been reported as a rare complication.[11]

To place the patient in the sitting position, three-point skull fixation is applied following induction of anaesthesia. Thigh-high compression stockings are applied to the legs, taking care to ensure they do not act as a tourniquet. The operating table is slowly flexed while cardiovascular parameters are closely monitored with the arterial pressure transducer at the level of the skull base. Intravenous fluid loading may be necessary during this manoeuvre.

The final position is between semirecumbent and full sitting with the feet at the level of the heart. Overflexion of the hips places traction on the sciatic nerve and should be avoided. The foot of the table is dropped 30° so the knees are flexed. The sitting position has been linked with common peroneal nerve injury. This may be due to direct compression by bandages at the fibular head or stretching of the sciatic nerve.[12] Care should be taken to avoid overflexion of the neck. There should be at least two finger breadths between the chin and the chest wall during inspiration. As with other positions, the tongue should be checked to ensure it does not protrude between the teeth. The arms are folded so that the hands rest on the lap. Pressure points at the elbows, lateral and medial aspects of the knees and heels should be carefully padded.

COMPLICATIONS OF THE SITTING POSITION

CARDIOVASCULAR

The sitting position is associated with venous pooling which results in significant hypotension. Studies using pulmonary artery flotation catheters have shown reductions in pulmonary capillary wedge pressure (PCWP) and cardiac index with compensatory increases in heart rate and systemic vascular resistance.[13] ASA III and IV patients have been shown to be more susceptible to reductions in blood pressure than ASA I patients.[14] Hypotension is exaggerated if the hips are not fully flexed and if intravascular volume is depleted. Reduction in venous return may be offset to some extent by wrapping the lower extremities.[15]

Positioning the head above the heart results in a local reduction in arterial pressure of 0.77 mmHg per centimetre of elevation.[16] To assess cerebral perfusion pressure (CPP) accurately, the arterial pressure transducer should be placed at the level of the skull base.

VENOUS AIR EMBOLISM

Air entrainment occurs when a vein is held open to atmosphere and venous pressure at the operative site is subatmospheric. Although air may be entrained at any time, it most commonly occurs during the first hour of surgery when the posterior fossa is being exposed. Entrainment can occur at pin sites, veins in muscle, diploic veins, emissary veins and intracranial venous sinuses. The cited incidence varies depending on the sensitivity of the detection device used. In studies where precordial Doppler monitoring is used, the incidence of VAE in the sitting position is 25–50%.[13] A study using the more sensitive transoesophageal echocardiography (TOE) has documented an incidence of 76%.[17] In a combined retrospective and prospective study, the incidence of VAE was found to be twice as high in the subpopulation of children compared with adults.[10] Furthermore, children are more haemodynamically compromised by VAE.[18]

The adverse effects of VAE can be attributed to local endothelial reaction and to mechanical obstruction of blood flow. At the level of the endothelium, an inflammatory response cascade is triggered by the release of endothelial mediators leading to the production of reactive O_2 molecules. These cause bronchoconstriction and pulmonary hypertension which lead to a reduction in venous return and cardiac output.[19] At a gross level, a bolus of air may act as an airlock which blocks right ventricular outflow with a subsequent reduction in venous return and cardiac output. This results in right ventricular failure and myocardial ischaemia and ultimately cardiovascular collapse.[20]

The impact of VAE on the patient is determined by the volume and rate of air entrainment. In dogs, a rapid massive infusion of 3 ml/kg of air results in near complete pulmonary obstruction. Right-sided pressures become elevated, right ventricular failure ensues and cardiac output falls.[21] The lethal dose of air in humans is not well documented.

Methods of detection

Precordial Doppler

Of the monitors which are non-invasive, practical and easy to use, the precordial Doppler is the most sensitive. Doppler systems generate an ultrasonic signal which is reflected by moving blood and cardiac structures. Air is a good acoustic reflector. When it passes through the heart, there is a clearly audible change in signal. As little as 0.015 ml/kg of intracardiac air can be detected.[22] The precordial Doppler is placed over the right parasternal border. Proper placement can be verified by rapid injection of agitated saline through a right atrial catheter.[23] The precordial Doppler does, however, have limitations. Use of cautery interferes with the signal. Most units have cautery suppression circuits so the probe is silent during surgical cautery. Intravenous mannitol crystals can mimic VAE.[24] Signals may be lost during inspiration, particularly in obese patients and in patients with abnormal chest wall configurations.

Transoesophageal devices

The disadvantages of the precordial Doppler are overcome by use of transoesophageal devices. A study comparing the sensitivity of the precordial Doppler with transoesophageal Doppler and echocardiography found that precordial placement detected injected micro-bubbles 10% of the time whereas transoesophageal placement had a 100% detection rate.[25] TOE has the added advantage of localizing air within the heart so that passage of air through a right-to-left shunt is detected early.[26] The disadvantage of TOE is that it is not specific for VAE and may give a false-positive signal in the presence of fat or blood emboli. TOE has been associated with recurrent laryngeal nerve palsy in patients undergoing craniotomy in the sitting position.[26] The invasive nature and cost of transoe-sophageal devices prohibit their routine use in posterior fossa surgery.

Exhaled gas analysis

Monitors of intermediate sensitivity are end-tidal (ET) CO_2 and N_2. With reduced lung perfusion in the presence of air, physiological dead space is increased and cardiac output decreased, resulting in a fall in $ETCO_2$. Where a bolus of air is entrained, the fall is abrupt. If there is slow entrainment, the fall in $ETCO_2$ is gradual. However, a reduction in $ETCO_2$ is non-specific since any fall in cardiac output, regardless of aetiology, causes a decrease in $ETCO_2$.

Changes in ETN_2 occur earlier than $ETCO_2$ and are specific for air. Entrained air releases and expels nitrogen through the lungs and, provided inspired gas does not contain N_2, there is an increase in ETN_2. Animal studies have shown that significant changes in $ETCO_2$ and ETN_2 are detected with 0.25 ml/kg of injected air.[27] To some extent, the degree of change provides an approximation of the magnitude of the VAE.

Central venous catheters

Another monitor of intermediate sensitivity is the pulmonary artery catheter (PAC).[28] In the event of VAE, central venous pressure (CVP) and pulmonary artery pressure (PAP) increase while PCWP decreases.[29] Aspiration of air from a central venous catheter positioned at the caval–atrial junction confirms the diagnosis of VAE.[18] Unfortunately, only small amounts of air can be aspirated from the orifice of a PAC.

Signs of impending cardiovascular collapse are arrhythmias, hypotension and pulmonary oedema. These are late, non-specific signs. The traditional 'mill-wheel' murmur is heard with the oesophageal stethoscope when large amounts of air are entrained. It too is a late sign and of little clinical use now that more sensitive monitors are available.

Since each monitor has its limitations, it is recommended that several monitoring modalities be used during surgery in which there is a risk of VAE. A precordial Doppler should be used in conjunction with at least one other monitoring technique.

Prevention of VAE

Reduction in the risk of VAE, and the potentially devastating complication of paradoxical air embolism (PAE), relies on careful surgical technique, vigilance on the part of the anaesthetist and clear communication between the anaesthetist and surgeon.

Pin sites have been identified as a source of air entrainment. The risk is reduced by wrapping them with Vaseline-impregnated gauze before elevating the patient's head.[38] Since bone is a site of entrainment, bone wax should be used liberally. Meticulous surgical technique is paramount.

The role of the anaesthetist is to maximize intravascular pressure safely. Intravenous fluid loading, wrapping the lower limbs and jugular venous pressure[39] are all effective means of preventing VAE. Spontaneous ventilation should be avoided since it generates negative intravascular pressure and the 'gasp' which is reported to occur with initial entrainment of air leads to further entrainment. Studies of the use of positive end-expiratory pressure (PEEP) have found that it does not reliably elevate intracranial sinus pressure.[39,40] Whether PEEP predisposes to PAE in at-risk patients is unclear. It has been shown that some patients with patent foramen ovale develop right-to-left shunting only when PEEP is used.[41] Other studies have shown that PEEP increases right atrial pressure (RAP) and PCWP to the same extent so the interatrial pressure gradient remains unchanged.[42,43] One animal study has shown an increase in right-to-left shunting across a septal defect at the time of discontinuation of PEEP.[44] Because PEEP decreases venous return and cardiac output and may cause RAP to exceed left atrial pressure (LAP), its use is not recommended in the sitting position.

Because nitrous oxide (N_2O) diffuses into air-filled spaces more rapidly than N_2 diffuses out, it increases the size of compliant air spaces. In dogs, the LD_{50} for a bolus injection of air during N_2O administration is one-third of that during anaesthesia where N_2O is not used.[45] A study in humans has reported that the use of N_2O does not alter the incidence of VAE or haemodynamically significant events provided it is discontinued as soon as venous air is detected.[8] For those anaesthetists who choose to use N_2O during neurosurgery, early detection of venous air entrainment is particularly important.

Treatment of VAE

In the event of VAE, the surgeon should be informed immediately, N_2O should be discontinued and the inspired concentration of O_2 increased to 1.0. The surgical field should be flooded with saline and the patient's head lowered to prevent continued entrainment of air. Right atrial catheter (RAC) aspiration is effective in reducing VAE morbidity.[46,47]

For optimal retrieval of air, a multiorifice, rather than single-orifice, catheter should be positioned with the tip 0.5 cm beyond the sinoatrial node.[48,49] The position should be confirmed radiographically or electrocardiographically.

Temporary jugular venous compression should be considered. It causes cerebral venous distension which may allow the surgeon to identify and repair a tear in a vein. Caution should be exercised since compression may be associated with inadvertent manipulation of the carotid artery or carotid sinus. Other therapies include administration of intravenous fluid, antiarrhythmics, inotropes and vasopressors as required. In the event of cardiovascualar collapse, external cardiac compression should be commenced immediately. Chest compressions may break up a large airlock.

Animal data show the lethal dose of injected air is doubled when the animal is positioned left side down.[21] This manoeuvre may not be feasible in the surgical setting. Changing the patient's position is probably only therapeutic if it promotes retrieval of air from the RAC.

PARADOXICAL AIR EMBOLISM

When air enters the systemic circulation, it triggers thrombus formation and causes critical ischaemia of distal tissues. The clinical outcome depends on the volume of air and the vascular bed affected. If air lodges in the coronary and cerebral circulations, the consequences may be life-threatening. The incidence of PAE complicating VAE is estimated to be 5–10%.[30]

Venous gas bubbles may cross to the systemic circulation through septal defects when pressure in the right side of the heart exceeds pressure in the left. Anatomically 2% of patients have interatrial septal defects and 25% have probe-patent foramen ovale on autopsy.[31] Functionally, a right-to-left atrial shunt has been demonstrated during release of Valsalva in 18% of healthy volunteers.[32] It has been shown that merely changing to the sitting position can reverse the interatrial pressure gradient in up to 50% of patients.[33]

Patients with functional or anatomical evidence of right-to-left shunt are clearly at risk of PAE in the event of venous air entrainment in the sitting position. However, PAE does not always occur when these conditions exist. Conversely, there have been reports of PAE in the absence of a cardiac septal defect.[34,35] Indeed, transpulmonary passage of air in the absence of a right-to-left shunt has been documented using TOE in a patient undergoing surgery in the sitting position.[36]

The probable explanation is that the filtering capability of the lung is overwhelmed by the volume of air entrained. The filtering capacity of the lungs is impaired by pulmonary vasodilators, in particular volatile anaesthetic agents.[37] Another possibility is the presence of pulmonary AVMs. However, these are rare.

Where it is suspected that VAE has been complicated by PAE, consideration may be given to hyperbaric oxygen therapy (HBO). The delivery of 100% O_2 at high pressures facilitates resorption of air bubbles and allows delivery of O_2 by diffusion mechanisms to tissues distal to arterial obstruction. There have been case reports of clinical improvement following HBO.[50] However, in the absence of strong evidence, it remains a controversial mode of treatment.

PNEUMOCEPHALUS

It appears that the presence of intracranial air is inevitable following posterior fossa surgery. A tension pneumocephalus occurs when this air expands to exert a mass effect on the brain. This is a potentially life-threatening complication of posterior fossa surgery which requires rapid diagnosis and treatment. A retrospective review of neurosurgery in the sitting position cites a 3% incidence of tension pneumocephalus.[12]

During surgery, use of diuretics, hyperventilation, blood loss, removal of a mass lesion and use of CSF drainage systems all contribute to brain shrinkage. As brain volume diminishes, air enters the epidural and dural spaces. Intraoperative use of N_2O exacerbates the situation by expanding the pneumocephalus. There have, however, been case reports of tension pneumocephalus when N_2O was not used or was discontinued 20–30 min prior to dural closure.[51,52] While avoiding N_2O may help, it certainly does not eliminate the problem.

The potential for tension pneumocephalus can be reduced by flushing the subdural space wth normal saline, minimizing use of diuretics and hyperventilation, ensuring adequate volume replacement and slowing CSF drainage. N_2O should be avoided for at least 14 days following posterior fossa surgery.[53]

Tension pnuemocephalus should be suspected in patients with neurological deficit following surgery in the sitting position. Air can be localized on CT scan and urgent aspiration via burr holes should be performed. Untreated tension pneumocephalus can result in brain herniation and has been associated with cardiac arrest.[54]

QUADRIPLEGIA

There have been reports of quadriplegia following surgery in the sitting position.[55] It is postulated that flexion of the neck in the anaesthetized patient stretches the cord and, especially if combined with hypotension, results in hypoperfusion of the spinal cord. It is likely that patients with degenerative spinal cord disease are particularly at risk of spinal cord ischaemia. The sitting position is relatively contraindicated in this at-risk group of patients.

CENTRAL NERVOUS SYSTEM MONITORING

SOMATOSENSORY EVOKED POTENTIALS (SSEPS)

SSEPs have been advocated as a means of monitoring potential spinal cord ischaemia as a result of excessive neck flexion in the sitting position.[55] Because SSEPs monitor the integrity of the dorsal sensory pathways, rather than anterior motor tracts, paralysis can occur in the absence of SSEP changes.[56] A major drawback of SSEPs is that they are sensitive to anaesthetic agents.

ELECTROENCEPHALOGRAPHY (EEG)

The EEG monitors spontaneous electrical activity in the cerebral cortex. Inadequate perfusion or oxygenation results in 'slowing' of the EEG, that is, reduced amplitude of higher frequency waves and increased amplitude of lower frequency waves. The EEG is susceptible to the effects of anaesthetic agents and hypothermia.

BRAINSTEM AUDITORY EVOKED POTENTIALS (BAEPS)

BAEPs are generated by delivering clicks to each ear and monitoring the response pathway from the auditory nerve to the pons and thalamus. They are relatively resistant to the effects of anaesthetic agents. It has been recommended that BAEPs monitoring be used whenever there is potential for brainstem injury, even if hearing is already diminished. Monitoring cranial nerve VIII helps preserve its function during acoustic neuroma surgery and microvascular decompression.[57]

ELECTROMYOGRAPHY (EMG)

Monitoring cranial nerve VII using evoked EMG reduces the risk of intraoperative damage during acoustic neuroma resection and microvascular decompression.[57] EMG monitoring requires that the patient not be fully paralysed.

SPONTANEOUS VENTILATION

Historically, the spontaneously ventilating patient was used as a monitor of brainstem function during posterior fossa surgery. The disadvantages of this technique were venous congestion secondary to hypercarbia and increased risk of VAE. There are those who believe spontaneous ventilation should be used as a means of detecting brainstem ischaemia during vertebral basilar surgery.[58] Most practitioners rely on more sensitive, but less specific, cardiovascular signs.

ANAESTHETIC MANAGEMENT

PREOPERATIVE EVALUATION

As well as the usual anaesthetic assessment, the preoperative evaluation should take account of the patient's neurological pathology and underlying cardiorespiratory function. The patient's mental status should be evaluated and preoperative neurological deficits documented. Evidence of lower cranial nerve pathology, specifically impaired gag reflex and history of aspiration pneumonia, should be sought (Figure 19.3). This has implications for airway protection in the postoperative period. Patients with a history of hypertension or cerebrovascular disease have impaired autoregulation in which case hypotension should be avoided.

The patient should be assessed as to their suitability for the proposed surgical position. Patients with cervical spine degeneration are not suitable for the sitting position. Obese patients are not suited to lying prone and consideration should be given to an alternative surgical position. Patients with known right-to-left shunts are at increased risk of PAE and should not undergo surgery in the sitting position. Given the lack of sensitivity of echocardiography and the fact that PAE can occur in the absence of a septal defect, routine preoperative screening echocardiography is not recommended.[59]

Patients are often dehydrated due to reduced oral intake, vomiting, use of diuretics and intravenous contrast administration. Provision should be made for intravenous fluid replacement in the preoperative period.

Premedication should include continuation of the patient's usual medications. Anxiolytic medication should be reserved for those patients who are neurologically intact.

INDUCTION

The goals of induction are to preserve cerebral perfusion pressure, avoid increases in intracranial pressure (ICP) and institute appropriate monitoring. In patients in whom control of blood pressure is important, an arterial catheter should be placed prior to induction. Other routine monitors include electrocardiography (ECG), non-invasive blood pressure (NIBP), ETCO$_2$ and pulse oximetry. The security and proper functioning of monitors warrants special attention in high-risk posterior fossa surgery.

Induction is achieved using an appropriate opioid, induction agent and muscle relaxant. In patients with poorly compliant brains it is important to avoid coughing at the time of intubation. Hypertension due to laryngoscopy can be obtunded using intravenous lignocaine, a short-acting β-blocker or opioid or a bolus of intravenous induction agent. An appropriately sized armoured endotracheal tube is inserted and secured immediately. This is an opportune time to insert a nasogastric tube in those patients who are likely to be ventilated postoperatively.

Following induction, a urinary catheter, temperature probe and RAC are inserted. To optimize the position of the RAC for aspiration of air, intravascular ECG can be used. If not done preoperatively, thigh-high compression stockings are applied to the legs in an attempt to limit venous pooling. In surgery where there is a risk of VAE, a precordial Doppler is applied to the anterior chest wall. Some anaesthetists also choose to insert a PAC in this situation. Central nervous system monitoring devices are instituted.

Application of head pins is a potent stimulus which elicits hypertension and tachycardia unless pretreated with accurate placement of local anaesthetic, an opioid or a bolus of intravenous induction agent.

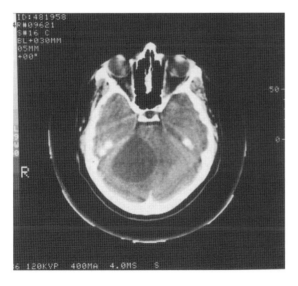

Figure 19.3   Large posterior fossa mass causing midbrain compression.

Hypotension can occur in the postinduction phase during positioning, particularly in frail, elderly patients. This needs to be treated promptly with intravenous fluids or vasopressors as appropriate.

The position of the endotracheal tube and the security of monitoring apparatus and intravenous lines must be rechecked once the patient is finally positioned.

MAINTENANCE

The aim is to reduce ICP while maintaining haemodynamic stability. The choice of anaesthetic agents is largely at the discretion of the individual anaesthetist. Many anaesthetists choose to avoid N_2O because of the problems associated with tension pneumocephalus and VAE. Some would minimize the use of inhalational anaesthetic agents because they facilitate the transpulmonary passage of air and because they interfere with SSEP monitoring. In procedures where EMG monitoring is used, muscle relaxants should be administered as an infusion to maintain partial paralysis or avoided altogether. In this situation, anaesthesia needs to be supplemented with an intravenous infusion of propofol or a short-acting opioid.

The usual practice is to ventilate patients undergoing posterior fossa surgery. This allows control of $PaCO_2$, thus reducing bleeding and ICP, and reduces the risk of venous air entrainment. Arterial blood gases should be checked once ventilation is established and then intermittently as required.

Mild hypothermia (34–36°C) is maintained intraoperatively. There is evidence from animal studies[60] and from observations in humans[61] that mild hypothermia improves outcome following a neurological insult. Mild hypothermia can be achieved with passive cooling. Patients usually need to be actively rewarmed to achieve a core temperature of 36°C at the time of emergence.

The administration of a diuretic, usually mannitol, prior to dural opening results in a large diuresis. Normovolaemia should be maintained using filling pressures as a guide. Glucose-containing solutions should be avoided since hyperglycaemia is known to aggravate ischaemic brain insults.[62] Blood loss should be recorded and the haematocrit measured periodically. The threshold for transfusion varies according to the underlying condition of the individual patient.

EMERGENCE

The management of emergence is determined by the patient's preoperative status and by intraoperative events. If the patient was neurologically intact preoperatively and has had an uneventful operative course, a smooth emergence is the goal. Ideally, coughing and straining should be avoided. An awake patient provides the best monitor of neurological function.

If there was preoperative compromise of airway reflexes or there has been extensive intraoperative manipulation around the brainstem, intubation and ventilation should be maintained postoperatively. The patient should remain intubated until there is evidence of return of a gag reflex. Occasionally positioning of the patient can result in swelling of the face and neck due to venous engorgement. Facial swelling can be indicative of swelling in the upper airway tissues. Where this is suspected, intubation should be maintained postoperatively until the swelling settles. When the ventilated patient is sedated, an ICP monitor may be the only means of monitoring the well-being of the brain.

CONCLUSION

Posterior fossa surgery poses a unique challenge for the surgeon and anaesthetist alike. It is important that the team be aware of the potential problems arising from the nature of the patient's pathology and surgical positioning. Care with positioning, meticulous surgical technique and vigilant monitoring help to minimize risk. Should a complication develop, it needs to be recognized early and treated appropriately. For these patients, the risk of complications continues into the postoperative period. Close monitoring after surgery is needed to ensure a safe outcome.

REFERENCES

1. Snell R. Clinical anatomy for medical students vol 1, 2nd edn. Little, Brown, Boston, 1981.

2. Petronio J, Walker M. Posterior fossa tumors. In: Rengachary S, Wilkins R (eds) Principles of neurosurgery, vol 1. Wolfe, London, 1994, pp 31.1–31.24.

3. Wilkins R. Cerebellar pontine angle tumors. In: Rengachary S, Wilkins R (eds) Principles of neurosurgery, vol 1. Wolfe, London, 1994, pp 30.1–30.7.

4. Drake CG, Friedman AH, Peerless SJ. Posterior fossa arteriovenous malformations. J Neurosurg 1986; 64(1): 1–10.

5. Spetzler RF, Martin NA, Carter LP, Flom RA, Raudzens PA, Wilkinson E. Surgical management of large AVM's by staged embolization and operative excision. J Neurosurg 1987; 67(1): 17–28.

6. Wen D, Haines S. Posterior fossa: surgical considerations. In: Cottrell J, Smith D (eds) Anesthesia and Neurosurgery, vol 1, 3rd edn, Mosby, London, 1994, p 330.

7. Coonan TJ, Hope CE. Cardio-respiratory effects of change of body position. Can Anaesth Soc J 1983; 30(4): 424–438.

8. Black S, Ockert DB, Oliver WC Jr, Cucchiara RF. Outcome following posterior fossa craniectomy in patients in the sitting or horizontal positions. Anesthesiology 1988; 69(1): 49–56.

9. Shenkin HN, Goldfedder P. Air embolism from exposure of posterior cranial fossa in prone position. JAMA 1969; 210(4): 726.

10. Matjasko J, Petrozza P, Cohen M, Steinberg P. Anesthesia and surgery in the seated position: analysis of 554 cases. Neurosurgery 1985; 17(5): 695–702.

11. Poppi M, Giuliani G, Gambari PI, Acciarri N, Gaist G, Calbucci F. A hazard of craniotomy in the sitting position: the posterior compartment syndrome of the thigh. Case report. J Neurosurg 1989; 71(4): 618–619.

12. Standefer M, Bay JW, Trusso R. The sitting position in neurosurgery: a retrospective analysis of 488 cases. Neurosurgery 1984; 14(6): 649–658.

13. Porter J, Pidgeon C, Cunningham A. The sitting position in neurosurgery: a critical appraisal. Br J Anaesth 1999; 82: 117–128.

14. Albin M, Babinski M, Maroon J et al. Anesthetic management of posterior fossa surgery in the sitting position. Acta Anaesth Scand 1976; 20: 117–128.

15. Marshall WK, Bedford RF, Miller ED. Cardiovascular responses in the seated position – impact of four anesthetic techniques. Anesth Analg 1983; 62(7): 648–653.

16. Ganong W. Dynamics of blood and lymph flow. In: Lange (ed) Review of medical physiology, 15th edn. Appleton and Lange, Norwalk, CA, 1991, pp 542–543.

17. Papadopoulos G, Kuhly P, Brock M et al. Venous and paradoxical air embolism in the sitting position. A prospective study. Acta Neurochir (Wien) 1994; 126: 140–143.

18. Cucchiara RF, Bowers B. Air embolism in children undergoing suboccipital craniotomy. Anesthesiology 1982; 57(4): 338–339.

19. Pfitzner J, Petito SP, McLean AG. Hypoxaemia following sustained low-volume venous air embolism in sheep. Anaesth Intens Care 1988; 16(2): 164–170.

20. Adornato DC, Gildenberg PL, Ferrario CM, Smart J, Frost EA. Pathophysiology of intravenous air embolism in dogs. Anesthesiology 1978; 49(2): 120–127.

21. Holt EP Jr, Webb WR, Cook WA, Unal MO. Air embolism. Hemodynamics and therapy. Ann Thorac Surg 1966; 2(4): 551–560.

22. Gildenberg PL, RP OB, Britt WJ, Frost EA. The efficacy of Doppler monitoring for the detection of venous air embolism. J Neurosurg 1981; 54(1): 75–78.

23. Tinker JH, Gronert GA, Messick JM, Michenfelder JD. Detection of air embolism, a test for positioning of right atrial catheter and Doppler probe. Anesthesiology 1975; 43(1): 104–106.

24. Losasso TJ, Muzzi DA, Cucchiara RF. Doppler detection of intravenous mannitol crystals mimics venous air embolism [letter]. Anesth Analg 1990; 71(5): 568–569.

25. Muzzi DA, Losasso TJ, Black S, Nishimura R. Comparison of a transesophageal and precordial ultrasonic Doppler sensor in the detection of venous air embolism. Anesth Analg 1990; 70(1): 103–104.

26. Cucchiara RF, Nugent M, Seward JB, Messick JM. Air embolism in upright neurosurgical patients: detection and localization by two-dimensional transesophageal echocardiography. Anesthesiology 1984; 60(4): 353–355.

27. Drummond JC, Prutow RJ, Scheller MS. A comparison of the sensitivity of pulmonary artery pressure, end-tidal carbon dioxide, and end-tidal nitrogen in the detection of venous air embolism in the dog. Anesth Analg 1985; 64(7): 688–692.

28. Bedford RF, Marshall WK, Butler A, Welsh JE. Cardiac catheters for diagnosis and treatment of venous air embolism: a prospective study in man. J Neurosurg 1981; 55(4): 610–614.

29. Marshall WK, Bedford RF. Use of a pulmonary-artery catheter for detection and treatment of venous air embolism: a prospective study in man. Anesthesiology 1980; 52(2): 131–134.

30. Young M. Posterior fossa: anesthetic considerations. In: Cottrell J, Smith D (eds) Anesthesia and neurosurgery, vol 1. Mosby, London, 1994, p 349.

31. Hagen PT, Scholz DG, Edwards WD. Incidence and size of patent foramen ovale during the first 10 decades of life: an autopsy study of 965 normal hearts. Mayo Clin Proc 1984; 59(1): 17–20.

32. Lynch JJ, Schuchard GH, Gross CM, Wann LS. Prevalence of right-to-left atrial shunting in a healthy population: detection by Valsalva maneuver contrast echocardiography. Am J Cardiol 1984; 53(10): 1478–1480.

33. Perkins-Pearson NA, Marshall WK, Bedford RF. Atrial pressures in the seated position: implication for paradoxical air embolism. Anesthesiology 1982; 57(6): 493–497.

34. Marquez J, Sladen A, Gendell H, Boehnke M, Mendelow H. Paradoxical cerebral air embolism without an intracardiac septal defect. Case report. J Neurosurg 1981; 55(6): 997–1000.

35. Tommasino C, Rizzardi R, Beretta L, Venturino M, Piccoli S. Cerebral ischemia after venous air embolism in the absence of intracardiac defects [see comments]. J Neurosurg Anesthesiol 1996; 8(1): 30–34.

36. Bedell EA, Berge KH, Losasso TJ. Paradoxic air embolism during venous air embolism: transesophageal echocardiographic evidence of transpulmonary air passage [see comments]. Anesthesiology 1994; 80(4): 947–950.

37. Katz J, Leiman BC, Butler BD. Effects of inhalation anaesthetics on filtration of venous gas emboli by the

pulmonary vasculature. Br J Anaesth 1988; 61(2): 200–205.

38. Cabezudo JM, Gilsanz F, Vaquero J, Areitio E, Martinez R. Air embolism from wounds from a pin-type head-holder as a complication of posterior fossa surgery in the sitting position. Case report. J Neurosurg 1981; 55(1): 147–148.

39. Grady MS, Bedford RF, Park TS. Changes in superior sagittal sinus pressure in children with head elevation, jugular venous compression, and PEEP. J Neurosurg 1986; 65(2): 199–202.

40. Zentner J, Albrecht T, Hassler W. Prevention of an air embolism by moderate hypoventilation during surgery in the sitting position. Neurosurgery 1991; 28(5): 705–708.

41. Cucchiara RF, Seward JB, Nishimura RA, Nugent M, Faust RJ. Identification of patent foramen ovale during sitting position craniotomy by transesophageal echocardiography with positive airway pressure. Anesthesiology 1985; 63(1): 107–109.

42. Pearl RG, Larson CP Jr. Hemodynamic effects of positive end-expiratory pressure during continuous venous air embolism in the dog. Anesthesiology 1986; 64(6): 724–729.

43. Zasslow MA, Pearl RG, Larson CP, Silverberg G, Shuer LF. PEEP does not affect left atrial-right atrial pressure difference in neurosurgical patients. Anesthesiology 1988; 68(5): 760–763.

44. Black S, Cucchiara RF, Nishimura RA, Michenfelder JD. Parameters affecting occurrence of paradoxical air embolism. Anesthesiology 1989; 71(2): 235–241.

45. Munson ES, Merrick HC. Effect of nitrous oxide on venous air embolism. Anesthesiology 1966; 27(6): 783–787.

46. Michenfelder JD, Martin JT, Altenburg BM, Rehder K. Air embolism during neurosurgery. An evaluation of right-atrial catheters for diagnosis and treatment. JAMA 1969; 208(8): 1353–1358.

47. Alvaran SB, Toung JK, Graff TE, Benson DW. Venous air embolism: comparative merits of external cardiac massage, intracardiac aspiration, and left lateral decubitus position. Anesth Analg 1978; 57(2): 166–170.

48. Bunegin L, Albin MS, Helsel PE, Hoffman A, Hung TK. Positioning the right atrial catheter: a model for reappraisal. Anesthesiology 1981; 55(4): 343–348.

49. Colley PS, Artru AA. Bunegin-Albin catheter improves air retrieval and resuscitation from lethal venous air embolism in upright dogs. Anesth Analg 1989; 68(3): 298–301.

50. Harvey WR, Lee CJ, Koch SM, Butler BD. Delayed presentation of cerebral arterial gas embolism following

proven intraoperative venous air embolism [see comments]. J Neurosurg Anesthesiol 1996; 8(1): 26–29.

51. Friedman GA, Norfleet EA, Bedford RF. Discontinuance of nitrous oxide does not prevent tension pneumocephalus. Anesth Analg 1981; 60(1): 57–58.

52. Toung T, Donham RT, Lehner A, Alano J, Campbell J. Tension pneumocephalus after posterior fossa craniotomy: report of four additional cases and review of postoperative pneumocephalus. Neurosurgery 1983; 12(2): 164–168.

53. Pandit UA, Mudge BJ, Keller TS et al. Pneumocephalus after posterior fossa exploration in the sitting position. Anaesthesia 1982; 37(10): 996–1001.

54. Thiagarajah S, Frost EA, Singh T, Shulman K. Cardiac arrest associated with tension pneumocephalus. Anesthesiology 1982; 56(1): 73–75.

55. Wilder BL. Hypothesis: the etiology of midcervical quadriplegia after operation with the patient in the sitting position. Neurosurgery 1982; 11(4): 530–531.

56. Lesser RP, Raudzens P, Luders H et al. Postoperative neurological deficits may occur despite unchanged intraoperative somatosensory evoked potentials. Ann Neurol 1986; 19(1): 22–25.

57. Linden R, Tator C, Benedict D et al. Electro-physiological monitoring during acoustic neuroma and other posterior fossa surgery. Can J Neurol Sci 1988; 53: 73–81.

58. Manninen PH, Cuillerier DJ, Nantau WE, Gelb AW. Monitoring of brainstem function during vertebral basilar aneurysm surgery. The use of spontaneous ventilation. Anesthesiology 1992; 77(4): 681–685.

59. Black S, Muzzi DA, Nishimura RA et al. Preoperative and intraoperative echocardiography to detect right-to-left shunt in patients undergoing neurosurgical procedures in the sitting position. Anesthesiology 1990; 72: 436–438.

60. Minamisawa H, Nordstrom CH, Smith ML et al. The influence of mild body and brain hypothermia on ischemic brain injury. J Cereb Blood Flow Metab 1990; 10(3): 365–374.

61. Shiozaki T, Sugimoto H, Taneda M et al. Effect of mild hypothermia on uncontrollable intracranial hypertension after severe head injury. J Neurosurg 1993; 79(3): 363–368.

62. Lanier W, Stangland K, Scheithauer B et al. The effects of dextrose infusion and head position on neurologic outcome after complete cerebral ischemia in primates: examination of a model. Anesthesiology 1987; 66: 39–48.

SECTION 4

NEUROSURGICAL AND NEUROLOGICAL INTENSIVE CARE

20

MANAGEMENT OF ACUTE HEAD INJURY: PATHOPHYSIOLOGY, INITIAL RESUSCITATION AND TRANSFER

Mark J. Abrahams, David K. Menon & Basil F. Matta

INTRODUCTION

Of all the injuries sustained in a traumatic event, head injury is frequently associated with the most devastating outcome. The patient often survives the accident only to end up with a major neurologic deficit. In addition to the stress this puts on the victims and their families, the economic costs are high because most of the injuries occur in the young during their working years.[1]

Better prehospital care, the institution of regional centres with new imaging techniques and the ready availability of multidisciplinary teams have improved the very poor outlook that was previously associated with head trauma. However, outcome continues to be affected by abnormal physiology in the immediate postinjury period.[2]

Anaesthetists are commonly involved in the management of patients who have suffered head injuries. Their role is in the emergency room protecting the airway and instituting resuscitation, in the operating theatre while treating the neurological injury (e.g. evacuating a haematoma) or other injuries (e.g. laparotomy for ruptured viscera) and in the intensive care unit. In this chapter, we review the pathophysiology of head injury and highlight new advances in the management of the severely head-injured patient.

PHYSIOLOGY OF CEREBRAL BLOOD FLOW

The human brain receives about 15% of the resting cardiac output but uses only 20% of the body's oxygen consumption. This translates into a mean cerebral blood flow (CBF) of about 50 ml/100 g/min and a mean cerebral metabolic rate for oxygen ($CMRO_2$) of 3.2 ml/100 g/min, with glucose as the main substrate (60 mg/100 g/min). Under normal circumstances regional CBF and metabolism are tightly coupled, with an increase in cortical activity leading to a corresponding increase in CBF. When oxygen delivery falls, $CMRO_2$ declines to basal levels (1.2–1.5 ml O_2/min/100 g) and there is an increase in anaerobic metabolism.

Brain tissue is particularly vulnerable to reductions in oxygen delivery because it has a high metabolic rate and no capacity to store substrate. It has to ensure that oxygen delivery is maintained at a constant level despite changes in the vascular and cranial environment. In the healthy, awake, normotensive individual, CBF is maintained at a constant level within the range of cerebral perfusion pressures (CPP) between 60 and 160 mmHg. This autoregulation is effected through direct variation in cerebral vascular resistance in response to alterations in the CPP. Since the CPP depends on the difference between mean arterial pressure (MAP) and intracranial pressure (ICP), changes to either can initiate autoregulation, i.e. a decrease in arterial pressure has the same effect on autoregulation as an increase in ICP. Although the exact mechanisms responsible for this very efficient process are not completely understood, it is likely that both myogenic and metabolic factors are involved. The process has been classically thought to occur in minutes but recent evidence suggests that, at least during small changes in blood pressure, it is complete in seconds.[3] The limits of autoregulation may be affected by disease processes and are modulated by sympathetic nervous system activity. α and β-blockade can change the lower limit of autoregulation (shift the curve to the left) and chronic hypertension increases the limits of autoregulation by shifting the curve to the right.[4] Autoregulation is also affected by the level of $PaCO_2$. Hypocapnia restores autoregulation when impaired and accelerates the process when present, while hypercapnia abolishes autoregulation and renders the cerebral circulation pressure passive.[5,6]

Arterial carbon dioxide tension is one of the most potent regulators of CBF. Within the range 3–10 kPa, CBF increases linearly by about 25% per kPa increase in $PaCO_2$. The effect of $PaCO_2$ on cerebral blood volume (CBV), however, is less pronounced. CBV changes by about 10% per kPa change in $PaCO_2$ in the healthy individual but recent evidence has suggested that the relationship between $PaCO_2$ and CBV is not predictable in the patient with brain injury. The cerebral blood volume constitutes only around 5% of the total intracranial volume but, since the brain is situated in an enclosed space, even a small change in CBV can have a profound effect on the ICP, particularly in those with reduced intracranial compliance.

Arterial oxygen tension has little effect on CBF in the physiologic range. However, high arterial oxygen tension (>100 kPa) can cause cerebral vasoconstriction, and PaO_2 below 7 kPa will cause cerebral vasodilatation which overrides any vasoconstriction due to hypocapnia. There is some evidence to suggest that CBF increases even during modest reductions in oxygen saturation.[7]

PATHOPHYSIOLOGY OF HEAD INJURY

When the head is struck, neurones and intracranial blood vessels are subjected to direct impact as well as flexion, extension and shearing forces as the brain moves inside the cranium. While most management issues focus on the treatment of raised intracranial pressure as a consequence of intracranial haematomas, contusions or brain swelling, it is important to realize that diffuse axonal damage may result in profound neurologic deficit without intracranial hypertension.

The *primary injury*, which is not treatable and can only be prevented, describes the damage that occurs at the time of initial impact. The amount of primary injury is dependent on the degree of force applied to the brain and is the principal factor that delineates a viable from a non-viable injury. Of the 1.1 million head injuries seen in hospital in Britain every year, 10,000 are severe.[1] Severe head injury renders the patient comatose from impact; those able to talk at any stage following the injury are unlikely to have sustained a substantial primary injury.

Secondary injury is the additional insult imposed on the neural tissue following the primary impact. Treatment is aimed at preventing secondary cerebral ischaemia and thereby reducing the incidence of patients with head injury admitted to hospital in a conscious state only to die later[8,9]. The main contributors to secondary ischaemia in the head-injured patient are:

- hypoxaemia;
- hypercapnia;
- hyperventilation;
- systemic hypotension;
- intracranial masses;
- intracranial hypertension;
- posttraumatic cerebral arterial spasm

REGULATION OF CEREBRAL BLOOD FLOW IN THE HEAD-INJURED PATIENT

In the healthy brain, local control mechanisms act to ensure that areas of the brain with higher metabolism are supplied with increased blood flow. This flow/metabolism coupling is produced by a combination of various factors, including hypoxic vasodilatation, the effects of changes in CO_2 concentration, the balance of autonomic nervous supply and the release of local metabolites, including prostaglandins, nitric oxide, calcium ions, potassium ions and adenosine. The effect of head trauma on CBF and cerebral metabolism is not entirely clear. Despite a reduction in absolute CBF, most patients who are comatose as a result of head injury (Glasgow Coma Scale (GCS) <9) have relative hyperaemia, with high CBF relative to metabolism.[10] However, in up to 90% of patients who die from head injury, lesions compatible with ischaemia are found at post-mortem.[11,12] This paradox is partly explained by the recent findings of a severe reduction in CBF occurring in the initial period (3–8 h) following injury. Over the next 24 h, this is followed by a gradual increase in CBF until eventually, cerebral metabolic needs are exceeded.[13,14,15] Furthermore, vasospasm, which occurs in 20–40% of patients with head injury,[16,17,18] may reduce CBF after this initial hyperaemic phase, with an increase in the incidence of non-contusion related cerebral infarction.[19] Thus, the change in the $CBF:CMRO_2$ ratio is by no means uniform in head-injured patients. The majority of the severely injured patients will suffer an initial decline in CBF, followed by a return to normal flow or relative hyperaemia and the flow may then decline again, particularly if vasospasm occurs. Both extremely low CBF and high CBF after head injury are associated with poor outcome.[14,20]

Head trauma impairs the mechanisms controlling CBF. Pressure autoregulation is commonly abolished following a severe head injury but this is not always indicative of poor prognosis.[21] In contrast, the complete absence of CO_2 reactivity with lack of vasoconstrictor response to barbiturates is associated with a poor outcome.[22] Cerebrovascular reactivity to CO_2 is often preserved but the magnitude of response may be reduced.[23]

MECHANISMS OF SECONDARY NEURONAL INJURY

Ischaemia may cause secondary injury by several different processes that increase the extent of damage to the central nervous system.[24] These include:

- accumulation of glutamate and aspartate, excitotoxic amino acids which interact with NMDA (N-methyl-D-aspartate) receptors and lead to intracellular accumulation of calcium ions;[25]
- activation of phospholipase;[26]
- breakdown of arachidonic acid;
- generation of free radicals;[27,28]
- lipid peroxidation.

The above processes can all contribute to eventual neuronal death. An understanding of the mechanisms involved may permit the development of pharmacological strategies that might help to prevent secondary neuronal injury.[29]

In the presence of a fixed energy supply, cellular outcome may be markedly affected by factors that modify energy demand. Thus hyperthermia,[30] coma, fits or excitotoxic neuronal activation can result in greater neuronal loss, while hypothermia and metabolic suppression may provide significant neuroprotection. Owing to the number of confounding factors present,[31] the mechanisms responsible for secondary neuronal injury are not easily studied in man. Much of the information has been obtained from animal models of focal ischaemia or craniocerebral trauma and extrapolation from these results to clinical situations must be undertaken with care.[32] The detection of an ischaemic penumbra with inactive but viable neurones and the use of reperfusion to rescue this tissue, which would otherwise have infarcted, suggests that these secondary mechanisms do exist.[33]

While ischaemic thresholds for cessation of electrical activity and cell death have long been recognized, it is increasingly obvious that other vital functions are inhibited at higher blood flow levels and may, over time, be responsible for cell death.

INTRACRANIAL PRESSURE

The normal intracranial contents can be divided into four compartments: tissue volume, interstitial waters, cerebrospinal fluid (CSF 75 ml) and blood volume (50 ml). Resting ICP represents the equilibrium pressure at which CSF production and absorption are in balance. The production of CSF remains constant as long as CPP remains adequate. CSF absorption is a passive process through the arachnoid granulations and increases with the increase in CSF pressure. In the resting adults the normal ICP is between 1 and 10 mmHg.

The 'four lump' concept describes most simply the causes of raised ICP inside the skull (which acts as a rigid box): cerebral oedema, CSF accumulation, vascular congestion or the presence of an intracranial mass. Any increase in volume in any of the four components will lead to a rise in ICP. This pressure–volume relationship is commonly referred to as the *intracranial compliance curve*. As cerebral perfusion pressure is determined by the difference between mean arterial blood pressure (MAP) and ICP, a high ICP will lead to cerebral ischaemia.

Small increases in mass may be compensated for, initially, by translocation of CSF into the spinal subarachnoid space and by compression of the venous blood volume. However, once this compensatory mechanism is exhausted, ICP rises steeply with further increases in intracranial content. As prolonged raised ICP is associated with a poor prognosis,[34–37] vigorous treatment is essential and should be instituted if ICP exceeds 25 mmHg for more than 5 min.

SYSTEMIC EFFECTS OF HEAD INJURY

Up to 65% of spontaneously breathing head-injured patients may be hypoxaemic, even though they may not appear to be in respiratory distress.[38] Hypoxaemia is associated with poor neurological outcome and should be promptly corrected.[35] The causes of the impairment in gas exchange may include:

- chest and abdominal injuries with flail segments, direct lung trauma, haemothorax and tracheobronchial disruption;
- aspiration of laryngeal and pharyngeal secretions due to impaired reflexes, with the adult respiratory distress syndrome developing 24–72 h later;
- fat embolism syndrome from long bone fractures;
- abnormal respiratory patterns as a result of cerebral hemispheric or basal ganglia damage;
- neurogenic alterations in residual functional capacity and ventilation/perfusion matching;
- acute neurogenic pulmonary oedema. This is rare, typically occurring 2–12 h after the injury, and usually resolves within a few hours.[39]

Brainstem compression, medullary ischaemia and raised ICP may cause severe elevations of blood pressure as a result of increased sympathetic activity following head injury.[40] This hyperdynamic response is responsible for the cardiac dysrhythmias and ECG abnormalities commonly seen after severe head injury[41,42,43] and such changes are severe enough to produce myocardial necrosis in up to 62% of those who die from an intracranial lesion.[43] The presence of these cardiovascular changes may complicate the management of the head-injured patient with cerebral hypoperfusion, as the use of inotropes may worsen the myocardial ischaemia. On the other hand, the presence of intracranial pathology may prohibit the use of venodilators because of their cerebral vasodilatatory effects.

With the exception of young children, in whom blood loss from scalp lacerations may lead to hypotension, low blood pressure in a patient with acute head injury is usually due to causes other than the head injury and requires prompt investigation and treatment.

Coagulation disturbances occur in up to 24% of patients with severe head injury and, when severe, are indicative of poor outcome.[44,45,46] The release of tissue thromboplastin may lead to widespread activation of the coagulation cascade and disseminated intravascular coagulation (DIC).[47] Hypothermia and large blood transfusion further increase the incidence of clotting abnormalities.[48] Therefore, coagulation studies should be performed routinely and replacement of clotting factors is advised.

Endocrine and electrolyte abnormalities often accompany severe head injury. Stress-induced β-adrenergic stimulation, respiratory alkalosis from hyperventilation and diuretic therapy may result in hypokalaemia.

Hyponatraemia is also common after head injury and may be associated with diminished, normal or increased extracellular fluid volume. It is important to diagnose which category the patient belongs to before treatment is initiated. Democlocycline, which impairs the effect of antidiuretic hormone (ADH) on the kidney, is used to treat the syndrome of inappropriate ADH secretion. The judicious administration of hypertonic saline may be necessary if the serum sodium concentration falls below 120 meq/l. In contrast, damage to the hypothalamic/pituitary axis my lead to a lack of ADH secretion and diabetes insipidus. Diabetes insipidus occurs in 1% of head-injured patients and can result in hypernatraemia due to the loss of large volumes of dilute urine (20 l/day). This hypernatraemia and polyuria is treated with the administration of DDAVP (desamino desarginine vasopressin) and 5% dextrose in water with careful monitoring of blood sugar levels. A more common cause of hypernatraemia, however, is the repeated administration of mannitol.

Severe head injury is accompanied by a significant stress response. The increase in the levels of circulating catecholamines and cortisol results in hyperglycaemia. If not treated, this will worsen neurological outcome.[49] The stress response is also associated with an increased risk of gastric ulceration and gastrointestinal bleeding. H2 antagonists or sucralfate are commonly used for prophylaxis.

MANAGEMENT OF HEAD INJURIES

The anaesthetist is normally involved in the management of those patients with moderate or severe injury and this chapter concentrates on the management of this group of patients. It is important, however, that any doctor is able to adequately assess the severity of head injury according to the history of injury and clinical signs and symptoms. A practical protocol for the assessment and management of the head-injured patient was recently outlined by Arienta et al[50] and is given in Box 20.1.

The management of the patient with moderate to severe head injury falls into three phases: initial resuscitation and transfer, intraoperative management, and intensive care and rehabilitation. This chapter concentrates on the initial resuscitation and intraoperative management of such a patient.

INITIAL RESUSCITATION

The importance of securing the airway and maintaining adequate oxygenation and blood pressure in the head-injured patient cannot be overemphasized. Secondary brain damage begins and continues to occur from the moment of impact and for every second that the patient is hypoxaemic or hypotensive. For this reason, it is essential that ambulance teams are trained properly, are aware of the need for aggressive treatment of hypoxia and hypotension in the head-injured patient and have the equipment and expertise to be able to start resuscitation at the scene of the accident. It has been shown that hypotension or hypoxia is present in the prehospital phase of care in approximately 30% of patients with head injuries.[51] Severely head-injured patients (GCS <8) are unlikely to be able to protect their airway and often have impaired gas exchange[52] and early use of endotracheal intubation may be necessary to maintain adequate oxygenation. An improvement in the incidence of mortality after severe head injury has been associated with 'in-field' intubation.[53] Accident and emergency departments must be forewarned of the impending arrival of a comatose patient and an anaesthetist should be available to intubate the trachea as soon as possible after arrival, if the airway has not been secured already. It is important to remember that a significant proportion of severe head injuries are associated with injuries to the cervical spine[54] and therefore, manual in-line stabilization of the neck during induction and tracheal intubation is essential.[55] If there is any doubt about the ability to intubate the trachea, because of either a difficult airway or significant facial trauma, the airway must be secured by surgical means. Nasal intubation is best avoided in the patient with basal skull fracture because of the risk of passing the endotracheal tube into the brain through the skull defect and because of the added risk of infection.[56]

Severely head-injured patients must be assumed to have a full stomach. Therefore, a rapid-sequence induction with a small dose induction agent followed by suxamethonium 1 mg/kg is mandatory. Apart from ketamine, which is contraindicated because of concerns about its effects on ICP, the choice of induction agent is not important as long as it is administered with care and large variation in blood pressure or significant hypotension is avoided. Thiopentone, propofol and etomidate are the main induction agents used at our centre. Lignocaine 1 mg/kg may be given as a useful adjunct in attenuating the cerebrovascular response to laryngoscopy and tracheal intubation.[57,58,59] Suxamethonium may result in a transient rise in ICP from increased CO_2 production and cerebral stimulation via afferent muscle activity.[60–63] However, the potential risk of hypoxaemia and hypercapnia far outweighs the risk of this transient increase in ICP. Furthermore, in sedated and mechanically ventilated patients with moderate to severe brain

Group A (minimal head injury GCS = 15)

- Patient is awake, orientated and without neurologic deficits and relates accident
- No loss of consciousness
- No vomiting
- Absent or minimal subgaleal swelling

The patient is released into the care of a family member with written instructions.

Group B (minor head injury GCS = 15)

- Patient is awake, orientated and without neurologic deficits
- Transitory loss of consciousness
- Amnesia
- One episode of vomiting
- Significant subgaleal swelling

The patient who has at least one of these characteristics undergoes neurologic evaluation and CT scan which, if negative, shortens hospital observation. If CT scan is not available, the patient has skull X-rays and is held for an observation period of not less than 6 h. If the skull X-rays are negative and a subsequent neurologic control is normal, the patient can be released into the care of a family member with written instructions. If the X-rays reveal a fracture, the patient undergoes CT scan.

Group C (moderate head injury or mild head injury with complicating factors GCS = 9–15)

- Impaired consciousness
- Uncooperative for various reasons
- Repeated vomiting
- Neurologic deficits
- Otorrhagia/otorrhoea
- Rhinorrhoea
- Signs of basal fracture
- Seizures
- Penetrating or perforating wounds
- Patients in anticoagulant therapy or affected by coagulopathy
- Patients who have undergone previous intracranial operations
- Epileptic or alcoholic patients

The patient with at least one of these characteristics undergoes a neurologic evaluation and a CT scan. Hospitalization and repeated scan, if necessary, within 24 h or prior to discharge.

Group D (severe head injury GCS = 3–8)

- Patient is in coma

Necessary resuscitation manoeuvres followed by neurological evaluation and immediate CT scan (prior to surgical intervention). Coma management.

Box 20.1   Practical Protocol for Management of Head-Injured Patients in the Emergency Department (modified from reference[50])

injury, suxamethonium has no clinically significant effects on ICP or the cerebral blood flow velocity.[64] The increase in serum potassium associated with the use of suxamethonium is an important consideration at later stages (>48 h after the initial injury), but not in the acute setting.[65]

Once the airway is secured, the lungs are mechanically ventilated to maintain mild hypocapnia (not less than 4 kPa) and adequate PaO_2. Oxygenation and ventilation are optimized and should be regularly verified by arterial blood gas analysis. The patient is best sedated and paralysed. There is no excuse for having the patient coughing or straining on the endotracheal tube. Clearly, not all patients with head trauma require tracheal intubation and the protocol used in our unit is outlined in Box 20.2.

The importance of maintaining systemic perfusion has recently been confirmed by the results from the American National Traumatic Coma Data Bank which demonstrated that systolic blood pressure <80 mmHg is a significant independent contributing factor to poor outcome.[66,67] The combination of an increased ICP and systemic hypotension leads to a reduction in CPP and cerebral ischaemia. Except for young children, in whom blood loss from a scalp wound is sufficient to cause hypotension, hypotension should prompt an investigation of sites of blood loss with immediate laparotomy or thoracotomy if necessary. Hypovolaemia may be masked by systemic hypertension secondary to intense sympathetic stimulation of the reflex response to intracranial hypertension.[68]

The increase in blood pressure is a compensatory response to maintain cerebral perfusion. Therefore, moderate levels of hypertension should not be treated but a blood pressure above the upper limit of autoregulation (mean arterial pressure >130 mmHg) must be actively treated, as it will increase CBV and ICP.

Although the effect of systemic hypotension on cerebral perfusion will depend initially on whether autoregulation is impaired or not, the final result will be a reduction in CBF. Hypotension will worsen cerebral perfusion in patients with impaired autoregulation as CBF is pressure passive. In contrast, in patients with intact autoregulation, hypotension will lead to cerebral vasodilatation with a resultant increase in ICP, a reduction in CPP and eventually decreased CBF.[69] Patients who are severely injured may exhibit 'false autoregulation', where the ICP changes by the same magnitude as systemic blood pressure, resulting in a constant cerebral perfusion pressure.[70]

The choice of fluid used for resuscitation is less important than the amount given. The use of glucose-containing solutions is discouraged unless hypoglycaemia is suspected, as hyperglycaemia (leading to lactic acidosis) has been shown to correlate with poor outcome after head injury.[49,71,72] Hyperglycaemia should be actively treated and blood glucose levels controlled with an infusion of insulin. Because the majority of head-injured patients receive mannitol, an adequate urine output is often a poor indicator of volume status in these patients. Central venous pressure monitoring is often very useful as an aid to

---

Immediately

- Coma (not obeying commands, not speaking, not eye opening, i.e. GCS = <8)
- Loss of protective laryngeal reflexes
- Ventilatory insufficiency as judged by blood gases:
  hypoxaemia (PaO_2 <13 kPa)
  hypercarbia ($PaCO_2$ >6 kPa)
  spontaneous hyperventilation causing $PaCO_2$ <3.5 kPa
  respiratory arrhythmia
- Uncontrolled seizures

Before start of journey to the neurointensive care unit

- Deteriorating level of consciousness (decrease in GCS by > 2 points since admission and not due to drugs), even if not in coma
- Bilaterally fractured mandible
- Copious bleeding into mouth (e.g. from a basal skull fracture)
- Seizures

Box 20.2   Indications for intubation and ventilation after head injury* (modified from reference[95])

*An intubated patient must also be ventilated, aiming for a PaO_2 >13 kPa and $PaCO_2$ of 4.0–4.5 kPa.

assessing intravascular fluid volumes and effectiveness of resuscitation and should be combined with the use of a pulmonary artery flotation catheter in the elderly, patients with heart disease and in those patients requiring inotropic support.

TRANSFER OF THE HEAD-INJURED PATIENT

Adequate resuscitation and a thorough reexamination of the patient must be completed before making decisions about further treatment priorities. Quality radiographs are taken of suspicious areas and CT scans arranged (Box 20.3). Blind burr hole exploration is rarely effective, can be harmful to the patient and delays the transfer of the patient and the initiation of definitive therapy. There is no longer any indication for this procedure in the modern accident and emergency department.

Once the patient has been stabilized, a decision can be made regarding transfer to a regional neurosurgical unit for further treatment (Box 20.4). Interhospital transfer of the head-injured patient is a potentially hazardous procedure and often poorly managed. Evidence suggests that the neurologically injured patient is at greater risk of cerebral ischaemia during transfer.[73] As the main causes of secondary brain damage are hypoxia, hypercarbia and cardiovascular instability, it is of vital importance to avoid any of these during transfer. The key to a successful and safe transfer involves:

- adequate resuscitation and stabilization of the patient prior to transfer;
- adequate monitoring during transfer with appropriate resuscitative equipment and drugs;
- the presence of an accompanying doctor with suitable training, skills and experience of head injury transfer;
- good communication between referring and receiving centres and an adequate, efficient and stable handover to the receiving team.[74,75]

- Confusion (GCS <14) persisting after the initial assessment and resuscitation
- Unstable systemic state precluding transfer to neurosurgical centre
- Diagnosis uncertain
- Fully conscious but with a skull fracture or following first fit (admit and consider CT scan)

Box 20.3   Indications for CT scanning in a general hospital

Without preliminary head CT

- Coma (not obeying commands) even after resuscitation and even without a skull fracture
- Deterioration in the level of consciousness of more than two GCS points or progressive neurological deficit
- Open injury, depressed skull fracture, penetrating injury or basal skull fracture
- Tense fontanelle in a child
- Patient fulfils criteria for CT but this cannot be performed within a reasonable time (3–4 h)

After CT scan in a general hospital

- Abnormal CT (preferably after neurosurgical opinion on electronically transferred images)
- CT normal but patient's progress unsatisfactory

Box 20.4   Criteria for neurosurgical referral of head-injured patients

---

The fundamental requirement during transfer is to ensure adequate tissue oxygen delivery and to maintain stable perfusion. The head-injured patient is at risk of respiratory compromise and this risk is increased during transfer. We would recommend that any patient with a significantly altered conscious level should be sedated, intubated and ventilated during transfer. There is no place for transferring unstable patients to neurosurgical units. A patient persistently hypotensive, despite resuscitation, must be investigated thoroughly and the cause of hypotension identified and treated prior to transfer. The transferring team must ensure that all lines and tubes are secured before transfer, that they have sufficient supply of drugs and portable gases and that there is enough power in battery-operated monitoring equipment for the duration of the journey.

Monitoring during transfer should be of a standard appropriate to a patient in intensive care and we would recommend that this should include invasive arterial blood pressure monitoring, central venous pressure monitoring, where indicated, and the use of capnography. The transferring doctor must have appropriate experience in the transfer of patients with head injuries, should be familiar with the pathophysiology and management of such a patient and with the drugs and equipment they will use. It is also of paramount importance to discuss the patient with the neurosurgical centre at an early stage, so that treatment priorities can be decided upon and that the receiving team is prepared for the arrival of the patient (Box 20.5). The

- Patient's age and past medical history (if known)
- History of injury
  Time of injury
  Cause and mechanism (height of fall, approximate impact velocity)
- Neurological state
  Talked or not after injury
  Consciousness level on arrival at A&E dept
  Trends in consciousness level after arrival (sequential GCS)
  Pupil and limb responses
- Cardiorespiratory state
  Blood pressure and pulse rate
  Arterial blood gases, respiratory rate and pattern
- Injuries
  Skull fracture
  Extracranial injuries
- Imaging findings
  Haematoma, swelling, other
- Management
  Airway protection, ventilatory status
  Circulatory status and fluid therapy (mannitol)
  Treatment of associated injuries (? emergency surgery)
  Monitoring
  Drug doses and times of administration

Box 20.5   What the neurosurgical centre needs to know at time of referral

care of the transferring doctor does not end at the door of the receiving hospital but continues until he or she ensures that the stability of the patient is maintained and a full and accurate handover to the receiving team is made. A copy of the neurosurgical transfer letter used in our region can be seen in Figure 20.1.

INTRAOPERATIVE MANAGEMENT

Head-injured patients may require anaesthesia for treatment of the primary neurological pathology or for the treatment of a non-neurological injury (e.g. fixation of compound fractures). The optimal timing of such operations is debatable and the decision to operate must be made only after thorough consideration by trauma, neurosurgical and neurointensive care teams. Recent evidence suggests that early long

bone fracture fixation may lead to a greater risk of intraoperative hypoxaemia and hypotension.[76] Since these are the principal factors contributing to secondary brain injury, the benefits of operating at an early stage after major trauma must be qualified by the potential for further damage to the brain.

For any operation on the head-injured patient, management priorities remain the avoidance of cerebral ischaemia, optimization of CPP and the prevention of intracranial hypertension.

Intraoperative care of the head-injured patient does not begin with knife to skin but should be a direct continuation of the resuscitation and stabilization process in the neurointensive care unit or the accident and emergency department. Transfer of the patient to and from the operating table must be achieved without subjecting the patient to hypotension or hypoxaemia. As the patient's head is inaccessible during the operation, the anaesthetist must ensure, before the patient is prepared and draped, that all the pressure points are padded, the eyes are protected, the endotracheal tube is secured and ventilation is adequate for maintaining good gas exchange. Venous drainage must not be obstructed with excessive neck rotation, ties or high inflation pressures. There is no point in employing pharmacological methods of controlling ICP to treat intraoperative brain swelling until these simple measures have been undertaken.

Because of the dangers of even short periods of cerebral hypoperfusion or hypoxia, it is essential that the patient is continuously and adequately monitored throughout the operation and throughout the transfer to and from the operating environment. Monitoring should include ECG, temperature, urine output, pulse oximetry and invasive systemic blood pressure. Special emphasis should be placed on end-tidal CO_2 monitoring as a means of continuously assessing the level of hyperventilation and a comparison with $PaCO_2$ is advisable. Central venous and/or pulmonary artery pressure monitoring, particularly in the elderly and in those with cardiac disease, will allow a more rational approach to fluid replacement, particularly in those patients requiring inotropic support to maintain an adequate CPP. In patients with neurological injury who require non-neurological surgical intervention, ICP monitoring is recommended especially if large intraoperative fluid shifts are possible. Intracranial pressure, cerebral venous oxygen saturation (SJO_2) monitoring and the use of transcranial Doppler (TCD) are discussed in detail in the respective chapters.

It is now accepted that head-injured patients do not have reduced anaesthetic requirements.[77,78] Inadequate

Neurosurgical Transfer Letter

Date/ Time Referral: _____   Referring Hospital: _____   Referring Doctor: _____

Receiving Neurosurgeon: _____

Patient Details: Hosp. No:

Name: _____

Address: _____

DOB:

GP:

Patient sticker if possible

Next of Kin: _____

Contact No: _____

Informed: Y / N

Named Medical Escort: _____

Named Nurse Escort: _____

Ambulance Crew Code: _____   Date/ Time of Transfer: _____

ADMISSION DETAILS

Head Injury ☐   Intracranial Haem ☐   Other ☐

History: _____

Positive findings on 1° survey & 2° survey / other clinical details: _____

Date/ Time of Transfer: _____   *(Provide details overleaf)*

PMH: _____   *(Provide details overleaf)*

Current Medication: _____   Allergies: _____

Observations:	at Scene:	Date	Time	GCS: E		V		M		BP		P		SpO_2
	on arrival A/E:	Date	Time	E		V		M		BP		P		SpO_2
	prior to intubation:	Date	Time	E		V		M		BP		P		SpO_2

INVESTIGATION BEFORE TRANSFER:

ABGs on arrival A/E: Time:	pO_2	pCO_2	H+/pH	FiO_2	Haem: Time:	Hb	PT	plats	G+S
Prior to Departure Time:	pO_2	pCO_2	H+/pH	FiO_2	Biochem: Time:	Na	K	Glucose	

Radiology: CxR: _____   Cx Spine: _____   Pelvic XR: _____

CT Scans: _____

Other: _____

ESSENTIAL TRANSFER CHECKLIST

Airway: None / ETT / Other

Ventilation: Spontaneous / IPPV

IV access: 2x 16g / CVP / Other

IA access: Radial / Brachial / Femoral

Urinary Catheter: Y / N

Orogastric / Nasogastric tube: Y / N

Chest drain(s):   Y / N

Sedation: Propofol mg/h: _____   Midazolam mg/h: _____

Analgesia: Fentanyl mg/h: _____

Paralysis: Atracurium mg/h: _____

Inotropes/ other drugs: _____

Mannitol 20% _____ mls time given: _____

Other iv fluids: _____

Documentation checklist:

Nursing charts: ☐   X-rays/ CT scans: ☐

Medical case notes: ☐   Other investigations (ECG, blood results): ☐

Valuables / Clothing: ☐

Significant events during transfer: _____

INTER HOSPITAL TRANSFER OBSERVATIONS

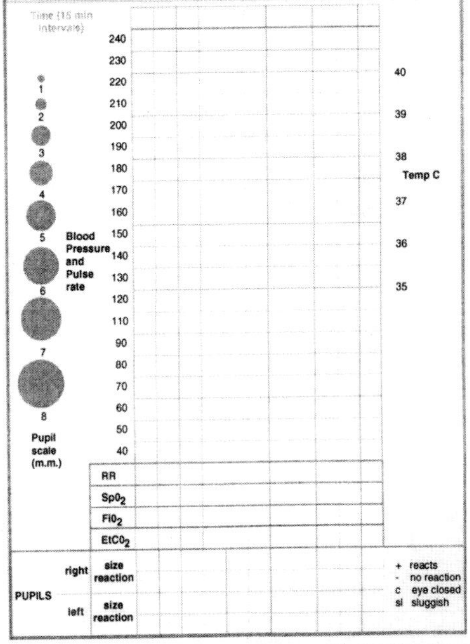

Time (15 min intervals)

Pupil scale (m.m.)

Blood Pressure and Pulse rate

240 230 220 210 200 190 180 170 160 150 140 130 120 110 90 80 70 60 50 40

40 39 38 Temp C 37 36 35

RR	
SpO_2	
FiO_2	
$EtCO_2$	

PUPILS   right   size / reaction   left   size / reaction

+ reacts
- no reaction
c eye closed
sl sluggish

Signed: _____   Print: _____   Grade: _____   Receiving Doctor: _____   Grade: _____   TIME: _____

Figure 20.1   A copy of the East Anglia neurosurgical transfer letter.

anaesthesia will allow the surgical stimulus to increase $CMRO_2$, CBF and ICP. The choice of anaesthetic agent and technique will depend on the patient's preoperative neurological status, his preoperative medical conditions and the presence of associated injuries. There is simply no evidence that a particular approach is better for anaesthetizing the patient with head injury. However, most commonly recommended methods have these goals in common:

- smooth induction without sudden or pronounced changes in blood pressure;
- maintenance of adequate CPP;
- preventing rises in $CMRO_2$, CBF and ICP;
- a rapid postoperative emergence, if desired.

The choice of maintenance agent should reflect these goals. In general, nitrous oxide and the inhalational agents are best avoided because of their effect on autoregulation, CBF and ICP.[79,80] Although nitrous oxide maintains autoregulation and CO_2 reactivity, it has been shown to stimulate cerebral metabolism, resulting in vasodilatation and increased CBF.[81] For this reason, its use in the head-injured patient is discouraged.

The inhaled volatile anaesthetic agents affect both CBF and autoregulation. The net effect of inhalational agents is to increase the CBF but their action on CBF is twofold. As all the inhalational agents tend to reduce cerebral metabolism, we would expect a corresponding reduction in CBF. The decrease in CBF, however, is overridden by a direct cerebral vasodilatory effect, partly mediated by nitric oxide. This vasodilatory effect increases with the dose of anaesthetic agent. Thus, although the increase in CBF produced by isoflurane, halothane and desflurane may be small at low doses, it is dose dependent and CBF may markedly increase at higher doses. This increase is further exaggerated when $CMRO_2$ is depressed, as may be the case in the head-injured patient.[80] Sevoflurane appears to be the "least" cerebral vasodilatory inhalational agent available at present.[82]

As blood pressure and CPP fluctuate in response to surgical stimulus, anaesthetic agents that maintain autoregulation and CO_2 reactivity will allow stable cerebral haemodynamics. Inhalational anaesthetics, with the exception of sevoflurane, impair both the ability to autoregulate (static autoregulation), and the rate of autoregulation (dynamic autoregulation) in a dose-dependent manner.[79] In addition, the inhalational agents impair CO_2 reactivity. In contrast, sevoflurane has been shown to maintain static autoregulation and preserves dynamic autoregulation and CO_2 reactivity better than the other commonly used volatile anaesthetic agents.[83] The reported epilepto-

genic side effects of enflurane prohibit its use in neuroanaesthesia.

Opioids have very little effect on CBF and metabolism but the newer synthetic opioids, fentanyl, sufentanil and alfentanil, have been shown to cause an increase in ICP in patients with head injury. This increase is thought to be secondary to respiratory depression and hypotension. These agents should therefore be used with great care to avoid systemic hypotension. Remifentanil, the recently introduced opioid agent with an ultra-short half-life, will probably affect ICP via its hypotensive effect.

We prefer to use a total intravenous anaesthetic technique of propofol and fentanyl infusions. Propofol reduces $CMRO_2$, CBF and ICP. It does not impair autoregulation and CO_2 reactivity, even at high enough doses to produce electroencephalographic isoelectricity.[84] The reduction in $CMRO_2$ with propofol anaesthesia may be neuroprotective. The patient's lungs are ventilated with O_2/air mixture to maintain mild hypocapnia. Although prolonged excessive hyperventilation is associated with poor neurological outcome, acute hyperventilation may be essential to reduce ICP in the head-injured patient.[85] Hypocapnia induces cerebral vasoconstriction and the resultant decrease in CBF and ICP may improve cerebral perfusion pressure. However, excessive cerebral vasoconstriction has been shown to cause cerebral ischaemia and hyperventilation must be used with great care. Should a $PaCO_2$ lower than 4 kPa be required, monitoring cerebral oxygenation with a jugular venous bulb catheter is advisable. Jugular bulb oximetry, though unable to detect local ischaemia, is a good indicator of the adequacy of CBF and global cerebral oxygenation. Hyperoxia can be used as a temporary measure to improve cerebral oxygen delivery during marked hyperventilation.[86,87]

Neuromuscular blockade should be maintained intraoperatively in all head-injured patients to prevent coughing or straining and the extent of neuromuscular block monitored with a neuromuscular stimulator.

The use of neuroprotective treatment regimens in the patient with moderate or severe head injury is of secondary importance to the maintenance of cerebral oxygenation, the avoidance of hypotension and the control of intracranial pressure. Hyopthermia has theoretical advantages in that it reduces $CMRO_2$, the production of cytokines, free radicals and glutamate and has been shown to be of benefit in animal studies.[88] Although conclusive outcome data are still lacking, a recent study in humans suggested that moderate hypothermia for 24 h was beneficial in improving outcome of head-injured patients with admission GCS of 5–7.[89] As hypothermia is not without its complications, mainly increased systemic vascular resistance and myocardial work and potential coagulation abnormalities, it cannot, therefore, be recommended as first-line treatment in head-injured patients. Hyperthermia, however, has been shown to adversely affect outcome and must be aggressively treated.[90]

As mentioned previously, the loss of pressure autoregulation in the damaged brain occurs frequently and results in the CBF varying directly with the patient's systemic blood pressure. Intraoperative hypotension can cause a marked reduction in the CBF and this reduction is reflected in significantly worse outcomes in those patients experiencing a prolonged fall (>5 min) in blood pressure during their operation. Pietrapaoli et al[91] demonstrated an 82% mortality in patients experiencing intraoperative hypotension, compared with a 25% mortality in those who remained normotensive. In addition, the duration of intraoperative hypotension was related directly to worsening outcomes. We would advocate, therefore, the use of early and sufficient resuscitation with intravenous fluids and blood and a low threshold for the appropriate use of inotropic support to maintain CPP.

The statistics in children with head injury also serve to emphasize the importance of the avoidance of hypoxia and hypotension. Pigula et al[92] showed a mortality of 22% in children with severe head injury with normal systemic blood pressures and PaO_2 levels on admission. However, in children who were hypotensive on admission, the mortality increased to 61% and, if the child was also hypoxaemic, mortality was closer to 85%.

The maintenance of normotension in the head-injured patient undergoing surgery is made more difficult by some of the problems and physiological effects associated with intracranial mass lesions. An acute intracranial lesion (subdural or extradural haematoma) with mass effect is normally accompanied by intense sympathetic stimulation leading to an increase in systemic vascular resistance. Surgical evacuation of such a lesion is commonly associated with an abrupt decrease in the blood pressure at the time of decompression. It is important to make sure that hypovolaemia is not concealed by this increased systemic vascular resistance. Patients who are able to compensate for hypovolaemia by systemic vasoconstriction and tachycardia may have a precipitous fall in blood pressure with cardiovascular collapse at the time of surgical decompression. Therefore, a high index of suspicion is needed in the management of those patients who are tachycardic and normotensive, with early initiation of vigorous fluid therapy, meticulous attention to the blood pressure and prompt treatment of hypotension with intravenous fluids and, if necessary, vasopressors at the time of decompression.

Although haemodilution reduces blood viscosity and may theoretically improve blood flow through the microcirculation, haemodilution therapy in patients with cerebral ischaemia has failed to support this contention.[93] Haemodilution does not produce an increase in tissue PO_2 and therefore cannot be recommended as a therapeutic manoeuvre in those at risk of cerebral ischaemia.[94] Blood transfusion is advocated for maintaining adequate cerebral oxygen delivery.

RECOVERY

Patients with severe head injury requiring surgery generally need continuing postoperative care in the neurointensive care unit and they should remain paralysed and ventilated at the end of the procedure. In patients with mild to moderate head injury (GCS between 12 and 15) undergoing evacuation of an epidural or subdural haematoma, it is not unreasonable to allow the patient to wake up at the end of the procedure. A rapid return to consciousness permits early clinical assessment and the detection of unexpected neurological deficit. This emphasis on rapid emergence makes the maintenance of haemodynamic stability difficult. Care must be taken to avoid excessive coughing and bucking which may cause not only a transient increase in ICP but, more importantly, an increased risk of venous bleeding. Uncontrolled hypertension on emergence may be responsible for intracerebral haemorrhage following neurosurgical procedures. Intravenous lignocaine (up to 3 mg/kg in divided doses) can be given during emergence to suppress coughing without significant effect on ventilation. Rises in blood pressure can be controlled with β-blockers. Finally, it is important to make sure that the patient is awake, can protect his or her airway, is able to maintain oxygenation and is normocapnic before extubation in order to avoid increases in ICP.

CONCLUSION

The principal aim of managing the severely head-injured patient is the prevention of secondary neuronal injury. The greatest impact on outcome is made by the institution of adequate and early resuscitation, by the availability and involvement of multidisciplinary teams and by the maintenance of adequate oxygenation and cerebral perfusion pressure throughout the entire posttraumatic period.

REFERENCES

1. Jennet B, McMillan R. Epidemiology of head injury. BMJ 1981; 282: 101–104.

2. Andrews PJD. What is the optimal cerebral perfusion pressure after brain injury? A review of the evidence with an emphasis on arterial pressure. Acta Anaesthesiol Scand 1995; 39(suppl): 112–114.

3. Aaslid R, Lindegaard K-F, Sorteberg W et al. Cerebral autoregulation dynamics in humans. Stroke 1989; 20: 45–52.

4. Edvinsson L, Owman C, Seisjo B Physiological role of cerebrovascular nerves in the autoregulation of cerebral blood flow. Brain Res 1976; 117: 518.

5. Paulson OB, Olesen J, Christensen MS Restoration of autoregulation of cerebral blood flow by hypocapnia. Neurology 1972; 22: 286–293.

6. Aaslid R, Newell DW, Stooss R et al. Simultaneous arterial and venous transcranial Doppler assessment of cerebral autoregulation dynamics. Stroke 1991; 22: 1148–1154.

7. Gupta AK, Menon DK, Czosnyka M, Jones GJ. Thresholds for hypoxic cerebral vasodilatation in volunteers. Anesth Analg 1997; 85(4): 817–20.

8. Lobato RD, Rivas JJ, Gomez PA et al. Head injured patients who talk and deteriorate into coma. Analysis of 211 cases studied with computerised tomography. J Neurosurg 1991; 75: 256–261.

9. Rockswold Gl, Leonard PR, Nagib MG Analysis of management in thirty-three closed head injury patients who 'talked and deteriorated'. Neurosurgery 1987; 21: 51–55.

10. Obrist WD, Langfitt TW, Jaggi JL, Cruz J, Gennarelli TA. Cerebral blood flow and metabolism in comatose patients with acute head injury. Relationship to intracranial hypertension. J Neurosurg 1984; 61(2): 241–253.

11. Graham DI, Adams JH, Doyle D. Ischaemic brain damage in fatal non-missile head injuries J Neurol Sci 1978; 39(2–3): 213–234.

12. Graham DI, Ford I, Adams JH et al. Ischaemic brain damage is still common in fatal non-missile head injury J Neurol Neurosurg Psychiatry 1989; 52(3): 346–350.

13. Bouma GJ, Muizelaar JP, Choi SC et al. Cerebral circulation and metabolism after severe traumatic brain injury: The elusive role of ischemia. J Neurosurg 1991; 75: 685–693.

14. Bouma GJ, Muizelaar JP. Cerebral blood flow, cerebral blood volume, and cerebrovascular reactivity after severe head injury. J Neurotrauma 1992; 09: S333–S348.

15. Marion DW, Darby J, Yonas H. Acute regional cerebral blood flow changes caused by severe head injuries. J Neurosurg 1991; 74: 407–414.

16. Weber M, Grolimund P, Seiler RW Evaluation of post-traumatic cerebral blood flow velocities by transcranial Doppler ultrasonography Neurosurgery 1990; 27(1): 106–112.

17. Martin NA, Doberstein C, Zane C et al. Post-traumatic cerebral arterial spasm: transcranial Doppler ultrasound, cerebral blood flow, and angiographic findings. J Neurosurg 1992; 77: 575–583.

18. Kakarieka A, Braakman R, Schakel EH. Clinical significance of the finding of subarachnoid blood on CT scan after head injury. Acta Neurochir (Wein) 1994; 129: 1–5.

19. Chan KH, Dearden NM, Miller JD. The significance of post-traumatic increase in cerebral blood flow velocity: a transcranial Doppler ultrasound study. Neurosurgery 1992; 30: 697–700.

20. Robertson CS, Narayan RK, Gokaslan ZL et al. Cerebral arteriovenous oxygen difference as an estimate of cerebral blood flow in comatose patients. J Neurosurg 1989; 70: 222–230.

21. Newell DW, Aaslid R, Stoos R et al. Evaluation of closed head injury patients using transcranial Doppler monitoring. In: Avezaat CJJ, Van Eijndhoven JHM, Maas AIR, Tans JTJ (eds) ICP VIII International Symposium. Springer-Verlag, Heidelberg, 1993, pp 309–312.

22. Schalen W, Messeter K, Nordstrom CH. Cerebral vasoreactivity and the prediction of outcome in severe traumatic brain lesions. Acta Anaesthesiol Scand 1991; 35: 113–122.

23. Cold GE. Cerebral blood flow in acute head injury. The regulation of cerebral blood flow and metabolism during the acute phase of head injury, and its significance for therapy. Acta Neurochir (Wien) 1990; 49: 1–64.

24. Siesjo BK. Pathophysiology and treatment of focal cerebral ischaemia. Part I: Pathophysiology. J Neurosurg 1992; 77: 169–184.

25. Mayer ML, Miller RJ Excitatory amino acid receptors, second messengers, and regulation of intracellular $Ca2+$ in mammalian neurones. Trends Pharmacol Sci 1990; 11: 254–260.

26. Smith WI, Borgeat P, Fitzpatrick FA. The ecosanoids: cyclooxygenase, lipoxygenase, and epoxygenase pathways. In: Vance DE and Vance J (eds) Biochemistry of lipids, lipoproteins and membranes. New comprehensive biochemistry. Elsevier Science Publishers, Amsterdam, 1991, pp 297–325.

27. Traystman RJ, Kirsch JR, Koehler RC. Oxygen radical mechanisms of brain injury following ischaemia and reperfusion. J Appl Physiol 1991; 71: 1185–1195.

28. McCord JM. Oxygen-derived free radicals in post-ischemic tissue injury. N Engl J Med 1985; 312: 159–163.

29. Faden AI, Salzman S. Pharmacological strategies in CNS trauma. Trends Pharmacol Sci 1992; 13: 29–35.

30. Wass CT, Lanier WL, Hofer RE, Scheithauer BW, Andrews AG. Temperature increases of >1°C worsens functional neurologic outcome and histopathology in

canine model of complete cerebral ischemia. J Neurosurg Anesthesiol 1994; 6: 305.

31. Molinari GF. Why model strokes? Stroke 1988; 19: 1195–1197.

32. Hsu CY. Criteria for valid preclinical trials using animal stroke models. Stroke 1993; 24: 633–636.

33. Memezawa H, Smith M-L, Siesjo BK. Penumbral tissues salvaged by reperfusion following middle cerebral artery occlusion in rats. Stroke 1992; 23: 552–559.

34. Miller JD, Becker DP, Ward JD et al. Significance of intracranial hypertension in severe head injury. J Neurosurg 1977; 47: 503–516.

35. Miller JD, Butterworth JF, Gudeman SK et al. Further experience in the management of severe head injury. J Neurosurg 1981; 54: 289–299.

36. Saul TG, Ducker TB. Effect of intracranial pressure monitoring and aggressive treatment on mortality in severe head injury. J Neurosurg 1982; 56: 498–503.

37. Marshall LF, Smith RW, Shapiro HM. The outcome with aggressive treatment in severe head injuries. Part II: Acute and chronic barbiturate administration in the management of head injury. J Neurosurg 1979; 50: 26–30.

38. Frost EAM. The pathophysiology of respiration in neurosurgical patients. J Neurosurg 1979; 50: 699–714.

39. Baigelman W, O'Brien JC. Pulmonary effects of head trauma Neurosurgery 1981; 9: 729–740.

40. Schulte AM, Esch J, Murray H et al. Haemodynamic changes in patients with severe head injury. Acta Neurochir 1980; 54: 243–246.

41. Hersch C. Electrocardiographic changes in head injury. Circulation 1961; 23: 853–860.

42. Miner ME. Cardiovascular effects of severe head injury. In: Frost EAM (ed) Clinical anesthesia for neurosurgery. Butterworth, Boston, 1991, pp 439–455.

43. Kolin A, Norris JW. Myocardial damage from acute cerebral lesions. Stroke 1984; 15: 990–995.

44. Piek J, Chestnut RM, Marshall LF et al. Extracranial complications of head injury. J Neurosurg 1992; 77: 901–907.

45. Kumura E, Sato M, Fukuda A et al. Coagulation disorders following acute head injury. Acta Neurochir (Wien) 1987; 85: 23–28.

46. Olson JD, Kaufman HH, Moake J et al. The incidence and significance of hemostatic abnormalities in patients with head injuries. Neurosurgery 1989; 24: 825–832.

47. Van Der Sande JJ, Veltkamp JJ, Boekhout-Mussert RJ et al. Head injury and coagulation disorders. J Neurosurg 1978; 49: 357–365.

48. Ferrara A, MacArthur JD, Wright HK et al. Hypothermia and acidosis worsen coagulopathy in the patient requiring massive transfusion. Am J Surg 1990; 160: 515–518.

49. Lam AM, Winn HR, Cullen BF et al. Hyperglycemia and neurological outcome in patients with head injury. J Neurosurg 1991; 75: 545–551.

50. Arienta C, Caroli M, Balbi S. Management of head-injured patients in the emergency department: a practical protocol. Surg Neurol 1997; 48: 213–219.

51. Wald S, Fenwick J, Shackford SR. The effect of secondary insults on mortality and long-term disability of severe head injury in a rural region without a trauma system. J Trauma 1991; 31: 104.

52. Gildenberg PL, Maleka M. Effect of early intubation and ventilation on outcome following head trauma. In: Dacey RG Jr et al (eds) Trauma of the central nervous system. Raven Press, New York, 1985, pp 79–90.

53. Pfenniger EG, Lindner KH. Arterial blood gases in patients with acute head injury at the accident site and upon hospital admission. Acta Anaesthesiol Scand 1991; 35: 148–152.

54. Crosby ET, Lui A. The adult cervical spine: implications for airway management. Can J Anaesth 1990; 07: 77–93.

55. Lam AM. Spinal cord injury and management. Curr Opin Anesthesiol 1992; 5: 632–639.

56. Grande CM, Barton CR, Stene JK. Appropriate techniques for airway management of emergency patients with suspected spinal cord injury. Anesth Analg 1988; 67: 714–715.

57. Bedford RF, Winn HR, Tyson G et al. Lidocaine prevents increased ICP after endotracheal intubation. In: Shulman K (ed) Intracranial pressure IV. Springer-Verlag, Berlin, 1980, pp 595–615.

58. Hamill JF, Bedford RF, Weaver DC et al. Lidocaine before endotracheal intubation: intravenous or laryngotracheal? Anesthesiology 1981; 55: 578–581.

59. Wojciechowski ZJ, Lam AM, Eng CC et al. Effect of intravenous lidocaine on cerebral blood flow velocity during endotracheal intubation. Anesthesiology 1992; 77: A194.

60. Lanier WL, Milde JH, Michenfelder JD. Cerebral stimulation following succinyl choline in dogs. Anaesthesiology 1986; 64(5): 551–559.

61. Lanier WL, Iaizzo PA, Milde JH. Cerebral function and muscle afferent activity following i.v. succinylcholine in dogs: the effect of pretreatment with defasciculating doses of pancuronium. Anesthesiology 1989; 71: 87–95.

62. Wright SW, Robinson GG, Wright MB. Cervical spine injuries in blunt trauma patients requiring emergent endotracheal intubation. Am J Emerg Med 1992; 10: 104–109.

63. Cottrell JE, Hartung J, Giffin JP et al. Intracranial and hemodynamic changes after succinylcholine administration in cats. Anesth Analg 1983; 62: 1006–1009.

64. Kovarik WD, Lam AM, Mayberg TS et al. Succinylcholine does not change intracranial pressure, cerebral blood flow velocity or the electroencephalogram in patients with neurologic injury. Anesth Analg 1994; 78: 469–473.

65. Frankville DD, Drummond JC. Hyperkalemia after succinylcholine administration in a patient with closed

head injury without paresis. Anaesthesiology 1987; 67: 264–266.

66. Chestnut RM. Secondary brain insults after head injury: clinical perspectives. New Horizons 1995; 3: 336.

67. Marmarou A, Anderson RL, Ward JD et al. Impact of ICP instability and hypotension on outcome in patients with severe head trauma. J Neurosurg 1991; 75: S59–S66.

68. Cushing H. Concerning a definite regulatory mechanism of the vasomotor centre which controls blood pressure during cerebral compression. Johns Hopkins Hosp Bull 1901; 126: 290–292.

69. Rosner MJ, Daughton S. Cerebral perfusion pressure management in head injury. J Trauma 1990; 30: 933–941.

70. Enevoldsen EM, Jensen FT. Autoregulation and CO_2 responses of cerebral blood flow in patients with acute severe head injury. J Neurosurg 1978; 48: 689–703.

71. Young B, Ott L, Dempsey R et al. Relationship between admission hyperglycemia and neurologic outcome of severely brain-injured patients. Ann Surg 1989; 210: 466–473.

72. Michaud LJ, Rivara FP, Longstreth WT Jr et al. Elevated initial blood glucose levels and poor outcome following severe brain injuries in children. J Trauma 1991; 31: 1356–1362.

73. Andrews PJD, Piper IR, Dearden NM, Miller JD. Secondary insults during intrahospital transport of head-injured patients. Lancet 1990; 335: 327–330.

74. Association of Anaesthetists of Great Britain and Ireland. Recommendations for the transfer of patients with acute head injuries to neurosurgical units. AAGBI, London, 1996.

75. Royal College of Surgeons of England. Report of the working party on the management of patients with serious head injury. RCS, London, 1988.

76. Jaicks RR, Cohn SM, Moller BA. Early fracture fixation may be deleterious after head injury. J Trauma 1997; 42(1): 1–6.

77. Todd MM, Weeks JB, Warner DS. A focal cryogenic brain lesion does not reduce the minimum alveolar concentration for halothane in rats. Anesthesiology 1993; 79: 139–143.

78. Shapira Y, Paez A, Lam AM, Pavlin EG. Influence of traumatic head injury on halothane MAC in rats. Anesth Analg 1992; 74: S282.

79. Strebel S, Lam AM, Matta BF et al. Dynamic and static cerebral autoregulation during isoflurane, desflurane and propofol anesthesia. Anesthesiology 1995; 83: 66–76.

80. Matta BF, Mayberg TS, Lam AM. Direct cerebrovascular effects of halothane, isoflurane and desflurane during propofol-induced isoelectric electroencephalogram in humans. Anesthesiology 1995; 83(5): 980–985; discussion 27A.

81. Matta BF, Lam AM. Nitrous oxide increases cerebral blood flow velocity during pharmacologically-induced EEG silence in humans. J Neurosurg Anesthesiol 1995; 7: 89–93.

82. Matta BF, Heath K, Tipping K, Summors A. Direct cerebral vasodilatory effect of sevoflurane: a comparison with isoflurane. Anesthesiology 1999 (in press).

83. Summors AC, Gupta AK, Matta BF. Dynamic cerebral autoregulation during sevoflurane anaesthesia: a comparison with isoflurane. Anesth Analg 1999; 88: 341–345.

84. Matta BF, Lam AM, Strebel S, Mayberg TS. Cerebral pressure autoregulation and CO_2-reactivity during propofol-induced EEG suppression. Br J Anaesth 1995; 4: 159–163.

85. Muizelaar JP, Marmarou A, Ward JD et al. Adverse effects of prolonged hyperventilation in patients with severe head injury: a randomised clinical trial. J Neurosurg 1991; 75: 731–739.

86. Matta BF, Lam AM, Mayberg TS. The influence of arterial hyperoxygenation on cerebral venous oxygen content during hyperventilation. Can J Anaesth 1994; 41: 1041–1046.

87. Thiagarajan A, Goverdhan P, Chari P, Somasunderam K. The effect of hyperventilation and hyperoxia on cerebral venous oxygen saturation in patients with traumatic brain injury. Anesth Analg 1998; 87: 850–853.

88. Xue D, Huang ZG, Smith KE et al. Immediate or delayed mild hypothermia prevents focal cerebral infarction. Brain Res 1992; 587: 66–72.

89. Marion DW, Penrod LE, Kelsey SF et al. Treatment of traumatic brain injury with moderate hypothermia. N Engl J Med 1997; 336: 540–546.

90. Wass CT, Lanier WL, Hofer RE, Scheithauer BW, Andrews AG. Temperature increases of $\geq 1°C$ worsen functional neurologic outcome and histopathology in canine model of complete cerebral ischemia. J Neurosurg Anesthesiol 1994; 6: 305.

91. Pietrapaoli JA, Rogers FB, Shackford SR, Wald SL, Schmoker JD, Zhuang J. The deleterious effects of intraoperative hypotension on outcome in patients with severe head injuries. J Trauma 1992; 33(3): 403–407.

92. Pigula FA, Wald SL, Shackford SR, Vane DW. The effect of hypotension and hypoxia on children with severe head injuries. J Paediatr Surg 1993; 28: 310–316.

93. Scandinavian Stroke Study Group Multicentre Trial of Haemodilution in Acute Stroke. Results in the total population. Stroke 1987; 18: 691.

94. Chan R, Leniger-Follet E. Effects of isovolaemic hemodilution on oxygen supply and electrocorticogram in cat brain during focal ischemia and in normal tissue. Int J Microcirc 1983; 2: 297–333.

95. Gentleman D, Dearden M, Midgley S, Maclean D. Guidelines for the resuscitation and transfer of patients with serious head injury BMJ 1993; 307: 547–552.

21

INTENSIVE CARE AFTER ACUTE HEAD INJURY

David K. Menon & Basil F. Matta

INTRODUCTION

Approximately 1.4 million patients suffer a head injury in the United Kingdom each year[1] and about 2500 of these suffer a severe head injury[2] (defined as a postresuscitation Glasgow Coma Score[3] ≤8) (Table 21.1). Head injury is responsible for 15% of deaths between 15 and 45 years[2] and is one of the most important causes of death in this age range. There is enormous variability in the inpatient case fatality rate for all head injuries (2.6–6.5%)[4] and for severe head injury (which ought to represent a more homogeneous subgroup of patients) from US and UK centres, with mortality ranging from 15% to over 50%.[5] Conversely, good outcomes, defined as a Glasgow Outcome Scale[6] of 1 or 2 (Box 21.1), vary from under 50% to nearly 70%.[5] Identification of the cause of such variability is important if overall outcome is to improve.

DETERMINANTS OF OUTCOME IN ACUTE HEAD INJURY: PRIMARY VS SECONDARY INSULTS

Little can be done about the extent of primary injury to the brain when patients present to intensive care following head trauma but the presence and severity of secondary neuronal injury, much of which is triggered by physiological insults to the injured brain, can be a major determinant of outcome.[7,8] Eloquent proof of the importance of such secondary neuronal injury is available from the 30–40% of patients who 'talk and die',[9] implying that the primary injury was, on its own, insufficient to account for mortality.

The most important physiological insults that affect outcome are listed in Table 21.2, and can be graded for severity with respect to their expected effect on secondary neuronal injury.[10,11] It is, however, essential to emphasize that rapid resuscitation and transport to definitive neurosurgical care are critical determinants of outcome.[11,12,13] The severity of physiological insults, both immediately after injury and during the ICU phase of the illness, can be related to outcome (Table 21.2).[10,11] Physiological insults are additive in their effect on outcome, both when multiple insults (e.g. hypoxia and hypotension) occur at the same time point or when the same insult occurs repeatedly (e.g.

---

1 = Good recovery
2 = Moderate disability
3 = Severe disability
4 = Vegetative state
5 = Dead

Many studies dichotomize the scale to good outcome (1 and 2) and poor outcome (3–5).

Box 21.1   Glasgow Outcome Scale

Table 21.1   Glasgow Coma Scale and Score

Parameter	15-point adult scale (from[3])		Paediatric scale*	
Eye opening	Spontaneous	4	As for adults	
	To sound	3		
	To pain	2		
	None	1		
Best verbal response	Orientated	5	Orientated	5
	Confused	4	Words	4
	Inappropriate words	3	Vocal sounds	3
	Incomprehensible sounds	2	Cries	2
	None	1	None	1
Best motor response	Obeys commands	6	Obeys commands	5
	Localizes pain	5	Localizes pain	4
	Flexion withdrawal	4	Flexion	3
	Flexion abnormal	3	Extension	2
	Extension	2	None	1
	None 1			
Maximum sum		15		14

*Simpson DA, Reilly PL. Paediatric coma scale (letter). Lancet 1982; ii: 450.

Table 21.2   Physiological insults following head injury and their relation to outcome

Insult	Significant relation to	
	Mortality	Grades within GOS
Duration of hypotension (SBP $\leq$90 mmHg)	Yes	Yes
Duration of hypoxia (SpO$_2$ $\leq$90%)	Yes	No
Duration of pyrexia (T$_{core}$ $\geq$38°C)	Yes	No
Intracranial hypertension (ICP >30 mmHg)	Yes	No
Cerebral perfusion pressure (CPP <50 mmHg)	Yes	No

Significance was demonstrated using a logistic regression model except for CPP, where this was not possible due to the confounding effects of ICP and MAP. However, a CPP <50 mmHg was shown to independently predict outcome using non-parametric statistics. Data are from ref[10], which showed that 91% of all patients had one or more physiological insults during the course of their ICU stay.

hypotension in the prehospital and ICU phases of the illness). The intensive care of head injury centres on avoiding, detecting and treating such physiological derangements in the expectation that outcome will be improved.

Targets for basic intensive care practice in this area have been widely debated and been the subject of systematic review, with the recent publication of guidelines in both the US and European literature.[14,15] These involve monitoring for secondary physiological insults and preventing or treating these. Novel neuroprotective agents may hold considerable promise in the future but their general failure in clinical phase III trials[16,17] suggests that these drugs are unlikely to materially alter outcome in the short term.

However, there appears to be much room for improvement in conventional clinical practice. A series of telephone and postal surveys suggest that basic recommendations for monitoring and general intensive care in severe head injury have not been consistently followed in many neurosurgical centres in the USA and UK. As an example, intracranial pressure (ICP) was monitored in only half the centres surveyed.[18,19,20] While preliminary results suggest that this situation may now be improving,[21] it is important to emphasize that the application of novel neuroprotective therapies is futile if stable cardiorespiratory and cerebrovascular physiology cannot be achieved.

PATHOPHYSIOLOGY IN ACUTE HEAD INJURY

The severity and type of impact will substantially influence the structural lesions that ensue as a result of head injury (Fig. 21.1). The acceleration-deceleration forces produced by falls and motor vehicle accidents can produce axonal dysfunction and injury, brain

contusions and axial and extraaxial haematomas. Such macroscopic injury is associated with microscopic and ultramicroscopic changes, including ischaemia, astrocyte swelling with microvascular compromise, blood–brain barrier disruption and inflammatory cell recruitment[16,22] (Fig. 21.2). These microscopic changes are underpinned by early, multiphasic gene activation and later recruitment of repair mechanisms. Several secondary neuronal injury processes have been classically associated with fatal brain trauma, the most consistent one of which is cerebral ischaemia.[24] Mechanisms involved in secondary neural injury include excitatory amino acid (EAA) release, intracellular calcium overload, free radical-mediated injury and activation of inflammatory processes (Fig. 21.3).[22–24] There is also good evidence now that there is a local inflammatory response in the human brain following a variety of insults,[16,25,26] with production of proinflammatory cytokines and adhesion molecule upregulation.[27,28] These changes result in early neutrophil influx and later recruitment of lympho-

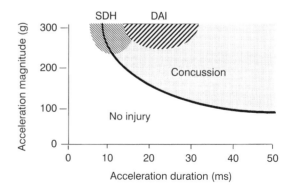

Figure 21.1   Effect of the duration and magnitude of acceleration/deceleration forces on the type of injury produced in the brain.

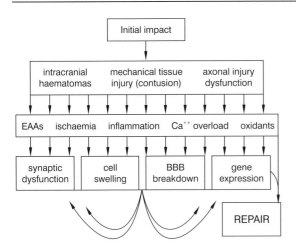

Figure 21.2 Sequential activation of injury processes in acute head injury.

cytes and macrophages and transformation of microglial cells into dendritic antigen-presenting cells.[29] These mononuclear cells may then contribute to the later stages of a prolonged inflammatory response, which may be associated with the laying down of amyloid. Indeed, head injury is a recognized risk factor for amyloid deposition in the brain and for Alzheimer's disease.[30,31] Further, the risk of these outcomes is related to an individual's apolipoproteinE (ApoE) genotype,[30,31] with an increased risk conferred by possession of the ApoEε4 genotype. Even more intriguingly, the ApoEε4 genotype has been shown to directly affect outcome in patients admitted with a severe head injury.[32] Identification of such genetic influences on outcome may enable us, in the future, to select high-risk patients for intensive neuroprotection strategies.

There is an intimate and continuing interplay between the processes described above. Intracranial haematomas may not only raise ICP and worsen cerebral hypoxia but may also be responsible for EAA release, inflammation and microvascular dysfunction. The microvascular dysfunction, in turn, may limit the ability of the injured brain to cope with minor variations in physiology, with elevation of the lower limit of autoregulation to a CPP of 60–70 mmHg, in contrast to normal individuals who tend to maintain cerebral blood flow down to CPP values of 50 mmHg. At later stages, the presence of extravascular blood may predispose to large vessel spasm, with the potential for distal hypoperfusion and ischaemia.

These varied consequences of a single structural pathology are well reflected by sequential changes in cerebrovascular physiology that are observed following head injury. Classically, cerebral blood flow (CBF) is thought to show a triphasic behaviour.[33] Early after head injury (<12 h), global CBF is reduced, sometimes to ischaemic levels. Between 12 and 24 h postinjury, CBF increases and the brain may exhibit supranormal CBF. While many reports refer to this phenomenon as hyperaemia, the absence of consistent reductions in cerebral oxygen extraction suggests retention of flow-metabolism coupling and a more appropriate label of hyperperfusion. CBF values begin to fall again several days following head injury and in some patients, these reductions in CBF may be associated with marked increases in large vessel flow velocity on transcranial Doppler ultrasound that suggest vasospasm.

These haemodynamic responses also define the vascular contribution to ICP elevation in time.[22] Immediately after head injury there is no vascular engorgement and though a transient blood–brain barrier (BBB) leak has been reported immediately after impact in experimental animals, this phenomenon is too shortlived to be clinically appreciated. Apart from surgical lesions (e.g. intracranial haematomas), ICP elevation during this phase is commonly the consequence of cytotoxic oedema, usually secondary to cerebral ischaemia. Increases in CBF and cerebral blood volume (CBV) from the second day postinjury onward make vascular engorgement an important contributor to intracranial hypertension. The BBB appears to become leaky between the second and fifth days posttrauma and vasogenic oedema then contributes to brain swelling. Unfortunately, patients vary enormously and different mechanisms responsible for intracranial hypertension may operate concurrently even within a single individual at any given time point. However, the discussion above does provide a useful basis on which to select initial 'best guess' therapy in an individual patient, especially when data from multimodality monitoring are also available to help guide therapy choices.

MONITORING IN ACUTE HEAD INJURY

None of the monitoring techniques and interventions that are widely used by specialist centres in severe head injury have ever been subjected to prospective randomized control trials. Indeed, some procedures such as ICP monitoring are now so widely accepted as being central to the management of patients with severe head injury that it may have become ethically impossible to mount a randomized trial addressing the efficacy of the procedure. However, the large body of

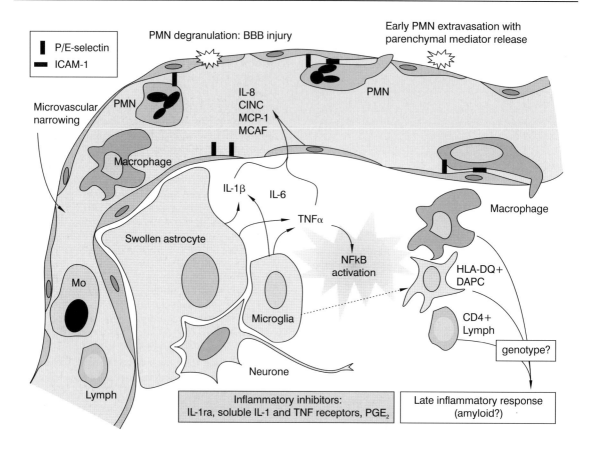

Figure 21.3 Induction of inflammatory responses following acute brain injury: TNFα, IL-1β and IL-6 are secreted by astrocytes and microglial cells, with later production of chemokines, including IL-8, cytokine-induced neutrophil chemotactic factor (CINC), monocyte chemoattractant protein-1 (MCP-1) and monocyte chemotactic and activating factor (MCAF, which attracts monocytes and macrophages). Leucocytes attracted by these chemokines subsequently interact with adhesion molecules such as P- and E-selectin and intercellular adhesion molecule-1 (ICAM-1). The initial cellular response is mainly polymorphonuclear (PMN) and later cellular responses predominantly consist of invading macrophages and CD4+ lymphocytes. These cells, along with microglia-derived HLA-DQ+ tissue macrophages with the morphology of dendritic antigen-presenting cells (DAPC), may be responsible for a sustained inflammatory response, the magnitude of which may show genetic polymorphism. TNF? also produces activation of the nuclear factor NFkB, which has wide ranging effects (from Menon DK. Cerebral protection in severe brain injury. Br Med Bull 1999 (in press).

clinical evidence that supports the use of many of these interventions provides a relatively strong basis for their recommendation as treatment guidelines.

DEFINING THERAPEUTIC TARGETS: A RATIONAL APPROACH TO SELECTING MONITORING MODALITIES

Basic physiology suggests the benefit of maintaining cerebral blood flow and oxygenation and these assumptions are confirmed by data from the Traumatic Coma Data Bank (TCDB)[11,34] and from other sources[10] which demonstrate the detrimental effects of hypotension (systolic blood pressure <90 mmHg) and hypoxia (PaO$_2$ levels < 60 mmHg (8 kPa)) in the early and later phases of head injury on outcome. Several studies that have addressed break points for cerebral autoregulation in patients with head injury have suggested preserved cerebrovascular autoregulation with maintenance of cerebral blood flow (CBF) at cerebral perfusion pressures above 60–70 mmHg.[9,35–37] Further, ischaemia is a consistent finding in fatal head injury[24] and retrospective studies from several groups have suggested that outcome is improved in patients who have fewer episodes of CPP or MAP reduction,[36] aggressive CPP management[38] or retained autoregulation.[39] There is, however, some emerging concern that relatively high perfusion pressures may contribute to oedema formation post-head injury and at least one group have focused on targeting relatively low cerebral perfusion pressures in order to minimize oedema formation.[40] Other small studies have shown that outcome may be worsened in patients who suffer episodes of jugular venous desaturation below 50%[41] or blood glucose elevation.[42] There appears to be general agreement that rises in body temperature may worsen outcome in acute brain injury.[16,43]

These findings make several points. First, they suggest that autoregulation may be impaired in these patients, since the CPP thresholds for loss of pressure autoregulation are higher than in healthy subjects. Second, they emphasize the importance of maintenance of cerebral perfusion pressure, rather than isolated attention to intracranial pressure as a therapeutic target. There are, however, data that show that ICP is an independent, albeit weaker, determinant of outcome in severe head injury,[43] with levels greater than 15–25 mmHg constituting an appropriate threshold for initiation of therapy.

MONITORING SYSTEMIC PHYSIOLOGY

The need to maintain cerebral oxygenation and CPP predicate the monitoring required to achieve these therapeutic targets. Consequently, monitoring of direct arterial blood pressure along with measurement of ICP are essential for computing and manipulating CPP. The need to rationally manipulate mean arterial pressure will also require the placement of a right atrial or pulmonary artery catheter as appropriate. Continuous pulse oximetry, regular arterial blood gas analysis, core temperature monitoring and regular measurement of blood sugar are also required in order to optimize physiology in these patients.

GLOBAL CNS MONITORING MODALITIES

While the monitoring described above may help to ensure the maintenance of optimal systemic physiology, detection of local changes in CNS physiology will require other tools. Commonly used bedside monitoring techniques in this area include transcranial Doppler ultrasound for non-invasive estimation of CBF, jugular venous saturation ($SjvO_2$) monitoring and monitoring of brain electrical activity. These techniques seek to estimate cerebral blood flow in the presence of an adequate CPP, estimate the adequacy of oxygen delivery to the brain and document the conse-

quences of possible oxygen deficit or drug therapy on brain function respectively.

INTRACRANIAL PRESSURE MONITORING[6,44]

The need to optimize CPP predicates the requirement of monitoring ICP in all patients with severe head injury. Clinical signs of intracranial hypertension are late, inconsistent and non-specific. Further, it has been shown that episodic rises in intracranial pressure may occur even in patients with a normal X-ray CT scan.[45] While intraparenchymal micromanometers (Codman, USA) or fibreoptic probes (Camino, USA) are increasingly being used instead of ventriculostomies due to ease of use and a lower infection risk, they are more expensive and do not permit CSF drainage for the reduction of elevated ICP.

In addition to static ICP elevation, patients with head injury may develop phasic increases in ICP, often triggered by cerebral vasodilatation in response to a fall in CPP (Fig. 21.4). 'A-waves' tend to occur on a high

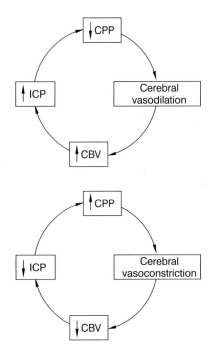

Figure 21.4   Vasodilatory/vasoconstrictor cascades (after Rosner). On the left, changes in cerebral blood volume (CBV) induced by vasodilatory responses to CPP reduction tend to increase ICP and further reduce CPP, resulting in a vicious circle. Conversely (right panel), CPP elevation will not only improve cerebral perfusion but also trigger autoregulatory vasoconstriction and reduce CBV and ICP.

baseline pressure and elevate ICP to 50–100 mmHg for several minutes, usually terminated by a marked increase in mean arterial pressure consequent to a Cushing response which results in catecholamine secretion. Shorter lived fluctuations lasting about a minute are referred to as B-waves. The frequency of both A and B-waves may be decreased by increasing MAP, thus preventing the reflex cerebral vasodilatory cascade that initiates CBV increases and ICP elevation.

TRANSCRANIAL DOPPLER (TCD) ULTRASONOGRAPHY

Reductions in middle cerebral artery flow velocity (MCA FV) provide a useful marker of reduced cerebral perfusion in the setting of intracranial hypertension but episodic rises in ICP may also be caused by hyperaemia, which may be diagnosed by *increases* in TCD FV. Transcranial Doppler ultrasonography can also be used as a non-invasive monitor of cerebral perfusion pressure. As the ICP increases and cerebral perfusion pressure correspondingly decreases, a characteristic highly pulsatile flow velocity pattern is seen. Continuing increases in ICP result first in a reduction and then loss of diastolic flow, progressing to an isolated systolic spike of flow in the TCD waveform and eventually to an oscillating flow pattern which signifies the onset of intracranial circulatory arrest.[37,46] The pulsatility index (PI) is one way of mathematically describing the waveform pattern and correlates more with cerebral perfusion pressure than with ICP.[47] This form of monitoring may become particularly useful in centres where ICP measurements are not routinely used (such as district general hospitals) or in patients in whom ICP monitoring is unavailable or may not be clearly indicated (e.g. mild closed head injury). Cerebral vasospasm results in *increases* in TCD flow velocity, as blood is pushed through narrow arterial segments into a widely dilated microvascular bed.[33,48–50]

The loss of cerebral pressure autoregulation and vasoreactivity to CO_2 are indicators of poor prognosis after head injury.[51,52] Classic tests of autoregulation involve recording TCD responses to induced changes in mean arterial pressure. Cerebral autoregulatory reserve is also assessed by the transient hyperaemic response test[53] (THRT). More recent algorithms constantly assess autoregulation by on-line calculation of changes in MCA FV in response to small spontaneous alterations in MAP.[39] Such analysis permits the on-line calculation of indices of cerebrovascular reactivity and compensatory reserve, which may allow prediction rather than recording of physiological behaviour, and facilitates the selection of patients for intensification of therapy.

JUGULAR VENOUS OXIMETRY

Classically right jugular venous oximetry has been used to assess the adequacy of CBF in head injury but a case can be made for targeting the side of injury or for using bilateral catheterization.[54] Reductions in $SjvO_2$ or increases in arteriojugular differences in oxygen content ($AJDO_2$) to greater than 9 ml/dl provide useful markers of inadequate CBF[55] and can guide therapy,[56] and $SjvO_2$ values below 50% have been shown to be associated with a worse outcome in head injury.[41] Conversely, marked elevations in $SjvO_2$ may provide evidence of cerebral hyperaemia. While $SjvO_2$ monitoring has been widely used in head injury, it is technically difficult. The use of continuous $SjvO_2$ monitoring with a fibreoptic catheter will detect episodes of cerebral desaturation associated with intracranial hypertension, hypocapnia, systemic hypotension and cerebral vasospasm but as many as half of the episodes identified as cerebral desaturation ($SjvO_2 < 50\%$) may be false positives.[57]

NEWER TECHNIQUES FOR BRAIN OXIMETRY

The major deficiencies of jugular venous oximetry are its invasiveness and the poor reliability of signal obtained. Other techniques that have been employed investigationally in acute head injury include near infra-red spectroscopy (NIRS),[57,58] direct tissue oximetry[59,60] and cerebral microdialysis.[61,62,63] These techniques are discussed elsewhere in this book.

CEREBRAL BLOOD FLOW MEASUREMENT

Despite the neuropathological evidence of ischaemia in fatal head injury, antemortem evidence of ischaemia from CBF studies was unconvincing in early studies.[64] CBF reductions were generally modest in the first few days following injury. Further, most patients exhibited $AJDO_2$ in the normal range, implying that the CBF reductions were appropriately coupled to decreases in cerebral metabolic rates for oxygen ($CMRO_2$).[64] Two different approaches have provided explanations for these observations. Ultra early (<12 h) CBF measurements after head injury have provided clear evidence that over 30% of patients exhibit global CBF reductions below commonly accepted ischaemic thresholds (<18 ml/100 g/min).[65] Later measurements in this study showed elevation of CBF to non-ischaemic levels by 24–48 h post-injury (Fig. 21.5).[65] These findings have been generally confirmed by other studies.[33] However, even at early time points, $AJDO_2$ remained relatively low despite a markedly low CBF (Fig. 21.5), with few patients demonstrating increases above 9 ml/100 ml.[33,65]

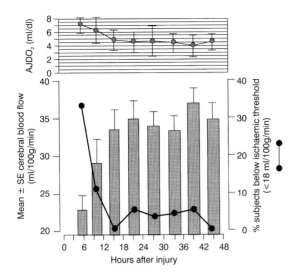

Figure 21.5 Global CBF (bars show means + standard error), percentage of patients below ischaemic threshold (solid circles and lines), and AVDO$_2$ (circles in upper panel) in the first 48 h following head injury (redrawn from data in reference[65]).

One explanation for the conflict between these clinical findings and the neuropathological evidence of ischaemia[66] may be found in the physiological heterogeneity in the injured brain. Both conventional monitoring methods and newer techniques are limited by the fact that they detect either globally averaged or highly localized abnormalities in cerebral physiology and may be unable to detect regional abnormalities in the metabolically heterogeneous injured brain.

IMAGING PHYSIOLOGY AND METABOLISM IN HEAD INJURY

The need to detect changes in regional physiology and the insensitivity of structural imaging changes (as detected by X-ray CT or conventional MRI) to early, reversible pathology have lead to the conclusion that there is a need to image physiology and metabolism in such patients. Marion et al[67] used stable xenon-enhanced CT to confirm that CBF values were reduced in the first 24 h following head injury. However, global CBF misrepresented regional CBF values in 48% of subjects and lobar or basal ganglia levels were often higher than might have been expected from global values.[67] They also demonstrated variations in global and regional perfusion patterns in different structural pathologies, with lowest perfusion in patients with diffuse swelling or bihemispheric contusions. Bouma et al[68] confirmed the presence of early ischaemia and demonstrated reductions in hemispheric

CBF on the side of intracranial haematomas. Several studies have demonstrated marked heterogeneity in perfusion patterns and CO$_2$ reactivity in the injured brain, especially in the vicinity of contusions.[67–69] In recent studies we have shown (Fig. 21.6) that moderate reductions in PaCO$_2$ (to 4.2 kPa in some instances) can decrease CBF to values below well-recognized ischaemic thresholds (<20 ml/100 g/min).[70] The development of these ischaemic areas is not reflected by reductions in jugular bulb oxygen saturations below commonly accepted thresholds for ischaemia (<55%). Recent interest has focused on increased uptake of the PET tracer ^{18}F-deoxyglucose around contusions and adjacent to haematomas, which are probably unaccompanied by increases in oxygen metabolism.[71,72] These data concur with previous animal studies and imply cerebral hyperglycolysis (anaerobic glucose utilization) and may represent metabolic changes associated with local epileptiform activity, high ECF glutamate or inflammatory activation.

MULTIMODALITY MONITORING

While individual monitoring techniques provide information regarding specific aspects of cerebral function, the correlation of data from several modalities has several advantages in head injury management. Integration of monitored variables allows crossvalidation and artefact rejection, better understanding of pathophysiology and the potential to target therapy.

THERAPY

ACHIEVING TARGET CPP VALUES

Most centres agree on the need to maintain cerebral perfusion by keeping CPP above 60–70 mmHg, either by decreasing ICP or by increasing MAP. While MAP is usually maintained with volume expansion, inotropes and vasopressors, the relative efficiency of each of these interventions in maintaining CPP has not been investigated. Indeed, we have no data on the safety of high doses of vasoactive agents in the presence of blood–brain barrier disruption. Drainage of CSF (where possible), mannitol administration, hyperventilation and the use of CNS depressants (typically barbiturates) have all been used to reduce ICP.

The debate in this area has focused on the means of optimizing CPP at a level above 70 mmHg (although some proponents would quote a substantial body of data to justify a target of 60 mmHg).[9,35–39,56] Rosner et al[38] have been the most enthusiastic proponents of the use of hypervolaemia and hypertension to increase MAP and induce secondary reductions in ICP. Cruz,[56]

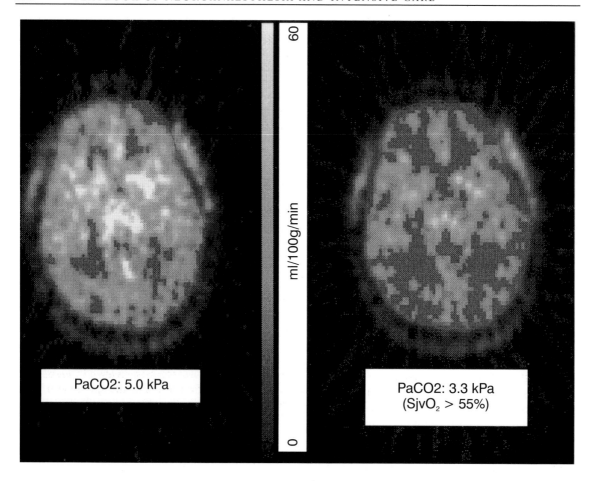

Figure 21.6   PET rCBF scan showing effect of hyperventilation in the first 24 h following head injury. Despite the maintenance of SjvO$_2$ at acceptable levels, hyperventilation results in marked increases in the volume of brain tissue (outlined) below an ischaemic CBF threshold (20 ml/100 g/min).

on the other hand, has proposed the use of 'optimized hyperventilation' (guided by SjvO$_2$ monitoring) to reduce ICP and hence increase CPP. It is likely that several different pathophysiological mechanisms coexist in individual patients and both approaches are likely to have a role if applied appropriately. It must be remembered that both hyperventilation and induced hypertension have clearly recognized systemic and cerebral side effects and their extent of use will also be limited by a risk:benefit ratio.[73]

The recent advent of intraparenchymal manometers or fibreoptic devices for measuring ICP has reduced infection risk but removed automatic access to ICP drainage in such patients. This change in practice bears review in the light of data quoted in the Brain Trauma Foundation guidelines for the management of severe head injury, which provide circumstantial evidence supporting the increased use of CSF drainage for ICP control.[5]

THE LUND PROTOCOL

In contrast to discussions above, publications from one centre[40,74] describe the use of a protocol that focuses primarily on the prevention and reduction of cerebral oedema rather than maximizing cerebral perfusion. This protocol accepts CPP values as low as 50 mmHg in adults, with reduction of mean arterial pressures using a combination of clonidine and metoprolol and reduction of cerebral blood volume with dihydroergotamine and low-dose thiopentone (used as a sedative). Plasma oncotic pressure was increased by transfusing albumin or plasma to maintain normal albumin levels. These papers report excellent results with this regime (8% overall mortality and 79% good outcome) which compare well with those from centres using conventional CPP-guided therapy. However, they used historical controls and there is some doubt as to whether the data are truly comparable to those obtained from other centres. In any case, their impressive outcome figures demand further investigation and it may well be that optimal CPP levels may vary widely, both between patients and at different stages after head injury in the same patient.[75]

VENTILATORY SUPPORT AND THE USE OF HYPOCAPNIA FOR ICP REDUCTION

It is generally agreed that patients with a GCS of ≤ 8 require intubation for airway protection and that such patients should receive mechanical ventilatory support in order to ensure optimal oxygenation and $PaCO_2$ control. Airway control and ventilation are also required for patients with ventilatory failure, central neurogenic hyperventilation or recurrent fits.

Hyperventilation, once the mainstay of ICP reduction in severe head injury, is now the subject of much debate.[76,77] The aim of hyperventilation is to reduce cerebral blood volume and hence ICP but this is accompanied by a reduction in global cerebral blood flow, which may drop below ischaemic thresholds.[41,56,64] Such ischaemia can be documented using jugular bulb oximetry and while conclusive data are not available, it is possible that these consequences may worsen outcome, especially when hyperventilation is prolonged or profound.[78] More recent studies have shown that hyperventilation may result in significant focal reductions in rCBF, shown by contrast-enhanced dynamic computed tomography or positron emission tomography,[69,70,79] which are undetected by global measures of cerebral oxygenation such as SjO_2 monitoring. In addition to concerns regarding ischaemia, hyperventilation may have only short-lived effectiveness in decreasing ICP due to compensatory reductions in cerebral extracellular fluid (ECF) bicarbonate levels, which rapidly restore ECF pH in normal subjects.[80] Although there is some evidence that these compensatory changes may be delayed after head injury,[64] it is likely that they will, over time, attenuate the effect of low $PaCO_2$ levels on vascular tone and result in rebound increases in cerebral blood volume and ICP when $PaCO_2$ is subsequently normalized. It has been suggested that the use of the diffusible hydrogen ion acceptor, tetra-hydro-aminomethane (THAM), may restore ECF base levels and cerebrovascular CO_2 reactivity. While such an approach has been shown to lower ICP and the need for intensification of ICP therapy after head injury, it does not alter outcome.[80]

FLUID THERAPY[81] AND FEEDING

Accurate fluid management may be complicated by continuing or concealed haemorrhage from associated extracranial trauma but every effort must be made to restore normovolaemia and prevent hypotension. Fluid replacement should be guided by clinical and laboratory assessment of volume status and by invasive haemodynamic monitoring but generally involves the administration of 30–40 ml/kg of maintenance fluid per day. The choice of hydration fluid is largely based on inconclusive results from animal data.[81] Fluid flux across the normal BBB is governed by osmolarity rather than oncotic pressure. Consequently, hypotonic fluids are avoided and serum osmolality is maintained at high normal levels (290–300 mosm/l in our practice) to minimize fluid flux into the injured brain. Dextrose-containing solutions are avoided since the residual free water after dextrose metabolism can worsen cerebral oedema and because the associated elevations in blood sugar may worsen outcome.[42] Some clinical data are now available to support these practices. Qureshi et al[82] used 3% saline in patients with brain oedema due to head injury and demonstrated a rise in plasma sodium and osmolality and at least temporary reduction in ICP and midline shift. Simma et al[83] reported that 1.6% saline, when compared to lactated Ringer's solution as maintenance fluid in head-injured children, resulted in lower ICP values, less need for barbiturate therapy, a lower incidence of acute lung injury, fewer complications and a shorter ICU stay. While these results are encouraging, it is important to balance them against imperfections in the design of both studies and potential side effects of hyperosmolar fluid therapy.[84]

Increases in plasma oncotic pressure might be expected to provide a distinct advantage in situations where blood–brain barrier disruption results in leak of sodium into the brain ECF.[81] Maintenance of oncotic pressure with albumin supplements is one of the cornerstones of the Lund protocol[40] and other authors have discussed the advantages of colloid use in this setting. Both albumin and gelatins have been used but the haemostatic disturbances produced by hetastarch may potentiate intracranial haemorrhage. Certain colloids (such as pentastarch) may be effective in reducing the cerebral oedema associated with cerebral ischaemic and reperfusion injury.[85] Agents which 'plug leaks' by acting as oxygen free radical scavengers and or by inhibiting neutrophil adhesion may be the resuscitation fluids of the future.[86]

Head-injured patients have high nutritional requirements and feeding should be instituted early (within 24 h), aiming to replace 140% of resting metabolic expenditure (with 15% of calories supplied as protein) by the seventh day posttrauma.[87] Enteral feeding is associated with a lower incidence of hyperglycaemia and may have protective effect against gastric ulceration, the incidence of which may be increased in these patients. Impaired gastric emptying, which is common in head injury, can be treated with prokinetic agents such as cisapride and metoclopramide.[88] In those who cannot be fed enterally, parenteral nutrition should be considered together with some form of prophylaxis against gastric ulceration (H_2 antagonists or sucralfate) and rigorous blood sugar control.

HYPEROSMOLAR THERAPY

Mannitol (0.25–1 g/kg, usually as a 20% solution) has traditionally been used to elevate plasma osmolarity and reduce brain oedema in the setting of intracranial hypertension.[89,90] In addition to its osmotic effects, mannitol probably reduces ICP by improving CPP and microcirculatory dynamics.[90,91] While it is reported to possess antioxidant activity, this is unlikely to be clinically important. Side effects include secondary increases in ICP when the BBB is disrupted, fluid overload from initial intravascular volume expansion and renal toxicity from excessive use. These can be minimized if its use is discontinued when it no longer produces significant ICP reduction, volume status is monitored and if plasma osmolality is not allowed to rise above 320 mosm/l.[90] Hypertonic saline solutions (7.5%) are currently being evaluated for small volume resuscitation and may improve outcome in comatose patients suffering from multiple trauma.[92] Recent reports also highlight the successful use of 23.4% saline for treatment of intracranial hypertension refractory to mannitol.[93] While more studies are required, it appears hypertonic saline will find a place in the treatment of brain swelling.[94]

SEDATION AND NEUROMUSCULAR BLOCKADE

Intravenous anaesthetic agents preserve pressure autoregulation and the cerebrovascular response to CO_2, even at doses sufficient to abolish cortical activity,[95,96] and decrease cerebral blood flow, cerebral metabolism and ICP.[96–99] While the reduction in flow and CBV are secondary to a reduction in metabolism, flow-metabolism coupling is not perfect and the decrease in CBF may exceed the corresponding decrease in $CMRO_2$, with a widening of the cerebral arteriovenous oxygen content difference.[100] Such uncoupled CBF reductions may be at least partially due to changes in systemic haemodynamics.

Barbiturates are now less commonly used for routine sedation, owing to the availability of other agents such as propofol which possess similar cerebrovascular effects but better pharmacokinetic profiles.[101] However, propofol can induce hypotension and

decrease in cerebral perfusion pressure. The lipid load imposed by a 20 ml/h continuous infusion of propofol must be taken into account in the calculation of daily caloric intake. In our hands, the use of 200 µg/kg/min propofol to produce burst suppression for long periods has often resulted in unacceptable levels of plasma lipids. These problems with lipid loading have been substantially ameliorated by the introduction of a 2% formulation of propofol.

Midazolam is often used in combination with fentanyl and propofol for sedating the patient with head injury. Midazolam reduces $CMRO_2$, CBF and CBV with both cerebral autoregulation and vasoreactivity to CO_2 remaining intact.[102,103] However, these effects are inconsistent and transient and even large doses of midazolam will not produce burst suppression or an isoelectric EEG. Opioids generally have negligible effects on CBF and $CMRO_2$. However, the newer synthetic opioids fentanyl, sufentanil and alfentanil can increase ICP in patients with tumours and head trauma[104] due to changes in $PaCO_2$ (in spontaneously breathing subjects) and reflex cerebral vasodilatation secondary to systemic hypotension.[105,106] These changes can be avoided if blood pressure and ventilation are controlled.[107–109]

Neuromuscular blockade in the head-injured patient receiving intensive care is currently the subject of much debate.[110–112] Neuromuscular blockers can play an important role in the head-injured patient by preventing rises in ICP produced by coughing and 'bucking on the tube'.[112] However, use of these agents is not associated with better outcomes, perhaps because of increased respiratory complications. Further, long-term use of neuromuscular blockade has been associated with continued paralysis after drug discontinuation[113] and acute myopathy,[114] especially with the steroid-based medium to long-acting agents. However, atracurium is non-cumulative and has not been associated with myopathy and theoretical concerns about the accumulation of laudanosine, a cerebral excitatory metabolite of atracurium, in head-injured patients have not been shown to be clinically relevant.[112]

ANTIEPILEPTIC THERAPY

Seizures occur both early (<7 days) or late (>7 days) after head injury, with a reported incidence of between 4–25% and 9–42% respectively.[115] Seizure prophylaxis with phenytoin or carbamazepine can reduce the incidence of early posttraumatic epilepsy but has little impact on late seizures, neurological outcome or mortality.[115,116] The incidence of posttraumatic seizures is greatest in patients with a GCS <10 and in the presence of an intracranial haematoma, contusion, penetrating injury or depressed skull fractures.[115] Since it is important to balance the possible benefit from seizure reduction against the side effects of antiepileptic drugs, such patients may form the most appropriate subgroup for acute (days to weeks) seizure prophylaxis following head injury.

CEREBRAL METABOLIC SUPPRESSANTS

Intravenous barbiturates have been used in the setting of acute head injury for ICP reduction for over 20 years.[117] While they clearly result in cardiovascular depression, increased ICU stay and increases in pulmonary infections, it appears that they have a significant role to play in patients whose problem is intractable intracranial hypertension that responds to intravenous anaesthetics.[118,119] They are administered as an intravenous infusion, titrated to produce burst suppression on EEG. One major disadvantage of barbiturates is prolonged recovery. This might suggest a role for other intravenous anaesthetics (etomidate and propofol) with more desirable pharmacokinetic profiles. However, the efficacy of these agents remains unproven and they have their own drawbacks. The adrenocortical suppression produced by etomidate has been well documented and the high doses of propofol required to achieve burst suppression (up to 200 μg/kg/min) necessitate the delivery of high lipid loads with resultant abnormalities in plasma lipid status.

NOVEL NEUROPROTECTIVE INTERVENTIONS

While a variety of novel pharmacological neuroprotective agents are currently under investigation, none of the drugs tested thus far in phase III trials have proved to provide benefit on an intention-to-treat basis.[16,17]

EXCITATORY AMINO ACID (EAA) ANTAGONISTS[17,120,121]

While the role of EAAs and protection by EAA antagonists have been documented in experimental head injury, early clinical studies have been disappointing. The prototype non-competitive glutamate antagonist acting at the NMDA receptor, dizocilpine (MK-801), never reached large-scale clinical trials because of fears regarding hippocampal neurotoxicity. More recent compounds have either been competitive or non-competitive antagonists, acted as allosteric modifiers of NMDA channel activity, acted at presynaptic sites to reduce glutamate release or at non-NMDA glutamate receptors. However, none of these has been proved to be effective in outcome trials.

CALCIUM CHANNEL BLOCKERS

Successful clinical trials of nimodipine in subarachnoid haemorrhage prompted trials of this agent in head injury. Recent studies have suggested that the agent may improve outcome in a subgroup of head-injured patients who have traumatic subarachnoid haemorrhage,[122,123] though this remains controversial.[124]

ANTIOXIDANTS

Animal studies have suggested a prominent role for free radicals in head injury and demonstrated protection by antioxidants. However, although initial clinical trials of polyethylene glycol-conjugated superoxide dismutase (pegorgotein) were encouraging,[125] a more recent large randomized outcome study has failed to demonstrate any benefit[126] and large phase III trials of the novel antioxidant tirilazad (which had proven efficacy in experimental models) have shown no improvement in outcome in clinical head injury.[127]

CORTICOSTEROIDS

A large outcome trial demonstrated small but significant benefit of early high-dose methylprednisolone in traumatic spinal cord injury.[128] Although isolated studies have reported benefit from steroids in acute head injury, a systematic review of the literature suggested that corticosteroids were ineffective or harmful in severe head injury.[129] However, a recent metaanalysis has reawakened interest in mounting a megatrial of early corticosteroid therapy in patients with head injury[130] but this approach is the subject of some debate.[131]

HYPOTHERMIA

Mild to moderate hypothermia (33–36°C) has been shown to be neuroprotective in animal studies which demonstrated improved outcome from cerebral ischaemia with small (1–3°C) reductions in temperature. Three early clinical studies demonstrated benefit from moderate hypothermia in head injury[132–134] and interim results from a large ongoing outcome trial have been encouraging, suggesting benefit in a subgroup of patients with GCS scores of 5–7.[135] There has been lively correspondence in various journals regarding the methodology and conclusions of this report[136–140] and publication of the final results of the study is awaited. Demonstration that temperature elevation can worsen outcome following brain injury[144] is particularly relevant in the context of findings that cerebral temperature tends to be above core temperature in the injured brain[143] and is more accurately estimated by brain tissue probes[141] or jugular bulb catheters.[142]

All patients with or at risk of intracranial hypertension *must* have invasive arterial monitoring, CVP line, ICP monitor and Rt SjO₂ catheter at admission to NCCU.

Aim to establish TCD and multimodality computer within the first six hours of NCCU stay.

Interventions in stage II to be targeted to clinical picture and multimodality monitoring.

Check whether the patient is in or may be a candidate for research protocols.

Guidelines may be modified at the discretion of the consultant in charge.

Treatment grades III and IV only after approval by NCC consultant.

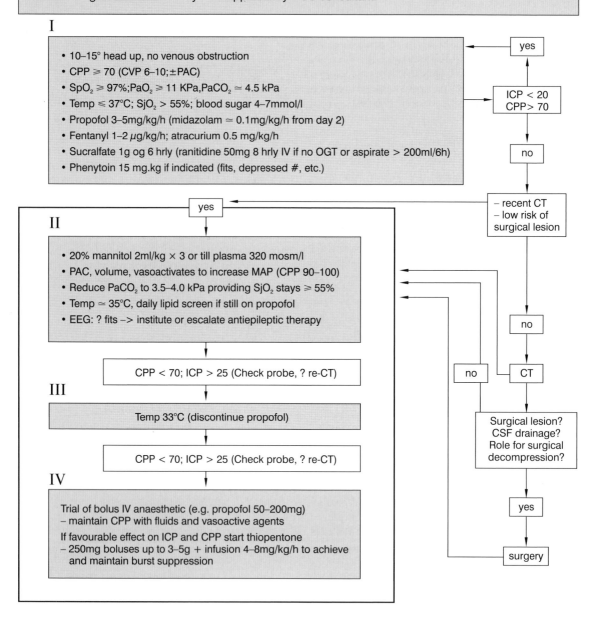

Figure 21.7   Addenbrooke's NCCU ICP/CPP management algorithm.

SEQUENTIAL ESCALATION VERSUS TARGETED THERAPY FOR THE INTENSIVE CARE OF HEAD INJURY

It is clear that a diverse range of pathophysiological processes operate in acute head injury and that there exist a wide range of therapeutic options, few of which have proven efficacy. One of two approaches may be used in the choice of therapy in such a setting. The first of these is to use a standard protocol in all patients and introduce more intensive therapies in a sequence based either on intensity of intervention or on local experience and availability. While such a scheme is simple, it does not provide for individualization of therapy in a given patient.

Alternatively, individual therapies can be targeted at individual pathophysiological processes. Examples are the use of hyperventilation in the presence of hyperaemia, mannitol for vasogenic cerebral oedema or the use of blood pressure elevation in the presence of B-waves. This intellectually appealing approach is hindered by the fact that pathophysiology is usually mixed, and global monitors of CNS physiology may miss critical focal abnormalities. Further, some interventions (e.g. hypothermia) work via multiple mechanisms and do not easily find a place in a strictly targeted therapy plan.

In practice, many established head injury protocols represent a hybrid approach. Initial baseline monitoring and therapy are applied to all patients and refractory problems are dealt with by therapy escalation, with the choice of intervention determined by clinical presentation and physiological monitoring. Often, interventions that are more difficult to implement or present significant risks (e.g. barbiturate coma) are used as a last resort. Figure 21.7 represents the ICP/CPP management protocol used in the neurosciences critical care unit (NCCU) at Addenbrooke's Hospital.

REFERENCES

1. Hodgkinson DW, Berry E, Yates DW. Mild head injury – a positive approach to management. Eur J Emerg Med 1994; 1: 9–12.

2. Jennett B, MacMillan R. Epidemiology of head injury. BMJ 1981; 282: 101–104.

3. Teasdale C, Jennett B. Assessment and prognosis of coma after head injury. Acta Neurochir (Vienna) 1976; 34: 45–55.

4. Fearnside MR, Simpson DA. Epidemiology. In: Reilly P, Bullock R (eds) Head injury. Chapman and Hall, London, 1997, pp 3–24.

5. Bullock MR, Povilshock JT. Indications for intracranial pressure monitoring. J Neurotrauma 1996; 13: 667–679.

6. Jennett B, Bond M. Assessment of outcome after severe brain damage. Lancet 1975; I: 480–484.

7. Jones PA, Andrews PJD, Midgley S et al. Measuring the burden of secondary insults in head injured patients during intensive care. J Neurosurg Anesthesiol 1994; 6: 4–14.

8. Mendelow DA, Crawford PJ. Primary and secondary brain injury. In: Reilly P, Bullock R (eds) Head injury. Chapman and Hall, London, 1997, pp 71–88.

9. Reilly PL, Adams RH, Graham DI, Jennett B. Patients who talk and die. Lancet 1997; ii: 375–377.

10. Jones PA, Andrews PJD, Midgley S et al. Measuring the burden of secondary insults in head injured patients during intensive care. J Neurosurg Anesthesiol 1994; 6: 4–14.

11. Chesnut RM, Marshall SB, Piek J et al. Early and late systemic hypotension as a frequent and fundamental source of cerebral ischaemia following severe brain injury in the Traumatic Coma Data Bank. Acta Neurochir 1993; 59(suppl): 121–125.

12. Mendelow AD, Gillingham FJ. Extradural haematoma: effect of delayed treatment. BMJ 1979; ii: 134.

13. Seelig JM, Becker DP, Miller JD et al. Traumatic acute subdural hematoma. Major mortality reduction in comatose patients treated within four hours. N Engl J Med 1981; 304: 1511–1518.

14. Bullock MR, Povilshock JT. Guidelines for the treatment of severe head injury – introduction. J Neurotrauma 1996; 13: 643–645.

15. Maas AIR, Dearden M, Teasdale GM et al. EBIC guidelines for management of severe head injury in adults. Acta Neurochir (Vienna) 1997; 139: 286–294.

16. Menon DK, Summors AC. Neuroprotection (including hypothermia). Curr Opin Anaesthesiol 1998; 11: 485–496.

17. Doppenberg EMR, Bullock R. Clinical neuroprotection trials in severe traumatic brain injury: lessons from previous studies. J Neurotrauma 1997: 14: 71–80.

18. Jeevaratnam D, Menon DK. Survey of intensive care of severely head injured patients in the United Kingdom. BMJ 1996; 312: 944–947.

19. Ghajar J, Hariri RJ, Narayan RK et al. Survey of critical care management of comatose, head-injured patients in the United States. Crit Care Med 1995; 23: 560–567.

20. Matta BF, Menon DK. Severe head injury in the United Kingdom and Ireland: a survey of practice and implications for management. Crit Care Med 1996; 24: 1743–1748.

21. Wilkins I, Matta BF, Menon DK. Management of comatose head injured patients in the United Kingdom: are we getting any better? J Neurosurg Anesthesiol 1998; 10: 280.

22. Bullock R. Injury and cell function. In: Reilly P, Bullock R (eds) Head injury. Chapman and Hall, London, 1997, pp 121–141.

23. Siesjo BK, Siesjo P. Mechanisms of secondary brain injury. Eur J Anaesthesiol 1996; 13: 247–268.

24. McIntosh TK, Smith DH, Meaney DF et al. Neuropathological sequelae of traumatic brain injury: relationship to neurochemical and biomechanical mechanisms. Lab Invest 1996; 74: 315–342.

25. McKeating EG, Andrews PJD. Cytokines and adhesion molecules in acute brain injury. Br J Anaesthesia 1998; 80: 77–84.

26. McKeating EG, Andrews PJ, Signorini DF, Mascia L. Transcranial cytokine gradients in patients requiring intensive care after acute brain injury. Br J Anaesth 1997; 78 : 520–523.

27. Fale A, Bacon PJ, Menon DK. Changes in circulating adhesion molecule levels following severe head injury. J Neurosurg Anesthesiol 1996; 8: 324.

28. Gupta AK, Thiru S, Bradley J et al. Delayed increases in adhesion molecule expression after traumatic brain injury in humans: preliminary results. J Cereb Blood Flow Metab 1995; 15: S33.

29. Holmin S, Soderlund J, Biberfield P, Mathiesen T. Intracerebral inflammation after human brain contusion. Neurosurgery 1998; 42: 291–299.

30. Zunarelli E, Nicoll JAR, Graham DI. Presenelin-1 polymorphism and amyloid beta-protein deposition in fatal head injury. Neuroreport 1996; 8: 45–48.

31. O'Meara ES, Kukull WA, Sheppard L et al. Head injury and risk of Alzheimer's disease by apolipoprotein E genotype. Am J Epidemiol 1997; 146: 373–384.

32. Teasdale GM, Nicoll JAR, Murray G, Fiddes M. Association of apolipoprotein E polymorphism after head injury. Lancet 1997: 350: 1069–1071.

33. Martin NA, Patwardhan RV, Alexander MJ et al. Characterization of cerebral hemodynamic phases following severe head trauma: hypoperfusion, hyperaemia and vasospasm. J Neurosurg 1997; 87: 9–19.

34. Chesnut RM, Marshall LF, Klauber MR et al. The role of secondary brain injury in determining outcome from severe head injury. J Trauma 1993; 34: 216–222.

35. Chan K, Dearden NM, Miller JD et al. Multimodality monitoring as a guide to treatment of intracranial hypertension after severe brain injury. Neurosurgery 1993; 32: 547–553.

36. PJD Andrews. What is the optimal perfusion pressure after brain injury – a review of the evidence with an emphasis on arterial pressure. Acta Anaesthesiol Scand 1995; 39(suppl 105): 112–114.

37. Chan KH, Miller JD, Dearden NM et al. The effect of changes in cerebral perfusion upon middle cerebral artery blood flow velocity and jugular bulb venous oxygen saturation after severe brain injury. J Neurosurg 1992; 77: 55–61.

38. Rosner MJ, Rosner SD, Johnson AH. Cerebral perfusion pressure: management protocol and clinical results. J Neurosurg 1995; 83: 949–962.

39. Czosnyka M, Smielewski P, Kirkpatrick P et al. Continuous assessment of the cerebral vasomotor reactivity in head injury. Neurosurgery 1997; 41: 11–19.

40. Eker C, Asgiersson B, Grande PO et al. Improved outcome after severe head injury with a new therapy based on principles for brain volume regulation and preserved microcirculation. Crit Care Med 1998; 26: 1881–1886.

41. Shienberg M, Kanter MJ, Robertson CS et al. Continuous monitoring of jugular venous oxygen saturation in head-injured patients. J Neurosurg 1992; 76: 212–217.

42. Lam AM, Winn HR, Cullen BF et al. Hyperglycaemia and neurological outcome in patients with head injury. J Neurosurg 1991; 75: 545–551.

43. Bullock MR, Povilshock JT. Intracranial pressure treatment threshold. J Neurotrauma 1996; 13: 681–683.

44. Bullock MR, Povilshock JT. Recommendations for intracranial pressure monitoring technology. J Neurotrauma 1996; 13: 685–692.

45. O'Sullivan MG, Statham PF, Jones PA et al. Role of intracranial pressure monitoring in severely head injured patients without signs of intracranial hypertension on initial computed tomography. J Neurosurg 1994; 80: 46–50.

46. Czosnyka M, Smielewski P, Kirkpatrick P et al. Monitoring of cerebral autoregulation in head-injured patients. Stroke 1996; 27: 1829–1834.

47. Czosnyka M, Matta BF, Smielewski P et al. Cerebral perfusion pressure in head-injured patients: a noninvasive assessment using transcranial Doppler ultrasonography. J Neurosurg 1998; 88: 802–808.

48. Chan KH, Dearden NM, Miller JD. The significance of posttraumatic increase in cerebral blood flow velocity: a transcranial Doppler ultrasound study. Neurosurgery 1992; 30: 697–700.

49. Martin NA, Doberstein C, Zane C et al. Posttraumatic cerebral arterial spasm: transcranial Doppler ultrasound, cerebral blood flow and angiographic findings. J Neurosurg 1992; 77: 575–583.

50. Aaslid R, Huber P, Nornes H. Evaluation of cerebrovascular spasm with transcranial Doppler ultrasound. J Neurosurg 1984; 60: 1: 37–41.

51. Bouma GJ, Muizelaar JP. Cerebral blood flow, cerebral blood volume and cerebral blood flow reactivity after severe head injury. J Neurotrauma 1992; 9(suppl 1): S333–S348.

52. Schal'en W, Messeter K, Nordstrom CH. Cerebral vasoreactivity and the prediction of outcome in severe traumatic brain lesions. Acta Anaesthesiol Scand 1991; 35: 113–122.

53. Smielewski P, Czosnyka M, Iyer V, Piechneik S, Whitehouse H, Pickard JD. Computerised transient

hyperaemic response test – a method for the assessment of cerebral autoregulation. Ultrasound Med Biol 1995; 21: 599–611.

54. Metz C, Holzschuh M, Bein T et al. Monitoring of cerebral oxygen metabolism in the jugular bulb: reliability of unilateral measurements in severe head injury. J Cereb Blood Flow Metab 1998; 18: 332–343.

55. Cruz J, Miner ME, Allen SJ et al. Continuous monitoring of cerebral oxygenation in acute brain injury: assessment of cerebral haemodynamic reserve. Neurosurgery 1991; 29: 743–749.

56. Cruz J. The first decade of continuous monitoring of jugular bulb oxyhemoglobin saturation: management strategies and clinical outcome. Crit Care Med 1998; 26: 344–351.

57. Kirkpatrick PJ, Smielewski P, Czosnyka M et al. Near-infrared spectroscopy use in head injured patients. J Neurosurg 1995; 83: 963–970.

58. Gopinath SP, Robertson CS, Grossman RG et al. Near infrared localisation of intracranial hematomas. J Neurosurg 1993; 79: 43–47.

59. Valadka AB, Gopinath SP, Contant CF et al. Relationship of brain tissue PO2 to outcome after severe head injury. Crit Care Med 1998; 26: 1576–1581.

60. Dings J, Jager A, Meixensberger J, Roosen K. Brain tissue PO2 and outcome after severe head injury. Neurol Res 1998; 20: S71–S75.

61. Bullock R, Zauner A, Woodward JJ et al. Factors affecting excitatory amino acid release following severe human head injury. J Neurosurg 1998; 89: 507–518.

62. Robertson CS, Gopinath SP, Uzura M et al. Metabolic changes in the brain during transient ischemia measured with microdialysis. Neurol Res 1998; 20: S91–S94.

63. Zauner A, Doppenberg EM, Woodward JJ et al. Continuous monitoring of cerebral substrate delivery and clearance: initial experience in 24 patients with severe acute brain injuries. Neurosurgery 1997; 41: 1082–1091.

64. Obrist WD, Langfitt TW, Jaggi JL et al. Cerebral blood flow and metabolism in comatose patients with acute head injury. Relationship to intracranial hypertension. J Neurosurg 1984; 61: 241–253.

65. Bouma GJ, Muizelaar JP, Choi SC et al. Cerebral circulation and metabolism after severe traumatic brain injury: the elusive role of ischaemia. J Neurosurg 1991; 75: 685–693.

66. Graham DI, Ford I, Adams JH et al. Ischaemic brain damage is still common in fatal non-missile head injury. J Neurol Neurosurg Psychiatry 1989; 52: 346–350.

67. Marion DW, Darby J, Yonas H. Acute regional cerebral blood flow changes caused by severe head injuries. J Neurosurg 1991; 74: 407–414.

68. Bouma GJ, Muizelaar P, Stringer WA et al. Ultra-early evaluation of regional cerebral blood flow in severely head-injured patients using xenon-enhanced computerized tomography. J Neurosurg 1992; 77: 360–368.

69. McLaughlin MR, Marion DW. Cerebral blood flow within and around cerebral contusions. J Neurosurg 1996; 85: 871–876.

70. Menon DK, Minhas PS, Herrod NJ, Cerebral ischaemia associated with hyperventilation: a PET study Anesthesiology 1997; 87: A176.

71. Bergsneider M, Hovda DA, Shalmon E et al. Cerebral hyperglycolysis following severe traumatic brain injury in humans: a positron emission tomography study. J Neurosurg 1997; 86: 241–251.

72. Menon DK, Minhas PS, Matthews JC et al. Perilesional F-18-deoxyglucose uptake following head injury: PET findings in patients receiving IV anesthetic agents. Anesthesiology 1998; 89: A342.

73. Chesnut RM. Hyperventilation versus cerebral perfusion pressure management: time to change the question. Crit Care Med 1998; 26: 210–212.

74. Asgeirsson B, Grande PO, Nordstrom CH. A new therapy of post-trauma edema based on haemodynamic principles for brain volume regulation. Intens Care Med 1994; 20: 260–264.

75. Schneck MJ. Treating elevated intracranial pressure: do we raise or lower the blood pressure? Crit Care Med 1998; 26: 1787–1788.

76. Bullock R, Povilshock JT. The use of hyperventilation in the acute management of severe traumatic brain injury. J Neurotrauma 1996; 13: 699–703.

77. Chesnut RM. Hyperventilation in traumatic brain injury: friend or foe? Crit Care Med 1997; 25: 1275–1278.

78. Muizelaar JP, Marmarou A, Ward JD et al. Adverse effects of prolonged hyperventilation in patients with severe head injury. A randomized clinical trial. J Neurosurg 1991; 75: 731–739.

79. Skippen P, Poskitt K, Kestle J et al. Effect of hyperventilation on regional cerebral blood flow in head-injured children. Crit Care Med 1997; 25: 1402–1409.

80. Wolf AL, Levi L, Marmarou A et al. Effect of THAM upon outcome in severe head injury – a randomized prospective clinical trial. J Neurosurg 1993; 78: 54–59.

81. Drummond JC. Fluid management of head injured patients. Acata Anaesthesiol Scand 1995; 39(S105): 107–111.

82. Qureshi AI, Suarez JI, Bhardwaj A et al. Use of hypertonic (3%) saline/acetate infusion in the treatment of cerebral oedema: effect on intracranial pressure and lateral displacement of the brain. Crit Care Med 1998; 26: 440–446.

83. Simma B, Burger R, Falk M, Fanconi S. A prospective, randomized, and controlled study of fluid management in clildren with severe head injury: lactated Ringer's solution versus hypertonic saline. Crit Care Med 1998; 26: 1265–1270.

84. Clark RSB, Kochanek PM. Pass the salt? Crit Care Med 1998; 26: 1161–1162.

85. Schell RM, Cole DJ, Schultz RL et al. Temporary cerebral ischemia. Effects of pentastarch or albumin on reperfusion injury. Anesthesiology 1992; 77: 86–92.

86. Prough DS, Kramer G. Medium starch please. Anesth Analg 1994; 79: 1034–1035.

87. Bullock R, Povilshock JT. Nutritional support of brain injured patients. J Neurotrauma 1996; 13: 743–750.

88. Spapen HD, Duinslaeger L, Diltoer M et al. Gastric emptying in critically ill patients is accelerated by adding cisapride to a standard enteral feeding protocol – results of a prospective, randomized, controlled trial. Crit Care Med 1995; 23: 481–485.

89. Paczynski RP. Osmotherapy. Crit Care Clin 1997; 13: 105–129.

90. Bullock R, Povilshock JT. The use of mannitol in severe head injury. J Neurotrauma 1996; 13: 714–718.

91. Rosner MJ, Coley I. Cerebral perfusion pressure: a hemodynamic mechanisms of mannitol and the pre-mannitol hemogram. Neurosurgery 1987; 21: 147–156.

92. Vassar MJ, Fischer RP, O'Brien PE et al. A multicentre trial for resuscitation of head injured patients with 7.5% sodium chloride. The effect of added dextran 70. The Multicenter Group for the Study of Hypertonic Saline in Trauma Patients. Arch Surg 1993; 128: 1003–1011.

93. Suarez JI, Qureshi AI, Bhardwaj A et al. Treatment of refractory intracranial hypertension with 23.4% saline. Crit Care Med 1998; 26: 1118–1122.

94. Prough DS, Zornow MH. Mannitol: an old friend on the skids? Crit Care Med 1998; 26: 997–998.

95. Pierce EC Jr, Lambertson CJ, Deutsch S et al. Cerebral circulation and metabolism during thiopental anesthesia and hyperventilation in man. J Clin Invest 1962; 41: 1664–1671.

96. Matta BF, Lam AM, Strebel S, Mayberg TS. Cerebral pressure autoregulation and CO2-reactivity during propofol-induced EEG suppression. Br J Anaesth 1995; 4: 159–163.

97. Herregods L, Verbeke J, Rolly G et al. Effect of propofol on elevated intracranial pressure. Preliminary results. Anaesthesia 1990; 43: 107–109.

98. Pinaud M, Lelausque J-N, Chetanneau A et al. Effects of propofol on cerebral hemodynamics and metabolism in patients with brain trauma. Anesthesiology 1990; 73: 404–409.

99. Van Hemelrijck J, Fitch W, Mattheussen M et al. Effect of propofol on cerebral circulation and autoregulation in the baboon. Anesth Analg 1988; 71: 49–54.

100. Vandesteene A, Trempont V, Engelman E et al. Effect of propofol on cerebral blood flow and metabolism in man. Anaesthesia 1988; 43: 42–43.

101. Beller JP, Pottecher T, Lugnier A et al. Prolonged sedation with propofol in ICU patients: recovery and blood concentration changes during periodic interruptions in infusion. Br J Anaesth 1988; 6: 583–588.

102. Forster A, Juge O, Morel D. Effects of midazolam on cerebral hemodynamics and cerebral vasomotor responsiveness to carbon dioxide. J Cereb Blood Flow Metab 1983; 3: 246–249.

103. Strebel S, Kaufmann M, Guardiola PM et al. Cerebral vasomotor responsiveness to carbon dioxide is preserved during propofol and midazolam anesthesia in humans. Anesth Analg 1994; 78: 884–888.

104. Sperry RJ, Bailey PL, Reichman MV et al Fentanyl and sufentanil increase intracranial pressure in head trauma patients. Anesthesiology 1992; 7: 416–420.

105. Albanese J, Durbec O, Viviand X et al. Sufentanil increases intracranial pressure in patients with head trauma. Anesthesiology 1993; 79: 493–497.

106. Trindle MR, Dodson BA, Rampil IJ. Effects of fentanyl versus sufentanil in equianesthetic doses on middle cerebral artery blood flow velocity. Anesthesiology 1993; 78: 454–460.

107. Mayberg TS, Lam AM, Eng CC et al. The effect of alfentanil on cerebral blood flow velocity and intracranial pressure during isoflurane-nitrous oxide anesthesia in humans. Anesthesiology 1993; 78: 288–294.

108. Weinstabl C, Mayer N, Richling B et al. Effect of sufentanil on intracranial pressure in neurosurgical patients. Anaesthesia 1991; 46: 837–840.

109. Weinstabl C, Mayer N, Spiss CK. Sufentanil decreases cerebral blood flow velocity in patients with elevated intracranial pressure. Eur J Anaesthesiol 1992; 9: 481–484.

110. Fahy BG, Matjasko MJ. Disadvantages of prolonged neuromuscular blockade in patients with head injury. J Neurosurg Anesthesiol 1994; 6: 136–138.

111. Wilson JA, Branch CL Jr. Neuromuscular blockade in head injured patients with increased intracranial pressure: continuous versus intermittent use. J Neurosurg Anesthesiol 1994; 6: 139–141.

112. Prielipp RC, Coursin DB. Sedative and neuromuscular blocking drug use in critically ill patients with head injuries. New Horizons 1995; 3: 456–468.

113. Partridge BL, Abraams JH, Bazemore C et al. Prolonged neuromuscular blockade after long-term infusion of vecuronium bromide in the intensive care unit. Crit Care Med 1990; 18: 1177–1179.

114. Griffin D, Fairman N, Coursin D et al. Acute myopathy during treatment of status asthmaticus with corticosteroids and steroidal muscle relaxants. Chest 1992; 102: 510–514.

115. Bullock R, Povilshock JT. The role of anti-seizure prophylaxis following head injury. J Neurotrauma 1996; 13: 788–793.

116. Schierhout G, Roberts I. Prophylactic antiepileptic agents after head injury: a systematic review. J Neurol Neurosurg Psychiatry 1998; 64: 108–112.

117. Bullock R, Povilshock JT. The use of barbiturates in the control of intracranial hypertension. J Neurotrauma 1996; 13: 799–802.

118. Eisenberg HM, Frankowski RF, Contant CF et al. High dose barbiturate control of elevated intracranial

pressure in patients with severe head injury. J Neurosurg 1988; 69: 15–23.

119. Rea GL, Rockswold GL. Barbiturate therapy in uncontrolled intracranial hypertension. Neurosurgery 1983; 12: 401–405.

120. Bullock R. Strategies for neuroprotection with glutamate antagonists – extrapolating from evidence taken from the first stroke and head-injury studies. Ann NY Acad Sci 1995; 765: 272–278.

121. Di X, Harpold T, Watson JC, Bullock MR. Excitotoxic damage in neurotrauma: fact or fiction? Restor Neurol Neurosci 1996; 9: 231–241.

122. Harders A, Kakarieka A, Braakman R et al. Traumatic subarachnoid haemorrhage and its treatment with nimodipine. J Neurosurg 1996; 85: 82–85.

123. European Study Group on Nimodipine in Severe Head Injury. A multicenter trial of the efficacy of nimodipine on outcome after severe head injury. J Neurosurg 1994; 80: 797–804.

124. Murray GD, Teasdale GM, Schmitz H. Nimodipine in traumatic subarachnoid haemorrhage – a reanalysis of the HIT-I and HIT-II trials. Acta Neurochir 1996; 138: 1163–1167.

125. Muizelaar JP, Marmarou A, Young HF et al. Improving the outcome of severe head injury with the oxygen radical scavenger polyethylene glycol-conjugated superoxide dismutase – a phase II trial. J Neurosurg 1993; 78: 375–382.

126. Young B, Runge JW, Waxman KS et al. Effects of pegorgotein on neurologic outcome of patients with severe head injury. A multicenter randomized control trial. JAMA 1996; 276: 538–543.

127. Marshall LF, Marshall SB, Musch B et al. Outcome of moderate and severe head injury in patients treated with tirilazad mesylate. J Neurosurg 1996; 84: 731.

128. Bracken MB, Shepard MJ, Collins WFJ et al. Methylprednisolone or naloxone treatment after acute spinal cord injury: 1 year follow-up data. Results of the second National Spinal Cord Injury Study. J Neurosurg 1992; 76: 23–31.

129. Bullock R, Povilshock JT. The role of glucocorticoids in the treatment of severe head injury. J Neurotrauma 1996; 13: 804–810.

130. Alderson P, Roberts I. Corticosteroids in acute traumatic brain injury: systematic review of randomised clinical trials. BMJ 1997; 314: 1855–1859.

131. Newell DW, Temkin NR, Bullock R, Choi S. Corticosteroids in acute traumatic brain injury. BMJ 1998; 316: 396.

132. Clifton GL, Allen S, Barrodale P et al. A phase II study of moderate hypothermia in severe brain injury. J Neurotrauma 1993; 10: 263–271.

133. Marion DW, Obrist WD, Carlier PM et al. The use of moderate therapeutic hypothermia for patients with severe head injuries: a preliminary report. J Neurosurg 1993; 79: 354–362.

134. Shiozaki T, Sugimoto H, Taneda M et al. Effect of mild hypothermia on uncontrollable intracranial hypertension after severe head injury. J Neurosurg 1993; 70: 263–268.

135. Marion DW, Penrod LE, Kelsey SF et al. Treatment of traumatic brain injury with moderate hypothermia. N Engl J Med 1997; 336: 540–546.

136. Hartung J, Cottrell JE. Editorial: statistics and hypothermia. J Neurosurg Anesthesiol 1998; 10: 1–4.

137. Marion DW. Response to 'Statistics and hypothermia'. J Neurosurg Anesthesiol 1998; 10: 120–123.

138. Cruz J. Hypothermia and brain injury. J Neurosurg 1997; 86: 911–912.

139. Shapira Y, Artru AA. Hypothermia to improve neurologic outcome after head injury in patients. J Neurosurg Anesthesiol 1998; 10: 55.

140. Marion DW. Treatment of traumatic brain injury with moderate hypothermia. J Neurosurg Anesthesiol 1998; 10: 55–56.

141. Rumana CS, Gopinath SP, Uzura M et al. Brain temperature exceeds systemic temperature in head injured patients. Crit Care Med 1998; 26: 562–567.

142. Crowder CM, Templehoff R, Theard A et al. Jugular bulb temperature: comparison with brain surface and core temperature in neurosurgical patients during mild hypothermia. J Neurosurg 1996; 85: 98–103.

143. DeWitt DS, Prough DS. Accurate measurement of brain temperature. Crit Care Med 1998; 26: 431–432.

144. Ginsberg MD, Busto R. Combating hyperthermia in acute stroke. Stroke 1998; 29: 529–534.

22

ICU OF PAEDIATRIC HEAD INJURY

Robert L. Ross-Russell

EPIDEMIOLOGY

The epidemiology of trauma has been discussed in Chapter 00. Traumatic head injury in England continues to be a major cause of morbidity and mortality. The incidence of paediatric head injury has been estimated at 200–300/100,000 children per year and although a larger proportion of these injuries are mild (86% versus 79% in adults), traumatic brain injury remains an important cause of disability and death, especially in older children and adolescents.[77]

PATHOPHYSIOLOGY

THE NORMAL CHILD

The anatomy and physiology of the normal human brain in relation to traumatic injury has been described in Chapter 00. In this chapter we will consider particular constraints and differences relevant to the child.

The infant head is proportionally larger that that of the adult and consequently proportionally heavier. Head control in this age group is less developed and this can affect the degree of injury, particularly following injuries involving significant flexion and extension. Relatively minor acceleration/deceleration forces may produce disproportionate injury due to the increased inertia of the head and its limited stability. The skull is thinner but also more flexible and can deform substantially without fracturing. The sutures are not fused and the anterior fontanelle is open for the first year or so of life. Because of the skull deformity, significant intracranial injuries can occur in the absence of bony damage and substantial intracranial injuries may be found with little or no external sign of injury. However, the brain is also better protected against raised intracranial pressure due to the ability of the skull to expand and this acts to reduce the risk of secondary injury due to cerebral oedema.[1]

The child's head shows features of both adulthood and infancy. Compared to the infant, neck support is greater and the relative size of the head is smaller, reducing the inertia of major flexion extension injuries. The skull is more rigid, however, reducing the capacity for the skull to tolerate increases in intracranial volume without increasing pressure. Damage to the spinal cord can be difficult to assess in young children.[2] The spine is more flexible than in adulthood and spinal cord injury is well recognized in patients with normal radiology.[3] Cervical injury is more frequent in children, possibly due to the relative size of the head, and complete dislocation and relocation of the spinal column may occur, with transection of the underlying cord but no radiographic evidence of damage.[2,3] Conversely, cervical spine X-rays may show pseudosubluxation of upper vertebrae in the normal child.[4]

There are other important anatomical differences in children. The larynx is conical and lies anteriorly compared to adults. This means that its narrowest point is at the level of the cricoid cartilage. There is relatively more mucosa in the hypopharynx and the adenoids are larger. All these factors tend to complicate the maintenance of a clear airway in children, increasing the risk of hypoxia in an obtunded child. The optimal positioning of a child's airway is therefore the neutral position and not with neck overextension as this may also compress the soft trachea.[5] Fractures of the ribs are uncommon due to their increased plasticity and significant pulmonary contusions may occur without bony injury. A more mobile mediastinum can also affect airway patency if, for example, an acute pneumothorax develops.

Physiological differences in breathing need to be accounted for. Respiratory rate varies with age and the closing volume of the lung is close to functional residual capacity. In infants with a strong expiratory effort (such as crying) the lungs may reach closing volume, giving rise to a shunt across occluded alveoli and rapid cyanosis. Maintaining a high inspired oxygen concentration is therefore important.

HEAD TRAUMA IN CHILDREN

Impact injury

Impact injury for the brain can be widespread and not just confined to impact points on the skull. The external damage may include scalp/facial injuries or skull fractures. Simple lacerations often bleed profusely but, after careful examination for foreign material, can usually be directly closed.[6] 'Degloving' injuries with significant avulsion are more difficult to treat and often require grafting. Significant facial injuries require a multidisciplinary approach involving plastic surgeons and maxillofacial input.

Skull fractures

As discussed above, the relative plasticity of the paediatric (and especially infant) skull means that relatively greater force is needed to produce a fracture. If present, therefore, a fracture should raise concern about underlying cerebral injury.[7] Some authors do query the value of routine skull X-rays which have been shown to be of little predictive value for severe injury.[8,9] The majority (around 90%) of skull fractures are linear.[10,11] These can be dramatic on X-ray with significant widening of the suture line (diastasis) although this is rarely a problem. Very occasionally, a persistently increasing gap is seen ('growing fracture' or leptomeningeal cyst) which may require surgical repair. Comminuted or depressed skull fractures suggest a greater degree of trauma and should be an indication for CT scanning.[12] Associated dural damage or cortical lacerations may be found in 50% of such fractures[12] and require surgical repair. Other indications for further investigation or treatment of simple fractures include a fracture over a major vessel (e.g. middle meningeal) or an open fracture with an associated scalp laceration. The latter clearly runs significant risk of CSF infection, although prophylactic antibiotics are not needed if the wound is clean.

Basilar skull fractures

These are not uncommon although again signify substantial trauma.[13,14] Their prognosis is usually very good.[15] They have certain characteristic signs, such as Battle's sign (mastoid bruising without direct trauma), blood behind the tympanic membrane, CSF otorrhoea or rhinorrhoea (which will test positive to glucose but is rare under five years of age)[16] or racoon eyes (periorbital bruising). Basilar fractures often produce more symptoms than other fractures[15] and nasal intubation (including nasogastric tubes) should be avoided in case of cribriform damage.[6] Meningitis may occur in patients with CSF leak[17,18] but prophylactic antibiotics are not recommended.[19,20]

Brain injury

Because the brain is suspended in CSF and has its own inertia, sudden deceleration of the skull results in the brain continuing to move and striking the inside of the skull. It may then rebound, causing contusions on the opposite pole of the brain ('contrecoup' injury). The anatomy of the skull increases the likelihood of particular injuries, with contusion especially likely around bony promontories (e.g. the sphenoidal ridges) or dividing membranes (falx cerebri and tentorium).

Direct damage to the brain can be broadly divided into contusions, haemorrhages or diffuse axonal injury. Contusions are caused by direct impact of brain on bone. They classically appear at the site of impact or directly opposite that point. Extradural haemorrhage is reportedly rare in childhood due to the close adherence between the dura and skull[21] although it can be found. When it is, the classic history of acute deterioration following lucid interval is much rarer in children and infants than in adults.[22,23] Prompt investigation with CT scan and surgical drainage leads to a good outcome. Subdural haemorrhage has a worse prognosis,[24,25] arising from bleeding points on the surface of the brain, and may frequently be associated with significant cerebral injury, especially when acute.[24] Chronic subdural haemorrhage is usually seen in younger children and may follow trauma, although the suspicion of non-accidental injury (NAI) should be raised in such cases.[26,27] Such cases may present with irritability and seizures and often with rather non-specific symptoms. Subarachnoid haemorrhage is common following trauma. Headaches, fever and vomiting are quite frequent but unless there is significant mass effect, conservative management is usually adequate.

Diffuse axonal injury

This is caused as a result of shearing forces involved in trauma. Classically, it involves the basal ganglia and thalamus and the corpus callosum. Shearing of axonal tracts and damage to fine bridging vessels occurs but early scans may show no abnormality. Raised ICP develops over 24–48 h and the long-term outcome can be devastating.[28,29] Such injuries are particularly seen after repetitive rotational injury such as severe shaking.[29,30]

RESUSCITATION

Emergency treatment of the head-injured child should follow algorithms common to the management of any trauma victim (Box 22.1). Resuscitation should be directed towards the prevention of secondary brain insult, the majority of which is related to anoxia, ischaemia or brain haemorrhage. Simple resuscitative priorities therefore remain the best approach to the child with head injury.

---

1. Provide airway
2. Protect cervical spine
3. 100% oxygen
4. IV access
5. Control external bleeding and replace loss
6. Assess conscious level and pupillary reaction
7. Elevate head (30%) in midline position
8. Minimize noxious stimuli
9. Plan further investigations and management

Box 22.1   Early management of paediatric head injury

ABCS

Following trauma, care of the airway and the cervical spine merit equal priority and stabilization of the cervical spine with sandbags/tape or trauma board immobilization should be initiated immediately in any child arriving in hospital following head or neck trauma.[5] In children who are combative, however, such immobilization may be detrimental and such children are better off left with a hard collar only or, if absolutely necessary, with no collar at all. Important anatomical differences between adults and children have been identified above and are of great importance when resuscitating so experienced paediatricians or paediatric anaesthetists should be used wherever possible.

One major priority in resuscitating the head-injured patient is the avoidance of ischaemia due to hypovolaemia. Early intravenous (IV) access is therefore needed and intraosseous access should be used if IV lines cannot be sited rapidly.[5] This technique can be used in children up to the age of eight using the upper tibia but any bone marrow access is acceptable.

In children, signs of shock can be more difficult to assess, as peripheral vasoconstriction protects blood pressure until late in shock. The most sensitive markers of shock are therefore measures of peripheral perfusion such as capillary refill time (<2 s), toe/core temperature difference (<2°C) and colour.

Early assessment of neurological damage should be simple. A graded assessment of conscious level (alert, voice responsive, pain responsive or unresponsive) coupled with pupillary reaction and any localizing features is usually adequate in the first assessment. This will allow early planning of investigations and imaging (Box 22.2). Subsequently a more detailed review and full examination (front and back) are needed.

The resuscitation process is one of constant review and reaction to problems as they arise. In view of this,

patients may go to theatre and subsequently arrive in intensive care before all elements of the process have been completed. Coordination between emergency care and ITU staff is therefore essential to ensure that a full assessment is properly completed.

FURTHER EVALUATION

Following resuscitation, careful evaluation and planning are required.

MANAGEMENT

PRINCIPLES OF MANAGEMENT IN THE INJURED BRAIN

These principles have been discussed in detail in Chapter 00. Specific differences in children and the effect this has on their management are discussed below.

GENERAL ISSUES

Following resuscitation and early intervention, the management of the traumatic head injury follows a systematic approach common to many intensive care problems.

Ventilation

Neurogenic pulmonary oedema (NPE) is common in adults and is most frequently seen in severe or fatal injuries.[31] Its aetiology is unclear but may result from an endothelial insult caused by a massive sympathetic outflow from an ischaemic brainstem.[32,33] Ventilation should be directed to ensure adequate oxygenation and positive end-expiratory pressure (PEEP) may be essential to counteract NPE or avoid atelectasis.[32,34] Theoretical adverse effects of PEEP on cerebral venous drainage need to be considered but in children under eight years of age the benefits of PEEP (2–4 cmH$_2$O) will almost always outweigh the risks.

Indications for skull X-ray	Indications for CT scan
<1 year	Skull fracture <1 year
LOC	Depressed skull fracture
Obvious fracture	Fracture over major vessel
CSF, otorrhoea/rhinorrhoea	Reduced level of consciousness (GCS< 12)
Battle's sign/racoon eyes	
Focal signs	
Suspected child abuse	

Box 22.2   Imaging in head injury

Physiotherapy and endotracheal suction can be very harmful to maintenance of cerebral perfusion and their use should be limited, with appropriate sedation/paralysis.[35,36]

Fluids

Conventionally, fluids have been restricted in this group of patients. However, the major goal in head-injured patients is the maintenance of adequate cerebral perfusion. Maintenance fluids should therefore be restricted to 60–80% of requirements. This should include all nutrition (see below) and drug infusions wherever possible. In small children (<2 years) it is important to include dextrose-containing fluids to avoid hypoglycaemia, but in older children and adults glucose solutions may exacerbate intracranial insult. Further supportive fluids (saline or colloid) may be needed in addition to this. Blood pressure should be maintained to ensure that the cerebral perfusion pressure is adequate. If this falls, fluids should be given to maintain central venous pressure at 7–10 cmH$_2$O and inotropes may be needed if this fails to maintain an adequate pressure. If inotropes are required consideration of myocardial dysfunction should be undertaken. This may be as a result of contusion, pericardial effusion or sepsis. Massive vasodilatation secondary to spinal trauma may also be seen, warranting vasoconstrictor therapy. Arrhythmias including ventricular arrhythmias or reentry tachycardias can be seen, especially if myocardial trauma has occurred, and acute lung injury may occur in isolated head injury and is associated with a poor prognosis.[37]

SPECIFIC ISSUES

Raised intracranial pressure (ICP) and ICP monitoring

As discussed above, one of the mainstays of neuro-logical intensive care in these patients is to sustain adequate cerebral perfusion.

In simple terms this requires a reduction in intracranial volume. As discussed earlier, mass effects from extradural or acute subdural haemorrhages require surgical drainage. In the more diffusely swollen brain, other measures have to be used but aggressive treatment can influence outcome unlike the situation following global hypoxic ischaemic damage.[38,39] Patients should be optimally sedated and paralysed although this can hamper the ability to assess neurological function. Midline positioning (to avoid obstruction to cerebral venous return) and 30° head elevation may also be helpful. Monitoring ICP can influence management and has been shown to affect outcome.[40]

Hyperventilation has been historically used but may in fact do more harm than good.[78] Initial responses do include a reduction in cerebral blood volume if CO$_2$ is lowered but continued hyperventilation diminishes this response[41] and outcome may be worse.[42] The CO$_2$ levels should therefore be maintained around 4–4.5 kPa although acute rises in ICP may be treated by brief reduction of CO$_2$ levels, using hand bagging.

Seizures

These occur in 5–10% of head-injured children, a higher incidence than reported in adults.[43,44] In severe head injuries, early seizures may occur in a third of patients[45] and are more common following depressed skull fractures or cortical laceration.[46] Late-onset seizures are less common. Children with preexisting seizures or who fitted in the early stages of their injury, together with at-risk patients (see above), can be put on prophylactic anti-convulsants (phenytoin or phenobarbitone). These should be continued for a few weeks following the injury at which time they can often be stopped.

Drug therapy

Specific drug therapies have met with limited success in the treatment of paediatric head injury. Diuretics such as frusemide and mannitol have been tried but long-term benefits in reducing cerebral oedema or improving outcome remain uncertain. Steroids and barbiturates have not been shown to be of uniform benefit in improving intracranial hypertension[47–50] and the latter may be positively harmful if blood pressure is lowered. A number of novel drug treatments are under current investigation.[51] Antioxidants, such as super-oxide dismutase (SOD), 21-aminosteroids and lazaroids can theoretically scavenge damaging oxygen radicals. Some experimental global ischaemia models have shown improved outcomes following treatment with albumin-binding SOD[52] but clinical evidence in trauma is as yet unavailable and similar mixed results with synthetic 21-aminosteroids have been reported.[53,54] Intracellular calcium accumulation has been strongly implicated as a factor in neuronal damage and calcium antagonists such as nimodipine have been used to treat postischaemic brain injury, especially after subarachnoid haemorrhage. There is no good evidence of a benefit following trauma. Similar interest in glutamate antagonists, blocking NMDA and non-NMDA receptors has yet to show clinical benefit.[55,56]

Hypothermia

This has been brought back into favour recently. Initial use of profound hypothermia did not improve outcome but recent work using mild hypothermia (32–34°C) has shown both experimental[57,58] and clinical benefits[59–61] although it has to be instituted rapidly.[58,62] Studies looking at core temperature and whole-body energy expenditure failed to show an effect of hypothermia on cerebral blood flow[63] and the relationship between whole-body energy expenditure and cerebral requirements is complex.[64,65]

NON-ACCIDENTAL INJURY (BOX 22.3)

Some of the most serious injuries and those with the greatest morbidity in paediatric intensive care relate to non-accidental injury (NAI).[66] Head injury in NAI usually relates to a combination of shaking and direct trauma (the 'shaken-impact' syndrome) and is most commonly seen in small infants.[67] The presentation is often very non-specific (e.g. poor feedings, 'off his feeds') but may include comatose infants.[29,68] Clinical findings often show signs of cerebral irritation, with large heads (often above the 90th centile).[29,68] Convulsions are common[69,70] and CT imaging shows diffuse injury to grey and white matter, often with sparing of the brainstem and basal ganglia.[26] Subdural haemorrhage is common[26] (but not necessarily due to NAI[71]) and there may also be blood along the falx or in the subarachnoid space.[27]

All such children should be examined for external bruising (which may often not be present), retinal haemorrhages (which are extremely suggestive of NAI) or other bony injury.[72] The prognosis in this group is extremely poor[30] with a very high morbidity in surviving children.[29,30] The injuries are predominantly due to shearing damage caused by the rotational element of the shaking[73] but some authors argue[68] that impact remains a major feature of serious damage.

Small children and especially premobile infants presenting with injuries should be considered as potential victims of NAI unless the history is clearly inappropriate.[72] Bruising is unusual in an infant who is not walking or crawling and significant cerebral or bony injury is rare following normal household accidents.[74–76]

REFERENCES

1. Lang DA, Teasdale GM, Macpherson P, Lawrence A. Diffuse brain swelling after head injury: more often malignant in adults than children? J Neurosurg 1994; 80: 675–680.

2. Osenbach R, Menezes A. Pediatric spinal cord and vertebral coloum injury. Neurosurgery 1992; 30: 385–390.

3. Pang D, Wilberger JE. Spinal cord injury without radiographic abnormalities in children. J Neurosurg 1982; 52: 114–129.

4. Connolly JF. DePalma's the management of fractures and dislocations, an atlas, 3rd edn. 1981.

5. Advanced Life Support Group. Advanced paediatric life support. BMJ Publishing Group, London, 1997.

6. Allen EM, Boyer R, Cherny WB, Brockmeyer D, Fan Tait V. Head and spinal cord injury. In: Rogers MC (ed) Textbook of pediatric intensive care. Williams and Wilkins, Baltimore, 1996, pp 809–857.

7. Bonadio WA, Smith DS, Hillman S. Clinical indicators of intracranial lesion on computed tomographic scan in children with parietal skull fracture. Am J Dis Child 1989; 143: 194–196.

8. Lloyd DA, Carty H, Patterson M, Butcher CK, Roe D. Predictive value of skull radiography for intracranial injury in children with blunt head injury. Lancet 1997; 349: 821–824.

9. Ong L, Selladurai BM, Dhillon MK, Atan M, Lye MS. The prognostic value of the Glasgow Coma Scale, hypoxia and computerised tomography in outcome prediction of pediatric head injury. Pediatr Neurosurg 1996; 24: 285–291.

10. Levi L, Guilburd JN, Linn S, Feinsod M. The association between skull fracture, intracranial pathology and outcome in pediatric head injury. Br J Neurosurg 1997; 5: 617–625.

11. Rosenthal BW, Bergman I. Intracranial injury after moderate head trauma in children. J Pediatr 1989; 115: 346–350.

12. Jamieson KG, Yelland JD. Depressed skull fractures in Australia. J Neurosurg 1972; 37: 150–155.

13. Henrick EB, Harwood-Nash DC, Hudson AR. Head injuries in children: a survey of 4465 consecutive cases

---

Features that may suggest NAI   *Investigations in suspected NAI*

1. Inappropriate history for injuries
2. <1 year
3. Rib fractures
4. Subdural haemorrhages
5. Retinal haemorrhage
6. Suspicious bruising

1. Photography
2. Retinal examination
3. Full skeletal survey
4. Clotting screen
5. Early involvement of child protection team

Box 22.3   Clues that suggest NAI and investigations that need to be triggered

at the Hospital for Sick Children, Toronto, Canada. Clin Neurosurg 1964; 11: 46.

14. Mealey JJ. Pediatric head injuries. Charles C Thomas, Springfield, 1968.

15. Einhorn A, Mizrah EM. Basilar skull fractures in children. Am J Dis Child 1978; 11: 1121–1124.

16. Jefferson A, Reilly G. Fractures of the flood of the anterior cranial fossa: the selection of patients for dural repair. Br J Surg 1972; 59: 585–592.

17. Lewin W. Cerebrospinal fluid rhinorrhoea, meningitis and pneumocephalus due to non-missile injuries. Clin Neurosurg 1964; 12: 23–52.

18. MacGee EE, Cauthen JR, Brackett CE. Meningitis following acute traumatic cerebrospinal fluid fistula. J Neurosurg 1970; 33: 312–316.

19. Klastersky J, Sadeghi M, Brihaye J. Antimicrobial prophylaxis in patients with rhinorrhoea or otorrhoea: a double blind study. Surg Neurol 1976; 6: 111–114.

20. Shulman K. Late complications of head injuries in children. Clin Neurosurg 1972; 19: 371–380.

21. Singounas EG, Volikas ZG. Epidural haematoma in a pediatric population. Childs Brain 1984; 11: 250–254.

22. Galbraith S, Teasdale G. Predicting the need for operation in the patient with an occult traumatic intracranial hematoma. J Neurosurg 1981; 55: 75.

23. Ceviker N, Baykaner K, Keskil S, Cengel M, Kaymaz M. Moderate head injuries in children as compared to other age groups, including the cases who had talked and deteriorated. Acta Neurochir Wien 1995; 133: 116–121.

24. Shenkin HA. Acute subdural haematoma: review of 39 consecutive cases with high incidence of cortical artery rupture. J Neurosurg 1982; 57: 254–257.

25. Britt RH, Hamilton RD. Large decompressive craniotomy in the treatment of acute subdural hematoma. Neurosurgery 1978; 2: 195–200.

26. Sinal AH, Ball MR. Head trauma due to child abuse: serial computerized tomography in diagnosis and management. South Med J 1996; 80: 1505–1512.

27. Zimmerman J, Bilaniuk LT, Bruce D, Schut L, Uzzell B, Goldberg HI. Interhemispheric acute subdural hematoma: a computed tomographic manifestation of child abuse by shaking. Neuroradiology 1978; 16: 39–40.

28. Sarsfield JK. The neurological sequelae of non-accidental injury. Dev Med Child Neurol 1974; 16: 826–827.

29. Haviland J, Ross Russell RI. Outcome after severe non-accidental injury. Arch Dis Child 1997; 77: 504–507.

30. Duhaime AC, Christian C, Moss E, Seidl T. Long-term outcome in infants with the shaking-impact syndrome. Pediatr Neurosurg 1996; 24: 292–298.

31. Weisman S. Edema and congestion of the lungs resulting from intracranial hemorrhage. Surgery 1939; 6: 722–729.

32. Kaufman T, Timberlake G, Voelker J, Pait TG. Medical complications of head injury. Med Clin North Am 1993; 1: 43–60.

33. Demling R, Riessen R. Pulmonary dysfunction after cerebral injury. Crit Care Med 1990; 18: 768–774.

34. Beckman D, Bean J, Baslock P. Neurogenic influence on pulmonary compliance. J Trauma 1974; 14: 111–115.

35. Prasad A, Tasker RC. Guide lines for the physiotherapy management of critically ill children with acutely raised intracranial pressure. Physiotherapy 1990; 76: 248–250.

36. Hsiang J, Chestnut R, Crisp C, Klauber M, Blunt B, Marshall L. Early, routine paralysis for intracranial pressure control in severe head injury: is it necessary? Crit Care Med 1994; 22: 1471–1476.

37. Bratton SL, Davis RL. Acute lung injury in isolated traumatic brain injury. Neurosurgery 1997; 40: 707–712.

38. Marshall LW, Smith RW, Shapiro HM. The outcome with aggressive treatment in severe head injuries, 1: the significance of intracranial pressure monitoring. J Neurosurg 1979; 50: 20–25.

39. Saul T, Ducker T. Effect of intracranial pressure monitoring and aggressive treatment on mortality in severe head injury. J Neurosurg 1981; 56: 498–503.

40. Pople IK, Muhlbauer MS, Sanford RA, Kirk E. Results and complications of intracranial pressure monitoring in 303 children. Pediatr Neurosurg 1995; 23: 64–67.

41. Muizelaar JP, Van Der Poel H, Li Z, Kontos H, Levasseur J. Pial arteriolar vessel diameter and CO_2 reactivity during prolonged hyperventilation in the rabbit. J Neurosurg 1988; 29: 743–749.

42. Muizelaar JP, Marmarou A, Ward J et al. Adverse effects of prolonged hyperventilation induced cerebral hypoxia. Am Rev Respir Dis 1980; 122: 407–412.

43. Cruz J, Miner M, Allen S, Alves W, Gennarelli T. Continuous monitoring of cerebral oxygenation in acute brain injury: assessment of cerebral hemodynamic reserve. Neurosurgery 1991; 29: 743–749.

44. Beni L, Constantini S, Matoth I, Pomeranz S. Subclinical status epilepticus in a child after closed head injury. J Trauma 1996; 40: 449–451.

45. Humphreys R. Complications of pediatric head injury. Pediatr Neurosurg 1991; 17: 274–278.

46. Ong LC, Dhillon MK, Selladurai BM, Maimunah A, Lye MS. Early post-traumatic seizures in children: clinical and radiological aspects of injury. J Paediatr Child Health 1996; 32: 173–176.

47. Dearden NM, Gibson J, McDowall DG, Gibson RM, Cameron M. Effect of high dose dexamethasone on outcome from severe head injury. J Neurosurg 1986; 64: 81–88.

48. Cooper P, Moody S, Clark WK et al. Dexamethasone and severe head injury: a prospective double-blind study. J Neurosurg 1979; 51: 307–316.

49. Marshall L, Smith R, Shapiro H. The outcome with aggressive treatment in severe head injuries, II: acute and chronic barbiturate administration in the management of head injury. J Neurosurg 1979; 50: 26–30.

50. Pittman T, Bucholz R, Williams D. Efficacy of barbiturates in the treatment of resistent intracranial hypertension in severely head-injured children. Pediatric Neuroscience 1989; 15: 13–17.

51. McIntosh T. Novel pharmacologic therapies in the treatment of experimental traumatic brain injury: a review. J Neurotrauma 1993; 10: 215–261.

52. Takeda Y, Hashimoto H, Kosaka F, Hirakawa M, Inoue M. Albumin-binding superoxide dismutase with a prolonged half-life reduces reperfusion brain injury. Am J Physiol 1993; 264: H1708–H1715.

53. Hall ED, Yonkers PA. Attenuation of postischemic cerebral hypoperfusion by the 21-aminosteroid U7400F. Stroke 1988; 19: 340–344.

54. Sutherland G, Haas N, Peeling J. Ischemic neocortical protection with U74006F – a dose-response curve. Neurosci Lett 1993; 149: 123–125.

55. Lanier WL, Perkins WJ, Karlsson BR et al. The effects of dizocilpine maleate (MK-801), an antagonist of the N-methyl-D-aspartate receptor, on neurologic recovery and histopathology following complete cerebral ischaemia in primates. J Cereb Blood Flow Metab 1990; 10: 252–261.

56. Vornov JJ, Tasker RC, Coyle JT. Delayed protection by MK-801 and tetrodotoxin in a rat organotypic hippocampal culture model of ischaemia. Stroke 1994; 25: 457–465.

57. Busto R, Dietrich WD, Globus MY, Valdes I, Scheinberg P, Ginsberg MD. Small differences in intraischemic brain temperature critically determine the extent of ischemic neuronal injury. J Cereb Blood Flow Metab 1987; 7: 729–738.

58. Carroll M, Beek O. Protection against hippocampal CA1 cell loss by post-ischemic hypothermia is dependent on delay of initiation and duration. Metab Brain Dis 1992; 7: 45–50.

59. Marion D, Obrist W, Carlier P, Penrod L, Darby J. The use of moderate therapeutic hypothermia for patients with severe head injuries: a preliminary report. J Neurosurg 1993; 79: 354–362.

60. Shiozaki T, Sugimoto H, Taneda M et al. Effect of mild hypothermia on uncontrollable intracranial hypertension after severe head injury. J Neurosurg 1993; 79: 363–368.

61. Clifton G, Allen S, Barrodale P et al. A phase II study of moderate hypothermia in severe brain injury. J Neurotrauma 1993; 10: 263–271.

62. Busto R, Dietrich WD, Globus MY, Ginsberg MD. Postischemic moderate hypothermia inhibits CA1 hippocampal ischemic neuronal injury. Neurosci Lett 1989; 101: 299–304.

63. Matthews DS, Bullock RE, Matthews JN, Aynsley Green A, Eyre JA. Temperature response to severe head injury and the effect on body energy expenditure and cerebral oxygen consumption. Arch Dis Child 1995; 72: 507–515.

64. Matthews DS, Matthews JN, Aynsley Green A, Bullock RE, Eyre JA. Changes in cerebral oxygen consumption are independent of changes in body oxygen consumption after severe head injury in childhood. J Neurol Neurosurg Psychiatry 1995; 59: 359–367.

65. Sharples PM, Stuart AG, Matthews DS, Aynsley Green A, Eyre JA. Cerebral blood flow and metabolism in children with severe head injury. Part 1: Relation to age, Glasgow coma score, outcome, intracranial pressure, and time after injury. J Neurol Neurosurg Psychiatry 1995; 58: 145–152.

66. Bax M. Sombre reading. Dev Med Child Neurol 1993; 35: 847–848.

67. Duhaime AC, Gennarelli TA, Thibault LE, Bruce DA, Margulies SS, Wiser R. The shaken baby syndrome. J Neurosurg 1987; 66: 409–415.

68. Duhaime AC, Alario AJ, Lewander WJ, et al. Head injury in very young children: mechanisms, injury types, and ophthalmologic findings in 100 hospitalized patients younger than 2 years of age. Pediatrics 1992; 90: 179–185.

69. Bonnier C, Nassogne M, Evrard P. Outcome and prognosis of whiplash shaken infant syndrome; late consequences after a symptom-free interval. Dev Med Child Neurol 1995; 37: 943–956.

70. Frank Y, Zimmerman R, Leeds NMD. Neurological manifestations in abused children who have been shaken. Dev Med Child Neurol 1985; 27: 312–316.

71. Howard MA, Bell BA, Uttley D. The pathophysiology of infant subdural haematomas. Br J Neurosurg 1993; 7: 355–365.

72. Hobbs CJ, Hanks HGI, Wynne JM. Child abuse and neglect: a clinician's handbook. Churchill Livingstone, Edinburgh, 1993.

73. Gilliland MG, Folberg R. Shaken babies – some have no impact injuries. J Forensic Sci 1996; 41: 114–116.

74. Johnson DL, Braun D, Friendly D. Accidental head trauma and retinal hemorrhage. Neurosurgery 1993; 33: 231–234.

75. Reiber GD. Fatal falls in childhood. How far must children fall to sustain fatal head injury? Report of cases and review of the literature. Am J Forensic Med Pathol 1993; 14: 201–207.

76. Wilkins B. Head injury – abuse or accident? Arch Dis Child 1997; 76: 393–396.

77. Ward JD. Paediatric head injury. In: Narayan RK, Wilberger JE Jr, Povlishock JT (eds) Neurotrauma. McGraw Hill, New York, 1996, pp 859–868.

78. Skippen P, Seear M, Poskitt K et al. Effect of hyperventilation on regional cerebral blood flow in head-injured children. Crit Care Med 1997; 25: 1402–1409.

23

INTENSIVE CARE MANAGEMENT OF INTRA-CRANIAL HAEMORRHAGE

Leisha S. Godsiff & Basil F. Matta

INTRODUCTION

Whereas nothing can be done about the primary brain injury associated with intracranial haemorrhage, secondary damage can be anticipated and prevented with good management. Regardless of the cause of the intracranial haemorrhage, common pathophysiological mechanisms exist. These include alterations in cerebral blood flow (CBF), impaired autoregulation, intracranial hypertension, cerebral arterial vasospasm with delayed ischaemic deficit, hydrocephalus and seizures. Many of the adverse events are associated with the release of compounds such as excitory amino acids and superoxide radicals that can promote further damage.[1,2]

Neurointensive care of patients with intracerebral haemorrhage aims to recognize, treat and prevent secondary cerebral ischaemia. This chapter discusses the common complications and basic management of patients with intracranial haemorrhage (ICH). It is not meant as a comprehensive review of more general intensive care issues.

PATHOPHYSIOLOGY

Cerebral perfusion pressure (CPP) represents the pressure gradient acting across the cerebrovascular bed and may be estimated using the formula:

$$\text{Mean CPP} = \text{mean arterial blood pressure (MAP)} - \text{mean intracranial pressure (ICP).}$$

Based on data obtained from head-injured patients, CPP >70 mmHg is generally considered adequate for most neurologically injured patients.[3,4] In common with most brain injuries, the processes which modulate CBF, namely autoregulation, vasoreactivity to carbon dioxide ($PaCO_2$) and flow-metabolism coupling, may be impaired in patients with intracranial haemorrhages. Therefore, blood pressure instability, changes in $PaCO_2$ and increases in metabolism may result in cerebral ischaemia.

ACUTE CARE ON ADMISSION

Once the patient with ICH is admitted to the neurointensive care unit, a detailed history and clinical examination are obtained. The information available is influenced by the nature of the admission: elective postoperative care or emergency.

For elective postoperative patients, the preoperative medical history and neurological state, operation performed, intraoperative drugs and fluids, post-operative instructions and problems encountered are usually available. For patients with subarachnoid haemorrhage (SAH), immediate postoperative problems encountered include brain swelling, bleeding into the operative site, fluid and electrolyte disturbances, hydrocephalus and cerebral vasospasm.

For emergency admissions, the mechanism of injury (traumatic or non-traumatic) will guide continued resuscitation, further investigations and treatment. This is of particular importance in patients who have suffered multiple trauma where an unrecognized cervical spine injury, tension pneumothorax or intra-abdominal haemorrhage may adversely affect outcome.[5]

The admission CT scan must be studied carefully for any factors that may be responsible for late neurologic deterioration. For example, patients with small extracerebral haematomas require careful observation as these may enlarge to cause a mass effect.[6] If there is any doubt a repeat CT scan is performed. Urgent evacuation of an extracerebral haematoma is generally required if there is a large volume of blood and midline shift. If the history is unclear, a SAH may have been the initial insult leading to the head injury and, when suspected, angiography is required.

SEDATION AND MUSCLE RELAXATION

There is no excuse for having a brain-injured patient coughing or straining on the endotracheal tube. Inadequate sedation increases cerebral stimulation, with concomitant increase in cerebral metabolism, CBF and ICP. Thus, it is of paramount importance to ensure adequate levels of sedation. However, assessing the level of sedation is difficult in these patients, because the cardiovascular signs are at best unreliable and muscle movements are usually prevented with neuromuscular blockade.

Intravenous anaesthetic and sedative agents reduce the cerebral metabolic rate, leading to a reduction in ICP. However, this is dependent on tight cerebral blood flow-metabolism coupling which may not be the case after brain injury. The main sedative agents used in our neurointensive care are propofol and midazolam. Both drugs approximate the ideal sedative by having a rapid and smooth onset of action, decreasing cerebral metabolism and ICP, preserving cerebral autoregulation and vasoreactivity to CO_2, allowing easy control of depth of sedation and providing windows for neurologic assessment.[7–10] However, propofol is not without its side effects. At high doses, it can induce hypotension with a decrease in cerebral perfusion pressure. The lipid load imposed by a 20 ml/h continuous infusion of propofol is not insignificant and must be taken into account in the daily caloric intake. In our hands, the use of 200 μk/kg/min propofol to produce burst suppression for long periods has often resulted in unacceptable levels of plasma lipids. The availability of the 2% propofol solution may help reduce the lipid load associated with its use.

Barbiturates are less commonly used for sedation and for the induction of cortical suppression, once advocated as a method of cerebral protection.[11] The reduction in barbiturate use may be attributed to the conflicting evidence about their efficacy in improving outcome, the increased risk of nosocomial infection and pneumonia, the cost of extended intensive care from the prolonged sedative effect and the availability of other agents (mainly propofol) with similar cerebrovascular effects but better pharmacokinetic profile than thiopentone.[12] In a recent survey, less than 5% of the units caring for head-injured patients in the UK routinely used barbiturates for sedation.[13]

Opioids generally have negligible effects on cerebral metabolism and CBF. However, the newer synthetic opioids fentanyl, sufentanil and alfentanil can increase ICP in patients with head trauma.[14,15] This increase, originally assumed to be secondary to an increase in CBF, is more likely to be the result of changes in $PaCO_2$ and/or systemic hypotension.[16,17] When blood pressure is carefully supported, there are no clinically relevant increases in ICP with intravenous administration of alfentanil or sufentanil.[18] Irrespective of the actual mechanism causing the increase in ICP, these observations underscore the importance of avoiding systemic hypotension.

Although neuromuscular blockade in patients receiving intensive care is controversial,[19,20] 94% of units caring for head-injured patients in the UK use atracurium or vecuronium routinely.[13] Neuromuscular blockers are used in conjunction with additional sedation to allow physiotherapy and therapeutic interventions to occur without increasing ICP further. They are also used to prevent shivering when hypothermia is employed in patients with a raise ICP. Although the prolonged use of neuromuscular blockers in intensive care patients has been associated with continued paralysis after drug discontinuation and acute myopathy,[21,22] these effects are more commonly associated with the steroid-based medium to long-acting agents. The most commonly used agent is atracurium, a quinolinium ester, which has not been associated with myopathy and is non-cumulative. Fears about the accumulation of laudanosine, a cerebral excitatory metabolite of atracurium, in head-injured patients without significantly compromised renal function are unjustified.

Neuromuscular blockers play an important role in the care of the brain-injured patient with reduced intracranial compliance. Coughing and "bucking on the tube" can result in an increase in ICP even when the patient is adequately sedated and hence, the administration of non-depolarizing muscle relaxants prevents such rises in ICP.[23] Coughing and related phenomena produce increases in intrathoracic and central venous pressure, thus increasing cerebral blood volume as well as increases in CBF from cortical stimulation by the afferent muscle activity.[24,25] Pulmonary toilet, frequent repositioning and suctioning can reduce the incidence of pneumonia and sepsis associated with the use of neuromuscular blockers.

It is difficult to identify seizure activity without monitoring the electroencephalogram (EEG) in sedated and paralysed patients receiving neurointensive care. Seizures increase cerebral metabolism, CBF and ICP and are associated with the release of excitatory amino acids, all of which can cause further cerebral damage. Data from head-injured patients suggest that those with reduced GCS (<10), haematoma contusion and depressed skull fractures are at greater risk for seizures. Seizures can occur following a SAH and lead to acute increases in blood pressure and rebleeding. When present, seizures should be controlled with anticonvulsants but there is currently no evidence to support the prophylactic use of anticonvulsants in this patient population and hence, they are not routinely administered at our institution.

FLUIDS, ELECTROLYTES AND NUTRITION

Fluid management is aimed at preventing hypotension and cerebral oedema. Large volumes of crystalloid, colloid and blood may be required for trauma patients. For non-trauma patients intravenous isotonic crystalloid solutions are preferred to maintain normal intravascular volume and plasma osmolality except when hypervolaemic, haemodilutional and hypertensive therapy is used to treat vasospasm.

Fluid replacement should be guided by blood pressure, pulse rate, urine output and the central venous and/or pulmonary artery occlusion pressure. The choice of fluid (colloid vs crystalloid) remains controversial. Colloids can expand the intravascular volume more efficiently but should the blood–brain barrier become disrupted, more cerebral oedema can occur. However, there is some evidence indicating that certain colloids (pentastarch) may be effective in reducing the cerebral oedema associated with cerebral ischaemic and reperfusion injury.[26] Those agents able to "plug leaks" by acting as oxygen free radical scavengers and/or by inhibiting neutrophil adhesion may be the resuscitation fluids of the future.[27] Anaemia will reduce cerebral oxygen delivery and effort should be made to maintain the haemoglobin concentration above 10 g/dl for optimal cerebral oxygen delivery.

Glucose-containing solutions are avoided because of the poor outcome associated with hyperglycaemia after head injury.[28,29] Furthermore, 5% dextrose solutions become hypotonic once the glucose is metabolized. Hypotonic solutions may cause more cerebral oedema and should be avoided.[30] Elevated blood glucose should be treated with insulin infusion.

Brain-injured patients have high nutritional requirements and feeding should be instituted early. Enteral feeding is preferred because it is simpler, is protective against gastric ulceration, the incidence of which may be increased in these patients,[31] and because of its beneficial effects on the immune system.[32] A nasogastric tube is used except in those patients with basal skull fractures when the orogastric route is utilized. In those who cannot be fed enterally, parenteral nutrition should be considered together with some form of prophylaxis against gastric ulceration (H$_2$ antagonists or sucralfate). There is some concern that altering gastric acidity with H$_2$ blockers creates an increased risk of aspiration pneumonia. However, although sucralfate does not alter the gastric pH it may affect the absorption of some oral drugs such as anticonvulsants.

Patients admitted to neurointensive care following brain injury are predisposed to electrolyte abnormalities as a result of the primary injury or secondary to the administration of osmotic diuretic. Electrolyte abnormalities, which may result in neurologic deterioration, can be avoided or treated early by the regular analysis of serum electrolytes.

Hyponatreamia

Patients with Na <130 mmol/l may be confused and irritable. If the plasma sodium is allowed to fall below 120 mmol/l, seizures and coma can result. Hyponatraemia may be iatrogenic (administration of hypotonic solutions), the result of cerebral salt wasting syndrome or syndrome of inappropriate secretion of antidiuretic hormone (SIADH).[33,34] In the cerebral salt wasting syndrome, patients are hyponatraemic with a reduced extracellular volume and therefore require fluid loading with normal saline. Only occasionally is hypertonic saline required but it should be used cautiously because if the serum sodium is corrected

too rapidly, there is a risk of central pontine myelinosis, cerebral oedema and seizures.

In SIADH, the plasma osmolality is low in the presence of an inappropriately high urine osmolality. Fluid restriction is required but hypotension must be avoided. Regular serum and urine osmolalities should be performed. Demeclocycline, which inhibits the action of ADH, may be required.

Hypernatraemia

Iatrogenic causes include the excess administration of hypertonic sodium solutions including total parenteral nutrition, osmotic diuretics or from overaggressive fluid restriction. Diabetes insipidus, resulting from the inadequate secretion of ADH and the inability to concentrate urine, is also a likely cause in this patient population. It is characterized by high urine output (>200 ml/h), low urine specific gravity (<1.005), low urine osmolality (<300 mosm/l) and plasma osmolality >295 mosm/l. Desmopressin acetate (DDAVP) is used to inhibit free water clearance. In severe brain injuries the presence of raised intracranial pressure and diabetes insipidus is associated with poor prognosis.

GENERAL CARE

Pressure sores should be avoided by the use of general skin care measures including regular turning. Fear about increasing ICP should not prevent high-quality nursing and physiotherapy. Chest physiotherapy, frequent turning, eye care and full hygiene care must be given. Frequent dressings of lines and catheter sites will minimize infection risk. Lignocaine, thiopentone, fentanyl, midazolam or propofol boluses may be used to reduce the response to physiotherapy and endotracheal suction.

Heparin and aspirin are not routinely used in this neurosurgical population for prophylaxis against deep venous thrombosis. Prophylaxis is restricted to the use of graduated compression stockings and passive or active exercises depending on the conscious level of the patient.

MONITORING

As many intensive care patients are sedated and ventilated, neurologic deterioration is difficult to detect clinically. Therefore, monitoring CBF, CPP and cerebral oxygenation are now important components of neurointensive care.[35,36]

Pulse oximetry, electrocardiography, invasive arterial blood and central venous pressures, temperature and urine output are routinely monitored in all patients admitted to our neurointensive care with intracerebral bleeds. A pulmonary artery catheter is used in elderly patients, those with cardiac disease and in poor-grade subarachnoid haemorrhage patients, especially if hypertensive, hypervolaemic, haemodilution therapy is contemplated.

Intracranial pressure is monitored with an intraventricular catheter or a subarachnoid bolt. Patients with an intracerebral bleed are at risk of developing raised ICP and in those with a GCS <9, ICP should be monitored. However, ICP monitoring in patients is not without its risks which include infection, intracranial haemorrhage and epilepsy. In our centre, SAH patients who remain of poor grade after resuscitation and/or have evidence of raised ICP on CT scan will have an ICP bolt inserted. A jugular bulb catheter measures jugular venous oxygen saturation and lactate and is used to monitor alterations in ventilation and blood pressure.[57,58] A cerebral function analysing monitor is used when seizures are suspected.

Other methods currently undergoing evaluation include near infrared spectroscopy, laser Doppler flowmetry and cerebral microdialysis which measures extracellular glutamate, pyruvate and lactate levels. An intraparenchymal probe, often sited at operation, measures cerebral oxygenation, carbon dioxide, pH and temperature and can be used in the ICU to guide postoperative care.

Laboratory investigations include regular full blood counts, coagulation, electrolyte, glucose and arterial blood gases. Serum and urine osmolalities are obtained if mannitol or diuretics are used or if diabetes insipidus is suspected.

SPECIFIC CONSIDERATIONS

INTRACRANIAL HYPERTENSION

ICP becomes elevated when one of the intracranial components (blood, brain, CSF) increases beyond the compensatory mechanisms. The normal ICP is between 1 and 10 mm Hg and active treatment is instituted when the ICP exceeds 20 mmHg.[37,38] Treatment is aimed at reducing cerebral oedema, cerebral blood volume (CBV) and CSF to maintain a CPP >70 mmHg. A more detailed account of ICP management can be found in Ch. 21.

General considerations

In the event of a neurological deterioration, such as the development of focal neurological signs, reduced level

Respiratory:	Obstructed airway
	Hypoxia
	Hypercarbia
	Excessive PEEP
Cardiovascular:	Hypertension
	Hypotension
	Hypovolaemia
Neurological:	Expanding haematoma
	Aneurysmal rebleed
	Hydrocephalus
	Cerebral oedema
	Seizures
Others:	Inadequate sedation
	Inadequate neuromuscular blockade
	Obstructed neck veins
	Pain
	Pyrexia
	Hyponatraemia

Box 23.1   Factors contributing to raised ICP

of consciousness or raised ICP, contributing factors (as shown in Box 23.1) need to be rapidly excluded before a CT scan is performed to rule out rebleeding, hydrocephalus or cerebral oedema.

Systemic hypotension, hypoxaemia, hypercapnia, impaired cerebral venous drainage and high intrathoracic pressures will increase CBV as a result of cerebral vasodilatation. Patients are best nursed in a 15° head-up position with the neck in the neutral position, thus ensuring that cerebral venous drainage is not obstructed.[11] The level of sedation is adjusted to avoid excessive stimulation during line insertion, endotracheal suctioning and physiotherapy. Ventilation is adjusted so that normoxia and mild hypocania are maintained (PaO$_2$ >11 kPa and PaCO$_2$ ~ 4.5 kPa). The excessive use of PEEP is avoided whenever possible as it may hinder cerebral venous drainage.[39] Permissive hypercapnia, tolerated in general intensive care patients with ARDS, may result in intracranial hypertension.

Marked Hyperventilation

Market hyperventilation (PaCO$_2$ level of <4.0 kPa) can be used to acutely reduce elevated ICP.[40] Hypocarbia induces a CSF alkalosis and cerebral vasoconstriction with a concomitant reduction in CBV, brain bulk and ICP. However, this effect is short-lived as compensatory mechanisms restore the CSF pH to normal within 24 h. The long-term use of marked hyperventilation is controversial as rebound increase in ICP can occur when normocarbia is restored and it is associated with poorer outcome.[42] Other organs are also affected by the resulting alkalaemia. Myocardial contractility may be reduced, coronary vasospasm can be precipitated and the oxygen dissociation curve is shifted to the left, impairing the release of oxygen to tissues. Hypocalcaemia and hypokalaemia may also be precipitated.

Hyperventilation is only effective in reducing ICP when the cerebral vasculature is responsive to changes in carbon dioxide tension. Cerebral vasoreactivity to CO_2 is often impaired in patients with brain injury and therefore, hyperventilation may be ineffective in reducing CBV and ICP.

Marked hyperventilation should not be used without monitoring cerebral oxygenation or CBF. We routinely use jugular venous oximetry (SJO_2) to guide hyperventilation in all neurologically injured patients admitted to our intensive care unit. The normal SJO_2 value is between 55% and 75%. An SJO_2 <55% implies increased cerebral oxygen utilization which can lead to cerebral ischaemia. Increasing the inspired concentration of oxygen can be a useful temporary measure to increase cerebral oxygen delivery during short periods of marked hyperventilation; however, it is preferable to increase $PaCO_2$ provided CPP is not compromised.[41]

Diuretics

Mannitol is used in doses of 0.25–1 g/kg to control ICP. It is an osmotic diuretic which reduces ICP by drawing fluid from the brain tissue into the vascular compartment. However, its initial action is thought to be independent of its diuretic effect. It may act by reducing blood viscosity which improves cerebral blood flow leading to cerebral vasoconstriction and a reduction in ICP.[42] Mannitol must be given carefully as rapid infusions have been shown to transiently increase cerebral blood flow and cerebral blood volume causes rises in ICP.[43] It can also precipitate pulmonary oedema in patients with poor myocardial function. Repeat doses of mannitol can be given until the serum osmolality reaches 315–320 mosm/l. Above this level there is a risk of systemic acidosis, renal failure and neurological deterioration. Mannitol is also thought to act as a free radical scavenger and inhibit CSF production.[44]

Frusemide, a loop diuretic, reduces ICP and although its mechanism of action is unclear, it might act via its ability to block chloride ion transport. It potentiates the effect of mannitol and also reduces the production of CSF. Diuretics can precipitate hypotension by depleting the intravascular volume and fluid balance must be carefully monitored to prevent this.

Temperature Control

Hyperthermia is avoided in patients with brain injury as the cerebral metabolic rate changes in proportion to body temperature. There is approximately a 5% increase in cerebral metabolism for each °C temperature rise. This increases CBF, CBV and ICP. Antipyretics and cooling blankets are used to treat the pyrexia and although blood in the subarachnoid space may be responsible, a source of infection must be excluded.

Conversely, hypothermia reduces cerebral metabolism, CBV and ICP. Patients with uncontrolled ICP may be cooled to 33°C.[45] Whenever hypothermia is used, muscle relaxants are required to prevent shivering.

Drainage of CSF

The removal of CSF via a ventricular drain reduces ICP, especially when hydrocephalus is present. When intracranial hypertension is mainly due to cerebral oedema, CSF drainage may only produce a temporary decrease in ICP as ventricular collapse prevents further CSF drainage.

Barbiturate Coma

In cases with intractable intracranial hypertension, an infusion of thiopentone can be used to achieve and maintain burst suppression of the EEG.[46,47] A loading dose of 3–5 g is given in incremental doses before an infusion is started at 4–8 mg/kg/h. Inotropes are likely to be needed to prevent hypotension. Patients whose ICP remains elevated have a poorer outcome than those who respond.[47]

Surgical decompression

Surgical decompression is required if there is uncontrolled cerebral oedema and the ICP remains persistently elevated despite aggressive medical therapy. Intracranial tissues or masses (haemorrhagic frontal or temporal lobes) may be resected and large bone flaps removed. This may cause further neurological damage and is normally only performed once other treatments to control ICP have failed.

CEREBRAL ARTERIAL VASOSPASM (DELAYED CEREBRAL ISCHAEMIA)

Delayed cerebral ischaemia secondary to cerebral arterial vasospasm is a leading cause of morbidity and mortality in patients who survive a subarachnoid haemorrhage (SAH)[48,49] and has also been described after severe head injuries.[50] Vasospasm is the result of the focal or diffuse narrowing of intracranial arteries confirmed by angiography. Although radiological evidence of vasospasm has been reported in up to 70% of angiograms performed within the first week of aneurysmal rupture, the incidence of clinically significant vasospasm approximates 20%.[48,51,52] The aetiology remains uncertain but appears to be related to the amount and distribution of blood in the subarachnoid space.[52,53] Several mediators have been postulated including oxyhaemoglobin, serotonin, histamine, catecholamines, prostaglandins, endothelin, angiotensin and lipid peroxidase.[53–55]

In the patient with SAH, the appearance of new focal neurological signs or a decrease in the level of consciousness may be an early sign of vasospasm. This is normally confirmed by CT scan and angiography. The onset of vasospasm is generally 3–5 days after the initial bleed, with a peak incidence at 6–8 days and duration of 2–4 weeks.[51] Patients present with focal or global neurological deficits, such as drowsiness, confusion and headache. A pyrexia and leucocytosis may also be present. Up to 14% patients with clinically significant vasospasm will die or have severe neurological deficits.[56]

Management of Cerebral Vasospasm

Diagnosis and monitoring

Cerebral angiography remains the gold standard for diagnosing vasospasm, which is seen as smooth constrictions in the cerebral vessels (Fig. 23.1). Vasospasm may be limited to the area surrounding the ruptured aneurysm or it may be widespread, when it is associated with poorer prognosis.[57] Although transcranial Doppler ultrasonography (TCD) is unreliable as a measure of CBF in patients with SAH because of vasospasm-associated changes in vessel diameter, it has become valuable for diagnosing vasospasm non-invasively prior to the onset of clinical symptoms. As the vessel diameter is reduced, for a given blood flow, red blood cell velocity (FV) increases. Hence, cerebral vasospasm is considered present when FV > 120 cm/s or the ratio between the FV in the middle cerebral artery (MCA) and the FV in the internal carotid artery (ICA) exceeds 3.[58,59] TCD is increasingly being used to diagnose vasospasm,[48] especially in sedated and ventilated patients, as it has the advantage of being a non-invasive bedside test. Wardlaw et al showed, in a prospective observational study, that routine TCD examinations made a positive contribution to the diagnosis of ischaemic neurological deficits in 72% of patients with this complication and led to altered management for the benefit of the patient in 43%.[60] More importantly, TCD results did not have any adverse influence on management or outcome.

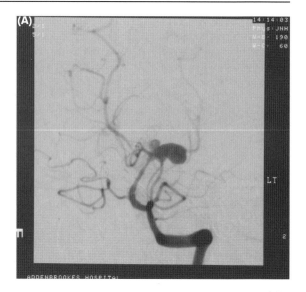

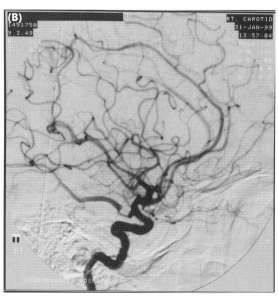

Figure 23.1   (A) The arrow points to a vasospastic segment of the basilar artery in a patient with a large basilar tip aneurysm. (B) The arrow indicates spasm in the posterior cerebral artery in a patient with basilar tip aneurysm.

In the sedated patient, the diagnosis of cerebral vasospasm relies on gross neurological signs, CT scan, cerebral angiography and TCD. Cerebral angiography and CT scan can only be performed intermittently, leaving TCD as the only way of diagnosing, judging the severity and the efficacy of treatment. The ratio of FV in the MCA to ICA should decrease with effective treatment. Needless to say, in order to rule out cerebral vasospasm by TCD, a thorough examination of the basal arteries is mandatory. Unfortunately, it is not possible to detect "small" vessel spasm. Our policy is to perform daily TCD examination in all patients with SAH. Initial impressions suggest that the incidence of TCD-diagnosed vasospasm is much higher than clinically significant vasospasm and therefore, we rarely escalate therapy purely on TCD findings alone. Cerebral angiography should be performed in any patient with clinically suspected vasospasm despite negative TCD findings. Other methods which can be used to diagnose vasospasm include single-photon emission tomography and positron emission tomography (PET).

Treatment

Early Surgery

There is a general belief that early surgery and the removal of blood reduce the risk of developing cerebral vasospasm.[61] The benefits of early surgery for SAH patients have been discussed in Chapter 14.

Hypertension, Hypervolaemia, Haemodilution Therapy (Triple H)

The aim is to optimize cerebral perfusion so that cerebral ischaemia progressing to infarction can be prevented. As autoregulation is often impaired, factors that increase the CPP are likely to increase blood flow to the ischaemic areas.[62,63] The use of triple H therapy has not been subjected to a prospective randomized controlled clinical trial but there is strong evidence to support its efficacy.[64] However, this treatment is not without complications which include pulmonary oedema, congestive cardiac failure, cerebral oedema, hypertensive cerebral bleeding and myocardial infarction as well as the risks associated with invasive monitoring.[65,66] It is performed only in the neuro-critical care setting and is continued until the neurological deficits resolve or complications from this treatment develop.

Triple H therapy aims to increase cerebral perfusion by increasing CBF and improving flow characteristics by haemodilution. The initial step is to increase cardiac output and blood pressure with aggressive volume expansion. In addition to maintenance fluids of 2–3 litres per day, colloids or packed red cells are used to obtain the following:

- haematocrit of 30–35%;
- pulmonary artery occlusion pressure of 14–18 mmHg;
- cardiac index of 4.5 l/m²/min;
- systemic vascular resistance index of 1400–2000 dyne/sec/cm⁻⁵;

- systolic blood pressure of 120–150 mmHg in unclipped and 160–200 mmHg in clipped aneurysms.

In younger patients it can be difficult to achieve these parameters as many develop a brisk diuresis in response to fluid loading. Parenteral desmopressin (1–4 μg) or fluorocortisone (0.1–0.2 mg/day) may be required.[67]

If after volume expansion the above parameters cannot be achieved or there is no improvement in neurologic status, inotropes (usually dopamine 2.5–15 μg/kg/min) are started. The use of appropriate ionotropes (dopamine, dobutamine and/or noradrenaline) is guided by a pulmonary artery catheter. In some cases, nimodipine may have to be withdrawn as it can interfere with attempts to induce hypertension.

PET has been performed in patients not responding to triple H therapy. The aim is to diagnose any hypoperfused areas which are not infarcted which will benefit from an improvement in blood flow. CBF values <20 ml/100 g/min have been found in the affected hemispheres of patients with symptomatic vasospasm and values <12 ml/100 g/min have been associated with irreversible changes.[68] The blood pressure is manipulated using ionotropes to see whether there is any increase in blood flow to these hypoperfused areas. This can be used to guide further blood pressure management on the intensive care unit.

Calcium Antagonists

Nimodipine, a dihydropyridine calcium antagonist, blocks the intracellular influx of extracellular calcium, preventing arterial smooth muscle contraction. It is more selective for cerebral than systemic vessels. In a number of prospective, randomized controlled trials, nimodipine was found to reduce morbidity and mortality from vasospasm in all patients with SAH irrespective of the grades.[69,70] Nimodipine's mechanisms of action are not fully understood as it does not appear to reduce the incidence of angiographic arterial narrowing. Postulated mechanisms of action include the dilatation of arteries at a microvascular level, neuronal protection at the membrane level and altering blood rheology to improve microcirculatory blood flow.

In our unit, nimodipine is routinely used in patients with SAH (60 mg 4-hourly PO). It can be given intravenously (1–2 mg/h) if the enteral route is not available but the dose may need to be reduced to prevent hypotension. Treatment is generally continued for three weeks.

Interventional Neuroradiology

Endovascular methods are considered if the CBF and clinical picture remain poor despite aggressive medical treatment. Low-pressure balloon angioplasty may be effective in reducing the severity of the vasospasm but there is a risk that the vessel may rupture and dissect with this technique.[72] When vasospasm is confined to small vessels or angioplasty is inappropriate, papaverine can be infused. Papaverine, a phosphodiesterase inhibitor, causes the accumulation of cyclic adenyl monophosphate within smooth muscle, leading to vasodilatation. The effects of papaverine may only last 12–24 h and repeat infusions may be necessary. However papaverine can precipitate systemic hypotension and intracranial hypertension so measures to support blood pressure and control ICP must be immediately available.[73]

Drugs under evaluation

As blood in the subarachnoid space precipitates cerebral vasospasm, it has been postulated that drugs which dissolve this blood clot may reduce the incidence of cerebral vasospasm and improve outcome. However, a recent trial using tissue plasminogen activator showed a reduction in angiographic vasospasm but no improvement in symptomatic cerebral vasospasm or neurological deterioration.[74] Other treatments that have been tried to prevent or treat vasospasm include tirilizad, a non-glucocorticoid 21-aminosteroid and potent free radical scavenger.[75] None has demonstrated significant efficacy in reducing vasospasm and improving outcome in SAH. In a retrospective study, patients taking aspirin[76] before their SAH had a reduced risk of delayed ischaemic deficit and therefore the use of aspirin postaneurysm clipping requires further study.

OUTCOME

The Glasgow Outcome Scale as shown in Table 23.1 can be used to assess the outcome for any brain disease.

Factors relating to outcome after SAH include the level of consciousness on admission, the amount of subarachnoid blood on CT scan, age and aneurysms of the posterior circulation. In the five-year period 1993–1998, patients admitted to our centre with an anterior circulation aneurysm who received a non-urgent operation (within 21 days of the initial event) were prospectively studied. The GOS was used to assess outcome at six months. Of the 391 patients studied, 44.7% had "early" surgery (day 1–3 postevent), 46.5% had "intermediate" surgery (day 4–10) and 8.8% "late" surgery (11–21). There were no significant differences between the groups in the demographics, site of the aneurysm and clinical condition of the patient. Early surgery did not adversely affect outcome, with a GOS at six months of 1–2 in 82.9%, 79.7% and 85.3% in the early, intermediate and late groups respectively. A favourable outcome (GOS 1–2) was achieved in 83.5% of patients less than 65 years and 73.3% in those over 65 years. There was a 6.5% rebleeding rate with a mortality of 63%. Only 0.5% occurred within three days of the initial event. Early surgery also reduced the total inpatient stay, with a mean time of 18.3, 20.4 and 31.7 days in the three groups respectively. These data have endorsed our view that, with appropriate preparation and support of the SAH patient, the timing of surgery

Table 23.1	Glasgow Outcome Score	
Grade	Description	Definition
1	Good recovery	Independent life with or without minimal neurological deficit
2	Moderately disabled	Neurological or intellectual impairment but is independent
3	Severely disabled	Conscious but totally dependent on others for daily activities
4	Vegetative survival	
5	Dead	

no longer influences surgical outcome. We therefore adopt an early surgery protocol to avoid the known effects of a rebleed.

REHABILITATION

The aim of rehabilitation is to return the patient to the maximum level of independence possible by reducing the effects of disease or injury on daily life. Rehabilitation is tailored to the individual patient's needs and should be assessed early on in the patient's admission. Indeed, some believe the prevention of secondary neuronal injury is part of the rehabilitation process. Those patients with minimal deficits require little rehabilitation. However, in patients with major deficits, initial efforts are focused on preventing the development of medical, musculoskeletal, bowel and bladder problems. After this, rehabilitation tries to provide the optimum medical, social and environmental conditions that will maximize the recovery process. Coping techniques and compensatory strategies will be taught to allow the patient to become as independent as possible.

Patients who survive a SAH will have a wide spectrum of cognitive and neurological deficits. Whilst many survivors function independently with few or no significant motor or sensory deficits one year after the event, many suffer from unrecognized subtle cognitive and emotional effects. These include confusion, amnesia, impaired judgement and emotional liability. Medical and nursing staff, family members, physiotherapists, occupational and speech therapists, psychologists and social services are all involved in the rehabilitation process. Some patients who have significant deficits but are well motivated with good social circumstances may benefit from transfer to a rehabilitation unit where they can continue to improve.

FUTURE DEVELOPMENTS

Whilst there has been an improvement in mortality rates for patients with an intracerebral haemorrhage, little has been effective in altering the high initial mortality in SAH patients. In those patients who survive the initial insult, early surgery has improved outcome by preventing rebleeding. However, future developments are focused on improving our understanding of the pathophysiological mechanisms behind secondary neuronal injury. Once these are better understood, a specific mechanism-targeted approach may improve outcome.

REFERENCES

1. Kajita Y, Suzuki Y, Oyama H et al. Combined effect of L-arginine and superoxide dismutase on the spastic basilar artery after subarachnoid hemorrhage in dogs. J Neurosurg 1994; 80: 261–268.

2. McCord JM. Oxygen derived free radicals in postischemic tissue injury. N Engl J Med 1985; 312: 159–163.

3. Chan KH, Miller JD, Dearden NM et al. The effect of changes in cerebral perfusion pressure upon middle cerebral artery blood flow velocity and jugular bulb venous oxygen saturation after severe brain injury. J Neurosurg 1992; 77: 55–56.

4. Rosner MJ, Rosner SD, Johnson AH. Cerebral perfusion pressure: management protocol and clinical results. J Neurosurg 1995; 83: 949–962.

5. Crosby ET, Lui A. The adult cervical spine: implications for airway management. Can J Anaesth 1990; 7: 77–93.

6. Knuckey NW, Gelbard S, Epstein MH. The management of "asymptomatic" epidural haematomas. A prospective study. J Neurosurg 1989; 70: 392–396.

7. Pinaud M, Lelausque J-N, Chetanneau A et al. Effects of propofol on cerebral hemodynamics and metabolism in patients with brain trauma. Anaesthesiology 1990; 73: 404–409.

8. Forster A, Juge O, Morel D. Effect of midazolam on cerebral hemodynamics and cerebral vasomotor responsiveness to carbon dioxide. J Cereb Blood Flow Metab 1990; 73: 404–409.

9. Matta BF, Lam AM, Strebel S, Mayberg TS. Cerebral pressure autoregulation and CO_2-reactivity during propofol-induced EEG suppression. Br J Anaesth 1995; 4: 159–163.

10. Strebel S, Kaufmann M, Guardiola PM et al. Cerebral vasomotor responsiveness to carbon dioxide is preserved during propofol and midazolam anesthesia in humans. Anesth Analg 1994; 78: 884–888.

11. Spetzler RF, Hadley MN. Protection against cerebral ischemia: the role of barbiturates. Cerebrovasc Brain Metab Rev 1989; 1: 212–219.

12. Artru AA, Shapira Y, Bowdle TA. Electroencephalogram, cerebral metabolic, and vascular responses to propofol anesthesia in dogs. J Clin Anesthesiol 1992; 4: 9–109.

13. Matta BF, Menon DK. Severe head injury in the United Kingdom and Ireland: a survey of practice and implications for management. Crit Care Med 1996; 24: 1743–1748.

14. Marx W, Shah N, Long C et al. Sufentanil, alfentanil and fentanyl: impact on cerebrospinal fluid pressure in patients with brain tumors. J Neurosurg Anesthesiol 1989; 1: 3–7.

15. Sperry RJ, Bailey PL, Reichman MV et al. Fentanyl and sufentanil increase intracranial pressure in head trauma patients. Anesthesiology 1992; 7: 416–420.

16. Albanese J, Durbec O, Viviand X et al. Sufentanil increases intracranial pressure in patients with head trauma. Anesthesiology 1993; 79: 493–497.

17. Trindle MR, Dodson BA, Rampil IJ. Effects of fentanyl versus sufentanil in equianesthetic doses on middle cerebral artery blood flow velocity. Anesthesiology 1993; 78: 454–460.

18. Mayberg TS, Lam AM, Eng CC et al. The effect of alfentanil on cerebral blood flow velocity and intracranial pressure during isoflurane-nitrous oxide anesthesia in humans. Anesthesiology 1993; 78: 288–294.

19. Fahy BG, Matjasko MJ. Disadvantages of prolonged neuromuscular blockade in patients with head injury. J Neurosurg Anesthesiol 1994; 6: 136–138.

20. Wilson JA, Branch CL Jr. Neuromuscular blockade in head injured patients with increased intracranial pressure: continuous versus intermittent use. J Neurosurg Anesthesiol 1994; 6: 139–141.

21. Partridge BL, Abraams JH, Bazemore C et al. Prolonged neuromuscular blockade after long-term infusion of vecuronium bromide in the intensive care unit. Crit Care Med 1990; 18: 1177–1179.

22. Griffin D, Fairman N, Coursin D et al. Acute myopathy during treatment of status asthmaticus with corticosteroids and steroidal muscle relaxants. Chest 1992; 102: 510–514.

23. Bedford RF, Durbin CG. Neurosurgical intensive care. In: Miller RD (ed) Anesthesia, 2nd edn. Churchill Livingstone, Edinburgh, pp 2253–2292.

24. Lanier WL, Milde JH, Michenfelder JD. Cerebral stimulation following succinylcholine in dogs. Anesthesiology 1986; 64: 551–559.

25. Minton MD, Grosslight K, Stirt JA et al. Increases in intracranial pressure from succinylcholine: prevention by prior non-depolarizing blockade. Anesthesiology 1986; 65: 165–169.

26. Schell RM, Cole DJ, Schultz RL et al. Temporary cerebral ischemia. Effects of pentastarch or albumin on reperfusion injury. Anesthesiology 1992; 77: 86–92.

27. Prough DS, Kramer G. Medium starch please. Anesth Analg 1994; 79: 1034–1035.

28. Young B, Ott L, Dempsey R et al. Relationship between admission hyperglycemia and neurologic outcome of severely brain-injured patients. Ann Surg 1989; 210: 466–473.

29. Lam AM, Winn HR, Cullen BF et al. Hyperglycemia and neurological outcome in patients with head injury. J Neurosurg 1991; 75: 545–551.

30. Kaieda R, Todd MM, Cook LN et al. Acute effects of changing plasma osmolality and colloid osmotic pressure on brain edema formation after cryogenic injury in the rabbit. Neurosurgery 1988; 24: 671–678.

31. Fabian TC, Boucher BA, Croce MA et al. Pneumonia and stress ulceration in severely head injured patients – a prospective evaluation of the effect of stress-ulceration prophylaxis. Arch Surg 1993; 128: 185–192.

32. Marshall WJ. Perioperative nutritional support. Care Critically Ill 1994; 10: 163–167.

33. Nelson PB, Sief SM, Maroon JC, Robinson AE. Hyponatremia in intracranial disease: perhaps not just the syndrome of inappropriate secretion of antidiuretic hormone (SIADH). J Neurosurg 1981; 55: 938–941.

34. Harrigan MR. Cerebral salt wasting syndrome: a review. Neurosurgery 1996; 38: 152–160.

35. Sloan TB. Does central nervous system monitoring improve outcome? Curr Opin Anaesth 1997; 10: 333–337.

36. Kirkpatrick PJ, Czosnyka M, Pickard JD. Multimodality monitoring in neurointensive care. J Neurol Neurosurg Psychiatry 1996; 60: 131–139.

37. Saul TG, Ducker TB. Effect of intracranial pressure monitoring and aggressive treatment on mortality in severe head injury. J Neurosurg 1982; 56: 498–503.

38. Marmarai A, Anderson RL, Ward JD et al. Impact of ICP instability and hypotension on outcome in patients with severe head trauma. J Neurosurg 1991; 75: 559.

39. McGuire G, Crossley D, Richards J, Wong D. Effects of varying levels of positive end-expiratory pressure on intracranial pressure and cerebral perfusion pressure. Crit Care Med 1997; 25: 1059–1062.

40. Warters RD, Allen SJ. Hyperventilation: new concepts for an old tool. Curr Opin Anaesth 1994; 7: 391–393.

41. Matta BF, Lam AM, Mayberg TS. The influence of arterial hyperoxygenation on cerebral venous oxygen content during hyperventilation. Can J Anaesth 1994; 41: 1041–1046.

42. Muizelaar JP, Wei EB, Kontos H et al. Mannitol causes compensatory cerebral vasoconstriction and vasodilatation in response to blood viscosity changes. J Neurosurg 1983; 59: 822.

43. Ravussin P, Archer DP, Tyler JL et al. Effects of rapid mannitol infusion on cerebral blood volume. A positron emission study in dogs and man. J Neurosurg 1986; 64(1): 104–113.

44. Schar A, Tsipstein E. Effect of mannitol and furosemide on the rate of formation of cerebrospinal fluid. Exp Neurol 1978; 69: 584.

45. Illievich UM, Spiss CK. Hypothermic therapy for the injured brain. Curr Opin Anaesth 1994; 7: 394–400.

46. Lee MW, Deppe SA, Sipperly ME et al. The efficacy of barbiturate coma in the management of uncontrolled intracranial hypertension following neurosurgical trauma. J Neurotrauma 1994; 11: 325–331.

47. Schalen W, Masseter K, Nordstrom CH. Cerebrovascular reactivity and the prediction of outcome in severe traumatic brain lesions. Acta Anaesthesiol Scand 1991; 35: 113.

48. McGrath BJ, Guy J, Borel CO et al. Perioperative management of aneurysmal subarachnoid hemorrhage: Part 2. Postoperative management. Anesth Analg 1995; 81: 1295–1302.

49. Kassell NF, Torner JC, Jane JA et al. The international co-operative study on the timing of aneurysm surgery. Part 1: overall management results: J Neurosurg 1990; 73: 18.

50. Weber M, Grolimund P, Seiler RW. Evaluation of post-traumatic cerebral blood flow velocities by transcranial Doppler ultrasonography. Neurosurgery 1990; 27: 106–112.

51. Weir B, Grace M, Hansen J et al. Time course of vasospasm in man. J Neurosurg 1978; 48: 173.

52. Mayberg M. Pathophysiology, monitoring and treatment of cerebral vasospasm after subarachnoid hemorrhage. J Stroke Cerebrovasc Dis 1997; 6(4): 258–260.

53. Fischer CM, Kistler JP, Davis JM. Relationship of cerebral vasospasm to subarachnoid hemorrhage visualized by computed tomography screening. Neurosurgery 1988; 19: 268–270.

54. Mayberg MR, Okada T, Bark TH. The role of hemoglobin in arterial narrowing after subarachnoid hemorrhage. J Neurosurg 1990; 72: 634–640.

55. Macdonald RL, Weir BKA. A review of hemoglobin and the pathogenesis of cerebral vasospasm. Stroke 1991; 22: 971.

56. Kassell NF, Sasaki T, Colohan A. Cerebral vasospasm following aneurysmal subarachnoid hemorrhage. Stroke 1985; 16: 562–572.

57. Saito I, Ueda Y, Sano K. Significance of vasospasm in the treatment of ruptured intracranial aneurysms. J Neurosurg 1977; 47: 412–429.

58. Aaslid R, Hubert P, Nornes H. Evaluation of cerebrovascular spasm with transcranial Doppler ultrasound. J Neurosurg 1984; 60: 37.

59. Lindegaard KF, Nornes H, Bakke SJ et al. Cerebral vasospasm after subarachnoid hemorrhage investigated by means of transcranial Doppler ultrasound. Acta Neurochirur 1988; 24: 81.

60. Wardlaw JM, Offin R, Teasdale GM et al. Is routine transcranial Doppler ultrasound monitoring useful in the management of subarachnoid hemorrhage? J Neurosurg 1998; 88(2): 272–276.

61. Hosoda K, Fujita S, Kawaguchi T, Shose Y, Hamano S, Iwakura M. Effect of clot removal and surgical manipulation on regional cerebral blood flow and delayed vasospasm in early aneurysm surgery for subarachnoid hemorrhage. Surg Neurol 1999; 51(1): 81–88.

62. Pritz MB, Giannotta SI, Kindt GW et al. Treatment of patients with neurological deficits associated with cerebral vasospasm by intravascular volume expansion. Neurosurgery 1978; 3: 364–368.

63. Kassell NF, Peerless SJ, Durward QJ et al. Treatment of ischemic deficits from vasospasm with intravascular volume expansion and induced arterial hypertension. Neurosurgery 1982; 11: 337–343.

64. Awad IA, Carter LP, Spetzler RF et al. Clinical vasospasm after subarachnoid hemorrhage: response to hypervolaemic hemodilution and arterial hypertension. Stroke 1987; 18: 365–372.

65. Dorsch NWC. A review of cerebral vasospasm in aneurysmal subarachnoid haemorrhage. Part II: Management. J Clin Neurosci 1994; 1(2): 78–92.

66. Shimoda M, Oda S, Tsugane R, Sata O. Intracranial complications of hypervolaemic therapy in patients with delayed ischemic deficit attributed to vasospasm. J Neurosurg 1993; 78: 423–429.

67. Hasan D, Wijdicks EFM, Vermeulen BJ. Hyponatremia is associated with cerebral ischemia in patients with aneurysmal subarachnoid hemorrhage. Ann Neuro 1990; 27: 106–108.

68. Powers WJ, Grub RL, Baker RP et al. Regional cerebral blood flow and metabolism in reversible cerebral ischemia due to vasospasm. Determination by positron emission tomography. J Neurosurg 1994; 62: 59–67.

69. Dorsch NWC. A review of cerebral vasospasm in aneurysmal subarachnoid haemorrhage. Part III: Mechanisms of action of calcium antagonists. J Clin Neurosci 1994; 1(3): 151–160.

70. Pickard JD, Murray GD, Illingworth R et al. Effect of oral nimodipine on cerebral infarction and outcome after subarachnoid haemorrhage. British Aneurysm Nimodipine Trial. BMJ 1989; 298: 636–642.

71. Duckwiler D. Balloon angioplasty and intra-arterial papaverine for vasospasm. J Stroke Cerebrovasc Dis 1997; 4: 261–263.

72. Linskey ME, Horton JA, Rao GF, Yonas H. Fatal rupture of the intracranial carotid artery during transluminal angioplasty for vasospasm induced by subarachnoid hemorrhage. J Neurosurg 1991; 74: 985–990.

73. Clouston JE, Numaguchi Y, Zoarski GH. Intraarterial papaverine infusion for cerebral vasospasm after subarachnoid hemorrhage. Am J Neuroradiol 1995; 16: 27–38.

74. Fidlay JM, Kassell NF, Weir BK et al. A randomized trial of intraoperative, intracisternal tissue plasminogen activator for the prevention of vasospasm. Neurosurgery 1995; 37: 168–176.

75. Kassell NF, Hayley EC Jr, Apperson-Hansen C, Alves WM. Randomized, double-blind, vehicle controlled trial of tirilazad mesylate in patients with aneurysmal subarachnoid hemorrhage: a cooperative study in Europe, Australia, and New Zealand. J Neurosurg 1996; 84: 221–228.

76. Juvela S. Aspirin and delayed cerebral ischaemia after aneurysmal subarachnoid hemorrhage. J Neurosurg 1995; 82: 945–952.

24

POSTOPERATIVE CARE IN THE NEUROINTENSIVE CARE UNIT

Helen L. Smith

INTRODUCTION

While the postoperative period is important in many areas of surgery, it can be a particularly critical phase for patients undergoing major neurosurgery. Many such patients may present preoperatively with specific risk factors including raised intracranial pressure, an altered sensorium and/or depressed airway reflexes. The further deterioration in physiological homoeostasis that occurs as a consequence of anaesthesia or surgery may additionally expose patients to the risk of respiratory compromise or cerebral ischaemia. Further, the brain is an unforgiving organ and there is an imperative to rapidly detect and correct alterations in systemic and cerebral physiology that could result in irretrievable neurological damage if left untreated. The major categories of patients who require intensive or high-dependency care following neurosurgical interventions are listed in Box 24.1.

PATIENT ASSESSMENT AND MANAGEMENT

On arrival in the ICU area, each patient requires full assessment with history, examination and relevant investigations. Good communication between theatre and ICU staff regarding any pertinent perioperative

---

Preoperative cardiorespiratory illness

Long surgery, large blood loss, coagulopathy, incidental hypothermia, unstable haemodynamics

Patients at risk of or documented to have intracranial hypertension

Patients requiring ventilation to provide stability for venous haemostasis

Patients requiring or recovering from a period of hypothermia induced for cerebral protection

Patients requiring postoperative intracranial pressure monitoring

Requirement for blood pressure manipulation as a part of:

    induced hypertension for CPP maintenance or as a part of triple H therapy

    induced hypotension for treatment of hyperaemia following carotid or AVM surgery

Box 24.1   Neurosurgical patients requiring postoperative intensive/high-dependency care

---

event is essential. The history should include admission diagnosis, surgery, problems with the surgery/anaesthetic and expected problems.

MONITORING

Clinical assessment and reassessment is the primary form of monitoring. Regular consultation is required between neurosurgeons and intensivists. Basic physiological monitoring required for all patients in the neurointensive care unit includes blood pressure, ECG monitoring, pulse oximetery and careful recording of fluid balance. Monitoring of hourly urine output is of particular importance since neurosurgical patients are at risk of large fluid shifts from urinary losses because of their illness (e.g. due to associated diabetes insipidus) or as a consequence of therapy with osmotic diuretics such as mannitol.

ARTERIAL BLOOD GASES AND INVASIVE BLOOD PRESSURE

An arterial line is required in all ventilated patients for the measurement of arterial blood gases. Direct arterial pressure measurement is indicated in patients who have undergone neurovascular procedures (clipping of ruptured aneurysms, resection of arteriovenous malformations and the early postoperative period following carotid endarterectomy), patients with haemodynamic instability or intracranial hypertension (in whom there is a risk of compromise of cerebral perfusion pressure) and patients requiring vasoactive agents for blood pressure control.

CENTRAL VENOUS PRESSURE (CVP)

CVP monitoring is needed for patients with large volume losses, cardiac disease, vasoactive infusions and hypotension or oliguria not readily responsive to fluid challenge. CVP monitoring may also be essential in the patient with pathological polyuria due to diabetes insipidus or the condition of cerebral salt wasting that occurs following subarachnoid haemorrhage. It must be remembered, however, that the CVP is an indirect measure of the intravascular volume status and is influenced not only by venous return but also by right heart compliance, pulmonary or right heart disease, intrathoracic pressure and posture.

PULMONARY ARTERY CATHETERIZATION

Pulmonary arterial (PA) catheterization offers several advantages over CVP monitoring in selected patients. Measurement of PA wedge pressure provides a more reliable index of left ventricular preload and intravascular volume status in the critically ill patient and the use of thermodilution catheters allows the measurement of cardiac output and calculation of systemic vascular resistance. These data are of particular benefit in patients with concurrent severe cardiorespiratory disease or severe sepsis. PA catheters are also valuable to guide the use of complex vasoactive interventions as part of cerebral perfusion pressure augmentation in intracranial hypertension or triple H therapy for vasospasm following subarachnoid haemorrhage.[1,2]

NEUROLOGICAL EXAMINATION

Patients recovering from neurosurgical procedures require careful monitoring of all aspects of neurological function so that early signs of bleeding or cerebral oedema can be detected. The neurological system should be reviewed with particular regard to the operation performed and the patient's preoperative neurological status. Regular neurological observations should be undertaken including the measurement of pupillary size and reaction, limb power and recording of Glasgow Coma Score.[3] Although originally designed to quantify the severity of a head injury, the Glasgow Coma Scale and Score (Box 24.2) allow categorization of patients with neurological dysfunction from other forms of brain injury and over a period of time act as a guide to any deterioration in a patient's neurological status.

Eye opening	
Spontaneous	4
To voice	3
To pain	2
None	1
Motor responses	
Obeys commands	6
Localizes pain	5
Normal flexion (withdrawal to pain)	4
Abnormal flexion (decorticate)	3
Extension (decerebrate)	2
None (flaccid)	1
Verbal responses	
Orientated	5
Confused conversation	4
Inappropriate words	3
Incomprehensible sounds	2
None	1

Box 24.2   The Glasgow Coma Scale

INTRACRANIAL PRESSURE MONITORING

Intracranial pressure (ICP) monitoring is indicated in all patients who have intracranial hypertension or are at risk of developing it. This is particularly true in patients who remain sedated and consequently cannot be assessed by regular neurological examination. While the technique used for ICP monitoring will vary between centres, it is essential that ICP measurements are related to mean arterial pressure (MAP) to provide continuous monitoring of cerebral perfusion pressure (CPP; where CPP= MAP–ICP). Many of the therapies available to treat neurosurgical patients are based on the reduction of ICP or optimization of CPP. These include a reduction in cerebral oedema by cerebral dehydration, administration of steroids, hyperventilation, blood pressure control, reduction of cerebral venous pressure, surgical decompression, cerebrospinal fluid drainage and hypothermia.

OTHER MONITORING MODALITIES

Transcranial Doppler ultrasound, jugular venous saturation monitoring, EEG and evoked potential monitoring are other modalities that may be useful in individual patients. Their use is dealt with elsewhere in this book.

INVESTIGATIONS

Routine postoperative tests – full blood count, clotting screen, urea and electrolytes – should be performed at the time of admission to the intensive care unit, along with arterial blood gases if the patient is ventilated or has a low oxygen saturation. A chest X-ray is indicated if the patient is ventilated, a central line has been inserted or gas exchange is abnormal. Neurological imaging procedures should be undertaken if there is deterioration in the patient's neurological state or rise in intracranial pressure.

ICU MANAGEMENT

AIRWAY AND VENTILATION

Examination of the respiratory system including airway patency and airway reflexes is required to define ventilatory requirements. Managing the airway is of primary importance. Any patient without the ability to protect or maintain the airway needs intubation and ventilation, as does a patient who is breathing inadequately. The patient should be placed in the neutral position as flexion or torsion of the neck can obstruct cerebral venous outflow and increase brain bulk and ICP.

Even mild hypoxia or hypercapnia can have important consequences in the neurosurgical patient. A rise in the $PaCO_2$ will result in cerebral vasodilatation and can raise intracranial pressure further. Hypoxia can lead to secondary brain injury. Cerebral ischaemia remains a common pathway to secondary brain damage in most critically ill neurosurgical patients.[4] Other indications for ventilation include haemodynamic instability, inadvertent postoperative hypothermia, sepsis and the need for controlled hyperventilation in order to reduce intracranial pressure, e.g. head injuries.

The rationale behind ventilation is to maintain oxygenation to the tissues and removal of carbon dioxide without damaging the lungs, interfering with venous return or raising intracranial pressure. While conventional ventilation strategies are generally applicable to neurosurgical patients, a few specific issues need attention. It is important to maintain $PaCO_2$ within tight limits (we use an initial target value of 4.5 kPa), since even mild hypercapnia can result in cerebral vasodilatation and rises in intracranial pressure. Conversely, profound hypocapnia may result in dangerous cerebral vasoconstriction and ischaemia (see Ch. 00). Since central ventilatory drive may be compromised by drugs or disease, this precludes, in many patients, the use of ventilatory modes (e.g. pure pressure support ventilation) that do not assure a near constant minute volume. Similarly, while mild arterial desaturation (SaO_2 <90%) is often well tolerated by non-neurosurgical patients, the resulting hypoxic cerebral vasodilatation can result in marked increases in intracranial pressure when the brain is non-compliant. We therefore tend to start with FiO_2 40%, tidal volume 10ml/kg, rate 12–16/min and PEEP 0–2.5 cmH_2O using controlled or synchronized intermittent mandatory ventilation. Parameters can be changed to optimize ventilation.

Tracheostomy may be indicated in those patients requiring long-term ventilation. Ideally, this should be performed using the percutaneous dilational technique where possible. In one study elective tracheostomy for selected patients with poor Glasgow Coma Scale scores and nosocomial pneumonia resulted in shortened ICU length of stay and rapid weaning from ventilatory support.[5]

HAEMODYNAMIC MANAGEMENT

The cardiovascular system needs to be reviewed with particular note of the need for further fluid replacement, vasoactive drugs and the possibility of the need for central venous or pulmonary artery catheter monitoring. The aim is to control haemodynamics and

ensure that any blood loss is replaced. Pulse and blood pressure with urine output and central venous pressure give a guide to the patient's haemodynamic state. Following assessment of the intraoperative blood loss and fluid replacement, the need for further blood or colloid replacement can be guided by these modalities in conjunction with the haematocrit. Fluid and electrolyte balance must be monitored closely with regular assessment of blood gases, urea and electrolytes. Glucose-containing solutions should be withheld from neurosurgical patients at risk of cerebral oedema or ischaemia, since the residual free water after glucose is metabolized will reduce plasma osmolality and accelerate cerebral oedema and since increases in blood sugar can worsen outcome in the ischaemic brain.[6]

GASTROINTESTINAL SYSTEM

Following examination, the early institution of enteral feeding should be considered, within the first 24 h if at all possible. While parenteral feeding may be needed in a small proportion of patients, it is essential that blood sugar and plasma osmolality be rigorously controlled.

Care needs to taken in the prevention and treatment of acute upper gastrointestinal bleeding. Gastric acid hypersecretion can be observed in patients with head trauma or neurosurgical procedures. Gastric mucosal ischaemia due to hypotension and shock is the most important risk factor for stress ulcer bleeding. The most important prophylactic measure is an optimized ICU regime aiming to improve oxygenation and microcirculation. Stress ulcer prophylaxis is indicated in patients at risk. This includes patients with severe head trauma, raised intracranial pressure and corticosteroid therapy. While it is generally recognized that enteral feeding substantially reduces the risk of erosive gastritis, high-risk patients will require additional cover with sucralfate, H_2 antagonists or proton pump inhibitors. The selection of drugs depends not only on efficacy but also on possible adverse effects and on costs. In this regard, the most cost-effective drug may be sucralfate.[7]

ANALGESIA, SEDATION AND MUSCLE RELAXATION

Pain most frequently occurs within the first 48 h after surgery but a significant number of patients endure pain for longer periods. The subtemporal and suboccipital surgical routes yield the highest incidence of postoperative pain. Postoperative pain after brain surgery is an important clinical problem.[8] For non-ventilated patients appropriate analgesia consists of codeine phosphate 30–60 mg up to six hourly im/po/ng, paracetamol 1 g six hourly po/ng/pr and diclofenac 100 mg pr up to 12 hourly (if no bleeding problem/renal insufficiency). Special measures may be needed to ensure adequate analgesia but this is not generally a problem for cranial surgery. Morphine sulphate can be given for spinal surgery where changes in the level of sedation are not a critical part of postoperative monitoring.

Sedatives are used to decrease anxiety and diminish awareness of noxious stimuli. Propofol offers particular promise in neurosurgical intensive care[9] and is particularly appropriate (in doses of 3–6 mg/kg/h) if overnight ventilation is required. If longer term ventilation is anticipated then midazolam up to 6 mg/h in an average adult may be used. When compared with midazolam, the quality of propofol sedation is better than midazolam and patients wake up significantly faster on discontinuation.[10] Prolonged or high-dose propofol usage presents problems of cost and lipid loading.

In ventilated patients analgesia with opiates should be used sparingly. The relative lack of pain in patients who have undergone cranial neurosurgery predisposes such individuals to the risk of prolonged respiratory depression and delayed weaning from mechanical ventilation. While low-dose fentanyl is commonly employed (1–2 µg/kg/h), there may be a role for shorter acting opioids such as alfentanil and remifentanil. This area requires further study. There appears to be no justification for withholding non-steroidal antiinflammatory agents for fear of haemostatic compromise and paracetamol, diclofenac and other non-opioid analgesics can be used for additional analgesia or antipyresis.

Neuromuscular blockade is sometimes required to facilitate ventilation and prevent increases in intracranial pressure associated with the patient breathing against the ventilator. These drugs should be used with caution because of their associated incidence of prolonged weakness or myopathy, the potential for neurotoxicity and their direct effect on outcome.[9] Since these problems appear to be most commonly reported with the long-acting or steroid-based neuromuscular blockers, atracurium is commonly used if paralysis is indicated.

POSTOPERATIVE COMPLICATIONS AND THEIR MANAGEMENT

Complications can be divided up into general and those associated with specific operations.

GENERAL

Cardiac arrhythmias, myocardial infarction and cardiac failure

Cardiac arrhythmias in the ICU are commonly due to underlying cardiac disease but may be precipitated or exacerbated by other factors including hypoxia, hypercarbia, drugs, electrolyte and acid–base balance. Such adverse factors may need to be corrected before treatment of the arrhythmia can be safe or effective. Postoperative myocardial infarction can be a complication in patients with ischaemic heart disease. Specific treatment with thrombolytic agents is precluded in the early postoperative period due to the risk of postoperative bleeding. Treatment consists of supportive therapy. Cardiac failure can be a complication in patients with preexisting myocardial disease.

Pulmonary emboli

Pulmonary embolism (PE) is a complication of deep vein thrombosis (DVT). It is a frequent cause of mortality in postoperative patients. The mortality in treated patients is significantly lower than in those undiagnosed or untreated. Hence prophylactic measures against DVT and early diagnosis and treatment of PE are important, especially in critically ill ICU patients. There are no clear data regarding the timing of initiating heparin therapy for DVT prophylaxis in patients who have undergone neurosurgical procedures but most units initiate low molecular weight heparin therapy between 24 and 48 h postsurgery. It is essential that non-pharmaceutical methods of reducing DVT risk (graduated pressure stockings, circulatory pumps, etc.) be used in all patients in the intra- and postoperative period. If patients do develop a DVT or PE systemic heparinization is contraindicated and it is often necessary to resort to a caval filter to prevent recurrence of PE.

Infection

Postoperative infections can be life threatening. Prevention has a much greater impact on reducing patient morbidity and mortality than treatment. Basic infection control is essential, with all staff washing hands on entry to the unit and on passing from one patient to the next. All invasive procedures should be carried out with full aseptic technique, gloves and gowns used. Patients with methicillin-resistant strains of staphylococcus should be isolated in a side room and barrier nursed.

A conservative approach to the use of antibiotics is indicated. Samples from CSF, blood, urine, sputum and lines taken out should be sent to the laboratory for microscopy and culture if there is any suspicion of infection. Antibiotics should be prescribed once the organism and its sensitivity are known. Therapy should be continued based on the clinical response observed.[11] If the patient is septic then antibiotics should be started in consultation with the microbiologist. Early involvement of the physiotherapist is needed for prevention and treatment of chest infections.

COMPLICATIONS SPECIFIC TO NEUROSURGICAL OPERATION

Management of raised intracranial pressure

Raised intracranial pressure is multifactorial and may be due to hydrocephalus, vascular congestion and/or cerebral oedema. Techniques for reducing ICP are aimed at the aetiological factor causing the ICP elevation. A patent airway, adequate oxygenation and hyperventilation provide the foundation of care in such patients.

The specific goals are:

- to limit oedema formation, maintain cerebral perfusion pressure and cerebral blood flow and maintain blood pressure in the normal range to optimize blood flow through non-autoregulated areas;
- to create an osmotic gradient toward the intravascular compartment;
- to eliminate obstruction to normal CSF flow or to prevent acute hydrocephalus.

There is no role for dehydration in patients with raised intracranial pressure, since cerebral hypoperfusion will worsen cerebral ischaemia and cause further increases in ICP by promoting cerebral vasodilatation. Reduction in vasogenic oedema can be achieved by using osmotic agents. Mannitol is the osmotic diuretic of choice for ICP reduction. This removes brain water more than the other organs because the blood–brain barrier impedes penetration of the osmotic agent into the brain, thus maintaining an osmotic diffusion gradient. In addition, it may improve cerebral perfusion via microcirculatory and rheological effects. Frusemide has been the loop diuretic most frequently used to lower ICP acutely and provides intracranial decompression by a diuresis-mediated brain dehydration, reduced CSF formation and resolution of cerebral oedema via improved cellular water transport.

Corticosteroids are effective in reducing vasogenic oedema associated with mass lesions (e.g. intracerebral tumour). Often neurological improvement will precede ICP reduction and is usually accompanied by some degree of restoration of previously abnormal blood–brain barrier. Steroids require many hours for their ICP effects to become apparent and are ineffective (and probably detrimental) in the setting of brain trauma and intracranial haemorrhage.

Lowering arterial $PaCO_2$ can increase cerebral vascular resistance and reduce cerebral blood volume, thereby reducing brain bulk and ICP. Aggressive hyperventilation has been used in the past but a real danger of severe vasoconstriction with resultant ischaemia may result from such a technique. Mild to moderate hyperventilation ($PaCO_2$ 4.0–4.5 kPa) may be relatively safe but is best employed with the safeguard of jugular bulb oximetry, which will provide warning of cerebral ischaemia.[12]

Changes in cerebral venous pressure can have a marked influence on ICP. Cerebral blood volume rapidly increases when cerebral venous return is impeded. Flexion or torsion of the neck can obstruct cerebral venous outflow and increase brain bulk and ICP. Large increases in central venous pressure can also increase ICP. Application of positive end-expired pressure (PEEP) or other ventilatory patterns that increase intrathoracic pressure can theoretically increase ICP but rarely do so in practice, since central venous pressures will dictate ICP only when ICP < CVP. While it is important to avoid unnecessary increases in intrathoracic pressure, there is no reason to withhold PEEP if it is required to optimize gas exchange. Muscle relaxation and sedation can indirectly reduce elevated ICP in patients by decreasing mean intrathoracic pressure and spikes in pressure caused by coughing.

Intracranial hypertension can be reduced by CSF drainage or by lowering CSF secretion rates, especially (but not exclusively) in the presence of hydrocephalus documented on imaging studies. The first of these two options is commonly employed in the perioperative period, typically by the use of an external ventriculostomy. While this allows the controlled and variable drainage of CSF and permits catheter flushing in the event of blockage, it is associated with a significant risk of infection and regular microbiological surveillance is mandatory.

Reducing the brain temperature lowers brain metabolism, cerebral blood flow, cerebral blood volume and CSF secretion rate with a resultant reduction in ICP. While the ability of induced hypothermia to reduce an elevated ICP is well documented, there is currently much debate as to whether hypothermia may be applied as a neuroprotective intervention in the absence of intracranial hypertension. There is no doubt at all that elevations in body temperature are severely injurious to the ischaemic or traumatized brain and aggressive treatment of pyrexia is essential in neurosurgical patients.

In the event of intractable intracranial hypertension with preserved electrical activity on EEG, the use of high-dose intravenous anaesthetics such as barbiturates or thiopentone, titrated to burst suppression, may reduce metabolic needs and result in cerebral vasoconstriction and ICP reduction.

Surgical removal of intracranial tissue or masses may be used for uncontrollable brain swelling. Besides reducing ICP, surgical decompression can reduce shifts in brain tissue that are associated with herniation and/or focal neurological dysfunction.

Intracranial bleed

Awake patients may suffer reductions in GCS and/or focal neurological deficits related to the site of bleeding. The level of consciousness is commonly altered early in the clinical course as mass effect impairs bilateral hemispheric or brainstem function. In sedated patients ICP monitoring may provide an early indication of postoperative intracranial haemorrhage, which should prompt early CT scanning for confirmation.

Seizures

Prolonged seizure activity produces irreversible cerebral damage, independent of any accompanying hypoxia and acidosis. Cell death is thought in part to occur as a result of the excessive metabolic demands and nutrition depletion in continuously firing neurones. Cerebral oedema and lactic acid accumulation ensue. Treatment with phenytoin (intravenous loading dose 15 mg/kg over 1 h, with maintenance at 3–4 mg/kg/day) is appropriate as a first line in the neuro ICU as, unlike other anticonvulsants in therapeutic doses, it does not cause significant depression of the conscious level.

Fluid and electrolyte imbalance

Both hypokalaemia and hypomagnesaemia are common in neurosurgical patients who have received mannitol and since they may predispose to cardiac arrhythmias, aggressive correction is advised.

Hyponatraemia in neurosurgical patients may be due to the syndrome of inappropriate antidiuretic hormone (SIADH) secretion. SIADH may accompany hypothalamic and cerebral lesions, including cerebral infarction, tumour, abscess, trauma or subarachnoid haemorrhage. Such patients present with a low plasma sodium and osmolality, preserved or expanded intravascular volume and a high urinary osmolality. Progressive symptomatology of headache, nausea, confusion, disorientation, coma and seizures is often observed when the plasma sodium falls below 120 mmol/l.

Treatment depends on the presence or absence of clinical manifestations, which may also relate to the speed of onset of hyponatraemia. In hyponatraemia of rapid onset, treatment with hypertonic saline may be needed. If the patient has seizures then rapid treatment of cerebral oedema is required. Outside the ICU SIADH commonly occurs as a consequence of drug therapy (chlorthiazide, chlorpropamide, cyclophosphamide, vincristine) or as a result of ADH secretion by tumours. While such patients are treated with fluid restriction, this approach is inappropriate in the setting of critically ill patients where maintenance of intravascular volume and cerebral perfusion is paramount. Since hyponatraemia may worsen cerebral oedema, we have a low threshold for treating SIADH with demeclocycline (300–1200 mg/day) when fluid therapy with normal saline does not restore plasma sodium to the normal range. Occasional patients who present with severe acute hyponatraemia, coma and fits may require hypertonic saline therapy. It is important not to elevate plasma sodium levels too rapidly in patients who have been chronically hyponatraemic, since this may predispose to the development of central pontine myelinolysis. In such patients plasma sodium should not be raised at a rate greater than 1 mmol/h or 12 mmol in any 24-h period.

Hyponatraemia in other neurosurgical patients, especially following subarachnoid haemorrhage, may be the consequence of 'cerebral salt wasting'.[13] Such patients present with a low plasma sodium and high urinary sodium and output and are usually fluid depleted. This syndrome may be the consequence of excessive secretion of brain natriuretic peptide and is treated with aggressive volume expansion with sodium containing crystalloid or colloid.

Many neurosurgical conditions, including trauma, intracranial hypertension, tumours, subarachnoid haemorrhage and brainstem death, can lead to diabetes insipidus. The relative lack or absence of ADH in these patients results in the passage of large volumes of dilute urine (up to 0.5–1 l/h) with the rapid development of hypovolaemia, plasma hyperosmolality and hypernatraemia. Diagnosis in the appropriate clinical setting is made by detection of a high plasma osmolality coupled with a low urinary osmolality and treatment is with des-amino d-arginine vasopressin (DDAVP; 1–8 μg boluses, repeated as required) and hypotonic fluids. Mild elevations in plasma sodium may be best left untreated, since they may help to minimize vasogenic oedema, and aggressive and rapid reduction of plasma sodium and osmolality in patients who have been chronically hypernatraemic may result in cerebral oedema.

INTRAHOSPITAL TRANSFER[14]

Imaging is important in the diagnosis of postoperative CNS deterioration. For some patients this will involve multiple journeys. Transfer of the patient from the neuro ICU to the CT scanner can be fraught with hazards.[15] Careful planning of the journey with appropriate monitoring, including the presence of an anaesthetist if the patient is ventilated or haemodynamically compromised, is essential. Communication with the imaging department is a priority to prevent any delays. Particular attention should be paid to assessment of the airway and the adequacy of intravenous access. As far as possible, the same degree of monitoring should continue with the patient from the ICU to the scanner. This includes pulse oximetry, ECG, blood pressure (invasive if arterial line in situ), intracranial pressure monitoring and capnography if available. Portable monitoring equipment with functioning batteries is required.

Care must be taken when moving the patient from the bed to the CT scanner to ensure that all lines remain intact and the endotracheal tube, if present, is not dislodged during transfer. If the patient is being ventilated a portable ventilator with full oxygen cylinder is required. In addition, equipment such as a self-inflating Ambu bag with oxygen tubing, a laryngoscope, spare endotracheal tube and drugs to facilitate reintubation should accompany the patient.

It is important for the patient to be as stable as possible during this period. Infusions required on the intensive care unit should continue, including appropriate doses of sedation, analgesia and muscle relaxant. Haemodynamic control in a ventilated patient can be difficult during transfer with periods of hyper/hypotension. Gentle movement, with carefully considered use of sedation, can help minimize this problem.[15] Resuscitative drugs should be carried with the patient.

During the time spent in the scanner careful attention must be paid to the patient's physiological state with particular regard to airway, breathing and circulation. Ideally, the scanning room should have its own anaesthetic machine, ventilator with a piped oxygen supply and suction apparatus with full moni-toring capabilities. Without this, the hazards of running out of oxygen from a cylinder during a long investigation and problems of running out of battery power on the monitors need to be borne in mind. Monitoring must continue throughout the procedure with the equipment being easily seen by the attending physician. Any intervention to stabilize the patient needs to take priority over the scanning procedure. Careful placement of the ventilator and ventilator tubing, drip stands and infusions is essential. The length of any tubing connected to the patient needs careful consideration, bearing in mind the movement required to actually scan the patient. Vigilance must be high at all times for potential hazards.

REFERENCES

1. Levy ML, Giannotta SL. Cardiac performance indices during hypervolaemic therapy for cerebral vasospasm. J Neurosurg 1991; 75: 27–31.

2. Kassell NF, Peerless SJ, Durward QJ, Beck DW, Drake CG, Adams HP. Treatment of ischaemic deficits from vasospasm with intravascular volume expansion and induced arterial hypertension. Neurosurgery 1982; 11: 337–343.

3. Teasdale G, Jennett B. Assessment of coma and impaired consciousness: a practical scale. Lancet 1974; 2: 81.

4. Dearden NM. Mechanisms and prevention of secondary brain damage during intensive care. Clin Neuropathol 1998; 17: 221–228.

5. Koh WY, Lew TW, Chin NM, Wong MF. Tracheostomy in a neuro-intensive care setting: indications and timings. Anaesth Intens Care 1997; 25: 365–368.

6. Sieber FE, Smith DS, Traystman RJ, et al. Glucose: a reevaluation of its intraoperative use. Anesthesiology 1987; 67: 72.

7. Tryba M, Cook D. Current guidelines on stress ulcer prophylaxis. Drugs 1997; 54: 581–596.

8. De Benedittis G, Lorenzetti A, Migliore M, Spagnoli D, Tiberio F, Villani RM. Postoperative pain in neurosurgery: a pilot study in brain surgery. Neurosurgery 1996; 38: 466–469.

9. Prielipp RC, Coursin DB. Sedative and neuromuscular blocking drug use in critically ill patients with head injuries. New Horizons 1995; 3: 456–468.

10. Ronan KP, Gallagher TJ, George B, Hamby B. Comparison of propofol and midazolam for sedation in intensive care unit patients. Crit Care Med 1995; 23: 286–293.

11. Reed RL. Antibiotic choices in surgical intensive care unit patients. Surg Clin North Am 1991; 71: 765–789.

12. De Deyne C, Van Aken J, Decruyenaere J, Struys M, Colardyn F. Jugular bulb oximetry: review on a cerebral monitoring technique. Acta Anaesthesiol Belg 1998; 49: 21–31.

13. Harrigan MR. Cerebral salt wasting syndrome: a review. Neurosurgery 1996; 38: 152–160.

14. Andrews PJD, Piper IR, Dearden NM, Miller JD. Secondary insults during intrahospital transport of head-injured patients. Lancet 1990; 335: 327–330.

15. Bekar A, Ipekoglu Z, Tureyen K, Bilgin H, Korfali G, Korfali E. Secondary insults during intrahospital transport of neurosurgical intensive care patients. Neurosurg Rev 1998; 21: 98–101.

25

MANAGEMENT OF ACUTE ISCHAEMIC STROKE

Liz A. Warburton

INTRODUCTION

The burden of stroke disease in the Western world is a significant problem. Stroke is the third most common cause of death behind heart disease and cancer and is the most common cause of disability in patients living at home. The United States spends approximately $67 billion on stroke per annum, with one-third spent directly in hospital and nursing homes.[1] In the UK stroke care accounts for 5% of the health service budget, much of which is directed to the care of disabled stroke patients.[2] The incidence of first stroke is approximately two per 1000 per year.[3] Despite advances in primary prevention such as effective hypertension screening, secondary prevention with antiplatelet therapy and carotid endarterectomy, it is unclear as to whether these measures have had an impact on overall stroke incidence.[4] Nevertheless in an ageing population stroke is a major health concern, as 75% of patients with ischaemic stroke are over 75 years old. In terms of research efforts, stroke has often been a 'poor third' when compared to the huge interest and research effort in ischaemic heart disease and cancer. However, over the last 10 years stroke has moved up the political agenda and has been the subject of two recent government Green Papers in the UK.[5,6] Research efforts are expanding and there is an increasing interest, particularly from the pharmaceutical industry, in the development of new acute treatments.

Given this accelerating interest, it is perhaps surprising that the most significant advance in the management of stroke in the last 5–10 years pertains to the process of service delivery with the improved organization of stroke services to provide coordinated care at every level. It is now recognized that a comprehensive stroke service should have a neurovascular clinic for the assessment of transient ischaemic attacks (TIAs) and 'mini-strokes', a stroke unit for the acute phase of care, with facilities for continued rehabilitation followed by secondary prevention.[7] The implementation of these changes and the introduction of thrombolytic therapy in some countries has now shifted the debate. Stroke physicians are beginning to ask whether there is a role for more intensive management for the majority of stroke patients in the acute stages and whether this will have an impact on stroke outcome.

This chapter will address the following issues based on the available evidence:

- Is there a role for more intensive care of acute stroke?
- If so what should be offered in terms of monitoring and therapy?

- In the light of the prevalence of stroke, these questions are of major importance to health-care systems as the impact on the costs of service delivery could be huge.

WHAT IS A STROKE UNIT?

The evidence for the efficacy of stroke units is now clear. Organized inpatient care has been shown to be more effective than conventional care for three major primary outcome measures: death, dependency and institutionalization.[8] On a stroke unit patients are more likely to survive, regain their physical independence and return home. All categories of stroke patients are shown to benefit and there is no reason to exclude patients on the basis of gender, age or stroke severity.[7] Stroke units are also effective in reducing the length of inpatient hospitalization. There have been many suggestions as to how organized stroke care can improve outcome. It is important to note that these benefits were found from reorganization of relatively 'low-tech' ward environments with no acute monitoring facilities, no new acute treatments and no increase in the amount of rehabilitation staff or sessions.[7] What seems to be important is the process of care for stroke patients. On a stroke unit, there can be standardized assessment and early management protocols, better prevention and treatment of the secondary medical complications and earlier active rehabilitation. The benefits of stroke unit care do not happen in the acute stages (when the neurological complications of stroke occur) but are seen in the first four weeks, i.e. when the medical complications of stroke and immobility occur.[7] Box 25.1 summarizes the essential components of the stroke units referred to in these studies.

The following discussion is in three parts: the first assesses the evidence base for the management of stroke on a general stroke unit. The second examines the case for more high-dependency management and the third the available evidence for managing acute stroke in a neurocritical care setting.

Stroke physician/neurologist
Nurses with an interest in stroke
Physiotherapists
Occupational therapists
Speech and language therapists
Dietician

Box 25.1   Essential components of a general stroke unit

ACUTE MANAGEMENT OF STROKE (0–48 HOURS): EVIDENCE-BASED SPECIFIC MANAGEMENT ON A GENERAL STROKE UNIT

ASPIRIN

Aspirin should be given as soon as possible after acute ischaemic stroke in an initial dose of 160–300 mg (patients with swallowing difficulties can be given aspirin via rectal suppository or nasogastric tube as the evidence suggests that aspirin confers an early benefit which is additional to the long-term secondary preventive actions.[9,10] Strictly speaking, aspirin should not be given until a CT brain scan has excluded a haemorrhage but recent pooled data from two large studies have shown that early use of aspirin does not confer a significant risk of worsening in a primary intracerebral haemorrhage and so can be given before the CT brain on clinical grounds. Aspirin 300 mg od should be continued for the first four weeks and then can be reduced to 75 mg od which is proven to be an adequate dose for effective secondary prevention.[11]

ANTICOAGULATION

Data from the International Stroke Trial (IST) and other randomized controlled trials do not support the routine early use of heparin in acute stroke.[12,13] This is because heparin has not been shown to affect mortality or incidence of second stroke but does increase the risk of early haemorrhagic stroke and major extracranial haemorrhage. Even in patients with atrial fibrillation or emboli from the heart, there was no net reduction in the risk of further stroke because the risk of haemorrhagic complications outweighed the reduction in early recurrent stroke.[10] These findings contrast with the clear benefit for secondary prevention of long-term anticoagulation in patients with atrial fibrillation.[14] It is unclear at what time following acute stroke anticoagulation should be started. In clinical practice it is usual that warfarin is not substituted for aspirin until two weeks following stroke onset to minimize the risk of haemorrhage. To date, studies on use of the low-molecular weight heparins and heparinoids in acute stroke provide no convincing evidence of long term benefit.[13]

OTHER GENERAL MEASURES

Deep vein thrombosis (DVT) is common following stroke and general measures should be taken to try and prevent it, i.e. ensuring optimal fluid balance, use of graded compression stockings and if the patient is still immobile after two weeks the use of low-molecular weight (LMW) heparins. Although the use of LMW heparin is shown to reduce thromboembolic complications, there is little evidence that this translates into a net reduction in the longer term rates of death or dependency.[13]

MANAGEMENT OF DYSPHAGIA AND ASPIRATION

Dysphagia can be complicated by aspiration, pneumonia and hypoxia, dehydration and poor nutrition. Pneumonia is one of the major causes of death in stroke in the second week. Improvements in the assessment and management of dysphagia may be one of the reasons why development of stroke units has been so beneficial to stroke patients.[7] Assessment of swallowing should be made before any food or fluid is given to the patient and testing for a gag reflex alone is an inadequate way of assessing a safe swallow.[15] The simple bedside assessment can be done by trained nurses with advice from speech therapists.[15] Initially, if there is any doubt about a patient's swallowing abilities then the patient should be put 'nil by mouth' (NBM) and an intravenous line put up. Dysphagia often improves significantly during the first week following stroke and so it is clinical practice to use a nasogastric feeding route after day 3 and then wait until about 10 days before deciding on whether a percutaneous endoscopic gastrostomy (PEG) tube is necessary.[16] Whether early feeding and nutritional support affect outcome in stroke is the subject of an ongoing randomized controlled trial (FOOD Trial – MS Dennis, personal communication).

MANAGEMENT OF 'EXTRACRANIAL' SEQUELAE: THE CASE FOR MORE 'MULTIMODAL' MONITORING AND STROKE HIGH-DEPENDENCY UNITS

Closer monitoring of parameters known to be deranged by acute stroke – such as blood pressure, ECG abnormalities, temperature, oxygen saturation and glycaemia – will only be worthwhile if the effect of the change in the parameter on the extent of ischaemic damage is known and it is shown that 'correction' of the given change has a beneficial effect on the ischaemic damage and subsequent outcome of the patient.

HYPERTENSION

High blood pressure is a sequelae of acute stroke[17,18] and is generally higher in patients with intracerebral haemorrhage. Of course there is a proportion of patients who are either chronically hypertensive or who have previously undiagnosed hypertension within this group. Usually, this acute blood pressure rise falls spontaneously over the first few days. Whether this initial hypertension should be treated is not known and there are no randomized controlled trials on which to base any recommendations. Theoretically, control of hypertension may reduce the risk of vasogenic oedema formation and also the risk of haemorrhagic transformation of the infarct. However, reductions in systemic blood pressure may actually worsen the ischaemic damage. It is known that collateral arteries dilate in response to acidosis in the ischaemic area and that the autoregulatory mechanisms controlling flow in these vessels are lost. This means that even modest reductions blood pressure can affect the rCBF and worsen the degree of ischaemic damage.[19,20] In one animal model, a reduction of only 5 mmHg shifted EEG patterns consistent with a reversible injury to activity indicating irreversible damage.[21] In three small human trials of calcium channel antagonists (IV and po nimodipine and IV nicardipine), there was evidence that functional status and early survival may have been worse in the treatment groups because the induced systemic hypotension increased the infarct volume.[22,23,24]

In view of this evidence, there is general agreement that in clinical practice antihypertensive medication should be withheld in the acute stages unless there is evidence of hypertensive encephalopathy, aortic dissection, cardiac failure or acute renal failure.[20] Only if the blood pressure readings exceed the upper limits of autoregulation (i.e. systolic > 220, diastolic >120) should the blood pressure be cautiously reduced to try to prevent vasogenic oedema formation and haemorrhagic transformation. The aim of therapy should be a moderate reduction in blood pressure over a day or so rather than minutes and usually an oral [gb]β[xgb]-blocker is sufficient. Nifedipine is often used in Europe but the disadvantage of this is unpredictability of response and the overshoot hypotension that can occur. Labetalol or enalapril are known to have minimal effects on cerebral blood vessels and can be tightly titrated. In the 'NINDS' trial of tPA in acute stroke,[25] a protocol for the management of hypertension was used with the aim of reducing the risk of haemorrhagic transformation; this has gained widespread acceptance in centres in the United States where thrombolysis protocols are used but has not been tested *per se* in any randomized controlled trial. A summary of the antihypertensives that may be used in acute stroke is shown in Table 25.1. Patients remaining hypertensive following the acute phase (i.e. week 2 post-stroke) should obviously be treated as part of a secondary prevention strategy.

HYPOTENSION

Low blood pressure is a less common finding in acute stroke but is often caused by volume depletion.[26] It seems appropriate to treat a systolic blood pressure of < 90 mmHg with plasma expanders or vasopressive drugs, based on the evidence in head injury patients, to ensure an adequate perfusion pressure.[27] There are

Table 25.1   Antihypertensive agents used in acute stroke

Drug	Dose	Onset	Duration	Adverse effects
Nifedipine	5–10 mg sublingual	5–15 min	3–5 h	Overshoot hypotension
Captopril	6.25–50 mg od oral	15–30min	4–6 h	Decrease in CBF hypotension
Enalapril	2.5–30 mg od oral	15–30 min	8–10 h	Not for use in renal failure
Nitroprusside	0.25–10 mg/kg/min IV	Immediate	1–5 min	Nausea, vomiting, muscle twitching sweating
Labetalol	20–80 mg IV bolus or 2 mg/min IV infusion	5–10 min	3–5 h	Vomiting, hypotension, dizziness nausea Not for use in respiratory disease

very few data about the risks and benefits of such an intervention in stroke patients but a recent study showed that pharmacological elevation of blood pressure with phenylephrine in acute stroke is safe and may be beneficial in certain patients.[28]

CARDIAC ARRHYTHMIAS

Abnormalities of the cardiac rate and rhythm are very common following stroke.[29] A small proportion of ischaemic strokes (approximately 5%) will be in patients presenting within six weeks of an acute myocardial infarction. It is not known whether continuous monitoring of the ECG is necessary in the acute stages of stroke. In one study a few patients were noted to develop a prolonged QT interval and ventricular repolarization changes that are significant risks for ventricular arrhythmias. This could certainly contribute to mortality as well as stroke extension due to arrhythmia-induced hypotension. Conversely, in other studies there were very few arrhythmias and very few cardiac sequelae, making the need for wholesale cardiac monitoring rather unnecessary.[30,31]

Perhaps the most important arrhythmia in terms of management and secondary prevention strategy is AF which occurs in about 17% of patients with stroke and in the majority precedes the stroke. This can be easily picked up by a 12-lead ECG and does not require monitoring unless the ventricular rate is uncontrolled.

OXYGENATION AND ABNORMALITIES OF RESPIRATION

In areas of cerebral ischaemia it has been shown that hypoxaemia does worsen ischaemic damage.[32] Many patients with stroke have abnormal respiratory function due to abnormal breathing patterns caused by the stroke itself. Also significant problems such as aspiration, atelectasis and pneumonia can be caused by the sequelae of the stroke. All these are potential causes of hypoxaemia and affect the oxygen availability to the brain. It would seem a pragmatic step to offer oxygen routinely to stroke patients, particularly those with abnormalities on pulse oximetry (oxygen saturations below 95%, for example). However, it is not known whether this would confer any benefit on subsequent outcome. Rather paradoxically in animal ischaemic stroke models and also *in vitro* studies there is evidence to suggest that excessive oxygen might increase the generation of free radicals, thereby enhancing lipid peroxidation and worsening outcome, especially during any reperfusion of thrombi.[33,34]

The disordered patterns of breathing are common and probably result from indirect or direct damage to the respiratory centre in the medulla. The most commonly observed abnormality is periodic hyperventilation-hypoventilation (Cheyne–Stokes respiration) observed in 12% of cases in one study and 53% in another.[35,36] In general these abnormal patterns do not necessarily imply a poor prognosis and are an acute phenomenon noted quite frequently in patients who subsequently make a good recovery.[35]

Several other abnormalities of respiratory pattern have been described, including complete and central sleep apnoea.[37] Often there is also evidence of chronic coexisting pulmonary disease and occasionally respiratory depression can be provoked by the overuse of sedative medication.

At the moment particularly in the UK there is very little routine monitoring of oxygen saturation on general stroke units, something which could easily be introduced onto general stroke units using pulse oximetry. There has been some recent success in using oximetry in high-risk patients in order to predict aspiration pneumonias but the central question about oxygenation and acute stroke remains unanswered. This is obviously an important area for further work as it would be a simple (and cheap) way to make a difference.

HYPERGLYCAEMIA

Hyperglycaemia occurs in up to 43% of patients with acute stroke (random blood sugar >8.0);. 25% of these have diabetes already and another 25% have a raised HBA1C, indicating latent diabetes. The acute rise in blood sugar in the remainder suggests this is a response to the stroke itself. The precise mechanism of this effect is not known but aetiological factors may be increased release of catecholamines and corticosteroids in response to cerebral ischaemia.[38,39,40]

There is a substantial amount of evidence from animal stroke models and patient studies that hyperglycaemia enhances ischaemic brain injury and worsens outcome.[38,39,42,43] Myriad detrimental effects have been demonstrated in experimental models of hyperglycaemia and cerebral ischaemia.[42,43] In the ischaemic brain anaerobic glycolysis occurs producing lactic acid from pyruvate. Hyperglycaemia enhances the entry of glucose into the brain and provides more substrate for this anaerobic glycolysis particularly within the ischaemic area. This results in an intracellular lactic acidosis which has detrimental effects on neurones, glial cells and endothelial cells. In neurones it exacerbates the biochemical events that precipitate irreversible cell damage by facilitating release of mitochondrial calcium. Patients who have hyperglycaemia following stroke have higher levels of neurone-specific enolase (NSE) an enzyme released from dying neurones compared with normoglycaemic patients.[44] Lactic acidosis also has a critical role in glial oedema inhibiting collateral flow and affecting the microcirculation . Astrocytes are damaged by the effects of hyperglycaemia and as a result, the nutritional and metabolic support to the neurones adjacent to the astrocytes fails. Hyperglycaemia also worsens the degree of acute blood–brain barrier breakdown.[41]

It would seem good clinical practice, therefore, to maintain tight glycaemic control with insulin and fluids if necessary (to aim for a blood sugar of 4–8) and to perform regular monitoring using BM stix. A randomized controlled trial is in progress to assess the impact of this approach on eventual outcome from stroke (CJ Weir, personal communication). One note of caution is that hypoglycaemia can worsen the neurological deficit so the blood sugar control should not be overdone.[42]

BODY TEMPERATURE

An elevated body temperature is an independent predictor of poor outcome from stroke.[45,46,47] In a recent human stroke study only 20% of the patients had a fever associated with an underlying infection demonstrating a central effect of cerebral ischaemia on body temperature.[47] The exact mechanism producing this effect is unknown but in animal models it is well known that neuronal damage is worsened by hyperthermia and reduced by hypothermia.[48] A possibility is that hypothermia may be neuroprotective because it reduces cerebral blood flow (rCBF) and improves the cerebral arteriovenous oxygen difference.[49,50] In the animal models, the timing of hypothermia appears crucial for its beneficial effects. To date, no effect of hypothermia has been observed in which hypothermia was induced one hour or more after ischaemia in animal models of global ischaemia. This obviously presents a problem in translating this to human stroke management.

However, based on the above evidence, it would seem that normothermia should be achieved following acute stroke, using antipyretics if necessary and that infections should be treated promptly and aggressively.[51,52] Whether hypothermia in acute stroke improves outcome remains a subject of debate.[51,52] Hypothermia is not without potential harmful side-effects: in moderate to deep hypothermia electrocardiographic changes and arrhythmias can be provoked and hypothermia increases the danger of infection. Also the effect on CBF can potentially become detrimental – particularly if CBF reaches critical levels that are found below 27 degrees.

BRAIN TEMPERATURE MONITORING

Knowledge about the differences between body temperature, jugular vein temperature and brain temperature is not very precise. In addition, it may well be that the temperature varies in different parts of the brain. For example, it has been shown that very early following stroke, the temperature in the ischaemic area is higher than in the unaffected hemisphere, and that after several hours this gradient shifts.[50] Hence much more work is required in this area to answer the question of what temperature measurement, and from where, correlates best with severity and outcome and, if hypothermia is neuroprotective in acute stroke.

SUMMARY

Table 25.2 summarizes the evidence for an increased intensity of monitoring following acute stroke. Using the available data, there is not enough evidence to support the immediate upgrading of general stroke units into higher dependency settings. However, there is certainly enough encouraging evidence to support further trials comparing the effect of acute stroke patients managed in this way with the usual general care. More specific research is required to investigate the effect of the individual components discussed above and, more generally, to assess the overall effect of this type of higher dependency management.

SPECIFIC TREATMENTS FOR ACUTE STROKE

THROMBOLYSIS TRIALS

The idea that reperfusion with a thrombolytic would affect outcome in acute stroke is not new. Small trials of thrombolysis were started almost 50 years ago but were virtually abandoned because of an increased risk of death.[53] However, there has been a resurgence of interest over the last 10 years, in part due to the widespread availability of CT scanning allowing for easy identification of brain haemorrhage and the success of thrombolytic therapy in cardiology.[54] Because the major beneficial effect of thrombolysis (clot lysis and reperfusion) and the major detrimental effect (haemorrhage) both occur spontaneously in acute stroke, there has been a move towards large randomized controlled trials (RCTs) to eliminate systemic bias in the analysis of the results. The most recent randomized trials of intravenous thrombolysis are shown in Table 25.3. Only one of these trials was unequivocally positive, i.e. the NINDS-rt-PA Stroke Study.[55] In this trial where patients were randomized within three hours of stroke onset (48% within 90

Table 25.2   Summary of the evidence for more intensive monitoring in acute stroke

Monitoring	Suggested intervention	Available evidence	Key references
Blood pressure	Aim to keep systolic <220 mmHg and diastolic <120 mmHg	No RCT evidence for risk/benefits of intervention. Relative hypotension known to reduce CBF in acute stages	17,20,23,25
Oxygen saturation	Aim to keep arterial saturation > 95%	Evidence of effect of oxygen on ischaemic brain limited. Probable benefit of monitoring in predicting aspiration pneumonias	35
Body Temperature	Aim to keep at 37 or less	Fever worsens outcome. No RCT evidence of benefit of induced *hypothermia*	47,50,51
ECG	Acute treatment of arrhythmias (particularly ventricular)	Incidence of beneficial interventions based on monitoring lacking. Sensible to monitor high risk cases	29,30,31
Blood glucose	Aim to keep glucose concentration 4.2–7.8 mmol/l with insulin pump if necessary (e.g. blood glucose > 15 mmol/l)	Hyperglycaemia worsens outcome. No RCT evidence of beneficial effects of tight control. Avoid hypoglycaemia	38,39,42

min), there was a trend towards neurological recovery at 24 h and at three months 50% of survivors had no or minimal disability compared with 38% of controls. However, the rate of symptomatic brain haemorrhages rose by a factor of 10 but despite this mortality at three months was the same in both groups. On the basis of this trial tPA was licensed for use in the USA in June 1996 and there are published guidelines for its administration.[25] However, partly because of the practical difficulties of the three hour time window both for patient time to presentation and logistic difficulties within hospitals in centres offering thrombolysis, only 5% of the strokes are eligible to receive it.

There remains considerable uncertainty, particularly in Europe, about the widespread use of thrombolysis especially as the recent European ECASS II Study did not show any definite benefits over placebo.[56] Therefore, outside the USA thrombolysis still remains an experimental treatment.

A systematic metaanalysis of 12 RCTs involving 3435 patients (still very small by cardiological standards) where thrombolysis was started within six hours has shown that thrombolysis reduced the proportion of patients who died or who remained dependent at the end of trial follow-up (i.e. at six months) and more so if therapy was started within three hours.[61,62] This treatment effect appeared clearer in those trials using tPA. However overall, patients given thrombolysis had an increased risk of death within two weeks and also by the end of follow-up. In one trial where there was a subgroup randomized to aspirin and streptokinase there was a highly significant interaction for the risk of haemorrhage.[57] Table 25.3 summarizes the results from the major trials of thrombolysis to date. Some of the debates resulting from these studies have tried to identify factors that will enable better patient selection for thrombolysis, i.e. to ensure that patients treated have the most to gain at the least risk possible.

Trial eponym and reference	Agent used	Dose	Stroke subtypes	Time from onset to treatment	Main effects
MAST-I[57]	Streptokinase	1.5 × 10 IU	Cortical	6 h	Excess of early deaths. Non significant reduction in death and disability in treatment group. Particularly high risk of haemorrhage in aspirin plus streptokinase subgroup.
MAST-E[59]	Streptokinase	1.5 × 10 IU	All	6 h	Stopped due to a twofold increase in odds of early death in treatment group
ECASS 1[60]	tPA	1.1 mg/kg	Cortical	6 h	Mortality higher in treatment group. Trends towards better outcomes in survivors, however
NINDS[55]	tPA	0.9 mg/kg	All	3 h	12% absolute increase in likelihood of good outcome at three months. No significant differences in mortality. Haemorrhage rate increased in treatment group by factor of 10
ASK[58]	Streptokinase	1.5 × 10 IU	All	4 h	Risk of early death increased. For the 0–3 h treatment subgroup there was a strong trend towards better outcome
ECASS 2[56]	tPA	0.9 mg/kg	Cortical	6 h	Non significant benefit in outcome at three months. Increase in haemorrhage rate but no significant increase in mortality

Table 25.3   Summary of intravenous thrombolysis trials.

Possible ways of improving patient selection for thrombolysis

Time window to treatment

One of the major differences in the NINDS Trial when compared to the other RCTs was the short time window to treatment and, in theory, it makes sense that a fresher thrombus occluding an artery is more likely to respond to lytic agents than an old more organized thrombus. However, data from functional imaging studies using positron emission tomography (PET) suggest that the therapeutic time window in terms of viable ischaemic but not infarcted brain may last less than one hour in some patients but up to 16 hours in others.[61,62] A simple imaging technique to detect ischaemic but still viable tissue in individual patients is urgently needed to help make these treatment decisions. If an area of salvageable brain was demonstrated then it would be easier to persuade patients to take the added haemorrhagic risk of the treatment. Developing MR technology looks promising in this respect.[63]

Predictors of brain haemorrhage and complications of thrombolysis

From the trials predictors of those more likely to haemorrhage are emerging. General predictive factors are time to treatment, the dose of thrombolysis, the initial blood pressure level and the severity of neurological deficit and Of ischaemia. More work is needed to delineate these indicators more precisely. Other potential complications of thrombolysis include reperfusion injury, arterial reocclusion and secondary embolization due to thrombus fragmentation.[64]

Problems of definition and intraarterial (IA) thrombolysis

One of the problems with IV thrombolysis is that it is not known whether the patient actually had an occluded artery at the time of treatment . The large IV trials have been non-angiographic and assumed that one large or small artery occlusion was present. From previous angiographic studies performed within 6–8 h of stroke this is the case in 75% of patients.[65] It is not known whether there is a differential response to IV thrombolysis in angiographically positive versus negative patients. One obvious advantage of IA thrombolysis is that it allows a more accurate selection of patients. Also it allows a higher local concentration of the drug. There have been some trials demonstrating success with IA thrombolysis for strokes within the posterior cerebral circulation[66] and a recent RCT of IA lysis using a prokinase showed good evidence of recanalization but too few patients were randomized to assess the impact on outcome[67] More studies are awaited with interest.

The impact of thrombolytic treatments on intensive care treatment of stroke

Should patients who are thrombolysed be managed on an intensive care unit? At the moment, this question remains open mainly due to the uncertainties surrounding thrombolysis itself. However, rather akin to the postthrombolysis management of myocardial infarction patients could easily have infusions of intravenous thrombolysis on a high dependency section of a general stroke ward. Protocols for the management of the infusion and potential complications such as hypertension and bleeding would help to ensure treatment was administered according to strict guidelines. IA thrombolysis may require a more intensive setting, particularly if there was a restless patient and a protracted angiographic procedure. This may necessitate an anaesthetic for the first 24–48 h although the proportion of patients in whom this would be applicable would probably be small.

NEUROPROTECTION FOR ACUTE STROKE

Table 25.4 summarizes the neuroprotective agents which have shown efficacy in animal ischaemic models and have been tested in phase II and III human

RCT's. To date, the results have been disappointing and there is much debate as to why promising results in animal studies have not translated into successful results in human stroke trials.[75,76,77] There are several possibilities: one may be the inclusion of stroke patients in trials on the basis of stroke rating scales rather than an objective assessment of the neuroanatomical and neurophysiological deficit. As most animal models involve cortical ischaemia in the MCA territory it would seem sensible to only include these strokes in the human studies. Unfortunately most rating scales assess the severity of the impairment and in most of the trials to date, no subgroup analysis based on neuroanatomical infarct site has been possible. Therefore, a potential benefit in cortical strokes may be diluted by the inclusion of other stroke syndromes (e.g. lacunar strokes with white matter ischaemia) in the analysis. It is interesting to note that in the CLASS Study,[73] where strokes were classified according to the Oxfordshire Community Stroke Project(OCSP) system, subgroup analysis demonstrated benefit in total anterior circulation strokes despite an overall negative result.

Another important consideration is the lack of a widely available imaging technique which demonstrates the existence of the ischaemic penumbra in an acute stroke patient. This is of crucial relevance to the efficacy of a neuroprotective agent. PET studies have shown that only around one-third of patients presenting 5–18 hours after onset have evidence of an ischaemic penumbra and in these patients the outcome is variable.[78] Also, in some patients the penumbral region is gone by one hour and in others it remains for up to 24 hours.[61,62,78] Therefore clinical trials of potential neuroprotective agents in the future will require more detailed phase II studies with carefully selected patient groups and functional imaging techniques of which there are several new possibilities, particularly perfusion and diffusion-weighted magnetic resonance imaging (PW and DW MRI).[63] More advanced imaging technology will also be important in defining evidence of beneficial effect with neuroanatomical and neurophysiological endpoints as well as clinical data.

INTENSIVE CARE MANAGEMENT OF ACUTE STROKE

CAUSES OF DEATH IN STROKE AND INDICATORS OF POOR PROGNOSIS

In the first few days following stroke, most patients who die do so as a result of the direct effects of the brain damage.[79] In brainstem strokes, the respiratory

Table 25.4 Neuroprotective agents tested or being tested in Phase 111 acute stroke trials

Agent and reference	Mode of action	Results
Nimodipine[22,69]	Calcium antagonist	Large RCTs did not demonstrate benefit. One suggested nimodopine induced hypotension was detrimental
Selfotel[68,70,76]	NMDA antagonist	Large RCTs stopped because of side effects/efficacy ratio
Cerestat[68,71,76]	NMDA antagonist	Side effects significant. Benefit unproven
Elipordil[68,76]	NMDA antagonist	Trials in progress
Magnesium[76]	NMDA antagonist	Trials in progress
Lubelozole[72,76]	Na channel antagonist and inhibitor of glutamate release	USA study showed benefit (5% reduced mortality and 7% increase in those with little or no disability. European study showed no benefits. Concerns over prolonged QT interval
Chlomethiazole[73,76,77]	Inhibitor of glutamate release	No significant benefit in large RCT (CLASS Trial). Some benefit in MCA stroke
Anti-ICAM-1 antibody (Enlimomab)[74]	Monoclonal antibody to ICAM-1 preventing leucocyte activation	High rates of fever, infection and poor outcome
CDP-choline (Citicholine)[75]	May prevent membrane breakdown and free radical production	Phase II studies promising. RCT trial in progress

centre may be affected by the stroke itself whereas in cortical infarctions the dysfunction of the brainstem results from displacement and herniation caused by vasogenic oedema and raised intracranial pressure (ICP). General predictors of an early death include Age, AF cardiac failure and ischaemic heart disease, diabetes, fever, incontinence, previous stroke and a depressed conscious level (e.g. Glasgow Coma Scale <9). Neurological features include a severe motor deficit, any visuospatial deficit and a large volume lesion with mass effect on CT. For a brainstem stroke, a decreased conscious level, conjugate gaze palsy, severe bilateral motor weakness, abnormal respiratory patterns and bilateral extensor plantars indicate a severe stroke and poor prognosis.[80,81] Having survived the first few days of stroke, subsequent deaths are most often caused by consequences of immobility the most common being pneumonia and pulmonary embolism followed by dehydration and renal failure, UTI's and sepsis and other comorbidities for example, ischaemic heart disease and cancer.

SEVERE STROKES AND INTENSIVE CARE

It is estimated that an intensive care setting for stroke might be appropriate for up to 10% of stroke patients because of life-threatening stroke with patients having many of the features discussed above.[83–86] Ostensibly, management of these patients would focus on respiratory care, cardiac care and intracranial pressure management. The stroke subtypes would most likely be acute and severe proximal middle cerebral artery (MCA) occlusions, basilar thromboses and space-occupying cerebellar infarctions or haematomas. Other patients who might benefit would be those with severe aspiration pneumonias and pulmonary emboli. If IA thrombolysis were to prove the most effective and safe means of clot lysis then it is likely that patients receiving this sort of management would be appropriate for this setting also, as they may well require ventilation for the procedure. For the majority of patients who will have a proximal MCA infarction the prognosis is poor.[81] 60% will die within the first year and 35% will be dependent on others for activities of daily living, leaving only 5% who will regain any form of functional independence.

RESUSCITATION DECISIONS IN STROKE PATIENTS

These issues in stroke at the present time remain controversial. Whether to ventilate a stroke patient or not and admit them to an intensive care unit depends on an objective assessment of each individual patient, the severity of the stroke and prospects for recovery, relevant comorbidities and, if possible, the wishes of the patient and their family. Often such patients are unable to give an informed decision themselves. There has been little specific work so far on resuscitation decisions in stroke patients.[82]

EVIDENCE FOR THE EFFICACY OF SPECIFIC MONITORING AND MANAGEMENT OF STROKE PATIENTS ON INTENSIVE CARE

There have been several small non-randomized studies of stroke intensive care units but to date, there is no good evidence that care in this setting has any beneficial impact on patient outcome.[83–86] What specific management strategies are possible and do they have any evidence base for benefit?

VENTILATION

Laryngoscopy and intubation may lead to a substantial haemodynamic response and may raise the ICP. Therefore short-acting agents such as thiopental (3–5 mg/kg) or propofol (1.5–3 mg/kg) are suggested along with a depolarizing neuromuscular blocking agent to avoid a reflex rise in the blood pressure and ICP during the procedure.[85,86] If artificial ventilation becomes necessary then it should initially be without positive end-expiratory pressure (PEEP) to minimize venous backflow. In general adequate sedation, volume controlled respiration, slight PEEP and prolongation of the inspiratory period are helpful. In addition a low pCO_2 leads to a fall in ICP by reduction in the intracranial blood volume.[86] It remains unknown as to whether ventilating and sedating in the context of acute stroke confers any neuroprotective benefit.

INTRACRANIAL PRESSURE MONITORING AND CONTROL

There are several mechanisms of ICP elevation in cerebrovascular disease that can exist independently or in conjunction. ICP is determined by the relative volumes of the cranial vault contents, i.e. brain 80%, blood 10%, CSF 10% and mass (variable %) the notion of the mass can encompass an infarction, haemorrhage, oedema, hydrocephalus and cerebral blood volume. ICP changes associated with particular cerebrovascular diseases include the accumulation of cytotoxic oedema, the volume or mass of parenchymal haemorrhage, obstructive hydrocephalus, as seen with intraventricular haemorrhage or cerebellar haemorrhage and infarction. The purpose of ICP monitoring is to try and prevent secondary cerebral injury or ischaemia. Large ischaemic cerebral infarctions can be accompanied by mass effect and elevated ICP which can cause additional infarction and herniation leading to brain death. To date, there have only been a few studies of ICP monitoring in stroke and these have not demonstrated any benefit.[87,88]

SPECIFIC MEDICAL TREATMENTS TO REDUCE RAISED ICP IN STROKE

Low molecular-weight hypertonic solutions such as glycerol, mannitol and sorbitol are used frequently to reduce brain water content by producing an osmolar gradient between brain and plasma and driving water from brain tissue into plasma.

Glycerol

This is a hyperosmolar agent said to reduce cerebral oedema and possibly increase CBF.[86] It can be given intravenously (125 or 250 ml of a 10% solution over one hour four times a day) or orally (50 ml of an 80% solution four times a day). Glycerol is metabolized by glycolysis within brain tissue and is cleared by the kidney. Volume overload, haemolysis and electrolyte disturbances are frequent problems associated with glycerol treatment[86] and renal function and central venous pressure (CVP) must be closely monitored during its administration. To date, there have been 10 RCTs of glycerol in acute stroke involving 593 patients.[89] From these trials it emerges that glycerol was associated with a marginally significant (42%) reduction in the odds of early death (95% CI: 6–64% reduction in the odds of death). However, at final follow-up early glycerol treatment was associated with only a non-significant 18% reduction in the odds of death (95% CI: 46% reduction to 23% increase). Therefore the use of glycerol cannot be recommended on the present evidence.

Mannitol

Mannitol 20% (0.25–0.5 g/kg every 4–6h) is an osmotic diuretic with a faster onset of action than glycerol. However, because equilibration between brain osmolality and plasma osmolality occurs, mannitol loses its effect after a few days. A reverse osmotic drive resulting in a marked rebound phenomenon may occur if treatment with mannitol is suddenly discontinued or reduced too rapidly. Electrolyte disturbances, renal dysfunction and hypovolaemia are known complications. The use of mannitol has not been tested in randomized controlled trials in stroke patients and therefore its use cannot be recommended in acute stroke.

DECOMPRESSIVE SURGERY

Cerebellar Infarction

Space-occupying cerebellar infarcts are caused by uni- or bilateral posterior inferior cerebellar artery (PICA) occlusion or by bilateral superior cerebellar artery (SCA) occlusion. Changes in consciousness can occur between days 2 and 4 and result from the compression of the fourth ventricle leading to occlusive hydrocephalus or from additional brainstem compression. The surgical decompression of cerebellar infarcts has been claimed to improve cerebral perfusion pressure (CPP) and also relieve obstructive hydrocephalus improving outcome in survivors. However, data from RCT's is lacking and results quoted are from open small case series. Also there is debate as to which patients should have surgery and at what point is the optimal time for surgical intervention.[90,91]

Large MCA Infarcts with massive oedema

Some patients with severe and extensive MCA infarction develop massive oedema and subsequent uncal herniation. They usually have severe hemiplegia and gaze palsies and show a rapid decline in conscious level with brainstem signs of herniation within 2–4 days after the onset of symptoms. This pattern of deficits has been referred to by some as the 'malignant MCA infarction'[92] and is mostly caused by occlusion of the distal internal carotid artery (ICA) or the proximal MCA trunk and is almost always associated with little or no collateral flow. This syndrome has a mortality of 80% and survivors are usually very disabled. If ICP monitoring is performed ICP values can exceed 30 mm.

Surgical decompression is claimed to be effective in reducing the ICP and preventing transtentorial herniation, the rationale being to allow expansion of the oedematous tissue away from the lateral ventricle, the diencephalon and the mesencephalon to reduce the ICP to increase the perfusion pressure and to preserve cerebral blood flow by preventing further compression of the collateral vessels. In an animal study it has been shown that animals treated within one hour and within 24 h of MCA stroke had a significantly reduced infarct size and improved outcome relative to controls.[93] In the literature to date there have been 111 hemicraniectomies performed for human MCA stroke during the last 50 years. It has been claimed that this method does have a beneficial effect on both mortality and morbidity in a trial of 32 patients. However, this trial was not randomized and included data from a non-randomized control group.[94] Obviously, more RCT's are required to assess the efficacy of this method. Also the selection criteria for patients will need to be better defined and at what point patients should have surgery.

HAEMODILUTION

Haemodilution is achieved by giving an infusion of dextran, hydroxyethyl starch or albumin.[95] Haemodilution can be achieved using this method and isovolemically by simultaneously removing several hundred mls of blood. The resulting effect is a reduction in whole blood viscosity and an increase in cerebral oxygen delivery, the theory being that this might be neuroprotective and reduce infarct volume. There have been 15 RCT's of haemodilution involving 2268 patients which have been reviewed.[95] No overall effect was seen on survival and, in the survivors, neurological outcome was similar in both groups with no subgroup deriving definite benefit.

SUMMARY AND CONCLUSION

There is no doubt that the management of stroke has been improved with changes towards organized stroke care on stroke units. Whether more intensive management and monitoring of acute stroke will provide the means for further improvement remains to be proven but evidence is accumulating that more intensive management of certain parameters may be indicated. The neurocritical care management of acute stroke and the benefit of specific monitoring modalities and interventions remain the subject of debate. More randomized controlled studies to assess the benefit of these expensive techniques assessing their impact particularly on the long-term outcome of stroke are required before more intensive management can be widely recommended. There is still no proven effective acute treatment for stroke although treatment with thrombolytic agents looks promising. It is likely that advances in this area as well as success in the search for effective neuroprotective agents will drive the management of acute stroke into the more intensive arena.

REFERENCES

1. American Heart Association. Heart and stroke facts. Statistical Supplement. 1995; pp 11–12.

2. Department of Health. Stroke rehabilitation. Effective Health Care 1992; 2: 1–11.

3. Bamford J, Sandercock P, Dennis M et al. A prospective study of acute cerebrovascular disease in the community: the Oxfordshire Community Stroke Project, 1981–1986. 1. Methodology, demography and incident cases of first ever stroke. J Neurol Neurosurg Psychiatry 1988; 51: 373–380.

4. Asplund K, Bonita R, Kuulasmaa K et al. For the WHO MONICA Project. Multinational comparisons of stroke epidemiology. Stroke 1995; 26: 355–360.

5. Department of Health. The Health of the Nation. HMSO, London, 1991.

6. Department of Health. A Healthier Nation. HMSO, London, 1998.

7. Dennis M, Langhorne P (eds). Stroke units: an evidence-based approach. BMJ Publishers, London, 1998.

8. Langhorne P, Williams BO, Gilchrist W et al. Do stroke units save lives? Lancet 1993; 342: 395–398.

9. CAST (Chinese Acute Stroke Trial) Collaborative Group. CAST: randomised placebo-controlled trial of early aspirin use in 20000 patients with acute ischaemic stroke. Lancet 1997; 349: 1641–1649.

10. International Stroke Trial (IST). A randomised trial of aspirin, subcutaneous heparin both or neither among 19 435 patients with acute ischaemic stroke. Lancet 1997; 349: 1569–1581.

11. Antiplatelet Trialists' Collaboration. Collaborative overview of randomised trials of antiplatelet therapy – 1: Prevention of death, myocardial infarction, and stroke by prolonged antiplatelet therapy in various categories of patients. BMJ 1994; 308: 81–106.

12. Counsell C, Sandercock P. Anticoagulant therapy compared to control in patients with acute presumed ischaemic stroke (Cochrane review). The Cochrane Library, Issue 2, Update software, Oxford, 1998.

13. Counsell C, Sandercock P. The use of low-molecular weight heparins or heparinoids compared to standard unfractionated heparin in acute ischaemic stroke (Cochrane review). The Cochrane Library, Issue 2. Update Software, Oxford, 1998.

14. Koudstaal P. Secondary prevention following stroke or transient ischaemic attack in patients with nonrheumatic atrial fibrillation: anticoagulant therapy versus control (Cochrane review). The Cochrane Library Issue 2. Update Software, Oxford, 1988.

15. Ellul J, Barer D. Detection and management of dysphagia in patients with acute stroke. Age Ageing 1993; 22(suppl 2): 17(abstract).

16. Raha SK, Woodhouse K. The use of percutaneous endoscopic gastrostomy (PEG) in 161 consecutive elderly patients. Age Ageing 1994; 23: 162–163.

17. Wallace JD, Levy LL. Blood pressure after stroke. JAMA 1981; 246: 2177–2180.

18. Fotherby MD, Potter JF, Panayiotou B, Harper G. Blood pressure changes after stroke; abolishing the white coat effect. Stroke 1993; 24: 1422.

19. Powers WJ. Haemodynamics and metabolism in ischaemic cerebrovascular disease. Neurol Clin 1992; 10: 31–48.

20. Powers WJ. Acute hypertension after stroke: the scientific basis for treatment decisions. Neurology 1993; 43: 461–467.

21. Date H, Hossmann KA, Shima T. Effect of middle cerebral artery compression on pial artery pressure, blood flow, and electrophysiological function of cerebral cortex of cat. J Cereb Blood Flow Metab 1984; 4: 593–598.

22. Wahlgren NG, MacMahon DG, De Keyser J, Indredavik B, Ryman T. Intravenous Nimodipine West European Stroke Trial (INWEST) of nimodipine in the treatment of acute ischaemic stroke. Cerebrovasc Dis 1994; 4: 204–210.

23. Lisk DR, Grotta JC, Lamki LIF et al. Should hypertension be treated after acute stroke? A randomised controlled trial using single photon emission computed tomography. Arch Neurol 1993; 50: 855–862.

24. Kaste M, Fogelholm R, Erila T et al. A randomised double blind placebo controlled trial of nimodipine in acute ischaemic hemispheric stroke. Stroke 1994; 25: 1348–1353.

25. Adams HP, Brott TG, Crowell RM et al. Guidelines for the management of patients with acute ischaemic stroke. A statement for healthcare professionals from a special writing group of the Stroke Council, American Heart Association. Stroke 1994; 90: 1588–1601.

26. Grotta JC, Pettigrew LE, Allen S et al. Baseline hemodynamic state and response to haemodilution in patients with acute cerebral ischaemia. Stroke 1985; 16: 790–795.

27. Reilly PL, Lewis SB. Progress in head injury management. J Clin Neurosc 1997; 4: 9–15.

28. Rordorf G, Cramer SC, Efird JT et al. Pharmacological elevation of blood pressure in acute stroke. Clinical effects and safety. Stroke 1997; 28: 2133–2138.

29. Oppenheimer SM, Hachinski VC. The cardiac consequences of stroke. Neurol Clin 1992; 10: 167–176.

30. Rem JA, Hachinski VC, Bourghner DR et al. Value of cardiac monitoring and echocardiography in TIA and stroke patients. Stroke 1985; 16(6): 950–956.

31. Mikolich JR, Jacobs WC, Fletcher GF. Cardiac arrhythmias in patients with cerebrovascular accidents. JAMA 1986; 246: 1314–1317.

32. Back T, Kohno K, Hossman K-A. Cortical negative DC deflections following middle cerebral artery occlusion and Kcl-induced spreading depression: effect on blood flow, tissue oxygenation and electroencephalogram. J Cereb Blood Flow Metab 1994; 14: 12–19.

33. Hori O, Matsumoto M, Maeda Y et al. Metabolic and biosynthetic alterations in cultured astrocytes exposed to hypoxia/reoxygenation. J Neurochem 1994; 62: 1489–1495.

34. Mikel HS, Yashes NV, Kempinski O et al. Breathing 100% oxygen after global brain ischaemia in Mongolian gerbils results in increased lipid peroxidation and increased mortality. Stroke 1987; 18: 426–430.

35. Nachtmann A, Siebler M, Rose G et al. Cheyne–Stokes respiration in ischaemic stroke. Neurology 1995; 45: 820–821

36. Turney TM, Garraway WM, Wishnant JP. The natural history of hemispheric and brainstem infarction in Rochester Minnesota. Stroke 1984; 15(5): 790–794.

37. Askenasy JJ, Goldhammer I. Sleep apnoea as a feature of bulbar stroke. Stroke 1988; 19: 637–639.

38. Oppenheimer SM, Hoffbrand BI, Oswald GA, Yudkin JS. Diabetes mellitus and early mortality from stroke. Br Med J 1985; 291: 1014–15.

39. Weir CJ, Murray GD, Dyker AG, Lees KR. Is hyperglycaemia an independent predictor of poor outcome after acute stroke? Results of a long term follow up study. BMJ 1997; 314: 1303–1306.

40. Van Kooten F, Hoogerbrugge N, Naarding P et al. Hyperglycaemia in the acute phase of stroke is not caused by stress. Stroke 1994; 24: 1129–1132.

41. Dietrich WD, Alonso O, Busto R. Moderate hyperglycaemia worsens acute blood–brain barrier injury after forebrain ischemia in rats. Stroke 1993; 24: 111–116.

42. Wass CT, Lanier WL. Glucose modulation of ischaemic brain injury: review and clinical recommendations. Mayo Clin Proc 1996; 71: 801–812.

43. Sjiesko BK. Pathophysiology and treatment of focal cerebral ischemia. Part 1: Pathophysiology. J Neurosurg 1992; 77: 169–184.

44. Sulter G, Elting JW, De Keyser J. Increased serum neurone specific enolase concentrations in patients with hyperglycemic cortical ischaemic stroke. Neurosci Lett 1998; 253: 71–73.

45. Castillo J, Martinez F, Leira R, JM et al. Mortality and morbidity of acute cerebral infarction related to temperature and basal analytic parameters. Cerebrovasc Dis 1994; 4: 56–71.

46. Hindfelt B. The prognostic significance of subfebrility and fever in ischaemic cerebral infarction. Acta Neurol Scand 1976; 53: 72–79.

47. Reith J, Jorgensen HS, Pedersen PM et al. Body temperature in acute stroke: Relation to stroke severity, infarct size, mortality and outcome. Lancet 1996; 347: 422–425.

48. Baker C, Onesti S, Barth K et al. Hypothermic protection following middle cerebral artery occlusion in the rat. Surg Neurol 1991; 36: 175–180.

49. Rosomoff H, Holoday D. Cerebral blood flow and cerebral oxygen consumption during hypothermia. Am J Physiol 1954; 179: 84–88.

50. Busto R, Dietrich W, Globus M-T et al. Small differences in intrahemispheric brain temperature critically determine the extent of ischaemic neuroneal injury. J Cereb Blood Flow Metab 1987; 7: 729–738.

51. Ginsberg MD, Busto R. Combating hyperthermia in acute stroke. A significant clinical concern. Stroke 1998; 29: 529–534.

52. De Keyser J. Antipyretics in acute ischaemic stroke. Lancet 1998; 352: 6–7.

53. Hommel M, Bogousslavsky J. Thrombolytics in acute cerebral ischaemia. Exp Opin Invest Drugs 1994; 3: 1011–1020.

54. Fibrinolytic Therapy Trialists (FTT) Collaborative Group. Indications for fibrinolytic therapy in suspected myocardial infarction: collaborative overview of early mortality and major morbidity results from all randomised trials of more than 1000 patients. Lancet 1994; 343: 311–322.

55. The National Institute of Neurological Disorders and Stroke rt-PA Stroke Study Group. Tissue plasminogen activator for acute ischaemic stroke. N Engl J Med 1995; 333: 1581–1587.

56. Hacke W, Kaste M, Fieschi C et al. Randomised double blind placebo controlled trial of thrombolytic therapy with intravenous alteplase in acute ischaemic stroke (ECASS 11). Lancet 1998; 352: 1245–1251.

57. Multicenter Acute Stroke Trial – Italy (MAST-1) Group. Randomised controlled trial of streptokinase, aspirin, and combination of both in treatment of acute ischaemic stroke. Lancet 1995; 346: 1509–1514.

58. Donnan GA, Davis SM, Chambers BR et al. For the Australian Streptokinase (ASK) Trial Study Group. Sreptokinase for acute ischaemic stroke with relationship to time of administration. JAMA 1996; 276: 961–966.

59. Multi-center Acute Stroke Trial-Europe Study Group. Thrombolytic therapy with streptokinase in acute ischaemic stroke. N Engl J Med 1996; 335: 145–150.

60. Hacke W, Kaste M, Fieschi C et al. For the ECASS Study Group. Intravenous thrombolysis with recombinant tissue plasminogen activator for acute hemispheric stroke. JAMA 1995; 274: 1017–1025.

61. Wardlaw JM, Warlow CP, Counsell C. Systematic review of evidence on thrombolytic therapy for acute ischaemic stroke. Lancet 1997; 350: 607–614.

62. Baron JC, von Kummar R, Del Zoppo GJ. Treatment of acute ischaemic stroke: challenging the concept of a rigid and universal time window. Stroke 1995; 26: 2219–2221.

63. Koroshetz WJ, Gonzalez G. Diffusion weighted MRI: An ECG for brain attack? Ann Neurology 1997; 41: 565–566.

64. Brott TG. Reopening occluded cerebral arteries. In: Bogousslavsky J (ed) Acute stroke treatment. Martin Dunitz, London, 1997, pp 109–148.

65. Fiesci C, Argentino C, Lenzi GL et al. Clinical and instrumental evaluation of patients with ischaemic stroke within the first 6 hours. J Neurol Sci 1989; 91: 311–322.

66. Mitchell PJ, Gerraty R, Donnan GA et al. Thrombolysis in the vertebrobasilar circulation: the Australian Urokinase Study (AUST): a pilot study. Cerebrovasc Dis 1997; 7: 94–99.

67. PROACT. A phase II randomised trial of recombinant pro-urokinase by direct arterial delivery in acute middle cerebral artery stroke. Stroke 1998; 29: 4–11.

68. Muir KW, Lees KR. Clinical experience with excitatory amino acid antagonist drugs. Stroke 1995; 3: 503–513.

69. Mohr J, Orgogozo J, Harrison M et al. Metaanalysis of oral nimodipine trials in acute ischaemic stroke. Cerebrovasc Dis 1994; 4: 197–203.

70. Grotta J, Clark W, Coull B et al. Safety and tolerability of the glutamate antagonist CGS 19755 (Selfotel) in patients with acute ischaemic stroke: results of a phase 11a randomised trial. Stroke1995; 26: 602–605.

71. Edwards D and the CNS 1102-008 Study Group. Cerestat (aptiganel hydrochloride) in the treatment of acute ischaemic stroke: results of a phase 11 trial. Neurology 1996; 46: A424.

72. Diener HC, Kaste M, Hacke P et al. For the LUB-INT-5 Lubelozole Study Group. Lubelozole in acute ischaemic stroke. Stroke 1997; 28: 271.

73. Chlomethiazole Acute Stroke Study Collaborative Group. The Chlomethiazole Acute Stroke Study (CLASS), II: results of a randomised controlled study of Chlomethiazole versus placebo in 545 acute stroke patients classified as total anterior circulation syndrome (TACS). Cerebrovascular Dis 1997; 7: 19.

74. Enlimomab Acute Stroke Trial Study Group. The Enlimomab Acute Stroke Trial Final Results. Neurology 1997; 48: A270.

75. Clark W, Warech S for the Citocholine Study Group. Randomised dose response trial of citicholine in acute ischaemic stroke patients. Neurology 1996; 46: A425.

76. Lees KR. Does Neuroprotection improve stroke outcome? Lancet 1998; 351: 1447–1448.

77. Muir KW, Grosset DG. Neuroprotection for acute stroke. Making clinical trials work Stroke 1999; 30: 180–182

78. Marchal G, Serrati C, Rioux P et al. PET imaging of cerebral perfusion and oxygen consumption in acute ischaemic stroke: relation to outcome. Lancet 1993; 341: 925–927.

79. Bamford J, Sandercock P, Dennis MS et al. The frequency, cause and timing of death within 30 days of a first stroke: the Oxfordshire Community Stroke Project. J Neurol Neurosurg Psychiatry 1990; 53: 824–829.

80. Britton M, de Faire U, Helmers C et al. Prognostication in acute cerebrovascular disease. Acta Med Scand 1980; 207: 37–42.

81. Bamford J, Sandercock PAG, Dennis MS et al. A prospective study of acute cerebrovascular disease in the community: the Oxfordshire Community Stroke Project 1981–86. 2. Incidence case fatality rates and overall outcome at one year of cerebral infarction, primary intracerebral and subarachnoid haemorrhage. J Neurology, Neurosurgery Psychiatry 1990; 53: 16–22.

82. Alexandrov AV, Bladin CF, Meslin EM, Norris JW. Do-not-resuscitate orders in acute stroke. Neurology 1995; 45: 634–640.

83. Kennedy FB, Pozen TJ, Gabelman EH et al. Stroke intensive care units – an appraisal. Am Health J 1970; 80(2): 188–196.

84. Pitner SE, Mance CJ. An evaluation of stroke intensive care: results from a municipal hospital. Stroke 1973; 4: 737–741.

85. Drake WE, Hamilton MJ, Carlsson et al. Acute stroke management and patient outcome: the value of neurovascular care units (NCU). Stroke 1973; 4: 933–945.

86. Hacke W, Schwab S, De Georgia M. Intensive care of acute ischaemic stroke. Cerebrovasc Dis 1994; 4: 385–392.

87. Woodcock J, Ropper AH, Kennedy SK. High dose barbiturates in non-traumatic brain swelling: ICP reduction and effect on outcome. Stroke 1982; 13: 785–787.

88. Frank JI. Large hemisphere infarction, deterioration and intracranial pressure. Neurology 1995; 45: 1286–1290.

89. Rogvi-Hansen B, Boysen G. IV glycerol treatment in acute ischaemic stroke. In: Warlow C, Van Gijn J, Sandercock P (eds) Stroke Module of the Cochrane Collaboration Database of Systematic Reviews. The Cochrane Library; Issue 3 Update Software, Oxford, 1995.

90. Rieke K, Krieger D, Adams H-P et al. Therapeutic strategies in space-occupying cerebellar infarction based on clinical, neuroradiological and neurophysiological data. Cerebrovasc Dis 1993; 3: 45–55.

91. Muffelmann B, Busse O, Jaub M et al. GASCIS-multicentre trial about space occupying cerebellar strokes. Cerebrovasc Dis 1995; 594: 240.

92. Hacke W, Scwab S, Horn M et al. Malignant middle cerebral artery infarction: clinical course and prognostic signs. Arch Neurol 1996; 53: 309–315.

93. Forsting M, Reith W, Schabitz WR et al. Decompressive craniectomy for cerebral infarction. An experimental study in rats. Stroke 1995; 26: 259–264.

94. Rieke K, Schwab S, Krieger D et al. Decompressive surgery in space occupying hemispheric infarction: results of an open, prospective study. Crit Care Med 1995; 23: 1576–1587.

95. Asplund K. Haemodilution in acute stroke. In: Warlow C, Van Gijn J, Sandercock P (eds) Stroke Module of Cochrane Collaboration Database of Systematic Reviews Update Software, Oxford, 1995

26

NEUROMUSCULAR DISEASE IN THE NEUROLOGICAL INTENSIVE CARE UNIT

Alasdair J. Coles

INTRODUCTION

Even in neurological intensive care units, neuromuscular disease is a relatively infrequent cause of admission. In Fink and Rowland's survey of 272 admissions to a New York neurological intensive care unit, only two patients presented with neuromuscular disease.[1] Yet it is important for intensivists to be familiar with at least the major neuromuscular diseases, namely the Guillain–Barré syndrome and myasthenia gravis, for failure to recognize eminent respiratory failure in these conditions and institute appropriate care remains an appreciable cause of unnecessary morbidity and mortality. The fall in the mortality of Guillain–Barré syndrome from 9–13% in early series[2,3] to the 5% of more recent series[4] is entirely attributable to improved intensive supportive rather than any specific therapy.

In the early 1970s, an account of neuromuscular diseases presenting with respiratory failure would have been sufficient for an analysis of neuromuscular disease on the neurological intensive care unit.[3] However, since that time, a family of neuromuscular diseases has been recognized that are acquired on the intensive care unit. After its first description in patients with asthma on steroid therapy, the entity of a critical illness necrotizing myopathy has been proposed.[5] Then, in the early 1980s, a diffuse axonal polyneuropathy that delayed weaning from non-neurogenic respiratory failure was described[6] and the designation 'critical illness polyneuropathy' emerged (although, in fact, it had been recognized as early as 1956[7]). Impairment of neuromuscular transmission, due to the prolonged action of neuromuscular blocking agents, was recognized in the early 1990s.[8] These neuromuscular complications of intensive care therapy are a significant cause of morbidity and usually delay discharge from the intensive care unit. They are the most common indication for electrophysiological studies in the intensive care unit; in a study of 92 patients with weakness in the intensive care unit requiring electromyography, 25 patients had preexisting neuromuscular disease that had prompted admission, 37 had acquired a 'critical illness myopathy' and 12 had a critical illness polyneuropathy.[9]

This chapter reviews briefly both those neuromuscular diseases presenting to the intensive care unit and those that may be acquired during intensive treatment of unrelated conditions. Within the first of these categories, particular attention is paid to the two most common neuromuscular causes of admission to the intensive care unit: Guillain–Barré syndrome and myasthenia gravis. Other similar reviews are available to the interested reader.[10–13]

NEUROMUSCULAR DISEASES PRESENTING TO THE NEUROLOGICAL INTENSIVE CARE UNIT

Rapidly progressive paralysis that includes the respiratory muscles is a frightening condition for patient and doctor alike. When faced with such a patient, the first step is to assess respiratory function. The physician's goal is to anticipate respiratory failure with sufficient time to organize admission to the nearest intensive care unit and institute therapy and plan elective intubation. Traditional bedside tests of vital capacity, such as the ability to blow out a candle or the duration of an exhaled breath, are useful only when spirometry is unavailable. Important physical signs are confusion, agitation and headache, which may indicate hypoxaemia; the use of accessory muscles of respiration and tachypnoea; paradoxical indrawing of the abdomen during inspiration, suggesting diaphragmatic paralysis; and the signs of right heart failure which may imply chronic respiratory failure.

The key investigation is vital capacity, which should be measured in all patients with an acute neuromuscular syndrome, regardless of the level of suspicion of respiratory compromise. Not only is the absolute measure of vital capacity important but also the rate of change in successive measures. The normal vital capacity is about 70 ml/kg. From the experience in Guillain–Barré syndrome, it is recommended that elective intubation be considered at 12–15 ml/kg or at 15 ml/kg if there is evidence of a progressive deterioration over the preceding 4–6 h.[14] For a 70 kg person, intubation should therefore be considered when the vital capacity has reached 1 l. Ideally, patients should be admitted to an intensive care unit well before intubation is necessary, with vital capacity at 20–30 ml/kg. A practical difficulty in measuring vital capacity arises in patients with a facial diplegia that causes weakness of the lips sufficient to compromise the seal necessary for accurate spirometry or bulbar weakness that allows nasal escape. The appropriate masks to correct these problems may not be available. Common errors in respiratory assessment of neuromuscular disease are the measurement of peak flow rates (which may be normal in patients with advanced neuromuscular respiratory failure) and reliance on serial arterial blood gases. The vital capacity may have fallen by 60% or so – to 25 ml/kg – before hypoxaemia is first measured and hypercapnia is seen usually only after a fall to 5–10 ml/kg.

Having secured safe ventilation, thoughts should turn to the cause of respiratory failure. The list of neuromuscular conditions that may cause acute respiratory failure is lengthy (Table 26.1), although in practice the principal causes are Guillain–Barré syndrome and myasthenia gravis, a detailed account of which follows. It is not always easy to arrive quickly at a clinical diagnosis. Physical signs may be confusing or misleading. For instance, it is relatively common to have difficulty distinguishing an acute myelopathy from a rapid polyneuropathy, despite the clearcut distinctions described in textbooks. Acute myelopathies may present with areflexia and an absent spinal cord level and bladder dysfunction is occasionally seen in Guillain–Barré syndrome. Investigations are usually necessary and those to consider urgently are spinal cord imaging, a creatinine kinase and electrophysiology.

Many myopathies and muscular dystrophies cause insidious respiratory failure when at an advanced stage. Ideally appropriate domiciliary ventilation will have been instituted long before ventilation on an intensive care unit is necessary but occasional such patients will present acutely because of a pulmonary infection that depletes a previously unnoticed dwindling ventilatory capacity. Finally, some neuromuscular disorders may require the attentions of an intensivist to protect the upper airways in bulbar failure rather than respiratory failure (Box 26.1).

GUILLAIN–BARRÉ SYNDROME

The eponym Guillain–Barré syndrome derives from the description of an acute ascending paralytic

Table 26.1	Differential diagnosis of respiratory failure due to neuromuscular disease	
Site	Disease	Clues to diagnosis
Spinal Cord	Transverse myelitis Epidural haematoma, abscess	Early sphincter disturbance, spinal cord level back pain
Motor neurone	Amyotrophic lateral sclerosis	Mixed upper and lower motor neurone signs, sensation normal
	Poliomyelitis	Flaccid paralysis, lymphocytic encephalitis, developing world
Acute polyneuropathy	AIDP (Guillain–Barré) Acute axonal polyneuropathy Porphyria Diphtheria	See text See text Abdominal pain, mental state disturbance, drugs Pharyngitis, cranial polyneuropathy, reduced pupillary accommodation
	Shellfish poisoning	Facial and limb paresthesiae, vomiting and diarrhoea
	Hypophosphataemia	Parenteral alimentation, cranial neuropathies, encephalopathy
Neuromuscular failure	Myasthenia gravis Lambert-Eaton myasthenia syndrome Hypocalcaemia Hypermagnesaemia Botulism	See text Autonomic disturbance, posttetanic potentiation Renal failure, drugs Encephalopathy, renal failure Tinned food, bulbar weakness and pupillary paralysis
	Organophosphate poisoning	Insecticides, cholinesterase inhibitors
Myopathy	Dermato- and polymyositis Myoglobinuric myopathy Hypokalaemic paralysis Trichinosis myositis	Ck very elevated, possible underlying malignancy Ck very elevated, drugs, toxins Thyrotoxicosis in Asian males Periorbital oedema, cardiomyopathy, trichinella on muscle biopsy
	Acid maltase deficiency	Acute-on-chronic respiratory failure, usually due to superadded infection
	Mitochoindrial myopathy	Acute-on-chronic respiratory failure, usually due to superadded infection
	Myotonic dystrophy	Acute-on-chronic respiratory failure, usually due to superadded infection
	Limb girdle muscular dystrophy	Acute-on-chronic respiratory failure, usually due to superadded infection

Myasthenia gravis
Polymyositis
Motor neurone disease (ALS)
Craniocervical Guillain–Barré syndrome
Botulism
Diphtheria

Box 26.1   Neuromuscular causes of acute laryngeal and bulbar failure

illness by Guillain, Barré and Strohl in 1916[15] (although Landry's 1859[16] account was earlier). On the basis of clinical criteria, electrophysiological characteristics and serum antiganglioside antibodies, several different variants of Guillain–Barré syndrome are now recognized; whether these are distinct disease entities or represent the spectrum of one pathogenic process is unclear and for practical purposes irrelevant. The prototypical form of Guillain–Barré syndrome is acute inflammatory demyelinating polyneuropathy, which occurs with an incidence of 1–2 cases per 100 000[17] affecting any age with no familial tendency or defined genetic susceptibility. Conventional diagnostic criteria for acute inflammatory demyelinating polyneuropathy are summarized in Box 26.2, derived from Asbury's work.[18,19]

Pathogenesis

In cases of acute inflammatory demyelinating polyneuropathy that come to postmortem, which necessarily represent the most severe cases, there is mononuclear cell infiltration and segmental demyelination of cranial nerves, dorsal and ventral nerve roots, dorsal root ganglia and peripheral nerves.[20] The

Clinical features required for diagnosis
Progressive motor weakness of more than one limb
Areflexia, usually complete, or distal areflexia with reduced biceps and knee jerks

Clinical features supportive of diagnosis
Progression
Relative symmetry
Mild sensory symptoms and signs
Cranial nerve involvement, especially facial weakness
Absence of fever
Autonomic dysfunction

Clinical features casting doubt on diagnosis
Marked, persistent asymmetry of weakness
Persistent bladder or bowel disturbance
More than 50 lymphocytes per ml in CSF
Sharp sensory level

Cerebrospinal fluid abnormalities in support of diagnosis
Elevated protein after the first week of the illness
Less than 10 lymphocytes per ml of CSF

Electrophysiological features in support of diagnosis
Three of the following four are required:
Reduction in conduction velocity in two or more motor nerves
Conduction block or temporal dispersion in one or more motor nerves
Prolonged distal latencies in two or more nerves
Absent or prolonged F waves in two or more nerves

Features that exclude the diagnosis
Current history of volatile substance abuse
Porphyria
Recent diphtheria
Lead neuropathy
Pure sensory syndrome

Box 26.2   Diagnostic criteria for Guillain–Barré syndrome

eventual distal preponderance of signs probably simply reflects the increased susceptibility of these nerves to disruption by virtue of their greater length. At first CD4+ T-cells dominate the infiltrate,[21] followed by macrophages which lie under the basement membrane of the nerve fibre, adjacent to the superficial lamellae of the nerve.[22] The myelin sheath is first disrupted at the node of Ranvier, where there is retraction and then myelin breakdown. In severe lesions, there is axonal degeneration as well. After the first week of illness, there are signs of Schwann cell proliferation and then remyelination of denuded axons, even while active demyelination persists in other areas.[23]

As Guillain–Barré syndrome is relatively common, many of the claimed antecedent infections may be attributable to chance. But there does appear to be robust evidence for a pathogenic role for prior infection with the herpesviruses CMV (in 15% of cases) and EBV.[24] Acute inflammatory demyelinating polyneuropathy may also occur at the time of primary infection with HIV as a seroconversion illness.[25] Evidence of *Campylobacter jejuni* infection has been found in up to 40% of patients with Guillain–Barré syndrome, often in the absence of a history of diarrhoea,[26] and in similar studies evidence of recent exposure to *Mycoplasma pneumoniae* has been found in 5%.[27] In their considered review, Arnason and Soliven concluded that the only additional established precipitants of Guillain–Barré syndrome were surgery and immunization with vaccines containing nervous tissue (such as old forms of rabies vaccine) and possibly lymphoma.[23]

A pathogenic mechanism of antecedent infection in Guillain–Barré syndrome is suggested by the presence of circulating antibodies against neural gangliosides. Epitopes on *Campylobacter jejuni* have been found that mimic ganglioside antibodies.[28–30] It is proposed that the immune response to the infection generates self-reactive antibodies that mediate the inflammatory demyelination.

Clinical features

Two-thirds of patients describe an antecedent illness of diarrhoea or a 'flu-like' upper respiratory tract infection with cough. The neurological illness starts 1–3 weeks later, usually after the antecedent symptoms have settled. The natural history of acute inflammatory demyelinating polyneuropathy is an evolution phase that is complete in two weeks in 50% and by four weeks in 90%,[31] followed by a plateau phase lasting less than four weeks in 85% and less than three weeks in 70%.[32] In a large, community-based study 33% of patients required ventilation acutely and 3% died in

the acute illness without ventilation. At one year, 13% of patients were dead, 14% were unable to walk and 7% were severely disabled.[31]

The usual presenting complaint is of symmetrical weakness. This commonly ascends from the legs to the arms and may be heralded by distal parasthesiae. For reasons that are not clear, interscapular back pain may be prominent as the first symptom. Later neuropathic pain may be a significant management problem, all too easily forgotten in the management of the paralysed patient. It is usual for patients to be areflexic at presentation. Proximal limb weakness is the earliest motor sign usually. Sensory abnormalities at presentation are less severe than might be expected from the complaints of dysesthesiae. Facial weakness is found in half of cases and oropharyngeal involvement is seen in 40%.[31]

Some 65% of patients with Guillain–Barré syndrome have impaired autonomic function. If this is expressed as a resting tachycardia treatment may not be required but bradycardia may lead to sinus arrest and the requirement for pacing.[33] Orthostatic hypotension can arise, due to diminished peripheral vascular tone. Hypotensive episodes may follow suctioning or intubation and persistent hypertension is also seen.

Variants of Guillain–Barré syndrome

Any number of clinical syndromes have been attributed to variants of acute inflammatory demyelinating polyneuropathy. The most robust candidates are the Miller Fisher syndrome and the pharyngeal-cervical-brachial variant. The Miller Fisher syndrome consists of the triad of ataxia, ophthalmoplegia and areflexia, without weakness.[34] Ventilatory support is not usually required but typical Miller Fisher patients may evolve into acute inflammatory demyelinating polyneuropathy syndromes and thus lead to respiratory failure. The presence of electrophysiological evidence of a demyelinating peripheral neuropathy in Miller Fisher syndrome supports the association with acute inflammatory demyelinating polyneuropathy. So too does the fact that such patients often have the anti-GMQ1b ganglioside antibody[29] that is also found in the 5% of patients with otherwise classic acute inflammatory demyelinating polyneuropathy who have an opthalmoplegia. In the pharyngeal-cervical-brachial variant, leg reflexes may be spared throughout the illness.[35] Intubation may be required to protect the airway.

In northern China, Japan and Mexico, an acute motor axonal neuropathy is more usually encountered than acute inflammatory demyelinating polyneuropathy.[36–38] Pathological studies show little inflammation and demyelination but macrophages accumulate at nodes of Ranvier and there is Wallerian degeneration.[39] In these patients there is a specific anti-ganglioside antibody, anti-GD1a, that is not found in acute inflammatory demyelinating polyneuropathy.[40] The prognosis for recovery is worse than for acute inflammatory demyelinating polyneuropathy.

Management of Guillain–Barré syndrome on the intensive care unit

Between 10% and 33% of patients with acute inflammatory demyelinating polyneuropathy will need admission to an intensive care unit.[41,42] This is predominantly to manage respiratory failure, although bulbar weakness, dysautonomia, sepsis and hypotension are also indications for admission. Ropper et al have made a careful clinical study of Guillain–Barré syndrome and highlight oropharyngeal weakness, as well as weakness of shoulder elevation and neck flexion, as harbingers of impending respiratory failure.[32] Ng et al noted in their patients that respiratory failure always paralleled limb and axial weakness and, furthermore, that bulbar weakness was always associated with ventilatory failure.[4]

Amongst a population of 79 patients with severe Guillain–Barré syndrome receiving intensive care, the mortality was 5% and the median duration of ventilation was 21 days.[4] Half the patients had respiratory tract infections and two patients required pacing for complete heart block; 20 patients developed severe persistent hyponatraemia due to the syndrome of inappropriate antidiuretic hormone secretion. Half the patients complained of pain that was resistant to simple analgesics and opiates; relief was obtained by the combination of an antidepressant and midazolam. Factors predicting a poor prognostic outcome were the duration of the plateau phase and the duration of ventilation. As well as mechanical ventilation, supportive treatment of Guillain–Barré syndrome should include monitoring for dysautonomia, rigorous physiotherapy to avoid contractures, eye care in patients with facial weakness, parenteral nutrition, analgesia and prophylaxis against DVT. The early involvement of speech therapists to facilitate communication is a boon to patients' morale, which usually fluctuates during the course of an intensive care unit admission. In discussion with patients who have recovered from Guillain–Barré syndrome, many report that they expected to die and that they did not believe their physicians' assurances of a recovery.

Two immunomodulatory therapies have proven efficacy in acute inflammatory demyelinating polyneuropathy: plasma exchange and intravenous immunoglobulin. Plasma exchange of 3–5 treatments, exchanging 200 ml/kg, in 245 patients reduced the time to recovery of ambulation from 85 days in controls to 53 days.[43] Three studies have now shown that intravenous immunoglobulin is as effective as plasma exchange in reducing the duration of disability and hospital stay.[44–46] In the largest of these studies,[46] there was a third arm of plasma exchange followed by intravenous immunoglobulin, which conferred no additional benefit. Once an improvement was seen in this study, only 1.6% of patients experienced an acute relapse. Intravenous immunoglobulin is easier to administer than plasmapheresis but it is expensive. Patients with dysautonomia or cardiovascular disease may tolerate intravenous immunoglobulin more easily but it is not without adverse effect: anaphylaxis, aseptic meningitis and renal failure are all reported and the potential dangers of transfusing a blood product should be recognized. Interestingly, despite the clear impact of immunotherapies on hospital stay and residual disability, the mortality rate of 5% in these studies is similar to that of series of untreated patients.

MYASTHENIA GRAVIS

In 1893, Jolly described a disease which he termed 'myasthenia gravis pseudoparalytica', pointing out that weakness increased with exercise and decreased with rest and that physostigmine might be an appropriate treatment.[47] Then in 1936, the therapeutic effect of thymectomy was noted.[48] Since then, there has been an outpouring of immunological studies on myasthenia gravis and its experimental counterparts, as it has become a prototypical organ-specific autoimmune disease. Despite this, the pathogenic link between thymic hyperplasia and the disease process remains mysterious.

Myasthenia gravis is an autoimmune disorder in which antibodies are directed against the acetylcholine receptor antibodies of the neuromuscular junction. The prevalence of 1–10 per 100 000 is made up of two broad populations: one mainly women in their 20s and 30s and one predominantly men aged between 50 and 70. A thymoma may occur in association with myasthenia gravis at any age; it is an absolute indication for a thymectomy although this will not influence the myasthenia gravis. In contrast, thymectomy is a disease-modifying treatment, especially in young women with thymic hyperplasia. The cardinal feature of myasthenia gravis is fatiguability; as movements are repeated, so the occupancy of acetylcholine receptors at the neuromuscular junction increases and less power is generated. The distribution of muscle weakness is also characteristic. In 70% of patients, there is ptosis and ophthalmoplegia due to weakness of some or all of the external ocular muscles. In 15%, weakness remains confined to the ocular muscles but the remainder develop generalized myasthenia within two years which usually presents as oropharyngeal or proximal limb weakness.[49] The progression from ocular to generalized disease commonly proceeds in a march from facial to bulbar weakness and then to truncal and limb muscles. The clinical diagnosis of myasthenia gravis is supported by a positive Tensilon test (see below), positive acetylcholine antibodies in 85% of patients with generalized myasthenia gravis[50] and a decremental response to repetitive stimulation on electromyography. The two classes of maintenance treatment are anticholinesterase inhibitors and immunomodulators, such as corticosteroids with or without azathioprine. It is common practice in the UK, but not the USA, to introduce corticosteroids slowly, because they may rarely cause an exacerbation of the disease.[51]

Myasthenia gravis in the intensive care unit

It is very rare for myasthenia gravis to present initially with such severity as to require intensive care. In a study of 1036 patients followed between 1940 and 1980, only 1% presented with dyspnoea.[52] There are two common situations in which intensivists encounter patients with myasthenia gravis. The first is during the pre- and postoperative management of patients undergoing a thymectomy. In some centres, even well patients are treated aggressively with plasma exchange prior to thymectomy. The procedure may be transcervical,[53] in which case there is a danger of leaving thymic tissue, or transsternal, which carries a slightly greater morbidity.[54] After the procedure, there is usually a dramatic symptomatic improvement within 24 h which lasts for a few days.

The most common presentation of myasthenia gravis to the intensive care unit is rapidly progressive bulbar or respiratory failure in a patient in whom the diagnosis has previously been established. This is usually due to a *myasthenic crisis* in which case the disease process has overwhelmed attempts at therapy. However, neuromuscular blockade can also be induced by excessive use of anticholinesterase inhibitors, which is termed a *cholinergic crisis*. In theory, these may be distinguished clinically by the muscarinic effects associated with a cholinergic crisis. A more robust discriminator is a Tensilon test. In a cholinergic crisis, the test dose of 1 mg of intravenous edrophonium increases weakness and provokes cramps, miosis, vomiting and diarrhoea. However, a reduction of weakness with 1–10 mg indicates a myasthenic crisis. In an acute situation, a controlled Tensilon test may be impractical and, furthermore, it

is claimed that myasthenic and cholinergic crises can coexist in the same patient and even the same muscle.[55] A pragmatic approach is to withdraw or at least reduce all anticholinesterase drugs in patients who proceed to more potent treatments or mechanical ventilation.

Myasthenic crises occur in 15–20% of patients with myasthenia gravis, most (74%) within the first two years of the disease and at a median of eight months after the onset of symptoms. It is more common in patients with a thymoma and carries a mortality of 10% due to comorbid medical illness. In two-thirds of patients a precipitating cause can be found, most commonly infection.[56] It is very important to identify any drugs that may have an anticholinergic effect (Box 26.3).

The indications for intubation and ventilation of the patient in myasthenic crisis are similar to those listed above for Guillain–Barré syndrome. Unlike in

---

Antibiotics
Neomycin
Kanamycin
Streptomycin
Gentamicin
Tetracyclines
Erythromycin
Polymixin
Ampicillin

Cardiovascular
β-Adrenergic blockers
Quinidine
Procainamide
Verapamil

CNS drugs
Chlorpromazine
Lithium
Morphine

Drugs for rheumatoid arthritis
D-penacillamine
Chloroquine
Quinine

Other
Lidocaine
Corticosteroids (see text)
Procaine
Gadolinium (contrast agent for MRI)

Box 26.3　Drugs that may exacerbate myasthenia gravis (from references[12,55])

Guillain–Barré syndrome, though, it would be expected that bulbar failure would precede respiratory failure and so accurate measurement of the vital capacity may be difficult. Having secured safe ventilation, initiated treatment of any provoking infections and withdrawn anticholinesterase and any drugs with anticholinergic effect, consideration should be given to acute disease-modifying treatment. The orthodox approach is plasma exchange. Various regimes have been tried, ranging from exchange of 5% of body volume every 2–15 days to daily exchanges of 2 l, and there is no absolute consensus.[57] Objective improvement may be noticed after a few days of plasmapheresis with a consequent fall in the acetylcholine antibody titre. Over recent years, intravenous immunoglobulin has been suggested as a treatment of the myasthenic crisis. But it has not yet acquired the established role in this condition as in Guillain–Barré syndrome.[58–60]

Once plasma exchange is stopped, the acetylcholine receptor antibody titre rises again within a few days, so it has no role in the long-term management of myasthenia gravis. It does, however, ameliorate a myasthenic crisis with sufficient time to correct its precipitating cause and initiate maintenance immunosuppression in the form of corticosteroids. Two schools of thought exist on the dosage of steroids in this situation. One, mindful of the potential of high-dose corticosteroids to transiently exacerbate myasthenia gravis, advocates the gradual increase of a low initiating dose (such as 10 mg prednisolone on alternate days). The other suggests that high doses (including giving pulsed intravenous methylprednisolone up to 2 g/day[61,62]) can be given abruptly because any such deterioration will occur in the controlled environment of the intensive care unit. Azathioprine is increasingly used to minimize the steroid dose required to control myasthenia gravis but it takes several months to exert its effect,[63] so has no place in the management of the myasthenic crisis.

NEUROMUSCULAR COMPLICATIONS OF INTENSIVE CARE

Neuromuscular illness may develop during the course of an admission to an intensive care unit and usually presents as a failure to wean patients off ventilation. The principal causes of such a syndrome are critical illness polyneuropathy, prolonged neuromuscular blockade and a necrotizing myopathy (see Box 26.4). Because such patients are often encephalopathic and treated with muscle relaxants and sedatives, clinical examination may be distinctly unrewarding. The presence of sensory symptoms points to a polyneuropathy, whereas their lack suggests either prolonged neuromuscular blockade or a myopathy. Reflexes may be both present or absent in critical illness polyneuropathy and the critical illness myopathies. Critical investigations are a serum creatinine kinase and neurophysiological examination of the nerves, which in skilled hands may include assessment of phrenic nerve conduction.[64]

CRITICAL ILLNESS NEUROPATHY

Critical illness polyneuropathy is a diffuse axonal polyneuropathy that most usually manifests as delayed weaning from ventilation. It was first recognized in 1956[7] and redescribed in the 1980s.[6,65] In a prospective study, electrophysiological evidence for a critical illness neuropathy was found in 70% of patients with sepsis and multiorgan failure.[66] Sepsis is its usual setting, although it has also been described in other conditions that promote multiorgan failure such as pancreatitis, trauma, burns and cardiovascular shock of any cause. These associations have raised the possibility that critical illness polyneuropathy is caused by some component of the inflammatory response such as nitric oxide and the Th1 cytokines IFN-γ and TNF-α. Some experimental studies lend support to this hypothesis,[67,68] but in morphological studies in man no inflammation is seen

Critical illness polyneuropathy	
Prolonged neuromuscular blockade	Non-depolarizing neuromuscular blockade
	Aminoglycoside antibiotics
Critical illness myopathy	Non-depolarizing neuromuscular blockade
	Steroids
Phrenic nerve palsy	Trauma, surgery
Guillain–Barré syndrome	Associated with e.g. mycoplasma pneumonia
Porphyria	Precipitated by drugs
Wound botulism	

Box 26.4   Neuromuscular causes of failure to wean from mechanical ventilation

but rather axonal degeneration and loss of dorsal root ganglia.[65] Unlike critical illness myopathy, drugs are not implicated in critical illness polyneuropathy. In patients who survive the precipitating illness, it pursues a monophasic course that usually recovers, over weeks in mild cases and over months in more severe.[69] There is no established treatment.

The physical signs of critical illness polyneuropathy are weakness and muscle wasting, usually with loss of deep tendon reflexes; however, the presence of reflexes does not exclude the diagnosis.[65] The face is usually spared clinically although may be involved electrophysiologically.[11] Often patients are receiving muscle relaxants and sedatives, in which case physical examination is largely unrewarding. The investigations of choice are nerve conduction studies, which usually show reduced compound muscle action potentials and sensory nerve action potentials, and electromyography, which shows fibrillations and positive sharp waves in proximal and distal muscles.[70]

A differential diagnosis that should tax the physician making the diagnosis of critical illness polyneuropathy – because of its potential implications for therapy – is Guillain–Barré syndrome, which may occur following surgery or sepsis. The clinical features that distinguish these conditions are the presence of facial weakness, raised CSF protein and conduction velocity slowing (indicating demyelination) in Guillain–Barré syndrome.[71] As noted above, though, there is a predominantly motor axonal variant of Guillain–Barré syndrome which may mimic critical illness polyneuropathy.

PROLONGED NEUROMUSCULAR BLOCKADE

In patients being treated with high doses of non-depolarizing neuromuscular blocking agents (pancuronium, vecuronium, atracurium), elevated plasma levels and abnormal decrement of the compound muscle action potential on repetitive stimulation may be found for up to 14 days after stopping the drug.[72] This may be due to impaired drug metabolism due to renal failure[8] or to the concomitant use of aminoglycosides and polypeptide antibiotics which increase the neuromuscular block.[73]

CRITICAL ILLNESS MYOPATHIES

It is probable that several different myopathies occur in the context of intensively treated patients. These range from mild disuse atrophy, in which there is loss of type II fibres and normal creatinine kinase, to a necrotizing myopathy in which there is elevation of the serum creatinine kinase. The latter was first seen in patients with

asthma treated using steroids and non-depolarizing neuromuscular blockade[5] and has been compared histologically to the myopathy seen in myasthenia gravis treated with high-dose steroids.[74] Electron microscopy shows a loss of thick filaments in the centre of muscle filaments so the syndrome has been called a thick-fibre myopathy. From these associations has emerged the concept that blockade of neuromuscular transmission accentuates the myopathic effect of steroids.[75] In Lacomis et al's series,[9] 34 of 92 patients studied electrophysiologically in a neurological intensive care unit had evidence of a myopathy acquired whilst on the unit. Of these, 27 had received intravenous corticosteroids and 28 non-depolarizing neuromuscular blockers. The diagnosis was based on the low motor amplitudes and normal sensory amplitudes.

REFERENCES

1. Fink ME, Rowland LP. Respiratory care: diagnosis and management. In: Rowland LP (ed) Merritt's textbook of neurology, 9th edn. Williams and Wilkins, Baltimore, 1995; pp 930–935.

2. McCleave DJ, Fletcher J, Cruden LC. The Guillain–Barré syndrome in intensive care. Anaesth Intens Care 1976; 4: 46–52.

3. O'Donohue WJ Jr, Baker JP, Bell GM, Muren O, Parker CL, Patterson JL Jr. Respiratory failure in neuromuscular disease. Management in a respiratory intensive care unit. JAMA 1976; 235: 733–735.

4. Ng KK, Howard RS, Fish DR et al. Management and outcome of Guillain–Barré syndrome. Q J Med 1995; 88: 243–250.

5. Griffin D, Fairman N, Coursin D, Rawsthorne L, Grossman JE. Acute myopathy during treatment of status asthmaticus with corticosteroids and steroidal muscle relaxants. Chest 1992; 102: 510–514.

6. Bolton CF, Gilbert JJ, Hahn AF, Sibbald WJ. Polyneuropathy in critically ill patients. J Neurol Neurosurg Psychiatry 1984; 47: 1223.

7. Olsen CW. Lesions of peripheral nerves developing during coma. JAMA 1956; 160: 39–41.

8. Segredo V, Caldwell JE, Matthay MA, Sharma ML, Gruenke LD, Miller RD. Persistent paralysis in critically ill patients after long-term administration of vecuronium [see comments]. N Engl J Med 1992; 327: 524–528.

9. Lacomis D, Petrella JT, Giuliani MJ. Causes of neuromuscular weakness in the intensive care unit: a study of ninety-two patients. Muscle Nerve 1998; 21: 610–617.

10. Bolton CF. Management of paralytic neuropathy in the intensive care unit. In: Latov N, Wokke JH, Kelly JJ, (eds). Immunological and infectious diseases of the peripheral nerves. Cambridge University Press, 1998.

11. Hund EF. Neuromuscular complications in the ICU: the spectrum of critical illness-related conditions

causing muscular weakness and weaning failure. J Neurol Sci 1996; 136: 10–16.

12. Bella I, Chad DA. Neuromuscular disorders and acute respiratory failure. Neurol Clin 1998; 16: 391–417.

13. Hughes RA. Management of acute neuromuscular paralysis. J Roy Coll Physicians Lond 1998; 32: 254–259.

14. Ropper AH, Kehne SM. Guillain–Barré syndrome: management of respiratory failure. Neurology 1985; 35: 1662–1665.

15. Guillain G, Barré J, Strohl A. Sur un syndrome de radiculonevrite avec hyperalbuminose du liquide cephalo-rachidien sans reaction cellulaire. Remarques sur les caracteres cliniques et graphiques des reflexes tendineux. Bull Soc Med Hop Paris 1916; 40: 1462.

16. Landry O. Note sur la paralysie ascendante aigue. Gaz Hebd Med Paris 1859; 6: 472,486.

17. Hankey GJ. Guillain–Barré syndrome in Western Australia, 1980–1985. Med J Aust 1987; 146: 130–133.

18. Asbury AK, Arnason B, Karp H, McFarlin D. Criteria for the diagnosis of Guillain–Barré syndrome. Ann Neurol 1978; 3: 565.

19. Asbury AK, Cornblath DR. Assessment of current diagnostic criteria for Guillain–Barré syndrome [see comments]. Ann Neurol 1990; 27(suppl): S21–24.

20. Kanda T, Hayashi H, Tanabe H, Tsubaki T, Oda M. A fulminant case of Guillain–Barre syndrome: topographic and fibre size related analysis of demyelinating changes. J Neurol Neurosurg Psychiatry 1989; 52: 857–864.

21. Honavar M, Tharakan JK, Hughes RA, Leibowitz S, Winer JB. A clinicopathological study of the Guillain–Barré syndrome. Nine cases and literature review. Brain 1991; 114: 1245–1269.

22. Brechenmacher C, Vital C, Deminiere C et al. Guillain–Barré syndrome: an ultrastructural study of peripheral nerve in 65 patients. Clin Neuropathol 1987; 6: 19–24.

23. Arnason BG, Soliven B. Acute inflammatory demyelinating polyradiculoneuronopathy. In: Dyck PJ, Thomas PK, (eds) Peripheral neuropathy. WB Saunders, Philadelphia, 1993.

24. Dowling PC, Cook SD. Role of infection in Guillain–Barré syndrome: laboratory confirmation of herpesviruses in 41 cases. Ann Neurol 1981; 9(suppl): 44–55.

25. Hagberg L, Malmvall BE, Svennerholm L, Alestig K, Norkrans G. Guillain–Barré syndrome as an early manifestation of HIV central nervous system infection. Scand J Infect Dis 1986; 18: 591–592.

26. Kaldor J, Speed BR. Guillain–Barré syndrome and Campylobacter jejuni: a serological study. BMJ 1984; 288: 1867–1870.

27. Goldschmidt B, Menonna J, Fortunato J, Dowling P, Cook S. Mycoplasma antibody in Guillain–Barré syndrome and other neurological disorders. Ann Neurol 1980; 7: 108–112.

28. Yuki N, Taki T, Inagaki F et al. A bacterium lipopolysaccharide that elicits Guillain–Barré syndrome has a GM1 ganglioside-like structure. J Exp Med 1993; 178: 1771–1775.

29. Yuki N, Taki T, Takahashi M et al. Molecular mimicry between GQ1b ganglioside and lipopolysaccharides of Campylobacter jejuni isolated from patients with Fisher's syndrome. Ann Neurol 1994; 36: 791–793.

30. Yuki N, Taki T, Takahashi M et al. Penner's serotype 4 of Campylobacter jejuni has a lipopolysaccharide that bears a GM1 ganglioside epitope as well as one that bears a GD1 a epitope. Infect Immun 1994; 62: 2101–2103.

31. Loffel NB, Rossi LN, Mumenthaler M, Lutschg J, Ludin HP. The Landry–Guillain–Barré syndrome. Complications, prognosis and natural history in 123 cases. J Neurol Sci 1977; 33: 71–79.

32. Ropper AH, Wijdicks EFM, Truax BT. Guillain–Barré syndrome. FA Davis, Philadelphia, 1991.

33. Krone A, Reuther P, Fuhrmeister U. Autonomic dysfunction in polyneuropathies: a report on 106 cases. J Neurol 1983; 230: 111–121.

34. Fisher M. An unusual variant of acute idiopathic polyneuritis (syndrome of ophthalmoplegia, ataxia and areflexia). N Engl J Med 1956; 255: 57.

35. Ropper AH. Unusual clinical variants and signs in Guillain–Barré syndrome. Arch Neurol 1986; 43: 1150–1152.

36. Ramos-Alvarez M, Bessudo L, Sabin AB. Paralytic syndromes associated with noninflammatory cytoplasmic or nuclear neuronopathy. Acute paralytic disease in Mexican children, neuropathologically distinguishable from Landry-Guillain–Barré syndrome. JAMA 1969; 207: 1481–1492.

37. McKhann GM, Cornblath DR, Ho T et al. Clinical and electrophysiological aspects of acute paralytic disease of children and young adults in northern China [see comments]. Lancet 1991; 338: 593–597.

38. Ho TW, Mishu B, Li CY et al. Guillain–Barré syndrome in northern China. Relationship to Campylobacter jejuni infection and anti-glycolipid antibodies. Brain 1995; 118: 597–605.

39. Sobue G, Li M, Terao S et al. Axonal pathology in Japanese Guillain–Barré syndrome: a study of 15 autopsied cases. Neurology 1997; 48: 1694–1700.

40. Ho TW, Willison HJ, Nachamkin I et al. Anti-GD1a antibody is associated with axonal but not demyelinating forms of Guillain–Barré syndrome. Ann Neurol 1999; 45: 168–173.

41. Andersson T, Siden A. A clinical study of the Guillain–Barré syndrome. Acta Neurol Scand 1982; 66: 316–327.

42. Winer JB, Hughes RA, Greenwood RJ, Perkin GD, Healy MJ. Prognosis in Guillain–Barré syndrome. Lancet 1985; 1: 1202–1203.

43. Mendell JR, Kissel JT, Kennedy MS et al. Plasma exchange and prednisone in Guillain–Barre syndrome: a controlled randomized trial. Neurology 1985; 35: 1551–1555.

44. Van Der Meche FG, Schmitz PI. A randomized trial comparing intravenous immune globulin and plasma exchange in Guillain–Barré syndrome. Dutch Guillain–Barré Study Group [see comments]. N Engl J Med 1992; 326: 1123–1129.

45. Bril V, Ilse WK, Pearce R, Dhanani A, Sutton D, Kong K. Pilot trial of immunoglobulin versus plasma exchange in patients with Guillain–Barré syndrome. Neurology 1996; 46: 100–103.

46. Anonymous. Randomised trial of plasma exchange, intravenous immunoglobulin, and combined treatments in Guillain–Barré syndrome. Plasma Exchange/Sandoglobulin Guillain–Barré Syndrome Trial Group [see comments]. Lancet 1997; 349: 225–230.

47. Jolly F. Uber myasthenia gravis pseudoparalytica. Berl Klin Wochenschr 1893; 32: 1.

48. Blalock A, Mason MF, Morgan HF. Myasthenia gravis and tumours of the thymic region: report of a case in which a tumour was removed. Ann Surg 1939; 110: 544.

49. Oosterhuis HJ. The natural course of myasthenia gravis: a long term follow up study. J Neurol Neurosurg Psychiatry 1989; 52: 1121–1127.

50. Yoshikawa H, Lennon VA. Acetylcholine receptor autoantibody secretion by thymocytes: relationship to myasthenia gravis. Neurology 1997; 49: 562–567.

51. Miller RG, Milner Brown HS, Mirka A. Prednisone-induced worsening of neuromuscular function in myasthenia gravis. Neurology 1986; 36: 729–732.

52. Grob D, Brunner NG, Namba T. The natural course of myasthenia gravis and effect of therapeutic measures. Ann N Y Acad Sci 1981; 377: 652–669.

53. Genkins G, Kornfeld P, Papatestas AE, Bender AN, Matta RJ. Clinical experience in more than 2000 patients with myasthenia gravis. Ann N Y Acad Sci 1987; 505: 1989.

54. Jaretzki A 3rd, Penn AS, Younger DS et al. "Maximal" thymectomy for myasthenia gravis. Results. J Thorac Cardiovasc Surg 1988; 95: 747–757.

55. Engel AG. Acquired autoimmune myasthenia gravis. In: Engel AG, Franzini-Armstrong C (eds) Myology, 2nd edn. McGraw-Hill, New York, 1994.

56. Thomas CE, Mayer SA, Gungor Y et al. Myasthenic crisis: clinical features, mortality, complications, and risk factors for prolonged intubation. Neurology 1997; 48: 1253–1260.

57. Anonymous. The utility of therapeutic plasmapheresis for neurological disorders. NIH Consensus Development. JAMA 1986; 256: 1333–1337.

58. Gajdos P, Chevret S, Clair B, Tranchant C, Chastang C. Plasma exchange and intravenous immunoglobulin in autoimmune myasthenia gravis. Ann N Y Acad Sci 1998; 841: 1998.

59. Howard JF Jr. Intravenous immunoglobulin for the treatment of acquired myasthenia gravis. Neurology 1998; 51: S30–36.

60. Jongen JL, Van Doorn PA, Van Der Meche FG. High-dose intravenous immunoglobulin therapy for myasthenia gravis. J Neurol 1998; 245: 26–31.

61. Arsura E, Brunner NG, Namba T, Grob D. High-dose intravenous methylprednisolone in myasthenia gravis. Arch Neurol 1985; 42: 1149–1153.

62. Lindberg C, Andersen O, Lefvert AK. Treatment of myasthenia gravis with methylprednisolone pulse: a double blind study. Acta Neurol Scand 1998; 97: 370–373.

63. Palace J, Newsom Davis J, Lecky B. A randomized double-blind trial of prednisolone alone or with azathioprine in myasthenia gravis. Myasthenia Gravis Study Group. Neurology 1998; 50: 1778–1783.

64. Bolton CF. AAEM minimonograph £40: clinical neurophysiology of the respiratory system. Muscle Nerve 1993; 16: 809–818.

65. Zochodne DW, Bolton CF, Wells GA et al. Critical illness polyneuropathy. A complication of sepsis and multiple organ failure. Brain 1987; 110: 819–841.

66. Witt NJ, Zochodne DW, Bolton CF et al. Peripheral nerve function in sepsis and multiple organ failure [see comments]. Chest 1991; 99: 176–184.

67. Redford EJ, Kapoor R, Smith KJ. Nitric oxide donors reversibly block axonal conduction: demyelinated axons are especially susceptible. Brain 1997; 120: 2149–2157.

68. Redford EJ, Hall SM, Smith KJ. Vascular changes and demyelination induced by the intraneural injection of tumour necrosis factor. Brain 1995; 118: 869–878.

69. Bolton CF, Young GB, Zochodne DW. The neurological complications of sepsis. Ann Neurol 1993; 33: 94–100.

70. Bolton CF, Laverty DA, Brown JD, Witt NJ, Hahn AF, Sibbald WJ. Critically ill polyneuropathy: electrophysiological studies and differentiation from Guillain–Barré syndrome. J Neurol Neurosurg Psychiatry 1986; 49: 563–573.

71. Spitzer AR, Giancarlo T, Maher L, Awerbuch G, Bowles A. Neuromuscular causes of prolonged ventilator dependency. Muscle Nerve 1992; 15: 682–686.

72. Barohn RJ, Jackson CE, Rogers SJ, Ridings LW, McVey AL. Prolonged paralysis due to nondepolarizing neuromuscular blocking agents and corticosteroids. Muscle Nerve 1994; 17: 647–654.

73. Argov Z, Mastaglia FL. Drug therapy: disorders of neuromuscular transmission caused by drugs. N Engl J Med 1979; 301: 409–413.

74. Panegyres PK, Squier M, Mills KR, Newsom Davis J. Acute myopathy associated with large parenteral dose of corticosteroid in myasthenia gravis. J Neurol Neurosurg Psychiatry 1993; 56: 702–704.

75. DuBois DC, Almon RR. A possible role for glucocorticoids in denervation atrophy. Muscle 1981; 4: 370–373.

27

BRAINSTEM DEATH AND MANAGEMENT OF THE ORGAN DONOR

Richard Seigne & Kevin E. J. Gunning

INTRODUCTION

From the earliest times the process of dying has preoccupied man. The definition and diagnosis of death itself, however, have changed over time. Although the absence of respiration, heart sounds and a palpable pulse was used to diagnose death, this diagnosis was not always certain and the fear of premature burial gave rise to a variety of means to alert watchers to any signs of life. One such device, invented by Count Karnice-Karnicki in 1897, consisted of a glass ball resting on the chest of the buried corpse that was attached by a tube to a flag and a bell above ground.

One of the earliest references to the idea of brain death was made in 1902 by Harvey Cushing who described how a patient with a cerebral tumour was kept alive by artificial respiration for 23 hours.[1] However, it was not until the introduction of cardiopulmonary resuscitation techniques and the development of intensive care units, where the circulation and ventilation could be maintained in patients who had suffered irreversible brain injury, that the traditional concept of death was challenged. In 1959, two French neurologists, Mollaret and Goulon,[2] used the term *coma dépassé* to describe 23 patients with irreversible brain damage who had the classic signs of brain death. These patients were unresponsive, apnoeic, poikilothermic and had developed diabetes insipidus. Although Mollaret and Goulon did not equate this state with death, all patients became asystolic within a short time. Other reports of *coma dépassé* noted the absence of cerebral blood flow.[3] These reports encouraged change from the traditional view that death occurred when the heart stopped to the philosophical concept of death being the permanent loss of consciousness and ability to breathe.

The Report of the Ad Hoc Committee of the Harvard Medical School on brain death,[4] published in 1968, stimulated greater interest in the concept of brain death. The report suggested that those patients who are unresponsive with absent spontaneous movement, spontaneous respiration and brainstem and deep tendon reflexes should be considered clinically dead, provided hypothermia and drug overdose had been excluded. Although a flat or isoelectric electroencephalogram was of value, the committee did not consider it mandatory.

Two neurosurgeons from Minneapolis proposed that to diagnose brain death, the coma should be the result of an irreparable intracranial lesion from a recognized cause.[5] Mohandas and Chou also made the important suggestion that irreversible damage to the brainstem

was the 'point of no return' and that without a functioning brainstem there is irreversible loss of function of the brain and the organism as a whole. The brainstem is responsible for consciousness and respiration. Lesions affecting the paramedian tegmental areas of the brainstem cause permanent coma because they damage the ascending reticular activating system. If the brain stem is irreversibly damaged, asystole is inevitable.[6]

The memorandum on brain death issued by the Conference of the Royal Colleges in 1976[7] laid down the conditions under which the diagnosis of brain death should be considered and described clinical tests for the diagnosis of brain death with certainty. In 1979, a further memorandum concluded: 'Identification of brain death means that the patient is dead, whether or not the function of other organs is still maintained by artificial means'.[8]

Death is now regarded as the 'irreversible loss of the capacity for consciousness, combined with the irreversible loss of the capacity to breathe'.[9] Death of the brainstem will produce this state and therefore brainstem death should equate with death of the individual.

The Uniform Determination of Death Act of 1981 in the United States defines death as follows:

> An individual who has sustained either (i) irreversible cessation of circulatory and respiratory functions, or (ii) irreversible functions of the entire brain, including the brainstem, is dead. Determination of death must be made in accordance with accepted medical standards.

This is now law in nearly all American states.

It is important to remember that the concept of brain death has evolved from changes in medical practice before organ transplantation had become established. The concept was not developed in order to fulfil the need for organ donation. The majority of the medical profession and general public now accept the concept of brain death; to prolong mechanical ventilation in a patient with a diagnosis of brainstem death (BSD) is futile and causes unnecessary suffering to the patient and their relatives.

The recognition and legal status of brain death in other countries is shown in Table 27.1.

MECHANICS OF BRAINSTEM DEATH

Brainstem death usually occurs after an irreversible rise in intracranial pressure (ICP) as a result of a supratentorial injury. It is commonly due to cerebral

Table 27.1   Examples of the medical and legal status of brain death

Country	BSD accepted by the medical profession as death	BSD legally accepted as death	Clinical criteria sufficient for diagnosis of BSD*
Australia	Yes	Yes	Yes
Belgium	Yes	Yes	Yes
Denmark	Yes	Yes	No
France	Yes	Yes	No
Germany	Yes	No	No
Holland	Yes	No	No
Italy	Yes	Yes	No
Japan	Yes	Yes	No
New Zealand	Yes	Yes	Yes
South Africa	Yes	No	Yes
Spain	Yes	Yes	No
UK	Yes	No	Yes
USA	Yes	Some states	Yes

*Diagnosis is based on clinical test only. EEG or cerebral angiography not required for diagnosis.

hypoxia, traumatic head injury, subarachnoid or intracerebral haemorrhage and bacterial meningitis. It may also be associated with primary brainstem pathology or other conditions that cause cerebral oedema and raised ICP (Table 27.2).

Classically, BSD secondary to a raised ICP is described as 'coning'. As ICP rises, a cone of brain tissue, usually the uncus or medial temporal lobe, will herniate through the tentorial opening. The midbrain lies within this opening, separated from the rigid tentorial margin by 1 mm. It is compressed against the margin by the cone of tissue or is 'strangled' between two cones of brain tissue. Unilateral or bilateral coning produces well-described patterns of injuries. As the brain is compressed, it becomes ischaemic in a rostro-caudal manner, i.e. diencephalon, midbrain, pons and finally medulla. Clinical signs are associated with this progression, but they may not be seen in all patients (Table 27.3).

Table 27.2   Causes of non-traumatic cerebral oedema

Diabetic ketoacidosis
Hepatic encephalopathy
(Pre) eclampsia
Water intoxication
Aspirin overdose
Malignant hypertension

In unilateral injuries, the lateral midbrain is compressed and the ipsilateral third cranial nerve is stretched or compressed as it runs over the tentorial margin, resulting in an ipsilateral dilated pupil that reacts to light. This is accompanied by ipsilateral decerebrate posturing. With increasing ICP the contralateral third cranial nerve is also affected and there is bilateral decerebrate posturing. If the ICP continues to rise, irreversible brain injury occurs.

Although the mechanisms responsible for BSD are widely accepted, they have been recently challenged by Fisher[10] who argued that the lateral displacement of the midbrain is the critical event producing BSD and that the herniation accompanies rather than causes this process. Following BSD nervous tissue undergoes pannecrosis throughout the cerebrum and brainstem. This is followed by autolysis despite a functioning cardiovascular system. There is no cerebral blood flow.[11] Part of the blood supply to the hypothalamus and the pituitary gland, particularly its posterior lobe, may continue for some time after BSD,[12] which may explain why panhypopituitarism is not a consistent feature of BSD.[13,14]

The descriptions of BSD highlighted above are based mainly on animal experiments under controlled conditions. Patients receiving intensive care are usually sedated and paralysed and are often being treated for intracranial hypertension with its associated complications so the classic rostrocaudal progression of cerebral ischaemia and associated signs may not be seen.

Table 27.3 Signs associated with a rising ICP	
Ischaemic area of brain	Signs
Diencephalon	Reduction in conscious level Small 1–3 mm pupils that react to light Paratonic rigidity, decorticate (flexor) posturing (bilateral corticospinal and extrapyramidal tract dysfunction) Periodic or Cheyne–Stokes respiration
Midbrain	Fixed, dilated or mid-position pupils Decerebrate (extensor) posturing
Pons	Cushing's reflex (see Physiological changes)
Medulla	Sympathetic storm (see Physiological changes) followed by sympathetic outflow failure Apnoea

PHYSIOLOGICAL CHANGES ACCOMPANYING BRAINSTEM DEATH

NEUROLOGICAL CHANGES

The motor and autonomic changes associated with the events preceding and accompanying BSD are described in the 'Physical causes' and 'Cardiovascular changes' sections respectively. Changes associated with the failure of the hypothalamic-pituitary axis have generated much interest in the last decade and are discussed in the 'Endocrine changes' section.

The temperature regulation centre in the hypothalamus is impaired following BSD and the patient becomes poikilothermic and hypothermic. Vasodilatation, intravenous fluid therapy and a low basal metabolic rate may exacerbate hypothermia.

CARDIOVASCULAR CHANGES

The cardiovascular and electrocardiographic (ECG) changes commonly associated with BSD are summarized in Table 27.4. These ECG changes are sometimes referred to as 'neurogenic', implying they do not indicate actual structural damage. As the ECG detects specific changes in the electrical activity of the heart, it is hard to see how the changes manifest in BSD are not the result of direct or indirect cardiovascular compromise.

Brainstem compression, medullary ischaemia and raised ICP may cause severe elevations of blood pressure. This hyperdynamic response mediated by the dramatic rise in catecholamines, the so-called 'sympathetic storm', is responsible for the cardiac dysrhythmias, ECG abnormalities, myocardial damage and functional renal impairment commonly seen after intracranial injury.[15] In animal models, BSD produces up to 750- and 400-fold rises in plasma epinephrine and norepinephrine levels respectively.[16,17] This sympathetic storm is well recognized clinically although the rise in catecholamine levels may not always be this dramatic.[18] Brainstem death in animals results in the release of noradrenaline from cardiac sympathetic fibres that produce interstitial concentrations far higher than the plasma levels at BSD.[19] Histological changes, which include petechial haemorrhages, contraction banding, coagulative myocytolysis, a loss of the linear arrangement of myofibrils, cytoplasmic banding and subendocardial necrosis, have been described after BSD.[16] This damage is not always associated with a rise in serum myocardial creatinine kinase concentration.

Cooper et al[20] describe an inhibition of mitochondrial function (cf. endocrine changes) resulting in a reduction in aerobic metabolic oxidative processes and a depletion of myocardial energy stores. These findings have been questioned by others.[21] White et al[22] demonstrated a marked uncoupling of β_1 and β_2-adrenergic receptors from adenyl cyclase and a reduction in the contractile response of the myocardium in brain-dead patients. They noted a lack of the receptor down-regulation found in chronic heart failure and suggested that the early implementation of β-blockade could attenuate the catecholamine-induced damage as described by Cruickshank.[23] Yoshioka[24] found that epinephrine had a reduced pressor effect in BSD patients, which was reversed by the concomitant administration of vasopressin. The overall result of these changes is a poorly functioning myocardium with poor myocardial perfusion and increasing myocardial dysfunction.

Table 27.4   Typical cardiovascular and ECG changes associated with BSD

Event	Result	Clinical change	ECG changes
Cerebral ischaemia	Vagal activation	Increased heart rate, cardiac output and blood pressure	Sinus bradycardia and bradyarrhythmias
Ischaemia in the pons sympathetic stimulation	Vagal activation and output and increased blood	Decreased heart rate, cardiac no ischaemia pressure → MAP (Cushing's reflex)	Sinus bradycardia,
Medullary ischaemia	Ischaemic vagal cardiomotor nucleus Unopposed sympathetic stimulation – 'storm'	Increased heart rate, cardiac output, blood pressure, vascular resistance and left atrial pressure (pulmonary oedema)	Sinus tachycardia, multifocal ventricular ectopics, marked ischaemia
Spinal cord ischaemia	Ischaemic sympathetic nuclei	Decreased heart rate, cardiac output, blood pressure and vascular resistance (spinal shock)	Sinus rhythm, reduced R-wave size, persistent ischaemic changes

The classic rostrocaudal progression of events may not develop in the clinical setting.

Following BSD, catecholamine levels fall. Together with relative hypovolaemia, hypothermia, autonomic dysfunction and the myocardial changes described above, this leads to a fall in cardiac output, systemic vascular resistance and mean arterial pressure.

Asystole usually occurs within 48 h without cardiovascular support but there is evidence that infusions of epinephrine and vasopressin can delay this for several weeks,[24] information that may be of relevance if organ donation is being considered.

PULMONARY CHANGES

During the sympathetic storm, the rapid rise in left atrial pressure (LAP) which may even exceed pulmonary artery pressure, in combination with an expanded lung blood volume (from an enhanced venous return and subsequent increased right ventricular output), may result in capillary disruption, protein-rich pulmonary oedema and interstitial haemorrhage.[20] This may lead to a deterioration in gas exchange and hypoxaemia.

ENDOCRINE CHANGES

Hypothalamic-pituitary axis

The discovery that BSD in animals is often followed by a decrease in plasma levels of T3, insulin and cortisol[20] has stimulated research on the hypothalamic-pituitary axis (HPA) during and after BSD, with mixed results.[12,13,17,25–28] Ill-defined hormone reference ranges in acutely ill patients, the use of free-standing hormone levels rather than their dynamic axis function and poor understanding of the interactions between various hormones probably accounts for the inconsistency of the results.

Posterior pituitary function

Neurogenic diabetes insipidus (DI) occurs in up to 84% of patients with BSD.[14] Polyuria >200 ml/h should alert the clinician to the possibility of DI. The serum osmolality is usually >310 mosmol/l with a urine osmolality of <200 mosmol/l. Electrolyte disturbances such as hypernatraemia, hypokalaemia, hypocalcaemia, hypophosphataemia and hypomagnesaemia occur rapidly without treatment.

Antidiuretic hormone (ADH) has intrinsic vasoconstrictive properties. Therefore, decreased levels of ADH may contribute to the cardiovascular instability associated with BSD. Replacement therapy has been shown to attenuate some of this instability in BSD patients.[32] Prolactin levels may be normal or low. The use of dopamine infusions in BSD patients may account for some of the low values that have been reported.[29]

Anterior pituitary function

There are conflicting reports regarding changes in anterior pituitary hormones following BSD.[14,29,30] Follicule stimulating hormone (FSH) and luteinizing hormone (LH) remain relatively unchanged. Circadian release of growth hormone (GH) and its

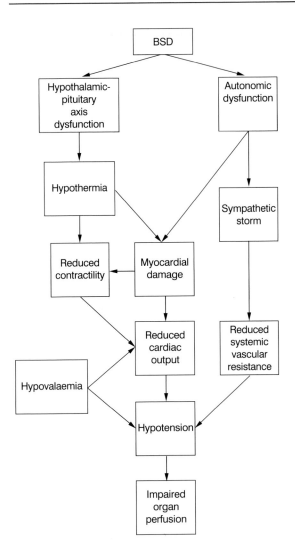

Figure 27.1 Cardiovascular effects of brainstem death

Table 27.5 Thyroid hormones levels in the sick euthyroid syndrome	
Hormone	Level
Total T_3	Increased
Free T_3	Decreased
rT_3	Normal or increased
Total T_4	Normal or decreased
TSH	normal

T_4 = thyroxine; T_3 = triiodothyronine; TSH = thyroid-stimulating hormone

associated with acute illness, results in impaired peripheral conversion of thyroxine (T_4) to triiodothyronine (T_3) and a rise in reverse T_3 (rT_3).

Although the exact significance of a reduced T_3 level is unknown, experimental work suggests an association with reduced myocardial function and an alteration in cellular mitochondrial metabolism from aerobic to anaerobic producing a lactic acidosis.[20] Furthermore, hypothyroidism reduces myosin Ca^{2+} activated ATPase activity and T_3 is probably an important regulator of Na^+/K^+ ATPase in the heart.[30] Although haemodynamics or metabolic acidosis is not improved by the sole administration of T_3 in BSD,[11,12,26,27] when used in combination with other hormones T_3 has been shown to result in cardiovascular and metabolic improvements which lead to an increase in the number of suitable organs for transplantation in potential donors.[20,25,29]

Insulin

A degree of peripheral resistance to insulin is common in BSD patients.[32] This may be aggravated by the increased level of catecholamines (endogenous and exogenous), the use of steroids and the concomitant acidosis often present.

RENAL CHANGES

The cardiovascular changes associated with BSD, vasoconstriction with subsequent reduced cardiac output, hypotension and hypovolaemia may result in renal damage.[32] Experimental evidence suggests that in BSD renal parenchymal cell integrity, as measured by cellular $Na^+:K^+$ ratio, is impaired.[33] Damage to renal cell parenchyma may be prevented (in animals at least) by the administration of T_3, cortisol and insulin independent of improvement in systemic haemodynamics.[33]

role in the stress response complicate interpretation of the changes seen in its levels after BSD.[12,14,29] Levels of adrenocorticotrophic hormone (ACTH) remain within the normal laboratory range after BSD.[12,14,30] Cortisol levels may also be 'normal' for non-stressed patients but this may indicate a relative deficiency, which might be uncovered with stress testing (short synacthen test). No relationship between cortisol levels and severe hypotension has been demonstrated.[14]

Thyroid hormones

Changes in thyroid hormone levels after BSD are similar to those found in patients with sick euthyroid syndrome (Table 27.5).[12–14,29] The syndrome, often

HEPATIC AND COAGULATION CHANGES

In an animal model of BSD, hepatic function remained unaffected by profound hypotension.[34] The arterial ketone body ratio did not change significantly, suggesting an adequate oxygen supply.

Fibrinolytic agents and plasminogen activators are released from damaged brain tissue into the circulation in patients with BSD and can cause coagulation defects, including disseminated intravascular coagulopathy. These defects may be aggravated by hypothermia.

METABOLIC CHANGES

Changes in oxidative processes have been demonstrated after BSD.[20] Reductions in plasma glucose, pyruvate and palmitate with parallel rises in lactate and fatty acids may indicate a shift from aerobic to anaerobic mitochondrial metabolism. This change could lead to reductions in cellular high-energy phosphates and thus cellular and organ function. Delivery-dependent oxygen consumption and high plasma lactate levels have been reported in BSD patients. It is not clear whether this is due to a reduction in tissue oxygen extraction or mitochondrial impairment.[21,35]

The possible complications of BSD are highlighted in Tables 27.6 and 27.7 and Figure 27.1 and 27.2.

DIAGNOSIS OF BRAIN DEATH

The criteria for the diagnosis of brain death published by the Honorary Secretary of the Royal Colleges and their faculties in the United Kingdom,[7] and the Harvard Report in the United States, became the basis for the confirmation of brain death in many other countries.[7] However, the exact criteria upon which brain death is diagnosed vary between countries, with

Table 27.6 Complications associated with BSD

Complication	Frequency	Contributing factors
Haemodynamic instability	Very common	Autonomic dysfunction Myocardial damage β-receptor dysfunction Hypovolaemia Hypothermia
Hypoxia	Common	Pulmonary oedema, retained secretions, atelectasis
Hypovolaemia	Common	Diabetes insipidus Endothelial damage Diuretics Hyperglycaemia Fluid restriction Haemorrhage
Hyperosmolality	Common	Diabetes insipidus
Hyperglycaemia	Common	Insulin resistance Acidosis Intravenous dextrose Endogenous and exogenous steroids Endogenous and exogenous catecholamines
Hypothermia	Common	Hypothalamic ischaemia Vasodilatation Reduced basal metabolic rate
Coagulation defects	Uncommon	Fibrinolytic agents Cytokines Plasminogen activators Hypothermia Transfused blood products

Table 27.7 Electrolyte disturbances associated with BSD	
Electrolyte disturbances	**Contributing factors**
Hypernatraemia	Diabetes insipidus
Hypokalaemia	Diabetes insipidus Insulin Diuretics Catecholamines Hyperventilation Endogenous and exogenous steroids
Hypomagnesaemia	Diabetes insipidus Diuretics
Hypocalcaemia	Diabetes insipidus Diuretics
Hypophosphataemia	Diabetes insipidus Diuretics Insulin

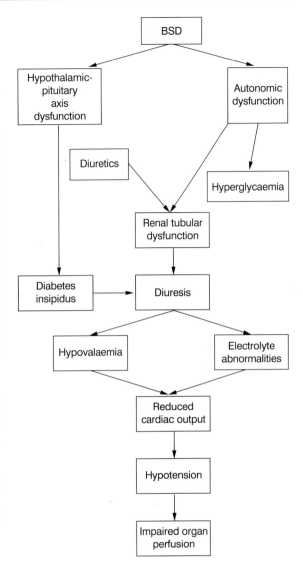

Figure 27.2   End-organ effects of brainstem death

some but not all countries requiring confirmatory tests of absent brain function, such as EEG or cerebral angiography. The diagnosis of BSD in the United Kingdom will be described in detail. A revision of the Code of Practice for the Diagnosis of Brainstem Death was published in 1998.[36]

There are three sequential steps in making the diagnosis of BSD. To avoid unnecessary testing and to eliminate the chance of making an incorrect diagnosis, it is *essential* that steps 1 and 2 are completed *before* beginning step 3.

STEP 1   PRECONDITIONS

The patient is deeply comatose and is being maintained on a ventilator because spontaneous ventilation had previously been inadequate or had ceased altogether. There should be no doubt that the patient's condition is due to irremediable brain damage of known aetiology.[7]

An accurate history of events before and after the onset of the coma is essential.

STEP 2   EXCLUSIONS

If the preconditions have been fulfilled, the necessary exclusions must be considered. These are to ensure that neither the state of apnoea nor the coma is contributed to or caused by a reversible condition. The major groups of conditions that may produce this clinical picture are:

- hypothermia, < 35°C;
- depressant drugs, both therapeutic and non-therapeutic;
- metabolic disorders, e.g. hyponatraemia;
- endocrine abnormalities, e.g. myxoedema.

Altered drug metabolism due to concurrent pathology or, less commonly, enzyme variants should be borne in mind at this stage. In the absence of toxicological screening, it has been suggested that three days is a reasonable time to allow potential drug effects to disappear.[37,38] Metabolic and endocrine abnormalities may be suspected from the history, examination and routine blood tests, i.e. full blood count, arterial blood gas, electrolytes and blood glucose measurements, although more sophisticated tests may be necessary. Certain abnormalities accompanying BSD (e.g. hypernatraemia) do not preclude the diagnosis of BSD.[38]

Specific conditions, such as the 'locked-in' syndrome and brainstem encephalitis (Bickerstatt's encephalitis or the Miller Fisher syndrome), may produce a clinical picture similar to that seen in BSD. When such conditions are suspected, BSD tests should not be undertaken as the patient does not comply with the precondition 'there should be no doubt that the patient's condition is due to irremediable brain damage of known aetiology.[37] The 'locked-in' syndrome is produced by a lesion in the pons which paralyses the limbs, respiratory muscles and lower cranial nerves. Patients are conscious and able to blink and produce vertical eye movements. Brainstem encephalitis may produce a comatose, areflexic, apnoeic patient, with motor and central nerve paralysis including internal and external ophthalmoplegia. Full recovery from brain encephalitis is possible.[39] Therefore, the importance of obtaining an adequate history consistent with the clinical picture together with strict adherence to the preconditions and exclusions before BSD testing cannot be overemphasized. If any doubt exists as to the cause of the patient's condition, BSD tests should not be performed.

STEP 3 THE TESTS

The tests should not be performed unless steps 1 and 2 have been fulfilled.

Who and when?

BSD tests should be performed by two medical practitioners who have been registered for more than five years and are competent in this field. At least one of the practitioners should be a consultant and neither practitioner should be a member of the transplant team. Two sets of tests should be performed; the two practitioners may perform the tests separately or together. The tests should be repeated to ensure no observer error has occurred. The timing of this second set of tests is a matter for the doctors involved but should be adequate for the reassurance of all those directly concerned.[40] The interval between the two sets of tests can be used to discuss the possibility of organ donation with the relatives if they have not already raised the subject.

How?

For confirmation of BSD, five tests of the brainstem reflexes and testing for apnoea are required (Table 27.8). The tests are easily performed at the bedside and have unambiguous endpoints. In the United Kingdom there is no requirement to perform cerebral angiography or electroencephalography for the confirmation of BSD.

Testing for apnoea

This test is considered positive if the patient does not exhibit any respiratory movements whilst disconnected from the ventilator despite a $PaCO_2$ of at least 6.65 kPa

Table 27.8 The five tests of reflexes		
Test	BSD criteria	Cranial nerves tested
1. A bright light is shone into both pupils	No reaction in either pupil	II and III
2. A strong stimulus is applied to the corneas	No blinking	V and VII
3. 20 ml of iced water is injected into both external auditory meatae	No eye movement	III, VI and VIII
4. painful stimulus is applied – supraorbital pressure†	No motor response in the cranial nerve distribution	III, IV, V, VI, VII, IX, X, XI and XII
5. suction catheter is passed into the trachea	No coughing or gagging	IX and X

*The tympanic membranes should first be visualized and seen to be intact.
†Spinal reflexes may be present.

(50 mmHg). The lungs are normally hypoventilated with 100% O_2 for 10 min prior to disconnection to achieve a $PaCO_2$ >6.6 kPa and to prevent hypoxaemia. Insufflation of oxygen at 6 l/min via a catheter passed into the trachea during disconnection will further reduce the risk of hypoxaemia during disconnection.

Common difficulties encountered when performing tests for BSD

The difficulties commonly encountered during BSD testing are summarized in Table 27.9.

Death is pronounced after the second set of tests but the legal time of death is recorded when the patient fulfils the first set of BSD criteria. When BSD has been diagnosed the relatives should be informed and the clinician should ensure that the relatives fully understand that death has occurred. If there is no absolute contraindication to organ donation, management of the patient should now be directed to preservation of organ function (Tables 27.10, 27.11).

The completion of the first set of BSD tests is a suitable time to discuss organ donation with the patient's relatives. In the United Kingdom, refusal by relatives accounts for the failure to donate organs in about 30% of potential organ donors. The local transplant coordinator should be contacted as soon as possible after the first set of BSD criteria have been fulfilled as they are experienced in dealing with bereaved relatives who are considering organ donation.

MANAGEMENT OF PATIENTS WITH BRAINSTEM DEATH

After permission for organ donation has been obtained from the patient's relatives, the intensivist in charge of the patient's care should contact the local transplant coordinator to discuss specific treatments which may be requested by the transplant team, e.g. hormone therapy. A continued high standard of nursing care, the use of invasive monitoring and prompt treatment to preserve organ function will increase the chances of successful organ donation. The patient management goals are similar to those before the diagnosis of BSD with the exception of specific measures to maintain cerebral perfusion pressure and oxygen delivery.

OPTIMIZE CARDIAC OUTPUT AND TISSUE OXYGEN DELIVERY

Cardiac output is optimized by volume loading guided by central venous and/or pulmonary artery wedge pressures. Blood, colloid and crystalloid solutions are used as appropriate to maintain the circulating volume. A combination of inotropes and peripheral vasoconstrictors is usually required to improve cardiac

---

Table 27.9   Common difficulties encountered when performing the tests for BSD

Difficulty	Advice
Patients with cataract(s)/false eye(s) and or disrupted tympanic membrane(s)	The published criteria are 'guidelines rather than rigid rules'. 'It is for the doctors at the bedside to decide when the patient is dead'.[40]
The patient is now hypothermic and/or has a metabolic disturbance, e.g. hypernatraemia	Abnormalities accompanying BSD do not preclude the diagnosis of BSD.[37] Although the exact temperature below which hypothermia is likely to be the cause of coma is uncertain, we do not perform BSD tests in patients whose core temperature is <35°C.
The patient has chronic obstructive pulmonary disease	A 'normal' set of arterial blood for that patient is obtained during disconnection and then the PaO_2 is allowed to fall by a further 1–2 kPa whilst observing for respiratory effort.[40]
Does the patient have other conditions that can account for the symptoms? (differential diagnosis)	Ensure the preconditions and exclusions have been strictly adhered to.

Table 27.10   Absolute contraindications to organ donation

	Contraindication	Notes
Legal	Coroner refuses consent	See Table 27.11
Moral	Patient directive, relative(s) refusal	
Age	>70 years	Corneas >90 years
Transmissible disease	Active bacterial, fungal, protozoan or viral infection	Includes patients in high-risk groups for HIV infection. Hepatitis C is not an absolute contraindication
Malignancy	Past or current diagnosis of malignancy including the following primary CNS tumours: Anaplastic astrocytoma (Grade III), glioblastoma multiforme, medulloblastoma, anaplastic oligodendroglioma, malignant ependymoma, pineoblastoma, anaplastic and malignant meningioma, intracerebral sarcoma, chordoma, primary cerebral lymphoma*	Exceptions: Low grade skin tumours e.g. basal cell carcinoma Carcinoma in situ of the uterine cervix Primary brain tumours that exceptionally spread outside the central nervous system
Hormone replacement	Treatment with human pituitary extract	
Organ specific		Discuss with transplant co-ordinator

*Council of Europe International Consensus Document: 'Standardization of Organ Donor Screening to Prevent Transmission of Neoplastic Disease' 1997.

Table 27.11   Referral to the coroner in the UK

The coroner should be informed if:

death is the result of an accident
death occurred intraoperatively or before recovery from anaesthesia
death is of unknown cause
death is the result of suicide
death is from violent or unnatural or suspicious cause
death is due to self-neglect or neglect by others
death is due to an abortion
the deceased was not seen by the certifying doctor either after death or within the 14 days before
   death
death occurred during or shortly after detention in police or prison custody
death may have been due to an industrial disease or related to the deceased's employment

Table 27.12   Physiological goals for heart or heart–lung donation

Criteria	Goal
Mean arterial pressure	>60 mmHg
Left ventricular stroke work index	>15 g/m^2
Cardiac index	>2.1 l/min
Pulmonary artery wedge pressure	12 mmHg
Central venous pressure	12 mmHg
Inotropic support	5 mg/kg/min

Table 27.13   Rule of 100s

Systolic blood pressure	>100 mmHg
Urine output	>100 ml/h
PaO$_2$	>100 mmHg
Haemoglobin	>100 g/l

contractility and to increase organ perfusion pressure. Although dopamine is the most commonly used agent, dobutamine, epinephrine and norepinephrine may be required depending on the cardiac index and systemic vascular resistance at the time. The transplant team may specify their most favoured regimen for organ preservation, as shown in Table 27.12.[28]

The 'rule of 100s' has been suggested as a guide to treatment (Table 27.13).

ADEQUATE OXYGENATION

As these patients are intubated and ventilated they are at risk of atelectasis, retained secretions and nosocomial pneumonia. Physiotherapy, aseptic tracheobronchial suction and low levels of positive end-expiratory pressure (PEEP) of 5 cmH$_2$O may be used to prevent basal atelectasis and improve gas exchange. Bronchoscopy may be necessary to facilitate clearance of secretions but care must be taken to avoid damaging the lungs if lung donation is being considered. To minimize the risk of barotrauma and volutrauma, the peak inspiratory ventilatory pressure should be kept below 35 cmH$_2$O and tidal volume less than 10 ml/kg. The lowest concentrations of inspired oxygen that give adequate haemoglobin saturation should be used to reduce the risk of oxygen toxicity. The end-tidal CO$_2$ should be kept within normal limits. However, this may be difficult as CO$_2$ production is low in brain-dead patients and dead space may have to be added to the ventilator circuit.

MAINTENANCE OF HOMEOSTASIS WITH FAILING AUTONOMIC AND HORMONAL SYSTEMS

Diabetes insipidus is treated with intravenous or subcutaneous boluses of desmopressin (DDAVP) 0.5–4.0 μg or, if the patient is hypotensive, intravenous vasopressin (AVP, Pitressin) 5–20 units. Repeat doses should be given to keep the urine output <200 ml/h. Rapid treatment is essential to prevent the development of electrolyte abnormalities and hypotension. Urine losses should be replaced with the appropriate crystalloid solution according to plasma and urine electrolyte measurements. Infusions of insulin should be used to maintain blood glucose concentrations within normal limits. By using a combination of hormone replacements, it is possible to increase the number of suitable donors (Table 27.14).

Hypothermia should be prevented by keeping the patient covered, the use of a warm air blanket, warmed fluids and humidification of the breathing circuit.

CONCLUSION

The change from the idea of a cardiovascular death to the concept of brain death arose as a result of advances in medical technology. Death of the brainstem, which can be reliably diagnosed by clinical tests, implies death of the whole brain and thus death of the individual. The preconditions that must be fulfilled before

Table 27.14   Hormone replacement combination (adapted from reference[29])

Hormone/drug	Dose
Methylprednisolone	15 mg/kg bolus
Triiodothyronine	4 μg bolus + 3 μg/h infusion
Antidiuretic hormone (pitressin)	1 IU bolus + 1.5 IU/h infusion
Insulin	Minimum 1IU/h – to maintain blood glucose of 6–11mmol/l
Epinephrine	1–5 μg/min – to maintain SVR 800–1200 dyne/s/cm^{-5}

a diagnosis of brainstem death can be considered are essential to prevent any errors in the diagnosis. Brainstem death results in a loss of homeostasis and therefore successful organ transplantation is only possible after careful management of the organ donor.[41]

REFERENCES

1. Cushing H. Some experimental and clinical observations concerning states of increased intracranial tension. Am J Med Sci 1902; 124: 375–400.

2. Mollaret P, Goulon M. Le coma dépassé (mémoire preliminaire). Rev Neurol (Paris) 1959; 101: 3–15.

3. Wertheimer P, Jouvet M, Descotes J. A propos du diagnostic de la mort du système nerveux – dans les comas avec arrêt respiratoire traités par respiration artificielle. Presse Med 1959; 67: 87–88.

4. Ad Hoc Committee of the Harvard Medical School. A definition of irreversible coma. JAMA 1968; 281: 1070–1071.

5. Mohandas A, Chou SN. Brain death – a clinical and pathological study. J Neurosurg 1971; 35: 211–218.

6. Jennett B, Gleave J, Wilson P. Brain deaths in three neurosurgical units. BMJ 1981; 28: 2533–2539.

7. Working Group of Conference of Medical Royal Colleges and their Faculties in the United Kingdom. Diagnosis of death. BMJ 1976; ii: 1187–1188.

8. Working Group of Conference of Medical Royal Colleges and their Faculties in the United Kingdom. Diagnosis of death. BMJ 1979; i: 3320.

9. Working Group of Conference of Medical Royal Colleges and their Faculties in the United Kingdom. The criteria for the diagnosis of brainstem death. J Roy Coll Physicians Lond 1995; 29: 381–382.

10. Fisher CM. Brain herniation: a revision of classical concepts. Can J Neuro Sci 1995; 22: 83–91.

11. Black PM. Brain death (first of two parts). N Engl J Med 1978; 299: 338–344.

12. Gramm HJ, Meinhold H, Bickel U et al. Acute endocrine failure after brain death? Transplantation 1992; 54: 851–857.

13. Powner DJ, Hendrich A, Lagler RG, Ng RH, Madden RL. Hormonal changes in brain dead patients. Crit Care Med 1990; 18: 702–708.

14. Howlett TA, Keogh AM, Perry L, Touzel R, Rees LH. Anterior and posterior pituitary function in brain-stem-dead donors. Transplantation 1989; 47: 828–834.

15. Kolin A, Norris JW. Myocardial damage from acute cerebral lesions. Stroke 1984; 15: 990–995.

16. Shivalkar B, Van Loon J, Wieland W et al. Variable effects of explosive or gradual increase of intracranial pressure on myocardial structure and function. Circulation 1993; 87: 230–239.

17. Chen EP, Bittner HB, Kendall SWH, Van Trigt P. Hormonal and haemodynamic changes in a validated animal model of brain death. Crit Care Med 1996; 24: 1352–1359.

18. Powner DJ, Hendrich A, Nyhuis A, Strate R. Changes in catecholamine levels in patients who are brain dead. J Heart Lung Transplant 1992; 11: 1046–1053.

19. Mertes PM, Carteaux JP, Taboin Y et al. Estimation of myocardial interstitial norepinephrine release after brain death using cardiac microdialysis. Transplantation 1994; 57: 371–377.

20. Cooper DKC, Novitzky D, Wicomb WN. The pathophysiological effects of brain death on potential donor organs, with particular reference to the heart. Ann Roy Coll Surg Engl 1989; 71: 261–266.

21. Depret J, Teboul J-L, Benort G, Mercat A, Richard C. Global energetic failure in brain-dead patients. Transplantation. 1995; 60: 966–971.

22. White M, Wiechmann RJ, Roden RL et al. Cardiac β-adrenergic neuroeffector systems in acute myocardial dysfunction related to brain injury. Circulation 1995; 92: 2183–2189.

23. Cruickshank JM, Neil-Dwyer G, Degaute JP et al. Reduction of stress/catecholamine-induced cardiac necrosis by β₁-selective blockade. Lancet 1987; 2: 585–589.

24. Yoshioka T, Sugimoto H, Uenishi M et al. Prolonged hemodynamic maintenance by the combined administration of vasopressin and epinepherine in brain death: a clinical study. Neurosurgery 1986; 18: 565–567.

25. Novitzky D, Cooper DKC, Reichart B. Hemodynamic and metabolic responses to hormonal therapy in brain-dead potential organ donors. Transplantation 1987; 43: 852–854.

26. Goarin J-P, Cohen S, Riou B et al. The effects of triiodothyronine on haemodynamic status and cardiac function in potential heart donors. Anesth Analg 1996; 83: 41–47.

27. Randell TT, Hockerstedt KA. Triiodothyronine treatment in brain-dead multiorgan donors – a controlled study. Transplantation 1992; 54: 736–738.

28. Wheeldon DR, Potter CDO, Oduro A, Wallwork J, Large SR. Transforming the 'unacceptable' donor: outcomes from the adoption of a standardized donor management technique. J Heart Lung Transplant 1995; 14: 734–742.

29. Harms J, Isemer FE, Kolenda H. Hormonal alteration and pituitary function during course of brain-stem death in potential organ donors. Transplant Proc 1991; 23: 2614–2616.

30. Power BM, Van Heerden PV. The physiological changes associated with brain death – current concepts and implications for the treatment of the brain dead organ donor. Anaesth Intens Care. 1995; 23: 26–36.

31. Galinanes M, Smolenski RT, Hearse DJ. Brain death-induced cardiac contractile dysfunction and long-term cardiac preservation. Rat heart studies of the effects of

hypophysectomy. Circulation 1993; 88(part 2): II–270–280.

32. Bensadoun H, Blanchet P, Richard C et al. Kidney graft quality: 490 kidneys procured from brain dead donors in one center. Transplant Proc 1995; 27: 1647–1648.

33. Wicomb WN, Cooper DKC, Novitzky D. Impairment of renal slice function following brain death, with reversibility of injury by hormonal therapy. Transplantation 1986; 41: 29–33.

34. Lin H, Okamoto R, Yamamoto Y et al. Hepatic tolerance to hypotension as assessed by the changes in arterial ketone body ratio in the state of brain death. Transplantation 1989; 47: 444–448.

35. Langeron O, Couture P, Mateo J, Riou B, Pansard J-L, Coriat P. Oxygen consumption and delivery relationship in brain-dead organ donors. Br J Anaesth 1996; 76: 783–789.

36. Cadaveric organs for transplantation. A code of practice including the diagnosis of brainstem death. HMSO, London, 1998.

37. Working Group of the Royal College of Physicians and the Conference of Medical Royal Colleges and their Faculties in the United Kingdom. Criteria for the diagnosis of brainstem death. J Roy Coll Physicians Lond 1995; 29: 381–382.

38. Pallis C. ABC of brainstem death. Diagnosis of brainstem death – I. BMJ 1982; 285: 1558–1560.

39. Al-Din ASN, Adnan JS, Shakir R. Coma and brain stem areflexia in brain stem encephalitis (Fisher's syndrome). BMJ 1985; 291: 535–536.

40. Robson JG. Brain death (letter). BMJ 1981; 283: 505.

41. The organ donor. Intensive Care Society, London, 1994.

SECTION 5

ANAESTHESIA FOR NEUROIMAGING

28

ANAESTHESIA FOR NEURORADIOLOGY

John M. Turner

The investigation of neurosurgical conditions by radiology began surprisingly early. Dandy (1918)[1] injected air into a lateral ventricle to allow its visualization by X-rays. Angiography followed in 1927 when Moniz[2] reported the injection of sodium iodide into a surgically exposed carotid artery, demonstrating the cerebral vessels. The technique was improved subsequently by percutaneous injection and the development of less toxic contrast agents and remains a mainstay of neuroradiology. Contrast studies of the ventricular system have lessened in number following the improvement of imaging techniques and the introduction of computed tomographic (CT) scans[3] and magnetic resonance imaging (MRI).

The demands made of anaesthetists in the X-ray department have changed considerably over the last 10 years as the techniques of imaging have changed and expanded. Improvement in imaging techniques and equipment has meant that very few neurosurgical patients require anaesthesia for diagnostic neuroradiology, but the continued development of interventional radiology, where some neurosurgical conditions may be treated in the X-ray department, makes new demands of the anaesthetist. The new procedures pose their own problems but usually share the dangers of anaesthesia and surgery in the operating theatre.[4,5,6]

DIAGNOSTIC RADIOLOGY

Some patients still require anaesthesia for diagnostic radiology:

- children;
- unconscious patients;
- movement disorders;
- adults with learning difficulties.

PROCEDURES

Angiography

The usual access to the cerebral vasculature is via a femoral arterial puncture. Under screening control, a catheter is advanced from the femoral artery to the arch of the aorta and the appropriate cerebral vessel entered. The catheter is placed in each of the major cerebral vessels in turn as indicated by the clinical presentation and injections of radiographic contrast are made to delineate the vascular anatomy of the lesion. Once the major vessels have been visualized in various projections, the catheter may be advanced into smaller vessels, where the detailed anatomy will be evaluated. Various patterns of catheter and guidewire are available to facilitate the process.

CT scan

Anaesthesia is only rarely required for a diagnostic CT scan. Children may require anaesthesia, especially if a high-definition scan is required, because they may be unable to lie still enough for good-quality images to be obtained.

MRI scan

The requirements for anaesthesia and sedation in MRI are discussed in Chapter 00.

Myelography

Imaging of the spinal cord has been greatly simplified by improvements in CT scanning and MRI. It is only occasionally necessary to perform a myelogram under general anaesthetic, especially for children. The practical problems centre around positioning the patient because in order to visualize the vertebral column and spinal cord, the radiologist tips the patient head up and head down, thus allowing the contrast agent to flow up and down the vertebral column. It is important to make sure that the patient is securely fixed and that cardiovascular function is preserved so blood pressure is maintained in the head-up position.

PROBLEMS OF ANAESTHESIA IN THE X-RAY DEPARTMENT

Neuroradiological procedures are associated with a significant morbidity and mortality.[7,8,9] Anaesthesia constitutes an additional hazard. There are a number of factors that add to the difficulties of the anaesthetist in the neuroradiological department:

- strange environment;
- hostile environment;
- bulky X-ray equipment;
- reduced lighting;
- patient movement;
- no skull decompression.

Strange environment

The neuroradiology department is best situated close to the neurosurgical operating theatre. It is, however, frequently part of the radiology department, so that expensive imaging equipment may be best used. This physical separation means that the X-ray staff may not be familiar with operating theatre disciplines and patient care. The anaesthetist must ensure that there is adequate, skilled help available and that the X-ray department staff are familiar with the requirements of anaesthesia. All the facilities available to the anaesthetist in the operating theatre are required and there should be a dedicated recovery area, staffed by appropriately trained nurses.

Hostile environment

The dangerous nature of X-rays is well known. The anaesthetist must know how to minimize personal exposure to radiation and advise any assisting personnel. The anaesthetist and any staff helping should wear 0.35 mm lead-equivalent aprons and avoid close exposure to the X-ray source. It is important, in minimizing exposure, to keep some distance away from the X-ray source as the inverse-square law determines the intensity of X-rays. It is also valuable, remembering that there is some scatter of X-rays, to keep behind the source of X-rays. The X-ray room should be so arranged that the anaesthetic machine and the monitoring equipment are easily visible from behind a lead glass screen and the anaesthetic team should take refuge behind the screen wherever possible. The importance of a clear line of sight from behind the screen is crucial; the anaesthetic machine, the lung ventilator and monitoring and also the endotracheal tube and its fixation must be clearly seen from the protected position.

Bulky X-ray equipment

The equipment required for X-ray is frequently expensive and bulky. In the neuroradiology room, surrounding the couch on which the patient lies, there will be the X-ray tube on its support (usually a balanced, motor-driven assembly), several monitors and computer controls. There may be automatic injectors. Careful planning is needed in setting up the room so that the X-ray equipment and the anaesthetic equipment do not impede each other. In particular, the X-ray tube, on its gantry, must be swung out of the way for induction of anaesthesia and at the end of the anaesthetic. It should be possible to move the tube assembly out of the way without delay in case of an emergency during a radiological procedure. Particular thought must be given to the likely movement required in the X-ray equipment (tube and couch) during an examination, so that such movement does not imperil the patient's life support systems.

Reduced lighting

Despite the improvement in screening techniques and display monitors, reduced lighting may be helpful for viewing X-ray monitors. The anaesthetic machine and anaesthetic monitors in use must be designed to be clearly visible in such circumstances.

Patient movement

The neuroradiologist performing cerebral angiography frequently needs to move the couch on which the patient lies, to clarify the vascular anatomy. During screening, the movement may be considerable and all connections to the patient (endotracheal and breathing tubes, monitoring cables, infusions) must not only be secure but arranged in such a way as not to impede the couch movement. Wherever possible, we mount equipment on the X-ray couch; if this is not possible, we ensure that there is adequate slack in cables, infusion lines or breathing tubes.

No skull decompression

In the operating theatre, the fact that the surgeon will be performing a craniotomy means that the brain is being decompressed and probably that CSF will be aspirated, so that the patient is to a certain extent protected from high ICP. In the X-ray room, the skull remains intact, so great care must be taken by the anaesthetist to avoid an increase in ICP in patients with space occupation.

ANGIOGRAPHY

In Interventional procedures a complex arrangement of catheters and guidewires may be used.[6,10] A large sheath (7.5 Fr gauge) is placed in the femoral artery and through it another catheter is passed into one of the major vessels, such as a carotid or vertebral artery. Finer catheters or guidewires, passed through main catheter, are used to access the vessel or lesion requiring treatment. Recent development of small catheters and guidewires has made the catheterization of small vessels a practical proposition.

The process is aided by modern digital radiographic techniques, where the bone and other non-vascular structures can be subtracted from the image. Another aid is the ability to make a 'road map' image. In this technique, the radiologist makes an injection of contrast into a major vessel, so outlining the vascular anatomy. This image is saved and computer techniques allow the live image obtained from screening to be superimposed on the saved image, so that the radiologist can see the position of the catheter relative to the vasculature. This facility helps the radiologist to advance the catheter along the cerebral vessels. It requires that no movement of the patient take place once the vessel anatomy has been visualized and stored; though, of course, repeated 'road map' injections may be made.

INTERVENTIONAL PROCEDURES

Interventional neuroradiology has advanced dramatically in recent years as improved imaging techniques and new tools for intervention have been developed. A wide variety of conditions, both intracranial and spinal, can be treated and sometimes the procedure is complete in itself. On other occasions, the procedure may be an adjunct to other forms of treatment. Intracranial aneurysms may be occluded completely (Fig. 28.1). A vascular tumour may be partially embolized before surgery in an attempt to reduce operative blood loss. It may be possible to obliterate an arteriovenous malformation (AVM), but commonly the AVM will be incompletely embolized to reduce its size and make it more amenable to surgery or radio-therapy. Dural venous malformations may also be completely embolized.

The tools and materials for interventional procedures are under rapid development. The treatment of intracranial aneurysms has recently been advanced by the development of the Guglielmi detachable coils (GDC).[11,12] These are coils of platinum wire attached to a stainless steel guidewire. The coil is manoeuvred into the aneurysm sac through a fine catheter and opens to hold itself in position. The position of the coil is checked, as it is important to ensure that there is no tendency for the coil to prolapse into the feeding vessel or to interrupt blood flow past the aneurysm. If the position is unsatisfactory, the coil can be removed. When the position is satisfactory, the connection between the guidewire and the platinum coil is fused (by passing an electrical current through the joint) so that the guidewire can be removed, leaving the coil in place. Several coils may be needed before the aneurysm is completely occluded but partial occlusion may allow recurrence of the subarachnoid haemorrhage. Giant aneurysms may be obliterated by coiling but occlusion of the feeding vessel by balloons is possible and may be combined with a subsequent extracranial-to-intracranial vascular anastomosis.[13]

Obliteration by coiling is not possible for all aneurysms. It may be impossible to reach the aneurysm with the catheter and the shape of the aneurysm must be such as to retain the coil within the aneurysmal sac.

Arteriovenous malformations can be treated in a number of ways, the main problems being presented by the morphology of the AVM. The AVM may have a dramatic appearance on angiography (Fig. 28.2), with many feeding vessels, multiple fistulae and large arteri-alized draining veins, through all of which the blood flow is extremely rapid. The high flow may be asso-ciated with the concomitant formation of an aneurysm.[14] Treatment is aimed at obliterating the fistulae in turn and because manipulating the catheter into each part of the AVM can be difficult, the

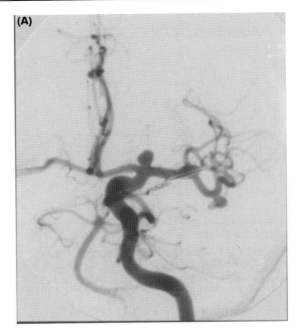

(A)

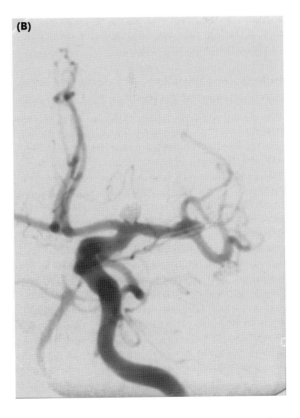

(B)

Figure 28.1 (A) Radiograph showing an aneurysm of the bifurcation between middle and anterior cerebral arteries. (B) Radiograph showing the obliteration of the aneurysm by Guglielmi detachable coils. Six coils were placed in all.

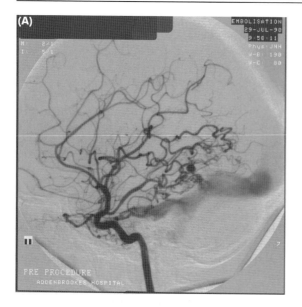
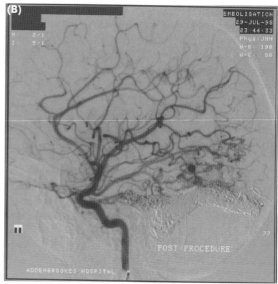

Figure 28.2   (A) Radiograph showing an arteriovenous dural fistula supplied mainly by the occipital artery but with feeders from middle cerebral artery and internal carotid artery. Aneurysmal dilatation is visible. (B) Radiograph showing the use of coils to produce a reduction in the high flow through the dural fistula.

procedure can be quite prolonged. Embolization therefore is frequently performed in several stages. Jaffar et al[15] suggest that embolization before surgical excision of an AVM reduces the intraoperative haemorrhage, making resection easier.

The position of the microcatheter used for the embolization is visualized radiographically and embolization is performed when the catheter feeds only the abnormal mass. Some units arrange anaesthesia or sedation so that the safety of the catheter placement can be checked[8] When testing is required, the sedation is reduced and a neurological examination relevant to the area under study is performed.[16] Sodium amylobarbital (30 mg) or lignocaine (30 mg), mixed with contrast, is given through the microcatheter. The neurological examination is repeated to determine any change in the patient's clinical state. While the testing is generally reliable, there are problems and false-positive results may occur if vigorous injection produces a reflux of the agent into normal vessels. False-negative results may occur if the flow to the AVM is so high that it carries the agent away quickly. Sodium amytal is used for investigation of grey matter, lignocaine for white matter.[17] Lignocaine may produce seizures if injected into the brain and it is suggested that, if it is to be used, amytal is injected first.

The usual material for embolization is contact adhesive (N-butyl-cyanoacrylate), which can be made up in various concentrations so that the rate of setting may be controlled between fast and slow. Other solid materials may be used for embolization, including balloons which may be detached from a catheter, Oxycel (oxidized cellulose) or pellets of materials such as silastic.[18,19]

The procedure may be helped in specific circumstances by the use of hypo- or hypercapnia or by induced hypo- or hypertension.

ANAESTHETIC TECHNIQUE

Patients should be seen and assessed for anaesthesia in the same way as for neurosurgery. Premedication is advisable, not least because many X-ray rooms, with a mass of complex, bulky equipment may be forbidding places to patients. Many patients are undergoing neuroradiological procedures or treatment because they have intracranial vascular pathology and therefore a sedative premedication producing a calm patient is of value because it minimizes hypertension produced by apprehension. Some patients (such as those with an AVM) may require several procedures before the treatment is completed and it is therefore essential to ensure that each procedure is not so unpleasant as to stop them returning for completion of the course of treatment.

Conscious sedation

The improvement in radiological techniques allows most diagnostic neuroradiological procedures to be performed under sedation with local anaesthesia as required. In interventional radiology, local anaesthesia with mild sedation allows the patient's conscious state to be monitored, which is of particular value if embolization is being performed near critical areas of the cerebral circulation. Any technique of sedation needs to relieve anxiety and pain and to provide such relief from discomfort that the patients lie still for prolonged periods of time. Young and Pile-Spellman[8] suggest that patients undergoing conscious sedation for interventional neuroradiology can only tolerate 4–5 h. The requirements of interventional neuroradiology are exacting in that when small vessels are being studied, patient immobility is vital. There are considerable problems with sedation and as well as patient discomfort during long procedures, they include the dangers of airway incompetence and of high $PaCO_2$, if the sedation is excessive. If an emergency occurs during a procedure being performed under conscious sedation, it is first necessary to secure the airway and ventilation before the cause of the emergency can be actively treated.

Several techniques are described for sedation. Young and Pile-Spellman[8] document their technique of neuroleptanalgesia with subsequent infusion of propofol. They begin with 2–4 µg/kg fentanyl and 2.5–5 mg droperidol intravenously, also using midazolam 3–5mg. During the procedure, they infuse propofol at low rates (10–20 µg/kg/min). They adjust the rate of propofol infusion to produce an unconscious patient with a clear airway. If neurologic assessment is required, then the propofol infusion rate may be turned down.

Manninen et al.[20] investigated two techniques of conscious sedation. All patients received 0.75 µg/kg fentanyl and midazolam 15 µg/kg before the procedure started. Conscious sedation was produced either by a second dose of midazolam (7.5–15 µg/kg) if required and then infusion of 0.5 µg/kg/min or by a bolus of propofol 0.25–0.5 mg/kg, followed by an infusion of 25 µg/kg/min. They aimed for a level of sedation, which they defined as producing a patient who was resting comfortably but easily rousable and alert to obey commands. There was general satisfaction with the technique of conscious sedation from both radiologists and patients. Complications were similar in the two groups. Of special interest is the incidence of movement which affected the procedure: 17 patients (there were 40 in the study) showed inappropriate movements or restlessness during critical periods. In only three patients did the restlessness occur during an angiographic series, requiring a rerun of the series.

Techniques of sedation were reviewed by Menon and Gupta.[21] They report many different sedative regimes, reflecting the difficulty of providing reliable sedation for children. They note the increasing use of propofol infusion for sedation during imaging either as the sole agent or in combination with other drugs.[22,23] They comment that many of the regimes involve sedative and anaesthetic drugs in doses that may produce airway, respiratory or cardiovascular compromise and that in some studies of sedation, the patients 'exhibited clinically significant falls in haemoglobin oxygen saturation, mean arterial pressure and respiratory rate'.

General anaesthesia

The use of general anaesthesia for interventional radiology has both advantages and disadvantages. The fact that the airway is protected and ventilation controlled is of value if there is a problem such as aneurysmal rupture or vascular occlusion. Alteration of $PaCO_2$ is easier under general anaesthetic, as is the use of controlled hypo- or hypertension.

The anaesthetic should aim to produce a stable blood pressure, with reduction of ICP in patients with intracranial space occupation and maintenance of cerebral perfusion. Interventional procedures may be quite long and special care should be taken to control the patient's temperature, to provide extra padding for pressure points, and to control fluids and airway humidity. The patients usually require urinary catheterization.

We induce anaesthesia with propofol or thiopentone and provide analgesia with a synthetic opioid, typically fentanyl or remifentanil. Muscle relaxation is achieved with an infusion of either atracurium or vecuronium. Anaesthesia is maintained with propofol infusion but as the degree of painful stimulation during the procedure is often quite limited, care must be taken in choosing drug dosage to avoid the development of hypotension.

Ventilation is controlled to produce moderate hypocapnia and the level of $PaCO_2$ checked by arterial blood gas estimation. The use of high-frequency jet ventilation (HFJV) is of considerable practical value in spinal interventional radiology because the high ventilation rates and low tidal volumes can be set so that they do not interfere with the use of the 'road map' image. The alternative, with conventional lung ventilators, is that ventilation must be halted repeatedly through the procedure, so that there are no ventilatory movements interfering with the acquisition of radiographic images.

Major procedures require the quality of monitoring used in the neurosurgical operating theatre.

Oximetry, direct intraarterial pressure, CVP and ECG are all required. Some workers suggest the use of the arterial catheter used by the radiologist for measurement of the arterial pressure.[8] We prefer to establish a line independent of the main investigating catheter. Central venous pressure measurement is useful not only for controlling fluid therapy but the central venous catheter may be used for administration of hypotensive agents, if indicated. Fluid overload from the flushing fluid used by the radiologist may also be detected.

DRUG EFFECTS

It has already been mentioned that, because the skull remains intact, great care is needed to avoid dangerous increases in ICP. It is interesting to recall that only recently, the use of vasodilating anaesthetic agents or of hyperventilation had a significant effect on the quality of radiographic films.[24]

When cerebral vasodilatation occurs, the bolus of contrast injected by the radiologist may not fill the arterial lumen so that the edge of the shadow produced by the contrast will not be sharp, because blood is travelling through the arteries at the same time. Vasoconstriction allows the contrast to fill the arterial lumen and therefore a sharper, clearer picture is obtained. The slowing of the cerebral circulation produced by hyperventilation has been valuable in allowing more films to be taken during the arterial phase of the angiogram. Indeed, Samuel et al[25] showed tumour vessels becoming more clearly defined when hyperventilation was instituted, so that normal cerebral vessels were constricted.

Current practice is to utilize digital processing of the X-ray image to enhance the quality of the radiographic films.

ANTICOAGULATION

Thrombus formation on intravascular catheters has been known for many years and the dangers of circulatory stasis when selective catheters are placed in small cerebral vessels are obvious. Heparinization should be used whenever there is selective catheterization of small intracranial vessels, which may result not only in endothelial damage but also in thromboembolic phenomena.

Monitoring of the level of anticoagulation varies from centre to centre. We measure APTT and PT after femoral arterial cannulation and give heparin IV (5000 units), so that the APTT is at least doubled. Measurements of APTT are repeated every hour.

BLOOD PRESSURE CONTROL

Controlled hypotension

Controlled hypotension is often of value during embolization of an AVM. An AVM may have a rich blood supply with an increased flow, so that materials injected into the feeding vessels of the AVM may pass straight through, carried by the fast flow, into the venous circulation. In this situation, slowing the blood flow by lowering the arterial pressure and simultaneously raising the venous pressure, to slow venous outflow, may allow materials such as glue to set within the AVM, rather than being carried straight through. The duration of hypotension required is usually short but several periods of hypotension may be needed for successive attempts at embolization. Before hypotension is used, the patient's fitness should have been confirmed and the anaesthetic and monitoring should be appropriate for induced hypotension.

The blood flow through the AVM is not under autoregulatory control so any reduction of MAP will be associated with a reduction in blood flow. The necessity for controlled hypotension and the level chosen can be estimated by observing the characteristics of the AVM as radiographic contrast is injected; if the contrast is carried through the AVM rapidly, some form of hypotension is likely to be of value. Young and Pile-Spellman[8] suggest that 'flow arrest' through the AVM needs to be achieved and they judge flow arrest by repeated contrast injections as the MAP is lowered.

Many agents have been used for inducing hypotension, which is easier to produce if the patient is anaesthetized, as Young and Pile-Spellman[8] confirm. In our practice, in which most of our patients are under general anaesthetic, we use a combination of a bolus of labetalol (10–20 mg) followed by infusion of 0.01% sodium nitroprusside (SNP) given through a central venous catheter. The choice of SNP is primarily because of its effectiveness and short duration of action.[26,27] It is possible that the cerebral vasodilatation produced by SNP may also be of value in reducing the flow through the AVM as CBF is diverted to the vasodilated normal cerebral vasculature. Sodium nitroprusside has been criticized as an agent because of the dangers of cerebral steal produced by the cerebral vasodilatation. Young and Pile-Spellman[8] point out that the extreme potency and rapidity of action of SNP mean that it is possible to make the patient unduly hypotensive and that, if the procedure is being performed with conscious sedation, the nausea and vomiting resulting from the hypotension 'can be disastrous'.

The main problems with SNP are associated with its potency and toxicity. It is easily possible to lower the

MAP too far with SNP. We choose to give SNP along a centrally placed venous catheter, so that the time lag between administration of the infusion and the lowering of blood pressure is kept to a minimum. The use of labetalol[28,29] before the SNP infusion starts avoids the development of a tachycardia in response to the production of hypotension and therefore makes the eventual achievement of hypotension much smoother. The short duration of hypotension means that toxicity is unlikely to occur.

Other agents that have been used for hypotension in this situation include esmolol, trimetaphan and nitroglycerin.[8]

The value of reducing the venous outflow from an AVM is undoubted but slowing the venous outflow from an AVM needs to be considered with care, because of the danger of causing considerable swelling of the AVM. Certainly, when the skull is open, neurosurgeons avoid obstructing venous blood flow from an AVM until they have isolated the feeding vessels. It is possible that distension of an AVM is limited when the skull is intact. The application of positive end-expiratory pressure (PEEP) is a time-honoured way of reducing cerebral venous flow and, in combination with controlled hypotension, effectively slows blood flow through an AVM. It must be remembered that application of PEEP during hypotension is potentially dangerous, because of the combined effect lowering cerebral perfusion. PEEP should only be applied for short periods and removed completely between embolization attempts.

MANIPULATION OF PaCO$_2$

Hyperventilation

We normally employ a moderate degree of hyperventilation (PaCO$_2$ 30–34 mmHg) because of the effect of hyperventilation on the quality of the vascular imaging.[25] The reduction in ICP is also of value when intracranial space occupation exists.

HYPERCAPNIA

Young and Pile-Spellman[8] recommend the use of deliberate hypercapnia when treatment of a venous malformation of the face or dural fistula is attempted by an injection into the venous circulation. In this situation they raise the PaCO$_2$ to 50–60 mmHg, so that the cerebral venous outflow is greater than the extracranial venous flow. This avoids the danger of the sclerosing agent or glue entering the intracranial venous drainage.

COMPLICATIONS

There is a significant morbidity associated with cerebral angiography. Earnest et al[7] list complications as new techniques were coming into use. In 1517 patients there was an overall complication rate of 8.5%, though neurologic complications were only 2.6%, with a permanent neurologic deficit in 0.33%. A more recent study[8] reported a total 30-day complication rate of 14% in 243 procedures; the rate for death and major complications was 1.2%.

Major vascular problems

The major vascular problems that complicate interventional neuroradiology are haemorrhage and cerebral infarction.

Intracranial bleeding, either from the rupture of an aneurysm or AVM or by perforation of normal vessels, takes place into the closed skull. The patient receiving conscious sedation may complain of headache, nausea or vomiting. The airway and ventilation need to be secured as appropriate in the clinical circumstances. If intubation is required it must be performed with adequate doses of intravenous induction agent and relaxant, so that further bleeding is not caused by hypertension on intubation. The use of thiopentone or propofol will in any case tend to limit the extent of the bleeding. If the bleed takes place under general anaesthetic, it is relatively easy to increase the dose of the intravenous hypnotic so that dangerous degrees of hypertension in response to the bleeding are avoided and to control arrhythymias which develop. Young and Pile-Spellman[8] recommend the immediate reversal of any heparinization, commenting 'the dispatch with which heparin is reversed may very well be the critical step between a good and a poor outcome from the bleed'.

Cerebral infarction results from vascular occlusion which may occur for a number of reasons, including thrombosis, and misplacement of injected material such as glue or equipment such as a balloon or coil. Vessels may also be blocked by a catheter. Subarachnoid haemorrhage is frequently associated with vascular spasm and the manipulation involved in placing a catheter to treat an aneurysm may also produce vascular spasm.

Treatment of a vascular spasm includes the induction of hypertension[30] so that perfusion through narrowed vessels is increased and flow along collateral vessels is maintained. With the vascular catheter in place, specific therapies can be used: vascular spasm may be treated by intraarterial injection of phentolamine or rogitine and occlusion of an artery can be treated by thrombolysis.

Contrast reactions

The injection of radiopaque contrast containing iodine is a central part of most radiological procedures. The contrast can be used intravenously (particularly in diagnostic scanning), intraarterially or intrathecally. The contrast agents have been associated with serious side effects but continued development is reducing the incidence of some toxicity. Older agents were ionic in nature and often hyperosmolar. The newer agents are non-ionic and have a lower osmolality. The incidence of serious reactions may be similar for both types of agents but non-ionic contrast agents have a lower incidence of moderate reactions. Patients with recognized sensitivity need steroid cover before contrast injection is undertaken.

The study by Manninen et al[20] also noted that 12 patients out of 40 complained of pain or moderate discomfort either during placement of the catheter or during embolization, when they experienced a hot sensation or headache.

CONCLUSION

Interventional radiology is under continuous and rapid development. The indications for interventional radiological procedures and their value in the treatment of neurosurgical conditions are constantly being reviewed. Evaluation of the common complications and their effective management must be part of the review, especially in relation to accepted therapies. New equipment and procedures are likely to be developed.

Anaesthesia is also likely to change quickly in the face of changing demands and this chapter is likely to be superseded very soon.

REFERENCES

1. Dandy WE. Ventriculography following the injection of air into the cerebral ventricles. J Neurosurg 1963; 20: 452.

2. Moniz E. L'encéphalographie artérielle; son importance dans la localisation des tumeurs cérébrales. Revue Neurol 1927; 2: 72.

3. Hounsfield GN. Computerized transverse axial scanning (tomography). Br J Radiol 1973; 46: 1016.

4. Luessenhop AJ, Spence WT. Artificial embolization of the cerebral arteries: report of use in a case of arteriovenous malformation. JAMA 1960; 172: 1153–1155.

5. Serbinenko FA. Balloon catheterization and occlusion of major cerebral vessels. J Neurosurg 1974; 41: 125–145.

6. Eskridge JM. Interventional neuroradiology. Radiology 1989; 172: 991–1006.

7. Earnest F 4th, Forbes G, Sandok BA et al. Complications of cerebral angiography: prospective assessment of risk. Am J Roentgenol 1984; 142: 247–253.

8. Young WL, Pile-Spellman J. Anesthetic considerations for interventional neuroradiology. Anesthesiology 1994; 80: 427–456.

9. Purdy PD, Batjer HH, Samson D. Management of hemorrhagic complications from preoperative embolization of arteriovenous malformations. J Neurosurg 1991; 3: 101–106.

10. Duckwiler G, Dion JE, Vinuela F, Bentson J. A survey of vascular interventional procedures in neuroradiology. Am J Neuroradiol 1990; 11: 621–623.

11. Guglielmi G, Vinuela F, Dion J, Duckwiler G: Electrothrombosis of saccular aneurysms via endovascular approach. J Neurosurg 1991; 75: 8–14.

12. Guglielmi G, Vinuela F, Duckwiler G et al. Endovascular treatment of posterior circulation aneurysms by electrothrombosis using electrically detachable coils. J Neurosurg 1992; 77: 515–524.

13. Ohman J, Heiskanen O. Cerebral revascularization: a review. Neurosurgery 1989; 25: 618–629.

14. Cunha E, Sa MJ, Stein BM, Solomon RA, McCormick PC. The treatment of associated intracranial aneurysms and arteriovenous malformations. J Neurosurg 1992; 77: 853–859.

15. Jaffar JJ, Davis AJ, Berenstein C, Choi IS, Kupersmith KJ. The effect of embolization with N-butyl cyanoacrylate prior to surgical resection of cerebral arteriovenous malformations. J Neurosurg 1993; 78: 60–69.

16. Purdy PD, Batjer HH, Samson D, Risser RC, Bowman GW. Intraarterial sodium amytal administration to guide preoperative embolization of cerebral arteriovenous malformations. J Neurosurg Anesthesiol 1991; 3: 103–106.

17. Rauch RA, Vinuela F, Dion J et al. Preembolization functional evaluation in brain arteriovenous malformations: the ability of superselective amytal test to predict neurological dysfunction before embolization. Am J Neuroradiol 1992; 13: 303–308.

18. Purdy PD, Batjer HH, Risser RC, Samson D. Arteriovenous malformations of the brain: choosing embolic materials to enhance safety and ease of excision. J Neurosurg 1992; 74: 217–222.

19. Germano IM, Davis RL, Wilson CB, Hieshima GB. Histopathological follow-up study of 66 cerebral arteriovenous malformations after therapeutic embolization with polyvinyl alcohol. J Neurosurg 1992; 76: 607–614.

20. Manninen PH, Chan ASH, Papworth D. Conscious sedation for interventional neuroradiology: a comparison of midazolam and propofol infusion. Can J Anaesth 1997; 44: 26–30.

21. Menon DK, Gupta AK. Anaesthesia and sedation for diagnostic procedures. Curr Opin Anesthesiol 1994; 7: 495–499.

22. Bloomfield EL, Masaryk TJ, Caplin A et al. Intravenous sedation for MR imaging of the brain and spine in

children: pentobarbital versus Propofol. Radiology 1993; 186: 93–97.

23. Martin LD, Pasternak LR, Pudimat MA. Total intravenous anesthesia with propofol in pediatric patients outside the operating room. Anesth Analg 1992; 74: 609–612.

24. Dallas SH, Moxon CP. Controlled ventilation for cerebral angiography. Br J Anaesth 1969; 41: 597.

25. Samuel JR, Grange RA, Hawkins TD. Anaesthetic technique for carotid angiography. Anaesthesia 1968; 23: 543.

26. Turner JM, Powell D, Gibson RM, McDowall DG. Intracranial pressure changes in neurosurgical patients during hypotension induced with sodium nitroprusside or trimetaphan. Br J Anaesth 1977; 49: 419

27. O'Mahony BJ, Bolsin SNC. Anaesthesia for closed embolization of cerebral arterial malformations. Anaesth Intens Care 1988; 16: 318–323.

28. Schroeder T, Schierbeck J, Howardy P, Knudsen L, Skafte-Holm P, Gefke E. Effect of labetalol on cerebral blood flow and middle cerebral arterial flow velocity in healthy volunteers. Neurol Res 1991; 13: 10–12.

29. Olsen KS, Svendsen LB, Larsen FS, Paulson OB. Effect of labetalol on cerebral blood flow, oxygen metabolism and autoregulation in healthy humans. Br J Anaesth 1995: 75: 51–54.

30. Young WL, Cole DJ. Deliberate hypertension: rationale and application for augmenting cerebral blood flow. Probl Anaesth 1993; 7: 140–153.

29

ANAESTHESIA FOR MAGNETIC RESONANCE IMAGING

Rowan M. Burnstein & David K. Menon

INTRODUCTION

The radiofrequency signals emitted when the nuclei of certain elements are placed in a strong uniform magnetic field and subjected to radiofrequency pulses at their resonant frequency forms the basis of nuclear magnetic resonance (NMR). Over the years it has become convenient to divide NMR into two separate branches: magnetic resonance imaging (MRI), which is based on the detection of signals from water and its application to the delineation of normal and pathological tissue, and magnetic resonance spectroscopy (MRS), which is mainly used for the detection of metabolites and uses signals from a variety of nuclei. In recent years the distinction between MRS and MRI has become blurred. Magnetic resonance imaging (MRI) is now clearly established as a valuable non-invasive imaging technique. It is particularly useful in imaging the central nervous system and the techniques of doing so and their applications continue to expand. Anaesthetists are increasingly involved in both anaesthesia and sedation for adults and children in this 'unfriendly' and often isolated environment and it is now possible to safely monitor critically ill patients for MRI. The use of high-strength gradient magnetic fields and radiofrequency waves during MRI poses particular problems for the anaesthetist and has major implications regarding patient safety.

In the last 15 years MRI research has focused on the development of different ways of interrogating the MR phenomenon by design of new pulse sequences and their application in particular clinical situations. Intrinsic to this has been the rapid advances in computer technology. Recent developments include functional MRI which allows visualization of local physiological changes within the brain that are associated with activation of the visual, motor and other brain systems. Magnetic resonance angiography (MRA) is being developed but has yet to supersede more traditional methods of angiography. Perhaps the most exciting area of MR is in application to the early diagnosis of stroke. Diffusion weighted imaging (DWI) and perfusion weighted imaging (PWI, obtained using rapid imaging after IV contrast administration) are new variants of MR which detect imaging changes within minutes to hours of ischaemia. Although still predominantly a research tool, MRS is finding clinical applications, particularly in the evaluation of tissue metabolism. MRI is increasingly used in conjunction with other imaging modalities, e.g. SPECT (single proton emission computed tomography) and PET (positron emission tomography) scanning, to improve anatomical and functional localization.

PHYSICAL PRINCIPLES OF MRI[1,2]

All atomic nuclei possess a charge (due to the presence of protons) and mass (due to the presence of neutrons and protons). Some nuclei also possess a property known as 'spin', which can be visualized as the nucleus rotating around its own axis. Just as a flow of electrons along a wire creates a magnetic field around that wire, so the rotation of neutrons and protons in a nucleus creates a local magnetic field and the nucleus behaves like a miniature bar magnet. Such nuclei are NMR sensitive. Hydrogen is the most sensitive of the biologically significant NMR-sensitive nuclei. Other MR sensitive nuclei include carbon, phosphorus, fluorine and sodium.

When these aligned nuclei are repeatedly subjected to a transient magnetic field oscillating at their resonant frequencies (typically in the radiofrequency range, between 20 and 120 MHz) they produce an MR signal. Clinical MR images are produced by mapping MR signal from hydrogen nuclei in tissue water, with the intensity of the signal being modified by the physico-chemical environment in tissues and modulated by the parameters used to produce the image. It is this variation in signal intensity that delineates anatomy and pathology ('contrast') in MR images. Signal from different parts of the imaged object are converted into pixels on an image by tagging them with spatially varying magnetic fields ('gradients') which enable the scanner to localize their position in space.

In summary, during MRI the subject is placed in a high-strength, static magnetic field. Radiofrequency magnetic fields are pulsed across the static magnetic field in order to elicit MR signal. This signal is spatially tagged by using gradient fields, which enable the scanner to allocate signal from different parts of the imaged object to individual pixels in the image. The resultant signal in each pixel is dependent on the concentration and physicochemical environment of tissue water, and variations in these parameters produce image contrast. This contrast can be modified by altering image acquisition conditions (which are defined by the pulse sequence).

While the natural image contrast produced during MR imaging can delineate anatomy and pathology, it is also possible to use an injectable MR contrast agent, which may provide further information about vascularity and blood–brain barrier integrity.

PRACTICAL ASPECTS OF MRI

MAGNETS AND FIELD STRENGTHS

Magnetic field strengths are measured in gauss (G) or tesla (T). 10,000 gauss equals 1 tesla. A refrigerator magnet usually measures 150–250 G. Field strengths used for MRI in clinical practice are usually 0.5–2 T with some newer systems as strong as 4T. Essentially the greater the static magnetic field, the better the spatial resolution but the greater the associated technical problems.

High-field MRI magnets (≥ 0.5T) are superconducting coils operating in liquid helium at 4.22°K. Older systems also contained liquid nitrogen (77.3°K). Lower field strength systems may employ resistive electromagnets or permanent magnets. A high-field whole-body magnet consists of a long tube, usually about 2 m in length. The hardware required for imaging and spectroscopy is contained within the magnet bore, leaving a free central bore of about 50–65 cm diameter in which the patient is positioned. The part of the body to be imaged may be placed in a smaller coil and positioned at the centre of the magnet. Once inside the magnet, access to the patient is limited; the part being imaged is approximately 1 m from the entrance to the magnet. Lower field systems may provide better patient access, as do some newer high-field magnets.

TIME CONSIDERATIONS

MR scans can take a considerable period of time to perform: 20 min to an hour or longer. Repeated data acquisitions, involving a variety of pulse sequences, are necessary to obtain the required information.

SOURCES OF INTERFERENCE DURING MRI

MRI signals are of very low intensity and interference occurs readily. The main sources of interference are high-frequency electromagnetic radiation (e.g. radio waves transmitted by FM radio stations) and interference arising from electrical equipment and monitoring devices. It is common practice to enclose the magnet in a radiofrequency shield or Faraday cage (Fig. 29.1). This may be built into the fabric of the room or immediately surround the magnet itself. Non-conductive devices such as ventilator tubing can safely traverse the Faraday cage, provided they are shielded at the point of entry by specially constructed copper-lined ports. However, any wires that traverse the Faraday cage act as aerials and feed noise in from the external environment. The electromagnetic noise that results may be so great that it is impossible to interpret the images.

In respect of monitoring equipment, this problem can be overcome in several ways. The equipment may be located at a safe distance from the scanner with long

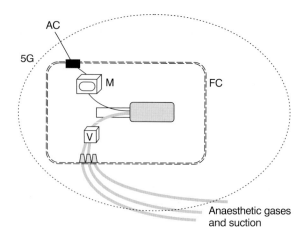

Figure 29.1   Layout of an idealized MR installation, showing the fringe field (in grey) extending beyond the boundaries of the Faraday cage (which excludes RF interference from the imaging suite). The 5 gauss (5 G) line is marked. AC power and gas pipes pass through specially designed ports in the cage (which may have filters incorporated in them). These supply power and anaesthetic gases to monitoring equipment (M) and ventilatory and anesthetic equipment (V).

monitoring leads which are filtered. Standard[3] or ECG-gated[4] bandpass electronic filters are the most commonly used. Care must be taken to ensure that filters are matched to specific monitors.[2] Alternatively, the monitor may be located closer to the scanner and an optical[5] or radio link[6] employed. Or the monitoring equipment may be housed in a smaller Faraday cage situated within the radiofrequency shield.[7]

Similarly, considerations apply to power sources for monitoring equipment. Mains wiring will carry interference into the Faraday cage unless it is adequately filtered and isolated. If this option is chosen it must be remembered that the small leakage currents present in π filters may activate isolation fault detectors in medical equipment even though the equipment may continue to function normally.[3] Alternatively, batteries may be used. These are usually strongly ferromagnetic and must be properly secured. Also, many devices operated by rechargeable batteries tend to switch off and blank their screens in the presence of magnetic gradients.[2]

Another source of interference during MRI is the presence of any large metallic mass in the vicinity of the magnet. This can subtly alter the magnetic field and degrade the quality of the images. Before each scan such sources of field inhomogeneity are compensated for by a process known as 'shimming'. Once the magnet has been shimmed it is vital that large metallic objects, like the anaesthetic machine, are not moved until scanning is complete. Other metallic objects, especially those which by necessity enter the scanner, can also degrade images. Anaesthetic apparatus,[2] including the valve on a laryngeal mask,[8] tattoos, cosmetics and implanted metallic objects have all been implicated. Patient movement is a potential source of poor-quality imaging in MRI.

FRINGE FIELDS (FIG. 29.1)

The field strength that characterizes a magnet is measured at the centre of the magnet, where it is maximal. However, the magnetic field extends beyond the magnet, gradually decreasing in strength. These magnetic fields surrounding the magnet are known as fringe fields. The strength of the fringe field is principally determined by the strength of the magnet and the distance from the magnet and will vary from one magnet to another. Newer, actively shielded magnets possess fringe fields which fall off more rapidly, although it is important to remember that the converse of this is also true; as one approaches the magnet the fringe fields rise rapidly.

Fringe fields are significant as they determine where ferromagnetic equipment may be located in relation to the magnet and how close patients with potentially ferromagnetic implants, such as intraocular foreign bodies and cerebral aneurysm clips, may get to the magnet. Electrical equipment, for example monitoring equipment, may malfunction in fringe fields, computer disks and magnetic tape may be erased and implanted electronic devices, such as pacemakers, may also malfunction or cease working altogether. In practice, it is important for the anaesthetist to determine where the 50 G and 5 G lines of the fringe field lie as these have various safety implications as outlined below.

SAFETY CONSIDERATIONS IN MRI

FERROMAGNETIC OBJECTS AND IMPLANTS

The attractive force of the magnet is considerable. There are anecdotal reports of impalement by runaway forklift trucks during construction near an MR imaging facility, as well as wheelchairs, fans, steeltipped shoes and nailclippers being attracted, to name just a few. Oxygen cylinders, identification badges, scissors and paging devices constitute a less dramatic but more frequent risk to patients. The attractive force on ferromagnetic objects becomes

significant at field strengths above 50 G. It is generally agreed that ferromagnetic objects that must be in the vicinity of the MRI suite, such as oxygen cylinders, should be stationed outside the 50 G line. Any person entering the suite must actively check for and remove any ferromagnetic objects from their person prior to entering.

Movement of implanted ferromagnetic objects under the influence of the magnet can be catastrophic. The problem is not as great as it first appears as most are non-ferromagnetic. However, it is imperative to determine whether or not an object is MRI compatible, particularly if it is in a vulnerable position. Of particular concern are cerebral aneurysm clips, shrapnel located adjacent to sensitive areas and intraocular foreign bodies. Individual objects can be tested with a powerful hand-held magnet. Lists of the properties of implants do exist.[11] However, it is worth being cautious of these as manufacturers have been known to change the composition of objects without notification. Some implanted ferromagnetic objects are safe, either because they are too small or they are firmly anchored in place by the surrounding tissue; for example, surgical clips that have been in for years. Most units have a comprehensive checklist for patients to complete prior to entering the scanning suite[2,9,10] (Fig. 29.2).

Metal detectors are too insensitive to play any role in screening patients prior to MR examinations[11] and safety demands obsessional attention to local rules and documentation. The risks involved in scanning patients with MR-incompatible implants are not trivial and too ready acceptance of implants in vulnerable positions can result in serious morbidity or mortality. Screening for intraocular foreign objects has caused controversy, since movement of a metal foreign body in the eye can cause vitreous haemorrhage and loss of the eye. If a patient has no symptoms and a series of plain radiographs of the orbits does not demonstrate a radiopaque foreign body, most centres would agree that an MR scan can be performed safely.[12] However, some units use thin-slice X-ray CT[13] for screening for intraocular foreign bodies.

Another major area of concern applies to aneurysm clips. While product information supplied with such implants will make statements regarding MR compatibility, it is important to recognize that repeated handling and sterilization can induce ferromagnetism in some previously non-magnetic alloys. It has been concluded by some authorities that only one of two criteria permit completely safe MR studies in a patient who has an intracranial aneurysm clip: a previous uneventful MR scanning *at the same field strength* or the

Wolfson Brain Imaging Centre MRI Screening Form

Important: this form should be completed carefully by/for all volunteers, patients & workers who will enter the MRI suite. The following items may be extremely hazardous or produce an artifact during the MRI scan. Please do not hesitate to ask for help in completing the list below.

Do you have any of the following:

Device category	YES (type)	NO	UNSURE
cardiac pacemaker			
aneurysm clips			
implanted cardiac defibrillator			
neurostimulator			
any biostimulator			
cardiac pacing wires			
cochlear implant			
any other internal electrodes			
implanted insulin pump			
Swan-Ganz catheter			
halo vest/metallic cervical (neck) fixation device			
any type of electronic, mechanical or magnetic implant			
hearing aid			
Intravascular coil, filter or stent			
implanted drug infusion device			
any foreign body, shrapnel or bullet heart valve prosthesis (artificial valve)			
any ear inplant			
penile prosthesis			
orbital/eye prosthesis			
surgical clips or staples			
long term line into a blood vessel			
intraventricular shunt			
artificial limb or joint			
orthopaedic implants (pins, plates etc)			
dentures or dental plates			
diaphragm/IUD (coil)			
Patches for drug delivery (eg HRT, angina, nicotine)			
tattoos or tattooed eyeliner			
implant held in place by a magnet			

Please mark on this diagram any metal in your body

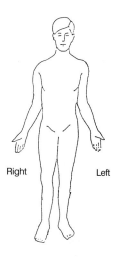

Right   Left

Have you ever worked as a machinist or metal worker?
Is there any possibility you could be pregnant?

I have read and understood this form and have had an opportunity to ask questions. This information is correct to the best of my knowledge.
Patient/volunteer/workers signature _____ date _____
Physicians signature _____
MRI staff signature _____

Figure 29.2   A sample checklist for screening for metallic implants prior to MR scans.

implant having been tested with a powerful hand-held magnet prior to application by the neurosurgeon.

Reference books and websites on the Internet provide useful information regarding a large range of other implants and devices. These are listed in Box 29.1.

NON-FERROMAGNETIC OBJECTS AND IMPLANTS

These must also be treated with caution, particularly if they are in close proximity to the region being scanned. As described earlier, they can distort or degrade the quality of the image. Further, the application of the oscillating radiofrequency field can lead to heating and burns from any metallic equipment or implants. Burns are the most common injury to patients associated with MRI.[10] Numerous first, second and third-degree burns have been described in relation to the use of monitoring equipment.[11,14,15] They result when a conductive loop is created between the patient's skin and a conductor, such as electrocardiographic leads or pulse oximeter probes. The risk of burns may be minimized by following some simple precautions.[2,11]

1. Check that the insulation on the surface coil and all monitoring wires and MR cables is intact.
2. Do not form large-diameter loops of wire or cross cables (heat generated in a conductive loop is typically greatest at the point where conductive materials cross each other). However, it is recommended to plait leads around each other so as to prevent large loops inadvertently forming in loose leads.
3. Remove any leads or wire not in use.
4. Separate all cables from skin (by padding if necessary).
5. Keep the cable and sensor as far away from the examination area as possible, e.g. place pulse oximeters on a toe for a patient whose head is being imaged.
6. Use only devices that have been tested to be MR compatible, both electronically and magnetically.
7. Burns have been caused when limb extremities in contact with each other form a conducting loop with a high-resistance region at the point of contact. Ensure that such contacts do not occur.

When patients have metallic implants it is standard practice to ask them to indicate if the area in question feels warm or uncomfortable. This is not possible in the anaesthetized patient. An assessment of risk should be obtained from the radiological staff in the MRI unit prior to the scan and the patient warned accordingly. Also, such potential sites must be checked for evidence of injury at the end of the procedure.

IMPLANTED ELECTRICALLY, MAGNETICALLY AND MECHANICALLY ACTIVATED DEVICES

MRI may interfere with the operation of such devices. There is also the potential for heating, which may result in burns, and image distortion, as already described. Cardiac pacemakers are the most common electrically activated device found in patients referred for MRI. Although MRI has been performed safely in patients with pacemakers,[16] fatalities have also been reported.[11] The acceptable safe level for exposure to magnetic fringe fields for patients with cardiac pacemakers are currently set at 5 G. At fields above this, the pacemaker will go into fixed rate mode. In these circumstances the delivery of a pacing spike on the upstroke of a T-wave following a spontaneously generated QRS complex can result in an R-on-T phenomenon and trigger ventricular fibrillation. Similar considerations apply to people with implanted cardiac defibrillators.

Other devices which may malfunction during MRI include implanted drug infusion systems, cochlear implants, bone growth stimulators and neurostimulators. In essence, MRI is contraindicated in any person who has one of these devices, unless it is known for absolute certainty that the device will function safely. Special precautions should be taken to establish a security zone in the vicinity of the MR suite. This should include warning signs and barriers to limit access to the area and to alert people with implanted devices which may be inactivated.

NOISE

The levels of noise permitted by regulatory bodies are clearly defined and MR systems should not exceed

Federal Drug Agency (USA)	http://www.fda.gov/cdrh/ode/primerf6.html
UK Medical Devices Agency	http://www.medical-devices.gov.uk/
International MR safety central website	http://kanal.arad.upmc.edu/mrsafety.html

Box 29.1   Useful Internet sites for information regarding MR safety

these.[2] Despite this, MRI is extremely noisy. The noise occurs during the rapid alterations of the magnetic currents within the gradient coils. These currents, in the presence of the static magnetic field, produce significant forces on the gradient coils, so causing them to impact upon their mountings.[11] The noise level is independent of the strength of the static magnetic field.[17] Temporary hearing loss has been reported following MRI,[18] although there are no substantiated reports of permanent loss.

To reduce acoustic noise, patients and technicians can be supplied with MRI-compatible earplugs. Antinoise techniques[19] have been described in which signals, opposite in phase from those produced by the scanner, are fed back into earphone covers. Repetitive gradient magnetic field noise is attenuated whilst verbal communication is maintained.

CONTRAST AGENTS

The contrast agents most commonly used for MRI are based on gadolinium. The incidence of side effects is low (2–4%), particularly as compared with iodinated contrast agents.[11] Reported side effects include headaches, nausea and vomiting, pain at the site of injection and hives. There have also been reports of transient elevations in serum iron and bilirubin levels which resolve within 24–48 h.[20] The incidence of anaphylaxis has been estimated at 1:100,000.[10] The safety of administering gadolinium-based agents to patients with impaired renal function has not been fully established. However, several studies suggest that it is well tolerated.[21,22]

CRYOGENS AND QUENCHES

Modern high-field (≥0.5 T) MRI systems are based on cryogenic magnets maintained in liquid helium at 4.22°K. Older systems also contained a cryostat buffer of liquid nitrogen at 77.3°K. Helium in its gaseous state is lighter than air and tends to rise to the top of a room whereas nitrogen has a similar density to air and stays at floor level. Losses due to evaporation are normally small. A sudden change in temperature of the magnet can result in a boil-off of cryogen, which is termed a *quench*. This has several implications. Available oxygen may be diluted. Asphyxiation can occur rapidly and with little warning.[11] The condensing vapour may result in frostbite or burns. The pressure inside the scanning room may be so great as to make opening doors impossible. In reality, such leaks occur gradually and can be difficult to detect. For this reason an oxygen monitor should be installed at an appropriate height in any room in which there is a cryogenic installation.

BIOLOGICAL EFFECTS OF MRI[11]

There is some controversy at present regarding safe limits of occupational exposure to static, gradient and RF fields involved in MR imaging, although it is possible that the next 12–24 months may see a consensus being achieved. The known facts regarding biological effects associated with MR are outlined below.

Effects of static magnetic fields

Data from human studies suggest that static magnetic fields do not have any significant deleterious biological effects at field strengths up to 2.5 T. The data regarding higher strength static fields (up to 4 T) are less clear. Volunteers exposed to such fields report a variety of symptoms, such as visual disturbances, metallic taste, nausea, vertigo, particularly when rapidly pushed into the magnet.[20]

Effects of rapidly switching gradient magnetic fields

Rapidly switching magnetic fields induce currents and voltages in patient tissues, the magnitude of which is determined by the resistance of the tissue, the cross-sectional area of induced current flow, the position of the tissue in relation to the end of the gradient coil and the rate of change of the gradient field with time.[11] Induced currents are greatest when there are large variations in the gradient over short time periods, i.e. in tissues located close to the ends of the gradient coils. The thermal effects that result from switching are clinically insignificant.[11] However, the electrophysiological consequences may be significant. Patients with underlying seizure disorders have had fits during MRI scans, although whether there is a causal relationship is unclear[11] Amputees have also reported an increase in phantom limb pain.[23] Peripheral muscle has been stimulated in gradient fields varying at 60 T/s. Extrapolation from this and other data suggests that it would require switching rates of 300 T/s or greater to induce ventricular fibrillation in normal myocardium.[2]

Effects of oscillating radiofrequency electromagnetic fields (B1 fields)

These fields also induce electric currents in tissues. In contrast to switching the gradients across the static field, application of the B1 field can have significant heating effects (although it does not have significant electrophysiological effects). There is particular concern over the effects on the eye and testes and in neonates. Data to date indicate that fears are unsubstantiated.[11] However, there is very little information regarding high-field magnets (4–5 T), which use 7–10 times as much radiofrequency energy as a 1.5 T system.

Carcinogenic and teratogenic effects

Although the evidence regarding the teratogenic effects of MRI is confusing and contradictory, it is safer than other equivalent forms of imaging that require ionizing radiation.[11] It is the imaging technique of choice in pregnant women where the alternative would involve exposure to ionizing radiation.[11] Many units limit occupational exposure during pregnancy. There does not appear to be any evidence that the fields used in MRI pose an increased risk for developing cancer.

MRI AND MONITORS AND OTHER ELECTRICAL EQUIPMENT USED DURING ANAESTHESIA

Reliable and accurate monitoring is an essential component for the safe examination of any individual undergoing MRI, but particularly for those who are unconscious or sedated. The problems associated with monitoring patients during MRI are listed in Table 30.1. The Federal Drug Administration in the USA (http: //www.fda.gov/cdrh/ode/primerf6.html) has provided useful definitions against which the performance of clinical equipment can be assessed in an MR environment. The terms 'MR safe' and 'MR compatible' are used to define equipment properties such that their possible use within an MR environment can be ascertained (see Table 29.1). The phrase 'MR safe' indicates that when a device is used in the MR suite it presents no additional risk to the patient, while the phrase 'MR compatible' indicates that a device is both MR safe and has been demonstrated to neither significantly affect the diagnostic quality of the imaging procedure nor have its operations affected by the MR scanning system. The criteria for labelling a device with

either of these terms cover its interactions with the static magnetic field (usually <2 T for clinical systems), magnetic field gradients used for image localization and the radiofrequency (RF) fields and signals used in MR image production and detection, respectively. In practice, many monitoring and infusion devices function normally at fields of 50 G or less but may be neither MR safe (since they present a projectile risk due to ferromagnetic components) nor MR compatible (since stray RF from the device may make imaging impossible). Some devices such as colour cathode ray screens may be distorted by fields that exceed 1–2 G, while monochrome screens function reasonably well up to 5 G. Liquid crystal display screens are not distorted.[25] Magnetic tape and computer disks are corrupted in fields greater than 30 G. Devices operated by rechargeable batteries may switch off and blank their screens. There are now integrated monitoring systems which have been developed specifically for use in MRI.

In evaluating monitors produced specifically for use during MRI, it is important to determine the conditions under which it has been tested. Monitors acceptable for use in low-strength magnetic fields may not function reliably in higher strength fields.[26] There are now numerous publications outlining the function of specific makes and models of monitoring equipment in the MRI environment.[11,26] It is not the purpose of this review to present these but to outline the general problems with the monitors and some of the solutions to such problems. Up-to-date lists of MR-compatible equipment are given on websites operated by MR equipment manufacturers such as GE (General Electric, USA).

ELECTROCARDIOGRAPHY (ECG)

The ECG shows significant changes within a static magnetic field.[27] Leads I, II, V1 and V2 are the worst affected, with changes in early T-waves and late ST segments which may mimic hyperkalaemia or

---

Table 29.1   Potential problems with medical devices in an MRI environment

MRI factor	Effect on/due to device	Possible problems
Static magnetic field	Torque on object	Tearing of tissues
Static magnetic field gradient	Translational force on object	Missile effect/tissue tearing
Gradient magnetic field	Induced currents	Device malfunction
RF field	Heating from RF currents	Burns
	*EM interference	Device malfunction
	*EM interference from device	Poor images and diagnosis
	Device in imaging volume	Poor images and diagnosis

*EM: electromagnetic.

pericarditis.[25] These changes are produced by currents that are induced in flowing aortic blood since it represents a conductive fluid moving in a magnetic field. These changes are directly related to the field strength and may make the ECG completely uninterpretable at fields above 4 T. The radiofrequency currents used during MRI also produce artefacts on the ECG due to current induction in ECG cables. Electrodes and leads which contain metal worsen ECG interference, as well as producing image artefacts. Carbon fibre leads are available, as are electrodes which do not cause interference. The relative length of ECG leads is critical to preventing gradient-induced artefacts and manufacturers advise against modifying ECG leads that are provided with MR systems.

There are several ways of improving ECG output during MRI. Low-pass filters (7–10 Hz) are incorporated into some commercial monitors.[28] A 'gated' ECG signal is obtained by subtraction of the MRI field and radiofrequency pulses from the measured ECG signal, leaving the net patient ECG signal.[26] The use of shielded cables, lossy transmission lines, telemetry and a fibreoptic system has also been described.[25] The recommendations of Dimick et al[29] and Wendt et al[30] include:

1. braiding or twisting the leads to reduce the loops across which potential differences can be generated;
2. placing ECG electrodes as close as possible to the centre of the magnetic field where the gradients should be changing the least;
3. keeping limb leads as close together as possible and in the same plane;
4. when using the chest leads, V5 and V6 are the least likely to develop and record artefacts.

Not all units routinely monitor the ECG during the MRI scan, relying on other monitors to measure the heart rate.[31]

PULSE OXIMETRY

Pulse oximetry has proved to be the most difficult monitor to adapt for MRI, because of both magnetic interference with the oximeter signal and degradation of the MR image by the pulse oximeter. Of particular concern is that patients have received burns from pulse oximeter probes.[32] Pulse oximetry systems based on fibreoptic technology are now available.[32] These devices operate without interference during MRI and it should not be possible for burns to occur as they do not contain metallic materials.[32,33]

CAPNOGRAPHY AND INSPIRED OXYGEN MONITORING

Standard capnographs have been used satisfactorily.[25,31] There is a maximum length of catheter (approximately 9 m) that can be used before the resistance to flow becomes too great and the machine alarms continuously.[31] The lag and alarm times are increased to about 10 s.[25] The long gas pathway results in a prolonged upslope, even in individuals with healthy lungs. However, trends in expired carbon dioxide can be observed and the respiratory rate estimated. MR-compatible gas monitors have made the use of such long sampling tubes unnecessary.

PRECORDIAL AND OESOPHAGEAL STETHOSCOPES

These may be unsatisfactory. Long tubing is required and with the noise that occurs during a scan, heart and breath sounds can be difficult to hear.

NON-INVASIVE BLOOD PRESSURE (NIBP) MONITORING

Satisfactory NIBP readings can be obtained from both a conventional manual sphygmomanometer and from standard automated systems.[11] Any ferrous connections between the cuff and tubing should be changed to nylon ones and the tubing lengthened as necessary.

INVASIVE BLOOD PRESSURE MONITORING (IBP)

IBP can be measured accurately.[34] The lead from the pressure transducer should be passed through a radiofrequency filter. The transducer should be as close to the patient as possible (within 1.5 m) to avoid the damping effect of excessively long saline-filled tubing.

INTRACRANIAL PRESSURE (ICP) MONITORING

ICP can also be measured accurately via a ventriculostomy. Parenchymal sensors present more of a problem but there are early reports of the safe use of a Codman microtransducer, monitored through a fibreoptic link (Fig. 29.3). Non-metallic subarachnoid bolts should be used to prevent undue interference with the image.

TEMPERATURE

Both peripheral and central temperature, can be measured accurately using temperature probes which incorporate radiofrequency filters,[25] although artefacts (e.g. induced eddy currents in the leads/probe causing heating) may distort the recording.[11] Fibreoptic systems with photoluminescent sensors are safe and reliable.[11]

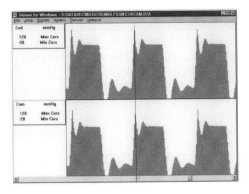

Figure 29.3 Validation of MR-compatible Codman ICP microtransducer (transduced through a fibreoptic link) against a standard Camino fibreoptic ICP probe (upper and lower panels, respectively) showing excellent concordance during simulated changes in pressure. (Figure courtesy of Dr M. Czosynka)

INTEGRATED MONITORING UNITS

Units designed specifically to function in high-strength magnetic fields have now been developed.[25] In the past, many departments have adapted existing equipment to form satisfactory integrated monitoring systems.[31,34] The availability of commercial systems for safe monitoring makes such home-made solutions completely unacceptable (Box 29.2). A typical MR system costs in excess of a million pounds and there seems little justification to avoid spending £30 000 to ensure safe anaesthesia in this context.

GENERAL ANAESTHESIA AND SEDATION FOR MRI

INDICATIONS

Anxiety/claustrophobia

Three to five percent of patients have been reported to terminate their MRI study due to anxiety or claustro-phobia.[35,45] Claustrophobia is particularly high in patients requiring brain MRI, as well as those with neurological diseases and those who have had previous scans.[45] Of those patients remaining awake for MRI, 12–14% will require some form of sedation to tolerate the procedure.[45] Non-pharmacological techniques, such as patient counselling, presence of a companion and the prone position can be explored before embarking on sedation. It is particularly important to provide patients with information about the sensations that will be experienced as providing patients with procedural information alone has been shown to be particularly anxiety provoking.[46]

Immobility

Patient movement during a scan degrades the final image with movement artefact and subsequent images may be affected. Infants, small children, confused and mentally ill patients may not be able to lie still for the requisite period.

Airway protection

This is necessary in unconscious and critically ill patients.

Control of ventilation

This is necessary to control $PaCO_2$ in some patients, e.g. head injuries, raised intracranial pressure.

CONSIDERATIONS FOR THE SAFE CONDUCT OF ANAESTHESIA FOR MRI

Anaesthesia for MRI requires modifications of anaesthetic techniques and equipment. The same standards of care apply to patients requiring sedation or general anaesthesia for MRI as apply to those in the operating theatre. Many imaging suites are constructed without thought for the need for general anaesthesia and require modification at a later date. This is far from ideal (see below).

Monitoring	MR Equipment Corporation, USA InVivo Corporation, USA Bruker GmbH, Germany
Anaesthetic equipment	Ohmeda, UK Drager, USA
Ventilators	Pneupac, UK
Infusion pumps	Mammendorfer Institut fur Physik und Medizin, Germany

Box 29.2   Representative list of manufacturers of MR-compatible anaesthetic equipment

Prior to instituting anaesthesia, it is essential to ascertain that there are no patient contraindications to MRI. The anaesthetist must also ensure that they are familiar with the MR installation, particularly the extent of the fringe fields and the location of resuscitation equipment.

Location of anaesthetic equipment

- Outside the magnetic field, i.e. outside the 50 G line, from where the attraction of ferromagnetic objects is unlikely to occur. Several metres of monitoring leads and ventilator tubing will be required and the risk of disconnection is increased.[25]
- Within the magnetic field. The anaesthetic machine and its components must be non-ferromagnetic. Once imaging has commenced, the machine cannot be moved as this will degrade the image. Any equipment used in the magnetic field must be tested for safe function in the MR environment.

Conduct of anaesthesia

Induction

Ideally this should take place outside the 50 G line with a dedicated anaesthesia machine/monitoring apparatus, etc. Standard Macintosh laryngoscopes are not ferromagnetic but do undergo a degree of torque in a strong magnetic field. Standard laryngoscope batteries are highly magnetic. Fibreoptic light sources or plastic laryngoscopes powered by paper-jacketed lithium batteries are available. Standard hospital trolleys are highly ferromagnetic and special trolleys should be used in the MR suite.

Sedation

The use of sedation, particularly in children, is controversial. More than 80% of toddlers are sedated for CT in some units.[36] Techniques employed for sedation of children include ketamine, barbiturates, benzodiazepines, high-dose chloral hydrate (50–150 mg/kg) and low-dose propofol infusions.[37,38] Sedation can safely be employed for MRI in children provided they are accompanied by trained personnel and are adequately monitored.[38] Supplementary oxygen should be given to sedated infants,[39] as well as any other patients requiring sedation for MRI.

Airway management

Controversy exists over the use of the laryngeal mask airway (LMA) for anaesthesia during MRI. Safe use has been reported,[40] but others consider the technique to be unsafe.[31] While LMAs reinforced with a metal spiral are ferromagnetic and produce substantial imaging artefact, newer reinforced LMAs contain a plastic spiral that can be used during MR studies. Where intubation is undertaken, use of a preformed endotracheal tube is preferable as once the head coils are in place, there may be little room for anything protruding from the mouth.

Maintenance of anaesthesia

Unless there is a specific indication, it is not absolutely necessary to ventilate patients for MRI. Both inhalational anaesthesia using halothane or isoflurane and total intravenous anaesthesia, with propofol, have been used successfully for spontaneously breathing and ventilated patients.[25,31,41]

Recovery

A suitable recovery area, equipped with monitoring equipment, suction apparatus, oxygen and trained staff, should be located outside the 50 G line.

Anaesthetic equipment

There are now numerous publications assessing the function of specific makes and models of anaesthetic equipment in the MRI environment.[25,26] It is not the purpose of this chapter to review these, but to outline the particular problems regarding the use of anaesthetic apparatus in the MRI suite. Past experience focused on the use of MR-incompatible anaesthetic machines and ventilators. Major problems with these included the need for long ventilator tubing which resulted in an increased risk of disconnection and concerns about increased expiratory pressures and compressible volume losses. Coaxial breathing systems were generally preferable as the number of lines running between the anaesthetic machine and the patient is reduced. Modified versions of the coaxial and non-coaxial versions of Mapleson D systems and T-pieces have been described.[25,31,42] Because of the long lengths of tubing, all these systems are cumbersome to store and must be checked meticulously before use. A particular concern is the resistance to respiration posed by such long tubing (up to 10 m), particularly in coaxial systems. However, the major cause of resistance in these circuits is the adjustable pressure relief valve.[42]

These issues have ceased to be active problems because of the availability of commercially constructed MR-compatible anaesthetic machines and ventilators, which can be sited close to the scanner. Vaporizers have been found to work satisfactorily during MRI.[3,43] Table 29.2 provides a representative (but not

Table 29.2   Representative list of manufacturers of MR-compatible anaesthetic equipment

Monitoring	MR Equipment Corporation, USA
	InVivo Corporation, USA
	Bruker, GmbH, Germany
Anaesthetic equipment	Ohmeda, UK
	Drager, USA
Ventilator	Pneupac, UK
Infusion pumps	Mammendorfer Institut fur Physik und Medizin, Germany

exhaustive) list of manufacturers who produce MR-compatible monitoring anaesthetic and ventilatory apparatus.

However, there continue to be problems with infusion devices, which may be ferromagnetic or malfunction or be inaccurate in fringe fields, although a number do function accurately.[26] Pumps must be supported on non-ferromagnetic poles. Needles and intravenous cannulae are usually non-ferromagnetic but should be tested first. Non-ferromagnetic suction apparatus should be available. The trolleys used for MR are very firm and should be suitably padded to prevent the development of pressure sores, especially for critically ill patients.

STRATEGIC ISSUES

Perhaps the most common continuing problems in connection with anaesthesia in MR enviroments pertain to a lack of strategic thinking when such facilities are being constructed. It is almost invariable for a claim to be made that the scanner will never be used for sedated, anaesthetized or critically ill patients. It is almost equally likely that this statement will be proved wrong within 12 months of opening the facility. It is therefore important that anaesthetists insist that they provide input when MR scanners are being planned or constructed. The provision of filtered AC power, piped anaesthetic gases and ports in the RF shield costs relatively little at the time of initial construction. Retrofitting these facilities after the scanner is operational may involve substantial costs and disruption to scanner use. It is equally important that a realistic assessment be made of needs for anaesthesia and supervised sedation during scans and resources identified (in terms of both money and people) to meet these needs.

INTERVENTIONAL MR[46-48]

There has been increasing interest in using MR to guide both minor and major surgical interventions (with procedures ranging from needle biopsies to craniotomies; Fig. 29.4). This use of MRI is classified as *interventional* (when MR imaging occurs while the procedure is underway) or *intraventional* (when the procedure is interrupted for repeated imaging to provide updates on the anatomy and extent of residual pathology). The latter approach may provide significant advantages in that surgical instruments need not be MR compatible. In anaesthetic terms, however, there is little difference between the two approaches, since anaesthesia and monitoring continue even when surgery ceases. However, both approaches substantially heighten patient risk when compared to anaesthesia for simple MR imaging, mainly because of the increased amount of people and hardware present in the MR suite, with an attendant increase in the risk of injury from ferromagnetic projectiles that have escaped screening.

INFORMATION RESOURCES

The rapid development of MR means that safe practice is dependent on up-to-date information regarding individual devices whose MR incompatibility may be responsible for serious morbidity or mortality. *If there is any doubt about the MR compatibility or safety of an implant or device, the assumption must be that it is unsafe.* It is important that the decision regarding the safety of an individual MR examination is taken by people who are well informed about the risks and

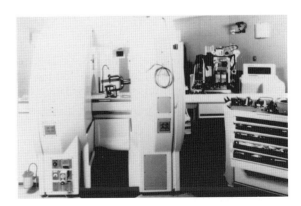

Figure 29.4   General Electric interventional MRI scanner showing double-doughnut magnet, with operator space between the two parts of the scanner. Note the trolley with MR-compatible instruments.

benefits of the procedure. Further, it is important that the responsibility for taking such decisions is clearly delegated to individuals within an organization. Several Internet sites provide useful information regarding individual implants or pieces of equipment. These are listed in Table 29.3.

CARDIOPULMONARY RESUSCITATION

It is impossible to resuscitate a patient in the bore of the magnet. The patient must be removed from the bore as speedily as possible and as far out of the fringe field as is practicable. In reality, this can be particularly cumbersome and the MRI suite staff must be well rehearsed. If the hospital cardiac arrest team is called, they must remove all ferromagnetic items from their person before entering the MRI suite.

Defibrillators should be kept outside the 5 G line. There is one report of a defibrillator failing at the edge of a magnetic field.[44] The leads to the defibrillator can be lengthened. This has not been shown to cause any decrease in the output.[25] The cathode ray oscilloscope trace on the defibrillator may be distorted but should still provide adequate clinical data. Common self-inflating resuscitators have no magnetic parts and can be used safely within the magnetic field. Similarly, a non-ferromagnetic suction unit should be available.

CONCLUSION

Anaesthesia for MRI has a multitude of potential hazards associated with it. However, with careful strategic planning, stringent safety procedures, compatible monitoring and anaesthetic equipment and a thorough understanding of the potential difficulties, anaesthesia for magnetic resonance studies can be relatively straightforward and rewarding and the information gained can be of high diagnostic quality.

REFERENCES

1. Gadian DG. Nuclear magnetic resonance and its application to living systems, 2nd edn. Oxford Science, Oxford, 1995.

2. Menon DK, Peden CJ, Hall AS, Sargentoni J, Whitman JG. Magnetic resonance for the anaesthetist. Part I. Anaesthesia 1992; 47: 240–255.

3. Karlik SJ, Healtherley T, Pavan F et al. Patient anaesthesia and monitoring at a 1.5T MRI installation. Magn Reson Med 1988; 7: 210–221.

4. Rokey R, Wendt RE, Johnston DL. Monitoring of acutely ill patients during nuclear magnetic resonance imaging; use of a time-varying filter electrocardiographic gating device to reduce gradient artifacts. Magn Reson Med 1988; 6: 240–245.

5. Henneberg S, Hok B, Wiklund L, Sjodin G. Remote auscultatory patient monitoring during magnetic resonance imaging. J Clin Monit 1992; 8: 37–43.

6. Rejger VS, Cohn BF, Vielvoyeg J, De Raadt FB. A simple anaesthetic and monitoring system for magnetic resonance imaging. Eur J Anaesthesiol 1989; 6: 373–378.

7. Boesch C, Martin E. Combined application of MR imaging and spectroscopy in neonates and children: installation and operation of a 2.35T system in a clinical setting. Radiology 1988; 168: 481–488.

8. Langton JA, Wilson I, Fell D. Use of the laryngeal mask airway during magnetic resonance imaging. Anaesthesia 1992; 47: 532.

9. Moseley I. Safety and magnetic resonance imaging. BMJ 1994; 308: 1181–1182.

10. Boutin RD, Briggs JE, Williamson MR. Injuries associated with MR imaging: survey of safety records used to screen patients for metallic foreign bodies before imaging (comment). Am J Roentol 1994; 162(1): 189–194.

11. Shellock FG, Kanal E. Magnetic resonance: bioeffects, safety and patient management. Raven Press, New York, 1994.

12. Shellock FG, Kanal E. MRI safety committee. Policies, guidelines and recommendations for MR imaging safety and patient management. J Med Reson Imaging 1991; 1: 97–101.

13. Mani RL. In search of an effective screening system for intraocular metallic foreign bodies prior to MR: an

---

Table 29.3	Useful inernet sites for information regarding MR safety
Federal Drug Agency (USA)	http://www.fda.gov/cdrh/ode/primerf6.html
UK Medial Devices Agency	http://www.medical-devices.gov.uk/
International MR Safety central website	http://kanal.arad.upmc.edu/mrsafety.html

important issue of patient safety. Am J Neuroradiol 1988; 9: 1032.

14. Kanal E, Shellock FG. Burns associated with clinical MR examinations. Radiology 1990; 175: 585.

15. ECRI. Thermal injuries and patient monitoring during MRI studies. Health Dev Alert 1991; 20: 362–363.

16. Gimbel JR, Johnson D, Levine PA, Wilkoff BL. Safe performance of magnetic resonance imaging on five patients with permanent cardiac pacemakers. Pacing Clin Electrophysiol 1996; 19: 913–919.

17. Hurwitz R, Lane SR, Bell RA, Brant-Zawadzki MN. Acoustic analysis of gradient coil noise in MR imaging. Radiology 1989; 173: 545–548.

18. Brummett RE, Talbot JM, Charuhas P. Potential hearing loss resulting from MR imaging. Radiology 1988; 169: 539–540.

19. Goldman AM, Gossman WE, Friedlander PC. Reduction of sound levels with antinoise in MR imaging. Radiology 1989; 173: 549–550.

20. Kanal E, Shellock FG, Talagala L. Safety considerations in MR imaging. Radiology 1990; 176: 593–606.

21. Haustein J, Niendorf H, Louton T. Renal tolerance of Gd-DTPA: a retrospective evaluation of 1171 patients. Magn Reson Imaging 1990(S); 8(S1): 43.

22. Haustein J, Niendorf H, Krestin G et al. Renal tolerance of gadolinium-DTPA/dimeglumine in patients with chronic renal failure. Invest Radiol 1992; 27: 153–156.

23. Yuh W, Fisher D, Shields R, Ehrhardt J, Shellock FG. Phantom limb pain induced in amputees by strong magnetic fields. J Magn Reson Imaging 1992; 2: 221–223.

24. National Radiological Protection Board. Board statement on clinical magnetic resonance diagnostic procedures. Documents of the NRPB, 1991, vol 2, no.1.

25. Peden CJ, Menon DK, Hall AS, Sargentoni J, Whitman JG. Magnetic resonance for the anaesthetist. Part II. Anaesthesia 1992; 47: 508–517.

26. Patteson SK, Chesney JT. Anaesthetic management for magnetic resonance imaging: problems and solutions. Anesth Analg 1992; 74: 121–128.

27. Mazrich R, Reicheck N, Kressel HY. ECG effects in high field MR imaging. Radiology 1985; 157(P): 219.

28. Rao CC, McNiece WL, Emhardt J, Krishna G, Westcott R. Modification of an anaesthetic machine for use during magnetic resonance imaging. Anaesthesiology 1988; 68: 640.

29. Dimick RN, Hedlund LW, Herfkens RJ, Fram EK, UTZ J. Optimizing electrocardiograph electrode placement for cardiac gated magnetic resonance imaging. Invest Radiol 1987; 22: 17–22.

30. Wendt RE, Rokey R, Vick GW, Johnston DL. Electrocardiographic gating and monitoring in NMR imaging. Magn Reson Imaging 1988; 6: 637–640.

31. Zorab JSM. A general anaesthesia service for magnetic resonance imaging. Eur J Anaesthesiol 1995; 12: 387–395.

32. Peden CJ, Daugherty MO, Zorab JS. Fibreoptic pulse oximetry monitoring of anaesthetized patients during magnetic resonance imaging. Eur J Anaesthesiol 1994; 11: 111–113.

33. Shellock FG, Myers SM, Kimble K. Monitoring heart rate and oxygen saturation during MRI with a fibre optic pulse oximeter. Am J Roentgenol 1991; 158: 663–664.

34. Taber KH, Thompson J, Covelar LA, Hayman A. Invasive pressure monitoring of patients during magnetic resonance imaging. Can J Anaesth 1993; 40: 1092–1095.

35. Quirk ME, Letendre AJ, Ciottone RA, Lingley JF. Anxiety in patients undergoing MR imaging. Radiology 1989; 170: 463–466.

36. Keeter S. Benator RM, Weinberg SM, Hartenberg MA. Sedation in pediatric CT: a national survey of current practice. Radiology 1990; 175: 745–752.

37. Vangerven M, Van Hemelrijk J, Wouters P, Vandermeersch E, Van Aken H. Light anaesthesia with propofol for children. Anaesthesia 1992; 47: 706–707.

38. Menon DK, Gupta AK. Anaesthesia and sedation for diagnostic procedures. Curr Opin Anaesthesiol 1994; 7: 495–499.

39. Fisher DM. Sedation of paediatric patients: an anaesthesiologist's perspective. Radiology 1990; 175: 613–615.

40. Frankville DD, Spear RM, Dyck JB. The dose of propofol required to prevent children from moving during magnetic resonance imaging. Anaesthesiology 1993; 79: 953–958.

41. Nixon C, Hirsch NP, Ormerod IEC, Johnson G. Nuclear magnetic resonance. Its implication for the anaesthetist. Anaesthesia 1986; 41: 131–137.

42. Rao CC, Krishna G, Baldwin S, Robbeloth R. Ohmeda (R) Fluotec-4 vaporizer output near MRI magnet. Anaesthesiology 1990; 73: A476.

43. Snowden SL. Defibrillator failure in a magnetic resonance unit. Anaesthesia 1989; 44: 359.

44. Murphy KJ, Brunberg JA. Adult claustrophobia, anxiety and sedation in MRI. Magn Reson Imaging 1997; 15: 51–54.

45. Melendez JC, McCrank E. Anxiety related reactions associated with magnetic resonance imaging examinations. JAMA 1993; 270: 745–747.

46. Gould SW, Darzi A. The interventional magnetic resonance unit – the minimal access operating theatre of the future? Br J Radiol 1997; 70: S89–97.

47. Lamb GM, Gedroyc WM. Interventional magnetic resonance imaging. Br J Radiol 1997; 70: S81–88.

48. Jolesz FA. Interventional and intraoperative MRI: a general overview of the field. J Mag Reson Imaging 1998; 8: 3–7.

Index